Molecular Biology in Medicine

D1264953

Molecular Biology in Medicine

EDITED BY

Timothy M. Cox MA MSc MD FRCP

Professor, Department of Medicine
University of Cambridge
Addenbrooke's Hospital, Cambridge

John Sinclair PhD

Lecturer, Department of Medicine
University of Cambridge
Addenbrooke's Hospital, Cambridge

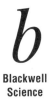

Blackwell
Science

© 1997 by
Blackwell Science Ltd
Editorial Offices:
Osney Mead, Oxford OX2 0EL
25 John Street, London WC1N 2BL
23 Ainslie Place, Edinburgh EH3 6AJ
350 Main Street, Malden
    MA 02148 5018, USA
54 University Street, Carlton
    Victoria 3053, Australia

Other Editorial Offices:
Arnette Blackwell SA
    224, Boulevard Saint Germain
    75007 Paris, France

Blackwell Wissenschafts-Verlag GmbH
    Kurfürstendamm 57
    10707 Berlin, Germany

    Zehetnergasse 6
    A-1140 Wien
    Austria

All rights reserved. No part of this
publication may be reproduced, stored in a
retrieval system, or transmitted, in any form
or by any means, electronic, mechanical,
photocopying, recording or otherwise,
except as permitted by the UK Copyright,
Designs and Patents Act 1988, without the
prior permission of the copyright owner.

First published 1997

Set by Excel Typesetters Co., Hong Kong
Printed and bound in Great Britain
at the Alden Press Ltd,
Oxford and Northampton

The Blackwell Science logo is a trade mark
of Blackwell Science Ltd, registered at the
United Kingdom Trade Marks Registry

DISTRIBUTORS

Marston Book Services Ltd
PO Box 269
Abingdon
Oxon OX14 4YN
(*Orders*: Tel: 01235 465500
             Fax: 01235 465555)

USA
Blackwell Science, Inc.
Commerce Place
350 Main Street
Malden, MA 02148 5018
(*Orders*: Tel: 800 759-6102
             617 388-8250
             Fax: 617 388-8255)

Canada
Copp Clark Professional
200 Adelaide St West, 3rd Floor
Toronto, Ontario
Canada, M5H 1W7
(*Orders*: Tel: 416 597-1616
             800 815-9417
             Fax: 416 597-1617)

Australia
Blackwell Science Pty Ltd
54 University Street
Carlton, Victoria 3053
(*Orders*: Tel: 3 9347 0300
             Fax: 3 9347 5001)

A catalogue record for this title is available
from the British Library

ISBN 0-632-02785-1

Library of Congress
Cataloging-in-publication Data

Molecular biology in medicine /
edited by Timothy M. Cox, John Sinclair.
      p.   cm.
    Includes bibliographical references and
      index.
    ISBN 0-632-02785-1
    1. Pathology, Molecular.
    I. Sinclair, John.   II. Cox, Timothy M.
    [DNLM: 1. Genetics, Medical.
    2. Transcription, Genetic.
    3. Molecular Biology.
    QZ 50 M71828 1997]
    RB113.M5854 1997
    616´.042—dc20
    DNLM/DLC
    for Library of Congress   96-21997
                                         CIP

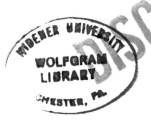
DISCARDED

WIDENER UNIVERSITY
WOLFGRAM
LIBRARY
CHESTER, PA.

Contents

Colour plates fall between pp. 214 and 215

List of contributors

Leslek K. Borysiewicz BSc, MB, PhD, FRCP

Professor of Medicine, University of Wales School of Medicine, Department of Medicine, Heath Park, Cardiff CF4 4XN

James Burnie MA, MSc, MD, MRCPath, MRCP

Professor of Medical Microbiology, University of Manchester, Medical School, Oxford Road, Manchester M13 9PT

Andrew Carmichael BA, BM, PhD, MRCP

MRC Clinician Scientist, Department of Medicine, University of Cambridge, Honorary Consultant Physician, Addenbrooke's Hospital, Cambridge CB2 2QQ

J. Michael Connor DSc, MD, FRCPEd, FRCPGlas

Professor of Medical Genetics and Director of the West of Scotland Regional Genetics Centre, Yorkhill, Glasgow G3 8RJ

Timothy M. Cox MA, MSc, MD, FRCP

Professor of Medicine (1962), University of Cambridge, Honorary Consultant Physician, Addenbrooke's Hospital, Cambridge CB2 2QQ

Graham Darby BSc, MA, PhD

Glaxo Wellcome Research and Development, Gunnels Wood Road, Stevenage, Herts SG1 2NY

Matthew J.C. Ellis BSc, MB PhD, MRCP

Assistant Professor of Medicine, Division of Medicine, Vincent T. Lombadi Cancer Center, Georgetown University, Washington DC, USA

Julian M. Hopkin MA, MSc, MD, FRCP

Consultant Physician, Churchill Hospital, Oxford OX3 7LT

Patricia M. Hurley MB, MRCOG

Consultant Obstetrician, John Radcliffe Hospital, Headington, Oxford OX3 9DU

Susan J. Kenwrick BSc, PhD

Lecturer, Department of Medicine, University of Cambridge, Addenbrooke's Hospital, Cambridge CB2 2QQ

Andrew M.L. Lever BSc, MD, FRCP, MRCPath

Lecturer, Department of Medicine, Fellow, Peterhouse College, University of Cambridge, Honorary Consultant Physician, Addenbrooke's Hospital, Cambridge CB2 2QQ

Ruth C. Matthews BSc, PhD, MD, MRCPath

Senior Lecturer, Department of Medical Microbiology, University of Manchester, Medical School, Oxford Road, Manchester M13 9PT

David B.G. Oliveira BA, MB, PhD, FRCP

Professor of Nephrology, Honorary Consultant Physician, St George's Hospital Medical School, Cranmer Terrace, Tooting, London SW17 0RE

Martin J. Page BSc, PhD

Unit Head, Oncology Unit, Glaxo Wellcome Research, Medicinal Research Centre, Gunnels Wood Road, Stevenage, Herts SG1 2NY

Timothy C. Peakman BSc, PhD

Group Leader, Gene Function Unit, Glaxo Wellcome Research, Medicinal Research Centre, Gunnels Wood Road, Stevenage, Herts SG1 2NY

Bruce A.J. Ponder BA, BM, PhD, FRCP

Professor of Clinical Oncology, Director, CRC Cancer Genetics Research Group, University of Cambridge, Addenbrooke's Hospital, Cambridge CB2 2QQ

Terence H. Rabbitts PhD, FRS

Protein and Nucleic Acid Chemistry Division, MRC Laboratory of Molecular Biology, Addenbrooke's Site, Hills Road, Cambridge CB2 2QH

Charles H. Rodeck DSc, FRCOG, FRCPath

Professor of Obstetrics and Gynaecology, University College London Medical School, Gower Street, London WC1

James Scott BSc, MB, MSc, FRCP

Professor of Medicine, Director, Department of Medicine, Royal Postgraduate Medical School, Hammersmith Hospital, Du Cane Road, London W12 0NN

John Sinclair BSc, PhD

Lecturer, Department of Medicine, University of Cambridge, Addenbrooke's Hospital, Cambridge CB2 2QQ

Karol Sikora MA, MB, PhD, FRCP

Professor of Oncology, Royal Postgraduate Medical School, Hammersmith Hospital, Du Cane Road, London W12 0NN

J.G. Patrick Sissons MA, MD, FRCP, FRCPath

Professor of Medicine (1987), Department of Medicine, University of Cambridge, Honorary Consultant Physician, Addenbrooke's Hospital, Cambridge CB2 2QQ

William B. Solomon AB, MD

Associate Professor, Department of Medicine, State University of New York/Health Science Centre at Brooklyn, 450 Clarkson Avenue, Box 50, Brooklyn NY 11203-2098, New York, USA

Edward G.D. Tuddenham   BSc, MD, FRCPath, FRCP

Professor of Haemostasis, MRC Clinical Sciences Centre, Royal
Postgraduate Medical School, Hammersmith Hospital, Du Cane
Road, London W12 0NN

Anthony P. Weetman   BMedSci, MD, DSc, FRCP

Professor of Medicine, University of Sheffield Clinical Sciences
Centre, Honorary Consultant Physician, Northern General
Hospital, Sheffield S5 7AU

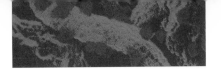

Preface

This book has been produced during an intellectual revolution in medical science from which there can be no retreat. The revolution is not a conceptual one but amounts simply to the realization that human physiological processes and the full spectrum of human disorders, congenital and acquired, are rapidly becoming susceptible to analysis in molecular terms. The techniques of molecular biology have evolved because of the need to understand the genetics of primitive organisms such as bacteria and phages, and also eukaryotic cells. It is a time of revelation in biology but given the ethos of medicine, the distractions of its practice and its pastoral demands, this excitement has neither been generally felt nor appreciated by established physicians or those in training.

Molecular biology is beginning to attack problems beyond those posed by the study of viruses or isolated cells, whether they be prokaryotes or eukaryotes. Its methods are now being applied to questions concerning the control of development and differentiation of whole tissues and organs, as well as the function of neural networks. Tumour formation, embryology and neurobiology, once subjects for observation, are now susceptible to decisive experiment, a triumph of analytical reductionism. Clearly, these advances bring with them implications for ethics in therapy as well as diagnosis—issues which are complex and which are themselves in a state of evolution.

Although the conceptual framework and lexicon of molecular biology is based upon the genetics of phage, yeast and bacteria, this probably does not explain the failure of many medical minds to grasp it. Simply the pace of discovery and the expansion of knowledge has been too rapid for full integration into training programmes and practice. By now, 20 years since methods for sequencing cloned genes have been developed, we already have novel reagents for the analysis, diagnosis and definitive treatment of human disease. These practical benefits have followed, with unprecedented rapidity, the tail of discovery.

The practice of medicine itself is changing and with it a self-conscious realization of its limitations and failure to influence favourably the demography of human disease. In response to a questioning public and a political climate obsessed with 'cost-effective' therapies, thoughtful doctors are increasingly conscious of ethical issues raised by contemporary 'high-tech' practices. Application of molecular genetics, especially in relation to predictive DNA testing for predisposition to conditions such as neurodegenerative disease or cancer, will precipitate arguably the most important ethical crisis that doctors, and the communities they serve, have ever faced. Although these are societal issues, they will be felt by nearly all practitioners of medicine and have relevance to this textbook.

Given the pace of discovery, none of the sections can be complete but the book reflects our desire to show how molecular biology is impinging on medicine and to indicate what lies ahead. Our contributors have not comprehensively revisited the historical framework of DNA and protein structure, molecular evolution, replication and microbial genetics: this is covered in undergraduate texts and, we feel, unrelated to our practical brief. However, our net has been cast wide to show the extent of scientific integration that is possible in medicine, and we have also tried to be honest about Pandora's box of genetic gifts. After the evils had issued from this beguiling goddess's box, hope alone remained to assuage the lot of man. There is now a molecular substance to this hope and we have attempted to demonstrate the extent to which it is tangible in medicine. The aim of this book has been to make introductions: to provide the curious student or practitioner with a basis to explore the medical potential of molecular biology; and still we hope to convey a real sense of wonder.

Acknowledgements

We thank our contributors for their co-operation and the efforts that they should be able to recognize in this version of the book.

No work of this kind can be produced without the dedication of a few professional enthusiasts who believe in publishing and work way beyond ordinary duties to see the task through. Peter Saugman of Blackwell Science had the courage to take us on and has left his splendid imprint on the completed work. We are especially grateful to Dr Andy Robinson, commissioning editor, who guided us almost from the beginning and worked tirelessly to help us realize our aims; he has become a true friend. By the same token, we were delighted when Jane Fallows, an old friend, took on the art work—an essential aspect of the book—and produced such excellent illustrations, often miraculously originating from apalling sketches! Julie Jones, our production editor, has brought the completed manuscript together and we are sincerely grateful for her uncompromising attention to detail.

We would also like to thank a whole host of academic reviewers (who shall remain nameless) for constructive criticism of each chapter, which has much improved the whole manuscript. In addition, we thank Jason Millington of University College and Middlesex Hospital Medical School for giving us the 'student's perspective' and Dr Vinod Achan of St George's Hospital for commenting as the 'junior doctor'. We trust that the book hits the mark.

Finally we thank Joan Grantham for secretarial forebearance over 7 years and for typing the entire manuscript accurately.

Chapter 1

Haemophilia: molecular biology at the centre of human disease

Editors' introduction

This introductory chapter sets the stage. It is the story of haemophilia from its time as a fatal disease of boys, best known to the Rabbis of antiquity, to the present day. Haemophilia is the paradigm of a human disease where the **application of molecular genetics** has already had tangible effects in **diagnosis** and in **therapy**.

The author has conveyed much of the optimism and excitement of molecular genetics as applied to medicine through his first-hand association with developments in this disease. Haemophilia has long been implicated as a cause of disability and death (see Plates 1–4, facing p. 214). Latterly, successful treatment of the condition by the administration of blood products had been complicated by life-threatening infections with **hepatitis viruses** and the **human immunodeficiency virus (HIV)**. The use of **recombinant methods** to manufacture a purified product for protein replacement has had a dramatic effect on the outcome of therapy for haemophilia, a therapy which is now free from the risk of viral transmission. This, and the diagnostic methods brought into clinical use only a few years after their initial discovery, is a landmark in the catalogue of benefits that have already accrued.

The following chapter is in the form of a light scientific narrative: it presumes some knowledge of the techniques and strategies used in molecular biology and the naive reader may not understand all the details on a first reading. We intend, nonetheless, that you will be swept along and that the tale will entice you to delve further: much of this book is about the issues encompassed in this chapter.

An ancient scourge solved by molecular biology

Zippori, Israel, second century

The Rabbi was puzzled. A young mother had come to him in great distress. Her first son had died after circumcision, performed with the usual practised skill at 8 days. Bleeding usually stopped after the operation in a few minutes, but her little boy had bled to death. The same sad end had befallen her second son. Here she was with her third boy child, now due to undergo the ritual that killed his older brothers. Rebbe Judah pondered: the law demanded circumcision, but in all circumstances saving life took precedence. He gave his verdict—dispensation from circumcision should be allowed in such cases. We know this because it is recorded in the Babylonian Talmud. Evidently, the Rabbis saw larger families with the problem, for the dispensation was later extended to maternal cousins of bleeders, showing remarkable insight into the pattern of sex-linked inheritance.

Cordoba, Moorish Spain, tenth century

The great surgical writer Khalaf Ibn Abbas, also known as Alsaharavius, visited a village where men were afflicted with uncontrollable bleeding from cuts and wounds. The problem was also evident in young boys of the village who sometimes bled to death after merely rubbing their gums. The sufferers generally died of haemorrhage but, Khalaf added, 'I have seen that the treatment of a cut is to quickly cauterize the place until

1

blood is held back. I have proof of this, for it was demonstrated in my presence'.

Philadelphia, New England, 1803

A Philadelphia physician, John Otto, heard about a family in which males bled for many days after trivial injury, becoming prostrated. He particularly noted that no females in the family were afflicted, although 'still capable of transmitting it to their male children'. Otto's report appeared in *The Medical Repository*, New York and was the first recognizable account of an inherited sex-linked bleeding syndrome in the modern medical literature. It aroused widespread interest and was soon followed by many similar family studies and case reports. The medical publishing bandwagon was rolling. By 1820, Nässe could compile a review and draw up a list of laws of inheritance. Significantly, he noted that women were never affected, that they could have affected or normal sons, and that their seemingly normal daughters could have affected sons. Despite available evidence from the Hay kindred (Fig. 1.1), he missed the fact that sufferers' daughters are always carriers, although correctly noting that their sons, if any, were normal. This

error was propagated by subsequent authors for almost a century, demonstrating the difficulty of correcting a mistake once it has appeared in print.

Wurzburg, Germany, 1820

In his inaugural dissertation, Hopff referred to four brothers who had each bled to death after trivial injury or in one case after rupture of a tumour in the thigh (evidently a haemophilic pseudotumour). He applied the curious term 'Haemophilie', literally 'blood lover' to these patients, a name which has stuck ever since.

The nineteenth century—clinical observations accumulate

Many more cases were described throughout the nineteenth century, culminating in a monumental review by Bulloch and Fildes (1911) which summarized almost 1000 cases and family reports, abstracting from them 224 pedigrees. This was in the heyday of the **eugenics movement** and the review was published by the Galton's eugenics laboratory as parts V and VI of their treasury of human inheritance series. Still influenced by Nässe,

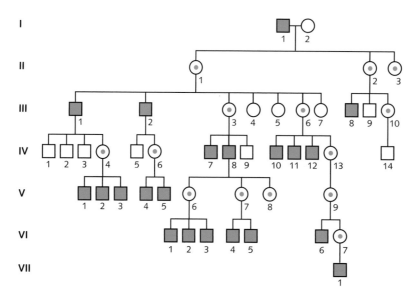

Fig. 1.1 Hay kindred of 'bleeders'. This family was first described in 1834 in the local guide book to a New England town (*History of Ipswich*) and later republished in the *Boston Medical and Surgical Journal* (1851). Osler reinvestigated the family in 1885. Strikingly, the affected males (filled-in squares) pass the bleeding tendency to their grandsons via carrier daughters (circles with inner dots). Despite this, the misconception that haemophiliacs could not pass on their illness to descendants persisted until 1911 (redrawn from pedigree 408 in Bulloch, W. and Fildes, *Eugenics Laboratory Memoir XII, Treasury of Human Inheritance parts V and VI, Haemophilia*). Hay, a physican who described the family, was married to one of the carrier females.

Bulloch and Fildes denied that a haemophiliac could pass the disorder to his descendants, despite the Hay family pedigree (Fig. 1.1) updated and illustrated in their review. However, they realized that the key to further progress in haemophilia lay in understanding the underlying blood disorder. Almroth Wright had shown in 1893 that haemophiliac blood was slow to clot, compared with normal blood, in a glass capillary. A case they studied together was a female haemophiliac, a possibility denied by Nässe and by Bulloch and Fildes. Later studies confirmed that this lady, who lived to be 90 and was restudied in the 1960s, actually had true haemophilia, being the offspring of a haemophiliac father and a carrier mother. This possibility was predicted and correctly explained by Bateson in 1909.

The twentieth century—modern genetics applied to haemophilia

Gregor Mendel's work had been rediscovered at the turn of the century and a new generation of experimental geneticists were enthusiastically applying Mendel's ideas to plant, animal and human heredity. Bateson, in his classic book *Mendel's Principles of Heredity* (1909), showed that colour blindness and haemophilia had

similar sex-linked inheritance. He saw the importance of the normality of affected men's sons and the carrier status of their daughters and drew up a scheme for sex-linked inheritance, essentially as shown in Fig. 1.2, that we still use today.

The most famous haemophiliac family in history was busy spreading its gene through the royal households of Europe at this time (Fig. 1.3). Queen Victoria was an obligate carrier of haemophilia, passing the defective gene on her X-chromosome to Leopold and to at least two daughters, Alice and Beatrice. Leopold's daughter Alice, an obligate carrier, had an affected son who died in childhood. The other affected males in this family all died without issue from haemorrhage, or in the Tsarvitch's case, met a violent end. The last definite carrier of the Royal Haemophilia died in 1980, but as her blood was not tested we still do not know if the underlying disorder in this family was type A or B (see p. 5). Early death without issue is in fact the commonest fate for untreated severely affected haemophiliacs and this fact was used by the geneticist Haldane in 1935 to predict the rate of spontaneous mutation causing the disease. By a brilliant *reductio ad absurdum* argument, he showed that new mutations must arise continuously to maintain the frequency of haemophilia in the general

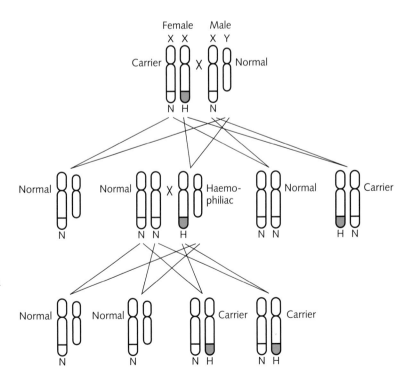

Fig. 1.2 X-linked inheritance. Three chromosomes are shown, a normal X (tip of long arm unshaded), an X bearing a mutant factor VIII gene (tip of long arm shaded) and a normal Y. A female carrier with a normal partner has four types of offspring with equal frequency: normal son, haemophiliac son, normal daughter and carrier daughter. A haemophiliac male has only two types of offspring: carrier daughters and normal sons.

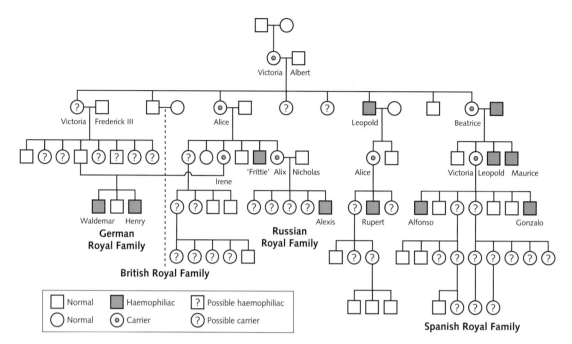

Fig. 1.3 The Royal Haemophilia. Queen Victoria was the first to carry haemophilia in this family having most likely received a mutant gamete from her normal father, Edward Duke of Kent. Her sixth child Leopold had severe haemophilia (it is still unknown whether it was A or B). He was the only bleeder male to live long enough to have children, including the obligate carrier Alice, whose son Rupert died of bleeding in childhood. At least two of Victoria's daughters were carriers, Alice and Beatrice, who passed the affliction to the German, Russian and Spanish Royal Families. The gene has almost certainly died out by now, due to the early death of affected males.

population. For if it were not so, given the rate of loss of mutant alleles, every male in the UK must have been a haemophiliac at the time of the Norman conquest. He concluded that about a third of mutations in any given generation must be of recent origin and likely to be heterogeneous. Both deductions, as we shall see, were to be triumphantly confirmed in the era of molecular genetics.

1911–1937   Early attempts to understand the coagulation defect in haemophilia

Back in 1911, however, attempts to understand the basic defect in haemophilic blood were running into difficulties. Working in Edinburgh, Addis took blood from normal and haemophiliac volunteers, anticoagulated it with sodium oxalate, so that the plasma could be separated, then allowed it to clot by adding calcium salts. The haemophilic plasma showed a much delayed clotting time, taking at least three times as long as normal plasma to form a clot after addition of calcium. He soon disproved Wright's idea that a deficiency of calcium caused the problem. With an extract of normal plasma made by

dilution and acidification he managed to correct the delayed clotting of the haemophiliac plasma. The fibrinogen content of the haemophiliac blood was normal and the corpuscles seemed to have normal amounts of thromboplastin—whatever that was. The prevailing blood coagulation theory of the day was that propounded by Morawitz in 1905: until very recently, you could see versions of it in physiology textbooks for medical students! This 'classical theory' supposes that coagulation is initiated by a mysterious thromboplastin from white cells which, in the presence of calcium ions, activates prothrombin to thrombin, which in turn converts fibrinogen to fibrin—thus forming the clot. The only constituent of this theory not tested for by Addis was prothrombin, which he was forced to conclude must be deficient in haemophilia. In the 1930s Armand Quick developed his 'prothrombin time' and showed it to be normal in haemophiliac blood. Thus an impasse had been reached. This was overcome by resurrecting Addis's experiments and by a new attack on theory. In 1937, Patek and Taylor in Boston showed again that a simple extract of plasma similar to Addis's corrected the defect in haemophilic blood, and they simply outflanked the

Table 1.1 Clinical severity versus factor VIII level.

Residual factor VIII (AHG) level	Bleeding manifestations
Less than 1% of normal	Frequent spontaneous bleeding into any tissue or organ, especially load-bearing muscles and joints. Early death from exsanguination common
2–5% of normal	Occasional spontaneous bleeds, bleeding after minor trauma
More than 5% of normal	Bleeding only after major trauma or surgery

Morawitz theory by calling the correcting factor antihaemophilic globulin (AHG for short; it did not acquire the name factor VIII until 1962).

1950–1965   Factor VIII defined and separated from factor IX

At Oxford in 1950 a highly important advance was made by Mersky and Macfarlane, who devised a sensitive specific assay for AHG. In retrospect this can be seen to be the essential prerequisite for efforts to purify the elusive factor missing from haemophiliacs' blood, that were to take another 30 years to reach a successful conclusion. Using the new quantitative AHG assay it was shown that the most severely affected patients had the lowest levels of or absent AHG, whilst milder cases had from 5% of normal upwards (Table 1.1).

In 1952, to everyone's surprise, it was found (by three groups independently in the USA and UK) that not all sex-linked haemophilia is due to AHG deficiency. About a sixth of such patients lack a different factor, so that the deficient plasmas cross-correct each other. The commoner type is haemophilia A or AHG deficiency, the rarer is haemophilia B or Christmas disease (named after one of the first patients to be described, who is still alive as it happens), now known as factor IX deficiency. Another surprise came the following year when French researchers found that AHG is deficient in the blood of patients with von Willebrand's disease, a bleeding disorder that affects males and females equally. How could a clearly X-linked defect also be part of an autosomal dominant disorder? The two conditions are also quite distinct clinically (Table 1.2). The solution to this puzzle would prove to be the key to the whole problem of haemophilia A, 20 years later.

In 1962 an international committee assigned Roman numerals to the clotting factors. AHG became factor VIII and the principle lacking in Christmas disease became factor IX (note that factor VI does not exist).

1950–1983   Development of plasma factor VIII concentrates for treatment

In the 1950s treatment for haemophilia, still a dreaded and usually fatal disorder, was developed, particularly by Macfarlane and colleagues at Oxford, where the first specialized centre for haemophilia treatment was set up. Supplies of human plasma were then very limited, and although plasma infusion was known to be effective for minor bleeding, its content of AHG was low preventing the attainment of high enough blood levels to treat major bleeding or to prepare the patient for surgery. Macfarlane therefore turned his attention to developing concentrates of AHG from animal blood, especially porcine and

Table 1.2 Comparison of haemophilia A with von Willebrand's disease.

	Haemophilia A	von Willebrand's disease
Inheritance	Sex-linked	Autosomal dominant or rarely recessive
Incidence	1:5000 males	1:1000 males and females
Clinical features	Joint bleeding Muscle bleeding Cerebral haemorrhage	Nose bleeds Menorrhagia Prolonged bleeding from cuts
Investigation	Factor VIII low or absent	Factor VIII low—never completely absent
	von Willebrand factor normal Bleeding time normal	von Willebrand factor low Bleeding time prolonged
Molecular genetics	Mutations at factor VIII locus Xq 28	Mutations at von Willebrand factor locus chromosome 12p12

bovine blood, available then as now in large quantities from the abattoirs. Although the concentrates he developed had the drawback of eliciting reactions and antibodies after repeated infusions, they saved many lives.

Gradually during the 1960s the plasma fractionation industry developed along commercial lines, with thousands of paid donors recruited to supply an internationally traded commodity—human plasma. The fractions derived from this, using technology developed by Cohn in the 1940s, included albumen, immunoglobulins, fibrinogen and later factor IX and factor VIII. The new factor VIII concentrates of the 1970s, although highly potent and convenient to use, were derived from large numbers of donors. Soon complications became apparent, particularly the presence of viruses. Hepatitis B was frequently transmitted, and by the late 1970s it was clear that a second hepatitis virus, C, was present in all factor VIII concentrates. Between 1979 and 1983 most commercial factor VIII concentrate also became contaminated with HIV, with the well-known tragic consequences for haemophiliacs. Subsequently, heat or solvent detergent treatment was developed to inactivate these viruses, making the concentrates considerably safer.

1965   The coagulation cascade hypothesis

The effort to understand blood coagulation as a biochemical process was hugely advanced in 1965 when Macfarlane proposed his cascade hypothesis and Davie and Ratnoff put forward a similar concept as the waterfall theory. With modification, the idea of enzymatic amplification (analogous to a photomultiplier cascade), by which an initial enzymatic step converts a second zymogen to an active form which in turn converts a third and so on, has been supported by increasingly sophisticated experiments. Figure 1.4 shows a modern concept of the coagulation cascade. Notice that factor VIII is a cofactor, not itself a proteolytic enzyme, which enhances the action of factor IXa on factor X in the middle step of the clotting cascade. From this (and the X-chromosomal location of the factor VIII and IX genes) it becomes obvious why haemophilia A and B are clinically indistinguishable.

1972–1982   Factor VIII and von Willebrand's disease: the puzzle resolved

The next major step in understanding haemophilia was taken in 1972 when Zimmerman, Ratnoff and Powell attempted to raise antibodies in rabbits against purified factor VIII. To their surprise the rabbit antibodies

detected an antigen that was reduced or absent in von Willebrand's disease, but always present in haemophilia A plasma. At first this entity was called factor VIII-related antigen. In 1975 Zimmerman and Edgington deduced that factor VIII coagulant activity and the new antigen co-purify, but are separate molecular entities. Because of its importance in von Willebrand's disease, the new antigen was soon redesignated von Willebrand factor antigen. Several groups (Hoyer in Connecticut, Bloom in Cardiff, Weiss in New York, amongst others) began to propose that factor VIII is an X-chromosome-encoded gene product and that the von Willebrand factor antigen is autosomally coded and somehow responsible both for maintaining the blood factor VIII level and for the bleeding time. Figure 1.5 illustrates this concept, in which factor VIII and von Willebrand factor circulate as a non-covalent complex. These clinically inspired ideas were to be completely vindicated as the tools of molecular biology became available to researchers in the 1980s and were applied to the problems of haemostasis.

In 1979, human factor VIII, completely free of von Willebrand factor, was purified by a group at the University of Connecticut (Tuddenham, Trabold, Collins and Hoyer).

1982–1984   Total purification and the race to clone factor VIII

In the early 1980s, the infant biotechnology industry was beginning to flex its muscles and look for projects with high potential earnings. The worldwide market for plasma-derived factor VIII concentrate, despite its increasingly manifest drawbacks, was worth several hundred million dollars annually. A recombinant factor VIII product, it was thought, could solve problems of quality and supply especially in relation to contamination with pathogenic viruses.

At least four industrial/academic partnerships were formed in 1982 to clone factor VIII, after a landmark conference in San Diego at which three groups announced total purification of factor VIII in sufficient quantity for biochemical characterization. The race was on. Figure 1.6 shows diagrammatically the procedure developed by the author's group at the Royal Free Hospital, London (Rotblat, O'Brien and Tuddenham). Very large quantities of starting plasma are first rather crudely reduced by cryoprecipitation to a solid chunk, retaining about half the factor VIII activity together with von Willebrand factor and huge amounts of other high molecular weight proteins such as fibrinogen and fibronectin. Indeed, for many years this crude prepara-

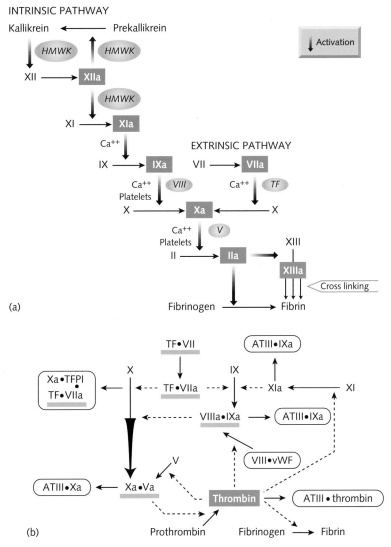

Fig. 1.4 The coagulation cascade. (a) A modified version of the scheme originally proposed by Macfarlane and by Davie and Ratnoff in 1964, in which the initiator is factor XII (top left). On binding to a surface, factor XII is reciprocally activated by kallikrein, then activates factor XI, which in turn activates factor IX and so on down to thrombin (IIa) which converts soluble fibrinogen to fibrin. Fibrin spontaneously polymerizes into a meshwork of fibres. Factor VIII is now known to be a cofactor for the activation of factor X by factor IXa. In this scheme, tissue factor initiation is added as an accessory or alternative pathway. Although the diagram is useful for interpreting coagulation screening tests performed *in vitro*, it has been realized more recently that tissue factor is in fact the physiological initiator, as shown in (b). (b) The current view of haemostasis. Coagulation is now seen as a network of interactions triggered by contact of blood with extravascular tissue factor. The initial conversion of factor X to Xa by the tissue factor/VIIa complex (TF·VIIa) leads to generation of small quantities of thrombin, which back-activate factor V and factor VIII. Rapid thrombin generation then proceeds with feedback to factor XI. Note that factor VIII bound to von Willebrand factor is inactive until proteolysed by thrombin.

tion, known as 'cryoprecipitate', was used to treat haemophilia—poor man's factor VIII concentrate maybe, but the only therapy available for more than a decade. The next step, a form of ion exchange chromatography, largely removes contaminating proteins but leaves factor VIII and von Willebrand factor with some hard-to-remove high molecular weight proteins. The next steps use immunoaffinity chromatography, first with monoclonal antibody to von Willebrand factor, then with a monoclonal antibody to remove fibronectin,

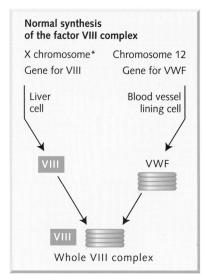
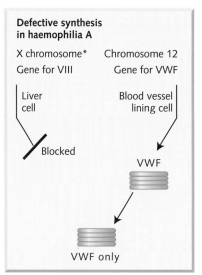
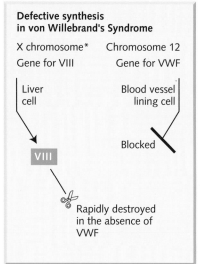

*Genes are distributed on 22 non-sex chromosome pairs and one sex chromosome pair. The X chromosome contains the genes encoding for VIII and IX.

Fig. 1.5 The factor VIII complex. The factor VIII and von Willebrand factor genes are on different chromosomes (X and 12) but the proteins produced naturally bind to each other in the blood and circulate as a high molecular weight complex (VIII.VWF). If either gene is non-functional factor VIII levels are low, but in von Willebrand's disease the whole complex is lacking, whereas in haemophilia A only factor VIII is lacking.

and finally a monoclonal antibody to factor VIII itself. The monoclonal antibodies were developed in collaboration with an immunologist at Royal Free Hospital, Dr Alison Goodall, and were the key to achieving total purity. Altogether, 10 000 litres of blood were processed batchwise through this procedure to yield about 20 mg of pure factor VIII, an odourless white powder. The specific activity of the final product was a staggering 5000 units/mg, implying that plasma contains only 200 ng/ml. This explains the long gap between Addis's experiments and our own results, since methods for isolating and manipulating such rare proteins were unavailable to earlier researchers. Zimmerman and Fulcher at the Scripps Clinic achieved a slightly lower level of purity — about 2000 units/mg — at the same time in 1982, and amazingly managed to obtain a patent on factor VIII of this and higher purity! With the backing of Armour Pharmaceuticals, this factor VIII patent survived several challenges and enabled Armour to settle out of court with the companies who successfully cloned factor VIII for a sum reputedly in excess of $200 million.

'A technical feat without parallel'

The factor VIII powder was freighted to Genentech Inc. in San Francisco where Gordon Vehar and his colleagues broke it down with the digestive enzyme trypsin and sep-

arated the fragments by reversed phase chromatography. The fragments were then subjected to automated Edman degradation to establish the sequence of amino acids of each peptide. One such fragment proved to have the sequence shown in Fig. 1.7. Dr Richard Lawn, a molecular biologist working at Genentech, was able to use this sequence to design an oligonucleotide probe by using the genetic code in reverse. Since more than one codon exists for all but two of the amino acids (the exceptions are methionine and tryptophan), a certain amount of guesswork and luck are needed to make a probe that closely matches the actual DNA sequence in the gene. The probe, a unique 36mer, was radiolabelled and applied to filters lifted from a gene library. The methods for making a human genomic library had been worked out by Lawn in Tom Maniatis' laboratory a few years earlier. Now they were applied in earnest to one of the most taxing gene cloning projects undertaken. The library was made using DNA from a cell line derived from an individual with four X-chromosomes, to enrich for the target sequences. The DNA was extracted, then partially digested with an enzyme that cuts rarely (the restriction endonuclease *Sau*3AI) and ligated into the vector phage λ charon 30.

Out of 500 000 recombinant clones from the charon phage library, 15 were selected by their ability to bind the radiolabelled synthetic oligonucleotide shown in Fig.

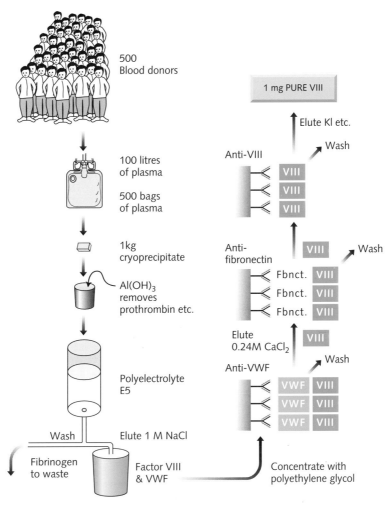

Fig. 1.6 Total purification of factor VIII from blood. The first step is a simple separation achieved by thawing frozen plasma at 4°C. The largest proteins in plasma are slow to dissolve leaving a precipitate of fibrinogen, von Willebrand factor, fibronectin and factor VIII amongst others. Adsorption to aluminium hydroxide removes other clotting factors such as prothrombin and factor IX. The resin polyelectrolyte E5 binds factor VIII and some von Willebrand factor allowing fibrinogen to flow through. Elution with concentrated salt yields a fraction very rich in factor VIII complex. This is then bound to a monoclonal antibody to von Willebrand factor immobilized on sepharose beads. After washing, the factor VIII is eluted with calcium chloride leaving the von Willebrand factor behind. The only remaining contaminant is fibronectin which is removed with another monoclonal antibody immobilized on Sepharose. Finally, the factor VIII is bound to a specific monoclonal antibody and the eluted product has 5000 units of activity/mg of protein and is 300 000-fold purified compared to plasma.

1.7 (second line). The DNA sequence of these clones contained overlapping sequences matching the predicted sequences and correctly specifying the first ten amino acids sequenced directly from the peptide. The last two codons diverged because, as it transpired, an exon–intron boundary had been reached (that between exon 16 and the downstream intron 16). Two strategies were then followed. Jane Gitschier, Dick Lawn and Terry Goralka cloned the gene by 'walking' along genomic libraries (see Box 1.1). Meanwhile, Bill Wood pieced together a DNA copy of mRNA (cDNA) from a cell line producing factor VIII message (see Box 1.2). Two large teams were involved in this work and incredibly they succeeded in cloning and mapping a gene of 26 exons spanning 185 kilobases, constructing a cDNA of 7.5 kilobases and demonstrating expression *in vivo*, in

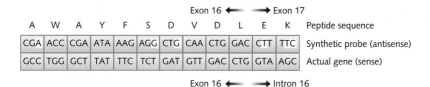

					Exon 16 ← → Exon 17							
A	W	A	Y	F	S	D	V	D	L	E	K	Peptide sequence
CGA	ACC	CGA	ATA	AAG	AGG	CTG	CAA	CTG	GAC	CTT	TTC	Synthetic probe (antisense)
GCC	TGG	GCT	TAT	TTC	TCT	GAT	GTT	GAC	CTG	GTA	AGC	Actual gene (sense)
					Exon 16 ← → Intron 16							

Fig. 1.7 One way to use a peptide sequence to clone a gene. The top line is the amino acid sequence in single letter code, obtained by Edman degradation of a fragment of pure factor VIII protein. Since the genetic code is degenerate more than one triplet of bases could code for each amino acid except for Trp(W) and Met(M). Therefore a guess has to be made. The synthetic probe matched the actual gene sequence at 27 out of 30 positions within exon 16. The match of course breaks down at the intron boundary, which we had no way of telling would fall within our peptide fragment of factor VIII protein. The radiolabelled probe bound to a colony of bacteria containing part of the factor VIII gene in a bacteriophage vector (see Box 1.1).

Genome Walking

Genomic libraries are made by digesting the total DNA extracted from thousands of cells of an organism with restriction endonuclease. Usually the restriction enzyme chosen is one whose target sequence recognizes a six nucleotide sequence in DNA, thus yielding fragments of, say, 5000–30 000 basepairs. The fragments are ligated into a vector consisting of the left and right arms of a bacteriophage. The assembled gene fragment/bacteriophage will now infect, replicate within, then lyse susceptible bacteria. The modification of this procedure that allows 'genome walking' is that the initial digestion of total DNA is deliberately incomplete, thus randomly overlapping fragments are generated. The library is screened by plating out bacteria thinly on a solid growth medium to form a lawn. The bacteriophages containing random fragments of DNA are now spread over the bacterial lawn at a density such that individual clear spots or plaques appear where each individual bacteriophage has initiated a cycle of infection and lysis.

A filter paper laid over the dish and picked up will bear a pattern of spots containing bacteriophage matching that on the plate, each containing copies of a single fragment of DNA. Next the DNA on the filter is fixed in place with ultraviolet light, then incubated with a radiolabelled probe matching part of the cloned DNA, such as a synthetic oligonucleotide probe corresponding to a factor VIII peptide. With luck this will bind to several spots on the filter paper, representing different clones overlapping the target sequence. The positive clones are then retrieved by matching the black spots on an X-ray film exposed to the probed filter to the pattern of clear spots on the original plate.

One can then 'walk' in either direction by mapping the inserted piece of DNA obtained in the first round of screening and selecting a new fragment as near as possible to either end. This new fragment is radiolabelled and used to probe the library again, and so on in repetitive rounds of screening. The mapping of the factor VIII gene required several different gene libraries and was achieved with eight walk probes after the initial oligonucleotide probe, yielding six overlapping phage clones and six cosmid clones (see figure below). The pile of X-ray films in Jane Gitschier's office generated by library screening and mapping the factor VIII gene was over 2 feet high at the end.

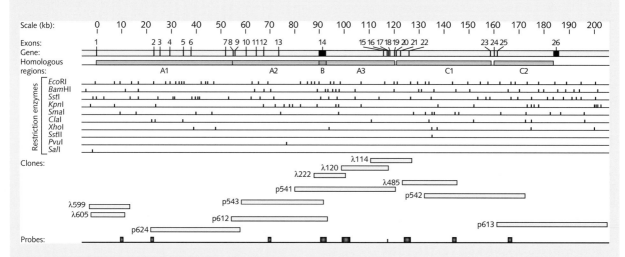

Fig. A Map of the human factor VIII gene. Bottom line, probes used for genome walking. λ599 etc.; phage clones; p.624 etc., cosmid clones. Restriction enzymes used to map individual clones were overlapped to generate the complete map.

Box 1.1

cDNA Cloning

A cDNA is a copy made with reverse transcriptase of processed mRNA, that is, a nuclear RNA transcript from which the introns have been spliced out so that only the protein-coding sequences are represented together with a short upstream sequence (5′ untranslated) and a downstream 3′ untranslated sequence including the polyA tail. Reverse transcriptase synthesizes from 3′ to 5′, so starting at sequences representing the carboxy-terminus of the protein. A particular problem in cDNA cloning factor VIII messenger was the rarity of the transcript, probably about 1 in 100 000 mRNA molecules in the liver. By screening large numbers of cell lines, Bill Wood found a tumour-derived lymphoid cell line producing significant amounts of factor VIII mRNA. This was a convenient source from which to extract messenger template for cDNA synthesis. The factor VIII message is too long to be reverse transcribed in one piece by reverse transcriptase, therefore synthetic primers were made progressively as the cDNA clones were sequenced, to push the transcriptase further 5′ in each round of synthesis. Eventually a cDNA 9 kilobases long was reconstructed from overlapping cDNA clones (see figure below). One of the factor VIII exons—number 14—is extremely large at 3100 basepairs, therefore a genomic clone, λ222, was used to provide this part of the protein coding sequence. The complete cDNA was then used to construct an expression vector (see Box 1.3).

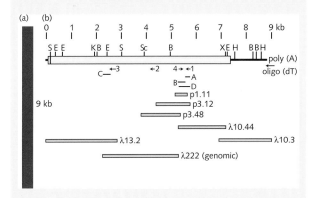

Fig. A Cloning the factor VIII cDNA.

Box 1.2

18 months. Every available technique of molecular biology was used. The editor of *Nature*, in which journal the results were published on 22 November 1984, described it as 'a technical feat without parallel'. Not only was the complete gene structure established, the largest and most complex then known, but the cDNA was used to direct synthesis of functional factor VIII in Chinese hamster ovary cells (see Box 1.3), by Bill Wood and his group, using a vector comprising several promoters and selection markers that have now become standard in the industry for protein synthesis. A third paper published in the same issue details results obtained by

Gordon Vehar and his team on the structure and function of factor VIII protein as purified heroically in the author's laboratory by Frances Rotblat and Don O'Brien. The purification scheme is outlined in Fig. 1.6.

The factor VIII gene and protein

A selection of these results is summarized in Fig. 1.8. At the top is a scale for the gene in kilobase pairs of DNA. Below this, the gene is represented by numbered shaded exons, separated by unshaded introns. It is obvious at once that the many exons are arranged within a large region of DNA (almost 0.1% of the whole X-chromosome) separated by some very large introns. One

Expressing Recombinant Factor VIII *in vitro*

Large post-translationally modified proteins like factor VIII cannot as a rule be successfully expressed in prokaryotes (bacteria) or lower eukaryotes (yeast, insect cells). Therefore mammalian cell lines are used, such as the two hamster cell lines Chinese hamster ovary (CHO) and baby hamster kidney (BHK). Both lines have been successfully transfected with virus-based vectors bearing the factor VIII cDNA, whereupon they synthesize functional factor VIII. The vector designed by Bill Wood (see figure below) consists of the following, starting from the top of the diagram: E, early promoter from the monkey virus SV40; AML, major late promoter from adenovirus; *Xho*I/*Sal*I etc., convenient restriction site for cloning; FVIII, the full length factor VIII cDNA; *Hpa*I to *Sst*I, part of hepatitis B untranslated region; DHFR, dihydrofolate reductase to enable selection. Using calcium phosphate the vector was introduced into BHK cells, which were then grown in methotrexate to select those expressing DHFR. Authentic factor VIII coagulant activity then appeared in the culture medium—cue for champagne all round and a press conference!

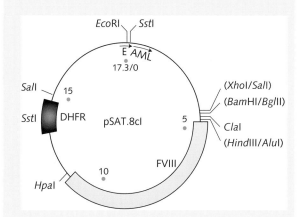

Fig. A Factor VIII expression vector.

Box 1.3

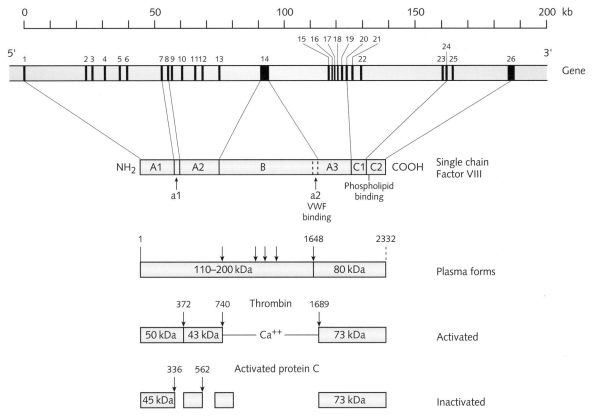

Fig. 1.8 Factor VIII gene and protein. The top line is a scale in kilobase pairs of DNA. The exons (protein-coding regions) of the factor VIII gene are shown as dark bands, the intervening non-coding regions are left unshaded. Lines connect the exons to the corresponding regions of the protein which they encode. For example, the A1 domain is encoded by exons 1 to 7. Two functions have been mapped to regions of the protein where indicated, namely binding to von Willebrand factor and to phospholipid. Factor VIII in plasma is virtually all in two chains due to proteolysis at sites indicated by an arrow in the fourth line. Thrombin attacks factor VIII where indicated in the fifth line to yield three-chain active factor VIII. Finally, activated protein C destroys active factor VIII by two cleavages adjacent to arginines at 336 and 562.

in particular, intron 22, is over 32 kilobases in length and will be referred to again later, as it contains the key to another mystery.

The exons are connected to a representation of the factor VIII protein which they encode, shown as a linear polypeptide. The cDNA encodes a 19 amino acid hydrophobic leader sequence that directs the protein for export out of the endoplasmic reticulum of the cell to the plasma, followed by 2332 amino acids, then a stop codon. The leader sequence is cleaved from the main segment by a signal peptide before or during release from hepatocytes, which are the main sites of synthesis *in vivo*, revealing the mature NH$_2$ terminus alanine–threonine–arginine etc. This sequence was determined directly from purified factor VIII protein, confirming the

assignment of the leader sequence peptide. A very interesting feature revealed by computer analysis of the protein sequence is the presence of repeating modules (A1,2,3 and C1,2) which are homologous to previously sequenced proteins. The three A domains strongly resemble in sequence the three A domains of caeruloplasmin, the blue copper-binding enzyme of plasma. However, caeruloplasmin consists solely of these domains, whilst factor VIII has a B domain inserted between the second and third copy of the A domains, and two C domains attached to the third A domain (Fig. 1.8, third line).

The C domains resemble in sequence the lectin (sugar-binding protein) discoidin, which is found in large amounts on the surface of slime moulds. Clearly a very ancient evolutionary link connects these proteins. More recently a protein binding to milk fat globules has been found, first in mice, then humans, that consists largely of C-type domains. This is a strong clue to the functional role of these domains in factor VIII. Most or all of the binding site for phospholipid resides within the C domains of factor VIII, enabling the protein to bind to platelets where it assembles the factor X-activating complex. The B domain is quite curious in several ways. First, it is not homologous to any other known protein sequence. Second, it is encoded entirely by a single very large uninterrupted exon, giving rise to speculation that this occurred by retrotransposition of a processed (i.e. spliced) mRNA. Reverse transcriptase-like sequences, called line elements, are widely dispersed in mammalian DNA and could provide the machinery for such a process. Third, the B domain of factor VIII is heavily glycosylated. Fourth, this entire region of factor VIII is snipped out and thrown away during the activation of factor VIII by thrombin. So what is it for? In brief, no one knows.

'Activation' and 'inactivation' in blood coagulation

All the circulating factors of the coagulation cascade share the property that, whether enzymes or cofactors, they exist in an inactive precursor form requiring proteolytic activation. A moment's reflection will show why this must be so, for if it were not, blood would be continuously clotting in the circulation. In the pathological situation of thrombosis this does occur, with dire consequences. The specific cleavages that activate factor VIII are performed by thrombin, as shown in the fifth line of Fig. 1.8. Mutation of the residues adjacent to the cleavage sites leads to inactive factor VIII in some cases of haemophilia as it later turned out (see below). Now the intricate balance of the haemostatic mechanism can be seen in the next step, which is *in*activation of factor VIII by activated protein C. Protein C is itself activated by thrombin, but only in the presence of a receptor located on the surface of blood vessel lining cells (endothelial cells). Hence the paradox that thrombin clots blood by converting fibrinogen to fibrin, but in the intact circulation acts as an anticoagulant by activating protein C. A chicken and egg-type paradox may be evident by now to the alert reader, namely, where does the thrombin come from? This problem continues to puzzle researchers: it is clear that a low rate of tickover in the cascade must and indeed does occur normally, as shown by sensitive assays which detect small amounts of activation fragments from factor X, prothrombin and fibrinogen in the blood of healthy people.

The function of factor VIII

With all this information about the linear structure and activation of factor VIII, do we know how it actually functions in the clotting cascade? The truthful answer must be — 'yes, but only vaguely'. It has been hard to work with the unstable macromolecule and no direct structural information on the polypeptide fold of the various modules is available. (Very recently the three-dimensional structure of caeruloplasmin has been solved and it is possible to build a plausible model of factor VIII based on that structure.) Enzyme kinetic studies of the effect of factor VIII on the activation of factor X by factor IXa show that the cofactor increases the V_{max} by 200 000-fold, with only a modest effect on K_m. Phospholipid itself lowers the K_m 3000-fold, which is interpreted to mean that phospholipid assembles factor VIII, factor IXa and factor X on its surface thereby increasing the local concentration, whilst factor VIII accelerates the enzyme–substrate interaction. Recently an allosteric effect on the active site of factor IXa induced by binding to factor VIII has been demonstrated. Suffice to say that a truly mechanistic explanation of the function of factor VIII is not yet available. This would be important to improve the design of new agents to treat haemophilia or to prevent thrombosis.

1985   Carriers of haemophilia and how to detect them

For every haemophiliac there are on average two heterozygotes and a larger number of women who might be heterozygote carriers since they belong to a kindred with haemophilia. An urgent question therefore may arise, often in the early stages of such a woman's pregnancy, who asks 'am I a carrier of the gene that killed my uncle, and if so, is this baby going to be affected as well?' Simple analysis of the pedigree will eliminate some women, and analysing the blood factor VIII level will identify most heterozygotes. However, in a minority of cases, because of random inactivation of either X-chromosome early in embryogenesis (a process called Lyonization, after Mary Lyon who first proposed that it should occur), a heterozygote may be operating the normal factor VIII genes in most of her liver cells and therefore have a normal factor VIII level. The pedigree analysis together with the blood factor VIII level, especially if measured together with the von Willebrand factor level, allow an estimate to be made of the likelihood that a woman is a heterozygote for the haemophilic gene. But odds in favour of heterozygosity give little confidence to a woman who knows that her child either is or is not going to be a haemophiliac. The problem may be resolved by linkage analysis using the natural variation that occurs in all genes, whether normal or bearing a mutation-causing disease. It is important to distinguish between these harmless polymorphic variants and disease-specific mutations. A polymorphic variant occurs by definition in 1% or more of the normal population. Very occasionally a disease-causing variation occurs at a polymorphic frequency, almost invariably because it provides some kind of selective advantage in the heterozygous state, whilst causing disease in homozygotes. The classic example of this is sickle cell disease, with cystic fibrosis a very probable counterpart in the northern hemisphere (the selective advantages being protection against malaria for the sickle cell gene and protection from cholera for the cystic fibrosis gene). Haemophilia confers no selective advantage and has never reached polymorphic levels, with one mysterious exception—factor XI deficiency amongst the Ashkenazi Jews—but that is another story.

The first useful polymorphic variation in the factor VIII gene turned up in intron 18, i.e. the intervening, untranscribed segment of genomic DNA lying between exons 18 and 19. Jane Gitschier searched specifically for variation in the pattern of fragmentation of the factor VIII gene produced by a battery of restriction enzymes used to digest DNA from a panel of normal individuals. Altogether 37 restriction enzymes recognizing different DNA sequences were tested. Only the enzyme *Bcl*I

showed a variation in fragment sizes detectable by Southern blotting (Fig. 1.9). The polymorphic site is in a DNA sequence which varies such that about 27% of factor VIII genes are not cleaved by *Bcl*I but 73% are cut by the enzyme in Caucasians (rates differ quite markedly according to ethnic group, as with many polymorphisms, e.g. blood groups). As a result the proportion of women who are heterozygous, that is to say have alleles of factor VIII that differ in sequence at this point, is $2 \times 0.27 \times 0.73 = 0.42$. The highest possible proportion for a simple diallelic marker is 0.5; therefore gene tracking is quite successful with this marker. The Mendelian inheritance of this marker, referred to as a restriction fragment length polymorphism, in reference to the method used to detect it, was established by studying members of several three-generation Mormon families from Utah.

Factor VIII gene tracking for real

An early approach to prenatal diagnosis of haemophilia using linkage methods was reported in 1978—this depended on the linkage of the factor VIII gene to the polymorphic locus for the blood enzyme glucose-6-phosphate dehydrogenase. However, this method is not generally informative and the first application of the tracking method in earnest came about when an Australian doctor, whose wife carried haemophilia, read our paper in *Nature*. Very early one morning the telephone rang in my bedroom. He explained the situation:

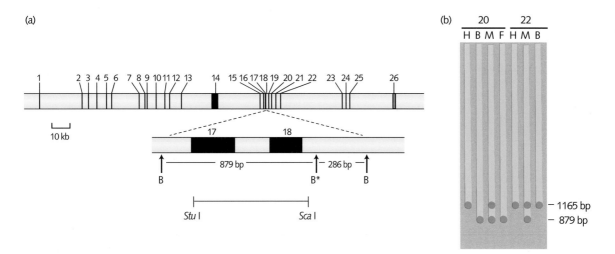

Fig. 1.9 The first polymorphism found in factor VIII. The enzyme *Bcl*I cleaves the factor VIII gene in about 60% of alleles at the point marked B*, yielding a fragment, detected by a Southern blot, of 879 basepairs. In the remaining 40% of

alleles no cut is made at B* and a fragment of 1165 basepairs is detected. This can be used to track a factor VIII allele through a family.

'My wife is pregnant with our first child; she is a carrier of severe haemophilia A. We could get a diagnosis at 18 weeks by fetal blood sample, but we couldn't face a termination at that stage. We'd rather stop the pregnancy now and wait until better methods are available. We've read that you have a new way of diagnosing haemophilia that would work on a chorion villus sample at 8 weeks. Can you help us? If not now, when?' I struggled to focus my mind on this desperate plea from 8000 miles away. 'Yes', I said, 'I think we can help.' The doctor described his wife's family—her haemophilic brother was alive and willing to donate blood, as were her parents and of course his wife, who was willing to undergo chorion villus sampling (CVS). Since CVS can only safely be performed up to 12 weeks' gestation there was very little time in hand for the first antenatal diagnosis of haemophilia A by linkage to be arranged. Several international phone calls later a batch of samples were on their way, frozen with solid CO_2, from Sydney to San Francisco. Jane Gitschier extracted the DNA from the blood and from the tiny piece of tissue taken from the placenta. The results of the Southern blot are shown in Fig. 1.10. To everyone's relief the result was clearcut and good news—the baby, a boy (sex established by karyotype), could not be affected as he had inherited his factor VIII gene, marked by the 1165 kilobase fragment, from his normal grandfather.

These results, and those of another family from the London area whose result was also good news, were published in a letter to the *Lancet*. This spin off from the factor VIII cloning project gave immediate benefit to families affected by haemophilia. Development of recombinant factor VIII for treatment was to take much longer.

1986   The first mutations causing haemophilia A identified

While screening for polymorphisms, Jane Gitschier used a large number of DNA samples from haemophiliacs that I sent her, and in a few of these abnormal Southern blot patterns appeared. Significantly as it turned out, these abnormal patterns were unique to individual patients and only detectable with the restriction enzyme *Taq*I (the first restriction endonuclease isolated from the bacterium *Thermus aquaticus*). This enzyme recognizes the sequence TCGA, a palindrome when you consider the opposite strands AGCT, containing the dinucleotide CG. Two of the patients from the first batch of samples showed a band shift due to loss of a *Taq*I site. Since the *Taq*I-digested DNA from the patients was probed with cDNA, the *Taq*I sites involved must lie within or immedi-

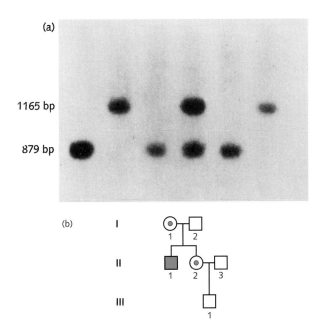

Fig. 1.10 The first antenatal diagnosis for haemophilia A. Southern blot demonstrating absence or presence of *Bcl*I cut site aligned vertically with family members in tree below. Individual I1 was known to be an obligate carrier as she had a brother with haemophilia and affected son II1. The carrier status of II2 was unknown and cannot be inferred from this analysis since her mother is 'uninformative', being homozygous for the presence of the *Bcl*I cut site. Fortunately however, the status of the fetus III1, sampled by chorion villus biopsy at 10 weeks' gestation, can be shown to be normal since he has the 1165 basepair allele derived from his normal grandfather I2.

ately flanking an exon. Further subcloning and sequencing located the mutation in patient H2 (Figs 1.10 and 1.11) to arginine codon 2209 in exon 24 of the factor VIII gene. Replacement of C by T in this codon destroys the *Taq*I site and creates a premature inframe stop codon (CGA → TGA)—a nonsense mutation, causing disease. Extra interest centres on this case, for the family study shows (Fig. 1.11) that the mutation has occurred *de novo* in the gamete supplied by his mother, only the second time such an event had been detected in human disease. In addition this patient had a very high titre of antibodies to factor ·VIII, which his immune system reacts to as foreign protein. These antibodies are still in use as a valuable reagent for immunological measurement of factor VIII (Fig. 1.12). The CG dinucleotide is the villain of this particular piece, for such pairs turn out to be the most important mutation hot spot in human genetic disease, accounting for one-third of all reported mutations, by the following mechanism. The cytosine on both sides of a CG dimer pair is methylated in the five

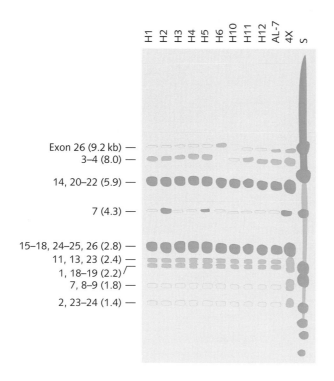

Exon 26 (9.2 kb) —
3–4 (8.0) —

14, 20–22 (5.9) —

7 (4.3) —

15–18, 24–25, 26 (2.8) —
11, 13, 23 (2.4) —
1, 18–19 (2.2) —
7, 8–9 (1.8) —

2, 23–24 (1.4) —

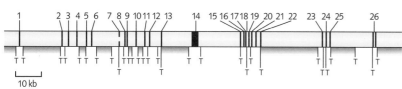

Fig. 1.11 Detection of the first mutations in haemophilia A. A Southern blot digested with the enzyme *Taq*I has been probed with a full length cDNA probe for factor VIII. The bands (hybridizing fragments) correspond to different exons of the gene as shown below. Most bands, due to similar sized fragments, represent several exons overlaid. The abnormal bands in lane H2 and H6 represent shifts due to loss of *Taq*I sites (see Fig. 1.12).

position of the pyridine ring. Spontaneous deamination of methyl-cytosine on the other strand converts it to thymidine. DNA repair mechanisms cannot of course recognize this as an abnormal base requiring replacement and therefore at the next round of replication the new T is matched to an A. By the same mechanism acting initially on the lower strand, G will be replaced by A on the other strand. Vivid proof of this mechanism can be obtained by inspecting any database of mutations in a large gene such as factor VIII. The Arg 2209 stop (a convenient shorthand for mutations) nonsense mutation had already been reported in six unrelated haemophiliacs with severe disease by 1991. Three of these patients had formed antibodies to factor VIII after treatment. However, the others had not, showing that other factors including perhaps immune response genes are involved in this particular complication of treatment. The same codon has also frequently suffered mutation on the other strand giving rise by CGA → CAA transition to a glutamine codon. Arg 2209 Gln had also been detected in at least 11 unrelated patients with moderate haemophilia A by 1991.

There are only five arginine codons in the factor VIII sequence that are also in *Taq*I sites and are therefore detectable by Southern blotting when mutated as in the examples above. Mutations at these sites together with large deletions also detectable by Southern blotting, the first examples of which were detected in the initial survey (Fig. 1.13), account for about 5% of severe haemophilia A: the rest of the mutations remain undetected by these rather crude methods.

Other arginine codons are not only potential hot spots, but also of functional significance, as they are adjacent to the essential activation cleavage sites recognized by thrombin or the inactivation sites used by activated protein C.

1987–1992   The polymerase chain reaction enables discovery of most mutations—but some are missing

This frustrating situation of knowing that a wealth of diversity existed (remember Haldane) but being unable to detect it was resolved by a dramatic advance in DNA

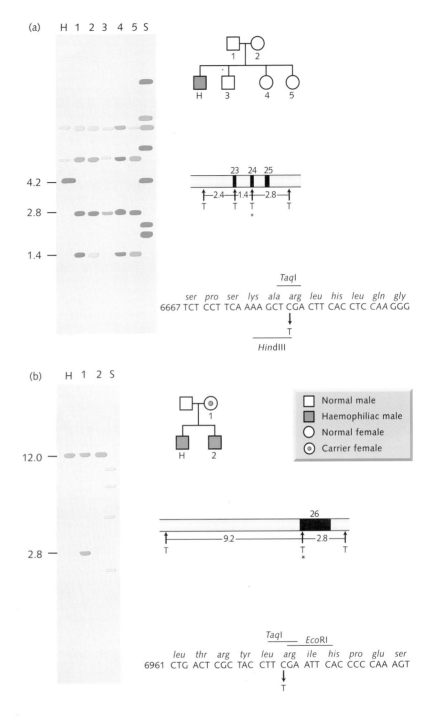

Fig. 1.12 Sequences of the first two point mutations identified in haemophilia A. Upper panel represents a family study on patient H2. The mutation destroying the *Taq*I site (TCGA) converts C to T, introducing a premature stop codon. The mutation is not present in his mother's peripheral blood white cells and is therefore due to a *de novo* mutation in the maternal germ line. The lower panel shows a similar mutation in exon 26 also introducing a premature stop codon.

technology—the polymerase chain reaction (PCR), which was invented by Kary Mullis (then at Cetus, another San Francisco-based biotechnology company). This technique allows selected segments of DNA to be enzymatically amplified in a few hours from genomic DNA—an advance which you would only fully appreci-

ate if you had spent 6 months trying to clone a piece of DNA from a patient's sample by standard methods only to fail, as I did with another gene at about this time, then succeeded with PCR (see Chapter 3 for details of PCR methodology).

A PCR-based technique enabled Jane Gitschier to go

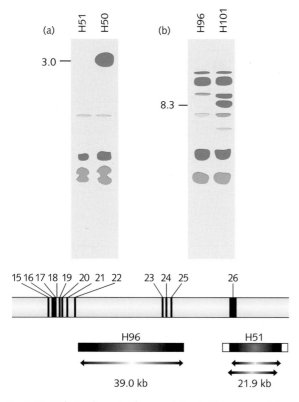

Fig. 1.13 Deletions causing haemophilia A. The extent of the two deletions, detected by aberrant fragments on the Southern blots, were mapped as shown by hatched bars.

back to some of my haemophilic patients' DNA and specifically screen the cleavage sites (Gitschier *et al.*, 1988). In brief, the short segments of DNA spanning the thrombin and protein C cleavage site were amplified by PCR from normal and patient DNA samples, then probed with a short piece of DNA that either matches the normal sequence or one of the two likely mutations (C → T or G → A as explained above). Two patients from about 100 screened proved to have a mutation as predicted (Fig. 1.14). One was in the arginine codon at position 336, next to the protein C cleavage site, converting it to a stop codon. No detectable factor VIII was present in his plasma. We speculated as to whether a missense mutation at this site, e.g. to a glutamine, would give rise to a circulating factor VIII protein resistant to inactivation, and therefore cause the patient to suffer from thrombosis, as is the case for deficiency of protein C itself. To date no example of this has been found, perhaps because there is a second protein C site (Fig. 1.8). (A mutation at the homologous site in factor V gives rise to activated protein C resistance and, being present in 4% of Europeans, is the single commonest cause of venous thromboembolism.) The other mutation identified by the survey caused a missense substitution of arginine 1689 by cysteine due to a C → T transition, again exactly as predicted. Now this patient's plasma contained normal amounts of factor VIII detected immunologically (using the antibody from the patient

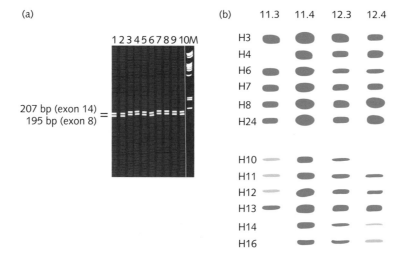

Fig. 1.14 Screening for mutations in the factor VIII gene using allele specific oligonucleotides. First a selected region of the factor VIII gene is amplified by PCR, demonstrated as the DNA sequences in the gel on the left. Then the PCR product is

bound to a filter and probed with a labelled oligonucleotide. Absence of an amplification product is due to mutation of a single base. In this way several novel mutations were discovered affecting the protease cleavage sites of factor VIII.

H2 with a premature stop codon 2209), but no factor VIII clotting activity. Don O'Brien therefore developed a modified and 500-fold scaled down scheme for purifying this variant molecule from a 500 ml blood sample generously donated by the patient (who happens to be a biochemist and very interested in the project). Sure enough the variant factor VIII light chain was totally resistant to thrombin cleavage at the light chain site (1689–1690), and furthermore could not be released from binding to von Willebrand factor by treatment with thrombin. This result supported other studies pointing to the segment of factor VIII between residues 1648 and 1689 as being essential for binding to von Willebrand factor, and showed that this thrombin cleavage is essential for simultaneous activation of factor VIII and for its release from the carrier molecule (Fig. 1.8). This study was the first to examine in detail a functional variant of factor VIII isolated from a patient's blood, and to explain mechanistically the bleeding condition that resulted from a particular missense mutation (O'Brien and Tuddenham, 1989). Further extensions of the PCR technique (see Box 1.4) led to the identification of most of the remaining mutations in mild and moderate haemophilia A, which turned out to be virtually all missense mutations, affecting the rate of protein synthesis, stability, protein function or any combination of these. The mutations in the severe cases (factor VIII less than 1%) were found in about half of the patients to be disabling lesions such as small inserts or deletions causing frameshift, splice junction alterations (in the canonical GT/AG), nonsense codons or large deletions. However, in half of the cases screened no abnormality at all could be found in the exons or flanking regions.

1992   The missing mutations

This mystery prompted several hypotheses but the explanation began to emerge when Jenny Naylor in Giannelli's laboratory at Guy's Hospital used a PCR-based method to amplify factor VIII cDNA obtained from peripheral blood lymphocytes. Now lymphocytes do not make detectable amounts of factor VIII but the transcription machinery seems to be prone to produce a few copies of mRNA from most genes in these cells, regardless of their usual tissue specificity. These apparently inconsequential or 'illegitimate' transcripts that result from 'leaky' expression of the factor VIII C gene in lymphocytes can be detected using the exquisite sensitivity of PCR—capable in the limit of 'detecting', or rather amplifying from a single template of cDNA obtained from mRNA by the action of reverse transcriptase. The clue that Jenny found was this: spliced mRNA represent-

---

Rapid DNA Scanning Techniques For Mutation Detection

Space does not allow any detail about these techniques, for which Michaelides *et al.* (1994) should be consulted.

1 Denaturing gradient gel electrophoresis (DGGE). Target DNA is PCR amplified then allowed to form heteroduplexes with normal DNA. The duplexes are electrophoresed through a denaturing gradient. Melting of the DNA duplexes occurs at a position characteristic of the sequence and strongly influenced by the presence of a mismatch. Upon melting, migration practically ceases because random coil, single-stranded DNA migrates much more slowly than double-stranded DNA. When the DNA is visualized on the gel after migration, any alteration in position from a normal control will indicate a sequence variation. The DNA is then recovered and sequenced.

2 Chemical cleavage. A target sequence is amplified and allowed to form heteroduplexes with normal DNA. In this case the DNA is end labelled with ^{32}P. The duplexes are then subjected to chemical modification with osmium tetroxide or hydroxylamine and then cleaved with piperidine. Only mismatches will be cleaved in this protocol, again revealing aberrant sequence by a cleaved band of lower molecular weight.

3 Single-stranded conformational polymorphism (SSCP). The target sequence is amplified by PCR, labelled with ^{32}P, melted by boiling, then rapidly cooled to allow single-stranded self-conformational structures to form, that are characteristic of a given sequence. Variation in these structures can be detected by electrophoresis in a non-denaturing polyacrylamide gel under carefully controlled conditions. Variants, if detected, are confirmed by directly sequencing the target DNA.

Box 1.4

---

ing exons 1 to 22 could be amplified, as could spliced mRNA covering exons 23 to 26, but try as she could no transcript crossing from exon 22 to 23 could be amplified. It seemed that the two halves of the message existed independently. Clearly the explanation for the missing mutations must lie in intron 22.

1993   The mystery of intron 22 solved

A few years earlier, Jane Gitschier and colleagues had discovered two small genes actually contained within intron 22 of the factor VIII gene, the first such 'intronic' genes to be found in a mammalian genome (subsequently other examples have cropped up, e.g. in the neurofibromatosis gene). These genes were named F8A and F8B to distinguish them from the standard gene name assigned to the whole locus F8C. F8A and F8B are transcribed in opposite directions from a CpG island—a common feature found upstream of many genes, especially 'housekeeping' genes active in many tissues. The function of these genes is unknown, indeed they appear to be expressed only as mRNA transcripts since no protein corresponding to the sequence of their open reading frames has been detected. Now F8A in intron 22 is not the only copy of this sequence; two more F8A genes were found nearer the tip (telomere) of the X-chromosome (see Fig. 1.15). Jane Gitschier reasoned therefore that a telomeric copy of F8A could cross over with the intronic copy. If this occurs the segment of DNA between the two F8A copies could be inverted, separating the factor VIII gene into two halves facing in opposite directions, giving rise to the two unconnected mRNA transcripts identified by Jenny Naylor. To prove this Jane Gitschier's group made a special probe to the F8A gene and showed by Southern blotting that a change in pattern, due to altered local environment of at least one F8A copy, occurred in all the patients whose mutation had not been detected elsewhere. As further confirmation they showed that the 5′ factor VIII message in these cases was attached to novel sequences, unrelated to factor VIII but which mapped to a region normally near the telomere of the X-chromosome — a situation which could only arise if a large inversion had moved the 5′ half of factor VIII nearer that region. Similar experiments by Jenny Naylor independently confirmed this remarkable mechanism. It is now clear from several confirmatory studies that nearly half of all patients with severe haemophilia A have this type of inversion, which must arise spontaneously at a remarkably high rate for a single type of genetic lesion. This mechanism is not unique to factor

VIII but no doubt arises due to the curious and indeed dangerous distribution of the F8A gene copies.

Thus in 1994 we could at last confidently approach a family-segregating haemophilia A expecting to find the underlying mutation after a few weeks' work. With this information one can then offer definitive carrier determination (or exclusion), and if requested antenatal diagnosis by CVS at 8–10 weeks' gestation. Indeed it has been proposed that national databases establishing the mutation in all known cases can be set up, to provide optimum genetic counselling and to gain the maximum scientific information concerning the mutational spectrum of a prevalent genetic disorder. This will also enable us to derive information about structure, function and synthesis of this vital protein from nature's own experimental databank.

1990–1993   Trials of recombinant factor VIII

The first demonstration of factor VIII activity in tissue culture was at a very low level.

Genentech soon sold their interest in the project to Cutter, a plasma fractionation company owned by German pharmaceutical giant, Bayer. Cutter painstakingly increased the level of expression in baby hamster kidney (BHK) cells to the point where a large-scale production process would be feasible. Although not officially published, this expression level is probably in the region of 1–2 mg factor VIII/litre or 5–10 activity units/ml of culture fluid. Allowing for losses it probably takes 200 litres of culture medium to produce the factor VIII needed by each adult haemophiliac each year. The pure recombinant factor VIII is stabilized with albumen. It was tested for efficacy first in dogs with haemophilia A in a colony kept for this purpose. It performed well in stopping bleeding from a standardized (capillary bed) wound, and had a reasonable half-life in their circulation. Fortunately canine von Willebrand factor binds and protects human factor VIII in the dog's circulation.

The first humans to receive recombinant factor VIII were a selected set of adult patients with severe haemophilia A. All went well, with several hundred infusions producing virtually no adverse side effects and proving highly effective in controlling or preventing bleeding. The next step was to try the product on previously untreated patients, mainly new diagnosed infants, who were all HIV-negative. This trial has also been successful, although a rather high rate of development of antibodies has been noted (almost 30%). Most of these antibodies have been of low titre and disappeared on further treatment. No exactly comparable group of patients given standard plasma-derived factor VIII is

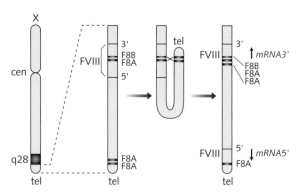

Fig. 1.15 The 'flip tip' inversion. About 40% of cases of severe haemophilia A are now known to have an inversion through their factor VIII gene. The putative mechanism of this prevalent mutation is shown. There are three copies of the small gene known of F8A, one within intron 22 of the factor VIII gene proper, and two more about 400 kb telomeric to the gene. During meiosis intrachromosomal crossover can occur, resulting in the two halves of the factor VIII gene being separated by 400 kb. This occurs most often during spermatogenesis as the distal portion of the X has nothing to pair with.

available so it is a moot point as to whether the recombinant protein is significantly more immunogenic than the plasma-derived factor VIII. Some studies of the plasma-derived treatment have shown similar rates of antibody development. Recombinant factor VIII produced by two companies (Baxter/Genetics Institute and Cutter/Genentech) has now been licensed for use in the USA and in Europe. Already haemophilia centre directors are preferring high-purity concentrate, whether plasma-derived or recombinant, for HIV-positive patients, because it preserves the CD4 counts compared to treatment with standard factor VIII concentrates. The latter appear to cause a steady fall in CD4 counts, thus potentially accelerating the onset of clinical AIDS.

Price comparisons, as in all other aspects of health care, are also influencing purchasing policy (no, the author has not been on a management course and hopes never to have to go on one!). Currently, high-purity plasma-derived factor VIII costs about 40 pence/unit, whilst recombinant factor VIII sells for about 65 pence/unit. The companies making the recombinant material also sell plasma-derived factor VIII, as well as all the other plasma-derived products. Anyone who owned a huge plasma fractionation plant, and all the plasmapheresis centres needed to supply its feedstock, would not want to see a sudden collapse in the plasma market induced by a dramatic fall in the price of factor VIII, the factor which currently supports and

Table 1.3 A brief history of factor VIII.

Date	Event
Second century	Rabbi Judah the Patriarch recognizes a hereditary disorder causing death after circumcision
Tenth century	Khalaf Ibn Abbas records a locally frequent male-specific bleeding tendency
1803	John Otto describes a family with bleeder males, and notes that females are not so afflicted
1820	Nässe summarizes the 'laws' of transmission but fails to note that affected males can transmit the disease (via carrier daughters)
1893	Almroth Wright shows that haemophilic blood is slow to clot *in vitro*
1909	Sex-linked inheritance explained by Bateson
1911	Addis prepares a fraction from normal plasma which shortens the clotting time of haemophilic plasma
1926	von Willebrand describes an autosomal dominant bleeding syndrome
1935	Haldane deduces that the incidence of haemophilia is due to a high rate of new mutations, and is genetically diverse
1937	Patek and Taylor isolate a correcting fraction from blood which they later call anti-hemophilic globulin (AHG)
1950	Specific assay for AHG devised by Merskey and Macfarlane
1953	AHG shown to be deficient in von Willebrand's disease as well as in haemophilia A by Larrieu and Soulier
1962	Roman numeral VIII assigned to AHG, defined as the factor deficient in haemophilia A
1965	Coagulation cascade hypothesis proposed by Macfarlane and by Davie and Ratnoff
1972	Zimmerman, Ratnoff and Powell measure an antigen related to factor VIII immunologically and show that it is low in von Willebrand's disease but normal in haemophilia A. At first called factor VIII-related antigen, but soon realized to be the von Willebrand factor
1973	Zimmerman and Edgington recognize that von Willebrand factor and factor VIII are independent molecular entities, although co-purifying
1979	Human factor VIII completely free of von Willebrand factor prepared by Tuddenham, Trabold, Collins and Hoyer
1982	Factor VIII cloning race entered by at least four biotechnology companies working with academic researchers
1984	Cloning and expression of factor VIII published simultaneously by two industrial/academic partnerships (Genentech/Royal Free Hospital and Genetics Institute/Mayo Clinic)
1985	Linkage analysis for haemophilia A achieved by using restriction fragment length polymorphism in the factor VIII gene
1986	First mutations in factor VIII gene identified
1991	Clinical trials of recombinant factor VIII
1993	Half of severe haemophilia A shown to be due to a unique inversion involving an intronic gene, F8A, and its extragenic copies
1995	Haemophiliac mouse models created by homologous recombination

Back to the future scenarios

1996–2000	Effective gene therapy vectors developed and tested in animal models
2000–2005	Clinical trials of gene therapy for haemophilia A
2005–	Widespread use of gene therapy for haemophilia A eliminates need for replacement therapy

effectively drives the economics of plasma collection and fractionation.

1995–2020   The future of factor VIII research

Are all the problems of haemophilia A solved? Is haemophilia research pretty much at the end of its golden age? What remains to be done?

The next items on the agenda are the following:

1 to determine the relative contribution of factor VIII mutational genotype and immune response genes to the development of inhibitory antibodies, so that effective prevention can be provided;

2 to develop gene therapy;

3 to solve the three-dimensional structure of factor VIII;

4 to work out the mechanism of factor VIII function;

5 to study the regulation of the factor VIII gene;

6 to examine the evolution of factor VIII.

Plenty to keep us busy for the next few years (Table 1.3).

History and personalities involved

The account of factor VIII research given above is not meant to be an exhaustive history. It is thoroughly biased towards the research programme of my own group and that of colleagues at Genentech. Jane Gitschier has continued her work at an academic institution (University of California, San Francisco, Howard Hughes Medical Institute).

Very similar and often exactly parallel work came from the laboratory of the Genetics Institute in Boston under Randall Kaufman and from Haig Kazazian's genetics group at Johns Hopkins in Baltimore. In some cases the work was competitive, as when racing for a biotechnological first, in others co-operative. Modern biomedical science is highly competitive, usually to the benefit of the end consumer, the patient, occasionally to his detriment, as when patents are used to extract huge settlements, ultimately paid for by the insurer or tax payer who supports health care.

The author is still in there, striving for the next 'first', sometimes elated, often frustrated, but carried forward by the incredible momentum of molecular biology in the late twentieth century.

Further reading

Bloom A.L., Thomas D., Forbes C. and Tuddenham E.G.D. (1994) *Haemostasis and Thrombosis*, 3rd edn. Churchill Livingstone, Edinburgh. This two-volume, multi-author reference book covers the broad sweep of basic science and clinical practice as applied to disorders of haemostasis which, in the form of thrombosis, are the most prevalent killers in Western societies.

Cooper D.N. and Krawczyk M. (1993) *Human Gene Mutation*. BIOS, Oxford. A survey of the whole of human inherited disease from the viewpoint of molecular genetics, focusing particularly on mechanisms of mutation.

Gitschier J., Kogan S., Levinson B. and Tuddenham E.G.D. (1988) Mutations of factor VIII cleavage sites. *Blood*, **72**, 1022–1028. The first detection of a mutation specifically affecting the function of factor VIII by altering a thrombin activation cleavage residue—Arg 1989 to Cys—and the first use of the polymerase chain reaction to analyse mutations in haemophilia A.

Haldane J.B.S. (1935) The rate of spontaneous mutation of a human gene. *Journal of Genetics*, **31**, 317–326. A classic paper in human genetics, the pure genius of logical thought applied to fairly sparse data to obtain a brilliant result.

Kazazian H.H., Tuddenham E.G.D. and Antonarakis S.E. (1994) Haemophilia A: deficiency of coagulation factor VIII. In: *The Metabolic Basis of Inherited Disease*, 7th edn (eds C.R. Scriver, A.L. Beaudet, W.S. Sly and D. Valle). McGraw Hill, New York. Further details of the molecular genetics, pathology and treatment of haemophilia A, in a book which is the acknowledged master reference for human inherited disease. Anyone interested in the molecular basis of human pathology and its alleviation should look at this book.

Kemball-Cook G. and Tuddenham E.G.D. (1997) The factor VIII mutation database on the World Wide Web: the haemophilia A mutation search test and resource site. HAMSTeRS update (Version 3.0). *Nucleic Acids Research*, **25** (in press). An exhaustive listing of all published mutations causing haemophilia A with over 500 different examples representing every type of genetic lesion, a review of the molecular pathology of Haemophilia A and a model structure of Factor VIII. Now accessible as a Web site at http://europium.mrcrpms.ac.uk.

Lusher J.M., Arkin S., Abildgaard C.F., Schwartz R.S. *et al.* (1993) Recombinant factor VIII for the treatment of previously untreated patients with haemophilia A. *New England Journal of Medicine*, **328**, 453–459. The first report of a large-scale trial of treatment for a blood disorder using recombinant protein as replacement therapy. A high incidence of antibodies against factor VIII was recorded (28%) but this may have been due to intensive surveillance. Most antibodies disappeared on further treatment.

Michaelides K., Schwaab R., Lalloz M.R.A., Schmidt W. and Tuddenham E.G.D. (1994) Mutational analysis: new mutations. In: *PRC II: A Practical Approach* (eds B.D. Hames and S.J. Higgins). IRL Press, Oxford. Full technical details on the methods now in use for rapidly detecting mutations. A cookbook for the molecular genetics of any organism.

O'Brien D.P. and Tuddenham E.G.D. (1989) Purification and characterization of factor VIII 1689 Cys: a non-functional cofactor occurring in a patient with severe haemophilia A.

Blood, **73**, 2117–2122. The first functional analysis of a mutant factor VIII protein isolated from the blood of a patient with haemophilia A.

Robb-Smith A. (1993) *Life and Achievements of Professor Robert Gwyn Macfarlane FRS, Pioneer in the Care of Haemophilics* [*sic*]. Royal Society of Medicine, London. A biography of the brilliant medical scientist who did so much to advance understanding of blood coagulation, and to apply that knowledge to the treatment of haemophilia, the disease which had inspired his researches in the first place.

Tuddenham E.G.D. and Cooper D.N. (1994) *The Molecular Genetics of Haemostasis and its Inherited Disorders*. Oxford Monographs in Medical Genetics No. 25. Oxford University Press, Oxford. Chapter 2 of this book covers the material of the present chapter in detail with references to the original literature.

Chapter 2

DNA, RNA and proteins

Introduction

Complex multicellular organisms are composed of different tissues (muscle, gut, brain etc.) whose individual characteristics are dependent on the specific proteins expressed in these cell types. Consequently, brain is distinguishable from muscle because of brain-specific proteins, and the differentiation and development of specific tissue is therefore dependent on the control of proteins synthesized by the cells within that tissue. These differentially expressed proteins may function in many ways: as structural components of the cell, or as regulatory proteins such as enzymes, cellular receptors or intracellular signalling proteins. It is the incorrect expression of such proteins, their expression in the wrong place, at the wrong time, or the production of abnormal levels of specific proteins or proteins with abnormal function which underpins all cellular disease with a genetic basis. Consequently, a complete understanding of the function of specific proteins and the control of their expression will help enormously in understanding disease.

All proteins are composed of chains of amino acids. The primary sequence (the order of amino acids) in a protein helps determine the way that protein folds and forms a three-dimensional structure, and hence its biophysical and biochemical character.

The cell nucleus contains all the information necessary to determine the spectrum of protein expression observed in different cell types. This information is encoded within the cell's chromosomes, in DNA, which acts as a template to define the order of amino acids within polypeptide chains. The regions of DNA which define proteins are termed genes and are present in specific sites on the chromosome. However, the deciphering of the DNA code into an amino acid sequence occurs on specialist cell organelles, the ribosomes, in the cell cytoplasm. Consequently, the nuclear DNA does not act itself as the template for ordering amino acids during protein synthesis. The information encoded within the DNA is first copied into RNA, in a process termed **transcription**, and then is transported out of the nucleus and onto the ribosomes where it is decoded to generate a primary amino acid sequence, by a process called **translation**.

The relationships between DNA, RNA and protein, known to date, are shown in Fig. 2.1. We will look at DNA, RNA and protein individually and then see how each fit into the complex mechanism of generating a functional protein from a gene.

DNA structure—the double helix

DNA is a variable polymer of four monomer units containing the purine bases adenine (A) or guanine (G), or the pyrimidine bases cytosine (C) or thymine (T), joined to a deoxyribose phosphate (Fig. 2.2)—the nucleotide. Individual monomer nucleotides are linked by a phosphodiester bond between the deoxyribose unit of neighbouring nucleotides in such a way that the 3′ carbon of the deoxyribose of one nucleotide links the 5′ carbon of the deoxyribose on the adjacent nucleotide. For this

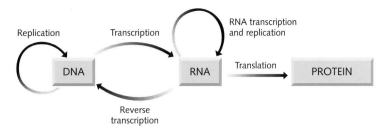

Fig. 2.1 DNA makes RNA makes protein. The one-way flow of information from DNA to protein was challenged by the discovery, in 1970, of reverse transcriptase, an enzyme capable of converting RNA to a DNA copy.

reason the phosphodiester linkages within the nucleotide chain have directionality (see Fig. 2.2).

After DNA is synthesized (see below) some of the purine and pyrimidine bases may be chemically modified. For instance, cytosine bases can become methylated to a 5-methyl-cytosine form and there is strong evidence that in higher eukaryotes the extent of DNA methylation may play a role in the regulation of expression of some genes (see Chapter 4).

DNA within a eukaryotic cell is predominantly present as a double-stranded helical structure (double helix) formed by two separate DNA polymers winding around each other. The two strands run antiparallel, which we will see later has important implications for the structure and function of DNA, such that the deoxyribose linkages of each strand run in opposite 5′–3′ orientations (see Fig. 2.3). The double helix is maintained by hydrogen bond pairing between nucleotide pairs on each strand of DNA, whereby A always pairs with T and G always pairs with C due to stereochemical constraints. Consequently, this complementary base pair rule means that the sequence of one DNA strand specifies the sequence of the other and it is this phenomenon which confers upon DNA the extraordinary biochemical properties necessary for replication, information decoding and repair.

The DNA sequence is a genetic code

The 5′–3′ sequential arrangement of these four nucleotides (adenine, guanine, thymidine and cytosine) in the polymeric chain of DNA is a direct code for the arrangement of amino acids in the protein that a specific DNA sequence encodes. One amino acid is encoded by the arrangement of three monomer nucleotides (the triplet codon). For instance, the amino acid methionine is coded for by the nucleotide triplet ATG. Consequently, as there are four monomers (A, T, G and C) and a triplet

codon comprises three of these, there are 64 possible codons. Of these 64, 61 specify a particular amino acid. The other three codons signal the end of a protein (stop codon). However, as there are only some 22 amino acids some of the 61 codons specifying amino acids are redundant, that is some different codons specify the same amino acid (see Table 2.1). For instance, the amino acid isoleucine can be coded for by the DNA sequence ATT, ATC or ATA. Whilst redundant, the code is never ambiguous, as one codon never specifies more than one amino acid.

Table 2.1 The genetic code.

First position (5′ end)	Second position				Third position (3′ end)
	U	**C**	**A**	**G**	
U	Phe	Ser	Tyr	Cys	U
	Phe	Ser	Tyr	Cys	C
	Leu	Ser	Stop	Stop	A
	Leu	Ser	Stop	Trp	G
C	Leu	Pro	His	Arg	U
	Leu	Pro	His	Arg	C
	Leu	Pro	Gln	Arg	A
	Leu	Pro	Gln	Arg	G
A	Ile	Thr	Asn	Ser	U
	Ile	Thr	Asn	Ser	C
	Ile	Thr	Lys	Arg	A
	Met	Thr	Lys	Arg	G
G	Val	Ala	Asp	Gly	U
	Val	Ala	Asp	Gly	C
	Val	Ala	Glu	Gly	A
	Val	Ala	Glu	Gly	G

For example: the codon AUG specifies methionine, whereas the codon GCA specifies alanine. UAA, UAG and UGA are translation termination signals.

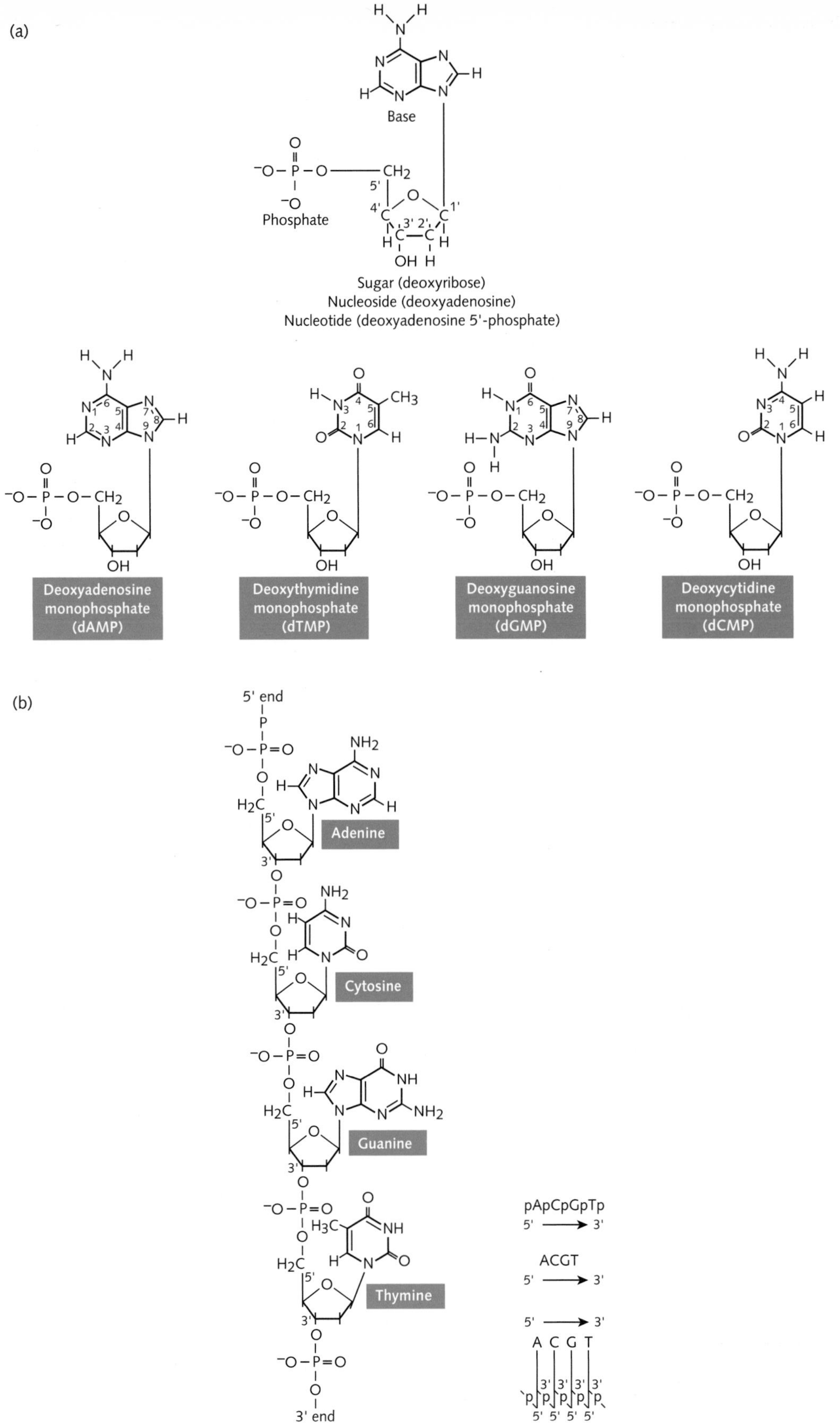

(a)

Base

Phosphate

5'
4'   1'
3' 2'
OH H

Sugar (deoxyribose)
Nucleoside (deoxyadenosine)
Nucleotide (deoxyadenosine 5'-phosphate)

Deoxyadenosine monophosphate (dAMP)

Deoxythymidine monophosphate (dTMP)

Deoxyguanosine monophosphate (dGMP)

Deoxycytidine monophosphate (dCMP)

(b)

5' end

Adenine

Cytosine

Guanine

Thymine

3' end

pApCpGpTp
5' ⟶ 3'

ACGT
5' ⟶ 3'

5' ⟶ 3'
A C G T

Fig. 2.2 Deoxynucleotides in DNA. DNA contains deoxynucleotides consisting of a specific heterocyclic nitrogenous base (adenine, guanine, cytosine or thymine) joined to a deoxyribose phosphate moiety. Adjacent deoxynucleotides are linked through their phosphate groups to form long polynucleotide chains (reproduced from Singer and Berg (1991)).

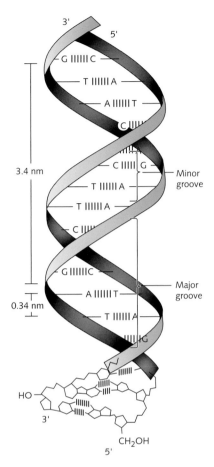

Fig. 2.3 Complementary basepairing between polynucleotide chains generates a double helix of complementary DNA strands, one 5′ to 3′ and the other 3′ to 5′, wrapped around each other (reproduced from Singer and Berg (1991)).

DNA is packaged as chromosomes

In eukaryotic cells, the bulk of the DNA is present in the nucleus as double-stranded linear molecules but mitochondria, present in the cell cytoplasm, also contain their own DNA which is present as a double-stranded, covalently closed circle. DNA does not exist free in eukaryotic cells, rather, it is complexed with proteins to form chromatin and this is compacted to generate structures called chromosomes. This condensing of the DNA is essential, as a human cell contains 23 chromosome pairs containing approximately 4×10^9 nucleotide pairs (often termed basepairs or bp) of DNA whose extended length would approach 1 m.

In the nucleus, chromatin consists of complexes of double-stranded DNA and five types of histone proteins: H1, H2a, H2b, H3 and H4. At the molecular level, isolated chromatin has a beaded structure, each bead result-

ing from a complex of 145 basepairs of DNA together with two molecules each of H2a, H2b, H3 and H4—the so-called nucleosome core. The beads or nucleosomes are separated by a single molecule of histone H1 (see Fig. 2.4). Nucleosomes are themselves compacted and condensed to form structures that have been termed solenoids, and these structures are then compacted even further with the aid of other non-histone chromosomal proteins to generate a single chromosome. Such structuring of the DNA into chromatin has profound affects on the ability of the chromatinized DNA to be transcribed, and requires complex regulation mechanisms (see Chapter 4).

RNA—a structural component of the cell and an intermediate between DNA and protein

There are a variety of RNAs present in the eukaryotic cell:

- messenger RNA (mRNA)
- transfer RNA (tRNA)
- ribosomal RNA (rRNA).

As well as mRNA, which consists of direct copies of protein-coding DNA sequences, eukaryotic cells also contain rRNA which is a structural component of ribosomes and tRNA which functions in transferring amino acids to growing polypeptide chains during protein synthesis and which is, like mRNA, coded for by DNA. RNA is about 10 times more abundant than DNA in a eukaryotic cell; of this RNA about 80% represents rRNA, 15% tRNA and less than 5% mRNA. Other minor species of RNA such as small nuclear RNA (snRNA) are also present.

Like DNA, RNA also consists of stretches of polynucleotides which include the adenine, guanine and cytosine bases found in DNA, but in RNA the thymine base is substituted for by the base uracil. In RNA, the purine and pyrimidine bases are joined not to a deoxyribose phosphate background but to a ribose phosphate background (hence the name ribonucleic acid). The ribonucleotide chains are linked by the same 5′ to 3′ phosphodiester bond seen in DNA. Most cell RNA is single-stranded but some viruses contain double-stranded RNA (see Chapter 13). The nature of RNA means that RNA sequences can form hybrids to both DNA and RNA if their sequences are complementary.

In the cell, mRNA is normally found associated with proteins in complexes called messenger ribonucleoprotein (mRNP) which package mRNA and aid its movement or transport to the cytoplasm where it is

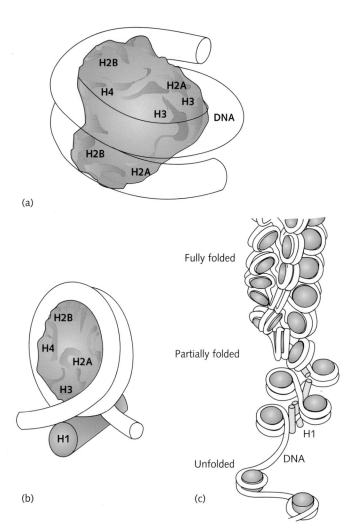

(a)

(b)

(c)

Fully folded

Partially folded

Unfolded

H1

DNA

Fig. 2.4 Histones package DNA into a higher order chromatin structure. (a) Approximately 145 basepairs of DNA are wrapped around an octamer of histones comprising two copies each of histones H1, H2A, H2B, H3 and H4. (b) These so-called nucleosome cores are linked along the polynucleotide chain by histone H1 and are folded into higher order chromatin generating a highly condensed solenoid structure (c) (reproduced from Singer and Berg (1991)).

decoded into a protein. rRNA is complexed with ribosomal proteins which generates a functional ribosome on which proteins are synthesized.

Proteins

Proteins, one of the structural bases of cells and cellular enzymes, contain one or more polypeptides which themselves consist of chains of polymerized amino acids, of which there are about 22. Each amino acid has a similar basic structure, containing a free amino group at one end and a free carboxyl group at the other. These are linked in polymers by a peptide bond between the amino- and carboxy-termini (see Fig. 2.6a) such that a polypeptide contains a free amino group at one end and a free carboxyl group at the other (hence the terms **amino**-terminal and **carboxy**-terminal ends of a protein). Each

amino acid also has a side chain which dictates the biochemical characteristic of that amino acid. For instance, sulphur-based amino acids such as cysteine can form disulphide bonds covalently linking polypeptide chains to themselves or to other distinct polypeptides (see Fig. 2.6b). Other amino acids can be modified, once in a polypeptide chain, by covalent addition of sugars or phosphate — so-called post-translational modification (see p. 35).

The primary sequence of a polypeptide will dictate the structure, function and biochemical nature of specific proteins.

Genes—DNA sequences that code for structural RNAs or proteins

Much has been written about the definition of a gene but

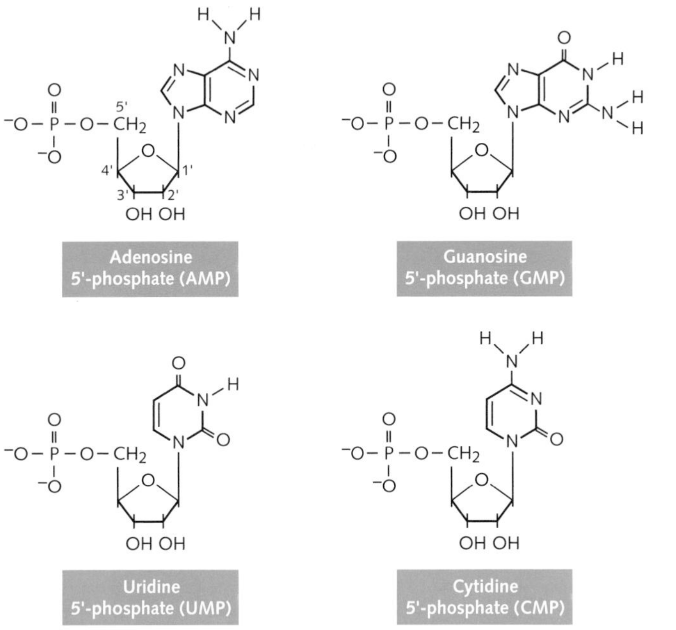

Fig. 2.5 Ribonucleotides in RNA. Like DNA, RNA contains four nucleotides, three of which, adenine, guanine and cytosine, are in common with DNA whilst the fourth, uracil, is specific for RNA. These nucleotides are linked to a ribose sugar and joined into chains by the same phosphodiester bonds seen in DNA.

it must be understood that a gene is a functional definition. The DNA sequences of a gene comprise 5′ promoter region, amino acid coding region, 3′ termination and processing signals, i.e. any DNA sequence which is necessary for correct expression of the gene in the right place at the right time — so-called **tissue-** and **temporal-specific expression**.

This knowledge came from molecular analyses which showed that the amount of DNA which functionally encodes a specific gene may be much larger than the size predicted by the amino acid sequence. For instance, the gene **promoter** comprises additional DNA sequences, often in front of (5′ to) the region of DNA encoding the protein, which contain signals necessary for regulated gene expression (see Chapter 4). Similarly, DNA after (3′ to) the amino acid-coding region may contain sequences which contain signals defining the end of the gene-coding region and which are necessary for correct stopping or **termination** of the RNA copy of the gene (the **RNA transcript**). This 3′ region may also contain signals which dictate whether the RNA is further modified by, for instance, **polyadenylation** (see below) to aid in its stability. By the late 1970s it also became apparent that the DNA sequences encoding a specific protein were not necessarily present in one uninterrupted, or **contiguous**, stretch of DNA, but that the DNA sequences which actually encoded information for the amino acid sequence of the protein — so-called **exons** — could be interrupted by regions of DNA sequence that were not involved in

coding for any amino acids — so-called **introns** or **intervening sequences** (see Fig. 2.7). In order for the mRNA copy of the gene to be formed, such introns in the RNA transcript must be removed and the exons joined back up in a process called **RNA splicing** to produce an mRNA transcript which can be transported to ribosomes and decoded to generate a protein. Consequently, analysis of specific RNA transcripts from a gene can result in a complex array of RNA transcripts, termed heterogeneous nuclear RNA (hnRNA), from a particular gene which reflect splicing intermediates of the primary transcript.

DNA replication

Cell division is an absolute prerequisite for growth, development and reproduction of all organisms. Consequently, as cells divide, it is essential that the chromosomes containing the cellular DNA are duplicated in order for daughter cells to contain a copy of the spectrum of genes required for cell structure and function. The complete replication of the cell's complement of chromosomes occurs upon cell division by a process termed mitosis, except when cells divide to form gametes during which a special cell division termed meiosis occurs (see Chapter 5).

The ability of DNA to copy itself faithfully is of fundamental importance to its role as the material of heredity. The double-strandedness of eukaryotic DNA and the

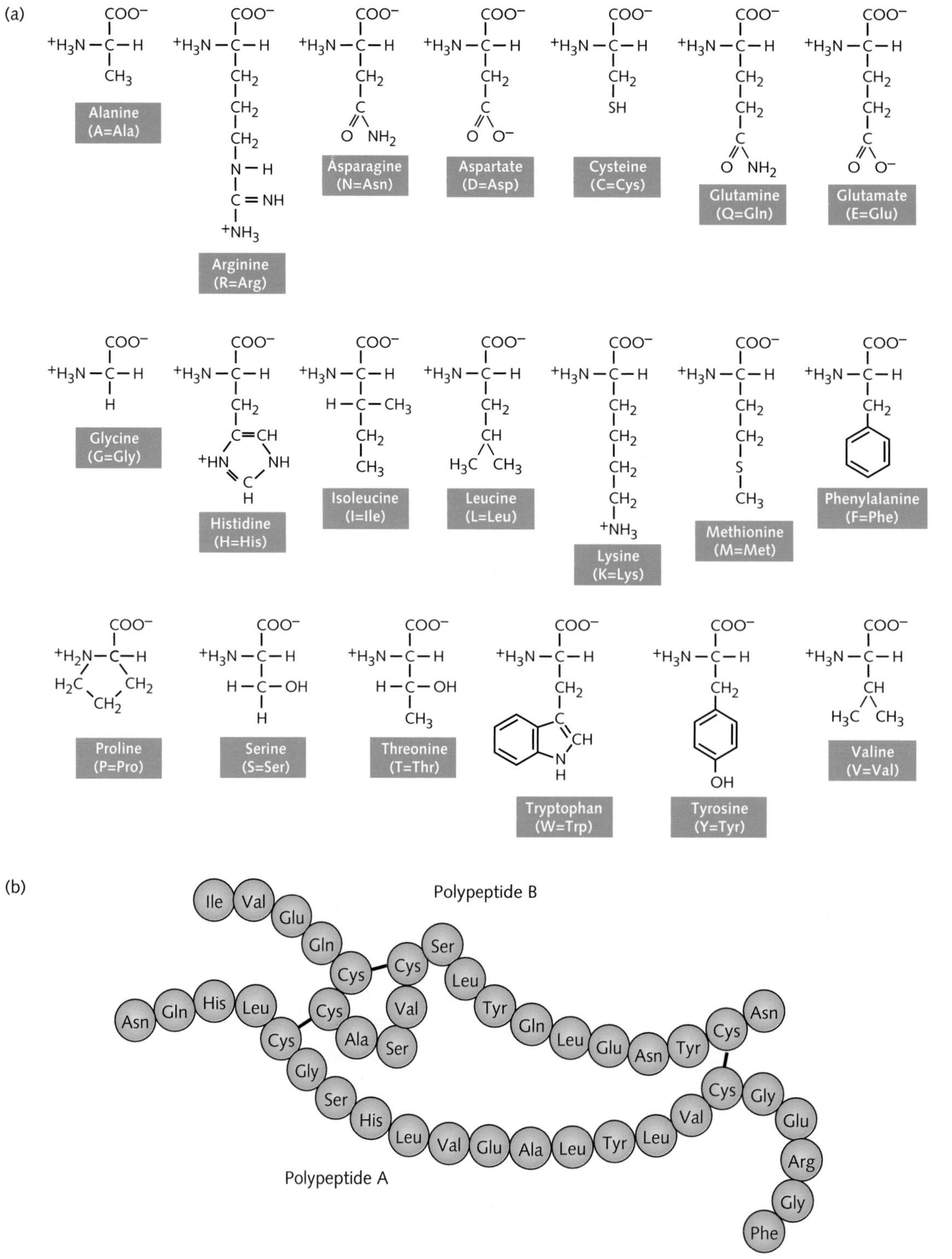

Fig. 2.6 Amino acids in proteins. (a) The most commonly occurring amino acids found in proteins are shown. Below each is given its full name as well as the routinely used one- and three-letter codes. (b) Chains of amino acids (polypeptides) can be linked by intramolecular and intermolecular disulphide bridges to generate covalent linkages between amino acids or one or more polypeptide chains, respectively (reproduced from Singer and Berg (1991)).

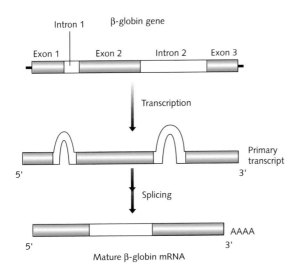

Fig. 2.7 Many genes contain regions of DNA which are not contiguous with their coding regions. The coding regions (exons) in the β-globin gene are bounded by non-coding regions (introns). Some genes may contain up to 50 introns varying in size from a few tens of basepairs to thousands of basepairs in length. Introns must be removed in order to generate a mature RNA. These are removed by splicing, resulting in a mature RNA containing continuous exonic sequences.

fact that the sequence of one strand dictates the sequence of the complementary strand lends itself to a mechanism of copying.

In DNA replication, the two parental strands of the DNA double helix are displaced and specific enzymes known as DNA polymerases make complementary daughter copies of each strand using the parental strand as a template (see Fig. 2.8). Since a replicated double-stranded DNA molecule contains one parental strand and one daughter strand of DNA, the process has been termed **semi-conservative replication**.

Replication does not just start anywhere on the DNA molecule, but at specific sites called **origins of replication**, and proceeds along the DNA molecule until the DNA is completely copied. As eukaryotic DNA replicates at about 10–100 nucleotide pairs second, to replicate the human genome of some 4×10^9 nucleotide pairs would take about 3 months. However, eukaryotic DNA contains multiple origins of replication at about every 20–30 kilobase pairs (kbp) and these long stretches of replicated DNA are eventually joined together to generate a complete daughter chromosome. In contrast, many DNA-encoded viruses have a single origin of replication consistent with their much smaller genome size (see Chapter 13).

DNA replicates via replication forks

DNA polymerases only add deoxyribonucleotide units to the 3′ hydroxyl group of a DNA strand. Consequently, synthesis of a new DNA strand must proceed in a 5′–3′ direction. For a double helix of DNA comprising two strands of DNA which run in opposite 5′–3′ directions, this results in the need for specialist mechanisms to extend DNA in two directions (**bidirectionally**) at the **replication fork** (see Fig. 2.8a): one in a 5′–3′ direction but the other in a 3′–5′ direction.

As shown in Fig. 2.9, the synthesis of a new daughter strand of DNA by DNA polymerase can proceed continuously in a 5′–3′ direction, using parental strand 1 as a copying template, from a single initiation event generating a daughter DNA molecule with 5′–3′ directionality. However, copying the second DNA strand from parental strand 2 continuously would require the addition of deoxyribonucleotide units in a 3′–5′ direction, which is not possible with DNA polymerase. Consequently, this is brought about by so-called **discontinuous DNA synthesis** requiring multiple initiation events along parental strand 2 which are then extended by DNA polymerase in 5′–3′ direction generating many short DNA sequences of 100–200 base pairs in length (**Okazaki fragments**) which must eventually be joined together to generate a continuous daughter strand.

As well as restrictions on the directionality of DNA polymerase, this enzyme can also only add deoxyribonucleotides to a pre-existing polynucleotide chain. It is now clear that the initiation event of DNA replication requires small RNA molecules (**primers**) which are complementary to DNA sequences around replication origins. DNA polymerase adds deoxynucleotides onto these primers, forming a complementary daughter strand using the parental strand as a template (see Fig. 2.9). The RNA primers are synthesized by special enzymes called **primases** and removed from the replicated DNA sequences by enzymes and replaced with equivalent DNA sequence. Okazaki fragments, therefore, require joining together by the enzyme **DNA ligase** to generate a continuous DNA strand.

Because eukaryotic DNA is associated with chromosomal proteins in chromosomes, a number of additional cellular enzymes are required to replicate chromosomal DNA. For instance, **DNA helicases** are required to separate parental DNA strands, and **single-stranded DNA-specific binding proteins** are needed to facilitate unwinding of DNA by binding to the single strands of the double helix as they become separated by the helicase enzyme. Similarly, other enzymes, such as **DNA topoiso-**

(a)

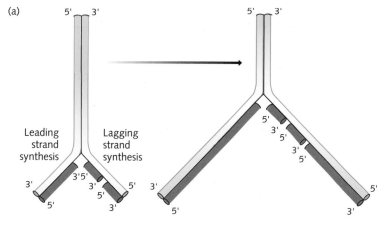

(b)

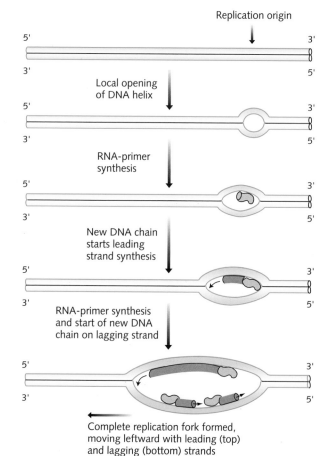

Fig. 2.8 Semi-conservative replication of DNA. (a) The two DNA strands act as templates from which to copy two new DNA strands; these are both synthesized in a 5' to 3' direction. (b) The leading strand is continuously synthesized whereas the lagging strand is synthesized as short Okazaki fragments and these are then joined together to generate a continuous DNA strand.

merase which nicks the double helix ahead of the replication fork, also help unwinding of the double helical DNA and allow unhindered progression of the replication fork down the chromosome (see Fig. 2.9).

DNA repair

The copying of DNA during multiple cell divisions is a process that is prone to errors. The frequency with which DNA polymerase incorporates the wrong deoxyribonucleotide unit when copying DNA is about one for every

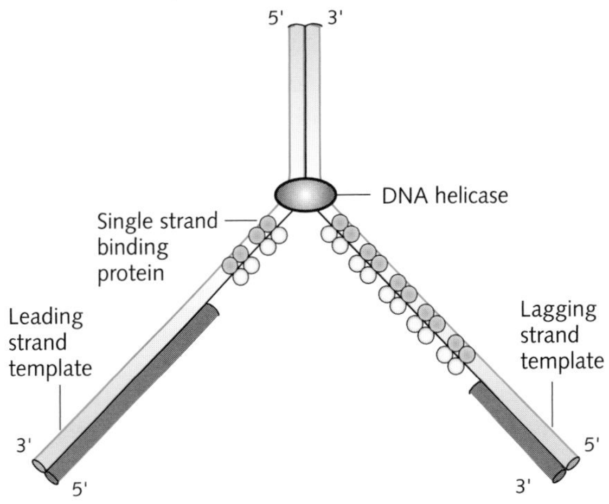

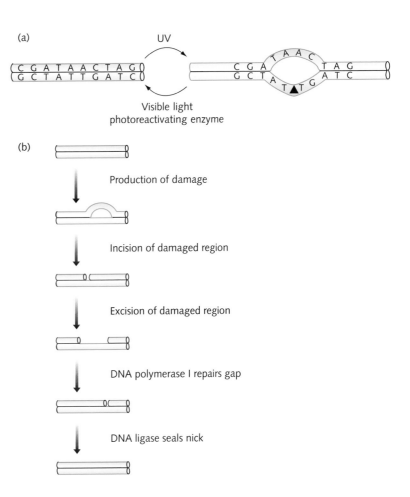

Fig. 2.9 DNA unwinding is required at the DNA replication fork. In order for the replication fork to proceed down the DNA duplex, cellular proteins, such as helicase and single-stranded DNA binding proteins, are required to keep the DNA duplex unwound. Similarly, in order for the fork to progress along the DNA strand, the supercoiling of the DNA must be relaxed and this is facilitated by DNA topoisomerase (reproduced from Singer and Berg (1991)).

Fig. 2.10 Replacement of damaged DNA— DNA repair. (a) DNA damaged by, for instance, ultra violet light can result in pyrimidine dimers which block DNA replication. (b) These can be repaired by excising the damaged DNA and replacing it using DNA polymerase (reproduced from Singer and Berg (1991)).

10^8 nucleotides copied. Similarly, many factors can result in the damage of DNA. Consequently, the ability to repair DNA is essential for the maintenance of a functional genome and is a continuous process in the dividing cell. Fortunately, the complementarity of eukaryotic DNA, whereby one strand specifies the sequence of the other, also means that the eukaryotic cell is able to repair such damage or misincorporations of nucleotides on one strand of the duplex. Chemicals can cause a variety of alterations of DNA structure, as well as ionizing radiation and ultra violet light. However, many of these alterations can be repaired by specific DNA repair enzymes. For instance, ultra violet light can cause dimerization between adjacent thymine residues on the same DNA strand such that these nucleotides are no longer able to pair with adenine residues on the complementary strand (Fig. 2.10). However, such modifications can be recognized by the cell, excised and then repaired using the complementary unmodified strand as a template for repair. Mutations in such DNA repair genes can result in the genetic defect known as xeroderma pigmentosum,

resulting in sensitivity to ultra violet light and increased susceptibility to a variety of skin cancers.

Copying DNA to RNA—transcription

Transcription — the copying of a DNA sequence into RNA — is carried out in the eukaryotic cell by specific **RNA polymerase enzymes** which use a DNA sequence as a template from which to synthesize a direct copy of the DNA as a ribonucleic acid. RNA synthesis is always in a 5′–3′ direction in which incoming ribonucleotide-5′ triphosphate is added stepwise to an elongating chain of RNA, catalysed by RNA polymerase enzyme (Fig. 2.11).

There are three types of RNA-dependent polymerase, called types I–III. Types I and III transcribe genes whose RNAs are not translated to proteins, such as rRNA and tRNA. Type II polymerase transcribes genes whose RNA is transported to the cytoplasm and decoded on the ribosome to generate a protein, and this RNA is mRNA. Polymerase II (but not I or III) transcripts have a modified 5′ end, referred to as the cap, which is added early on in transcription, and a modified 3′ end, containing stretches of polyadenylic acid residues. This **polyadenylation** is not encoded in the gene but is added post-transcriptionally at a specific site (the polyadenylation signal) 3′ to the translation termination signal (Fig. 2.12). Capping and polyadenylation are believed to increase the efficiency of translation and stability of the mRNA, respectively. However, it should be noted that not all polymerase II transcripts are polyadenylated, for instance mRNAs encoding histone proteins have no poly(A) tails.

A consensus polymerase II-transcribed gene is shown in Fig. 2.12. They generally include a 5′ promoter/regulatory region which may contain DNA sequences that bind specific cellular proteins involved in gene regulation (see Chapter 4), a coding region which may or may not

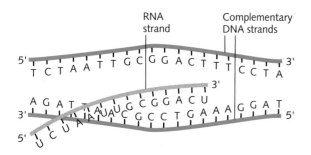

Fig. 2.11 Transcription—copying DNA into RNA. A region of DNA is made partially single-stranded by local melting of the DNA duplex and RNA polymerase binds to the DNA and uses it as a template to make an RNA copy of the DNA strand.

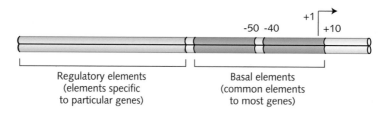

Fig. 2.12 The structure of a typical RNA polymerase II-transcribed gene. Generally, genes transcribed by RNA polymerase II have a promoter regulatory region that can be divided into two domains. One contains the so-called basal promoter which often contains a TATA element, or if not an initiator element. This basal promoter binds general

transcription factors, such as RNA polymerase II, present in all cell types. The level of activity of the basal promoter is regulated by binding of cell-specific factors to the second domain which contains DNA sequences recognized by these gene-specific cell factors.

include introns, and a 3′ region which specifies termination signals and whether the transcript should be polyadenylated. Transcription from this gene generates a primary transcript which is processed by addition of a 5′ cap, excision of introns and splicing together of exons as well as polyadenylation to generate a fully processed mRNA transcript.

Introns are prevalent amongst genes of higher eukaryotes but absent from most bacteria. They can be found in all types of eukaryotic genes, type I, II or II transcribed, and can vary in size from 10–20 to hundreds of thousands of basepairs in length. Common to most introns are specific DNA sequences at their 5′ and 3′ borders, the so-called 5′ and 3′ **splice junctions**. In mRNA, the splice junctions are well conserved and necessary for the splicing reaction. Splicing involves association of the primary transcript with snRNAs and small nuclear ribonuclear proteins (snRNPs). This complex is thought to form on the intron and facilitate the excision of the intron RNA and subsequent joining of the exons. Such mature transcripts are then transported from the nucleus for translation as mRNP complexes.

Decoding mRNA to protein—translation

The mechanism by which a mRNA transcript is decoded into the correct protein sequence (its **cognate protein**) is termed **translation** and takes place on specialized organelles in the cytosol, known as ribosomes. The eukaryotic ribosome is an 80 S particle (as defined by sedimentation behaviour) and comprises a small (40 S) and a large (60 S) subunit. The small subunit consists of an RNA molecule of approximately 1900 nucleotides and about 35 accessory proteins and the large subunit comprises three RNA species of 120 (5 S), 160 (5–8 S) and 4800 (28 S) nucleotides together with about 50 accessory proteins. These rRNAs are polymerase I-transcribed genes.

Amino acids cannot interact directly with a triplet codon specifying it on the mRNA. They are positioned onto the mRNA transcript by the specialized tRNA molecules, which are polymerase III-transcribed. There is a family of different tRNAs and each one specifically interacts with one specific amino acid. Each also carries three nucleotides (the **anticodon**) which are complementary to the mRNA sequence specifying that amino acid (see Fig. 2.13). Consequently the anticodon on a specific tRNA which is, in turn, linked to a specific amino acid recognizes an mRNA codon and positions the amino acid on the mRNA transcript via this tRNA adapter molecule— this is the so-called adapter hypothesis. The tRNA associated with its cognate amino acid is termed the aminocyl tRNA. One tRNA can in some cases recognize more than one triplet codon because the base at the 5′ end of tRNA anticodons can be a modified form of adenine, called inosine, which can base pair with several types of bases at the 3′ end of the codon (see Fig. 2.13). This 'wobble' concept explains why there are not 61 different tRNAs and defines the rules which allow multi-codon translation by a single tRNA (see Table 2.1).

Translation initiation starts by dissociation of the 80 S ribosome which depends on accessory proteins, known as eukaryotic initiation factors (eIFs). The 40 S subunit, in association with other eIFs, then binds a special initiator aminoacyl tRNA, which in eukaryotes is a methionine-linked tRNA (tRNAI$_{met}$). For this reason, most eukaryotic proteins start with the amino acid methionine, encoded in the DNA by an ATG triplet codon. This complex then binds to the cap region at the 5′ end of an mRNA and the 40 S subunit complex scans down the mRNA in a 5′–3′ direction until it comes to an AUG codon in the mRNA which specifies the amino acid methionine and the start of translation. The sequence of triplet codons beginning with the initiator ATG codon, which encode a protein, has been termed the **open reading frame** (ORF) of translation. Whilst no specific sequences specify a correct initiation codon, nucleotides around the AUG codon may influence the efficiency of initiation. The complex of 40 S subunit, initiation amino acid tRNA and cofactors then combines with the 60 S subunit and translation of successive triplet codons down the mRNA transcript occurs; whereby amino acids, brought to the ribosome complex via their specific tRNA adapters and positioned on the mRNA complex by codon–anticodon matching, are linked by peptide bonds thus elongating the peptide chain. Successive additions of amino acids (**chain elongation**) carry on until a stop codon is encountered on the mRNA transcript resulting in release of the polypeptide chain (Fig. 2.13c).

Post-translational modification of polypeptide chains

For many proteins the synthesis of the primary polypeptide chain is not sufficient to generate a functional protein. Polypeptides must be folded into correct two- and three-dimensional structures and in some cases must be associated with other proteins in order to generate a functional product. Similarly, many proteins contain covalently modified amino acids, for example modified by phosphorylation (addition of a phosphate group), glycosylation (addition of carbohydrate groups),

(a)

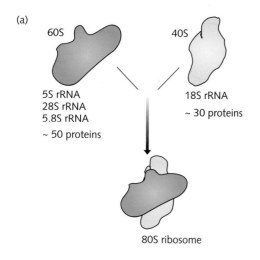

(c)

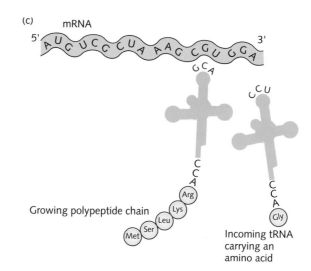

(b)

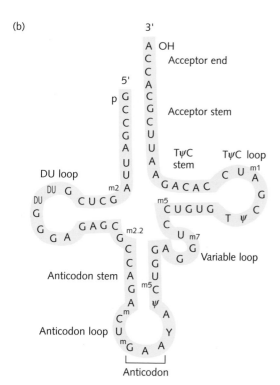

Fig. 2.13 (a) The eukaryotic ribosome, the cellular organelle responsible for translating an mRNA copy into its cognate protein, is composed of two subunits, a large subunit of 60 S and a small subunit of 40 S. The large subunit contains three rRNAs (5 S, 5.8 S and 28 S) as well as 50 ribosomal proteins. The small subunit contains an 18 S rRNA and 30 proteins. (b) The structure of tRNA. All tRNAs resemble a clover leaf structure. They contain the anticodon complementary to and, hence, specific for individual tRNA species. (c) At the ribosome, triplet codons of the mRNA molecule basepair with their corresponding anticodons on the tRNAs. Each tRNA is physically associated with a specific amino acid which is then incorporated into the growing polypeptide chain.

myristylation (addition of fatty acids), acetylation (addition of acetyl groups) or are non-covalently associated with, for example, metal ions. Furthermore, some neuropeptides and hormones are synthesized as a large inactive precursor and the so-called polyprotein must be cleaved to generate a functionally mature protein, as is seen for insulin (see Chapter 14). This allows an additional level of control of the protein's function.

Targeting proteins to their sites of action

The eukaryotic cell contains a number of intracellular organelles bounded by specific membranes, e.g. nuclei, mitochondria, Golgi bodies, lysosomes etc. These organelles perform specific functions within the cell and require certain proteins in order for them to carry out these functions. Obviously, many proteins produced in the cytoplasm on the ribosomes need to be 'directed', somehow, to their correct cellular sites of action.

Proteins that are destined for certain organelles and the cytosol (aqueous portion) of the cytoplasm are synthesized on free cytosolic ribosomes, whereas proteins that are destined to travel to membrane structures such as the Golgi bodies, plasma membrane and lysosomes are synthesized on ribosomes associated with the cellular **endoplasmic reticulum** (ER). The ER, a series of membranes which permeates the cell and surrounds the ER lumen, has two forms: rough ER which is ribosome associated, and smooth ER which has no ribosome association. Proteins synthesized on membrane-bound ribosomes are transported through the ER lumen and contain a hydrophobic stretch of amino acids (the signal sequence) at the amino-terminal end (the end encoded by the 5′ end of the DNA), presumably to assist transport of the protein through the hydrophobic lipid layers of the cell membrane. Transport from the ER-associated ribosome to the ER lumen occurs by specific interactions between this polypeptide signal sequence, a signal sequence recognition particle (SRP) of complexed proteins and a signal sequence recognition particle receptor (SRP-R) present on the ER; such that the SRP binds the signal sequence of the polypeptide and this is 'captured' by the membrane-bound SRP-R which steers the protein through the ER to the ER lumen (see Fig. 2.14). The signal sequence is then specifically cleaved off the mature protein by a specific enzyme that can cleave amino acids within a protein (**endopeptidase**) inside the ER lumen.

However, not all signal peptides are amino-terminal in the protein to be transported or cleaved after transport, nor do all transported proteins contain a recognizable signal sequence. Other factors involved in the correct targeting of proteins across membranes involve so-called **molecular chaperones** such as the heat shock proteins (so called because they increase in production upon cellular stress such as increased temperatures) which help protein folding and translocation.

Proteins destined for secretion, lysosomes or plasma membranes pass through the Golgi apparatus via vesicles that bud off from the ER. Other proteins, destined for intracellular organelles such as the nucleus and mitochondria, are synthesized on free ribosomes and transported to their sites of action by unknown mechanisms. Similarly, some organellar proteins are encoded by DNA within the organelle. For instance the mitochondrion contains DNA which can encode specific mitochondrial genes and whose mRNAs are translated on mitochondrial ribosomes (see Chapter 5).

Evidence is also accumulating to indicate that amino acid sequences within the primary protein sequence may, in some proteins, define their localization. For instance, defined amino acid sequences present in some proteins are essential for correct nuclear localization.

Inhibitors of transcription and translation

Whilst not necessarily therapeutic due to relatively high toxicity, a number of compounds have been defined

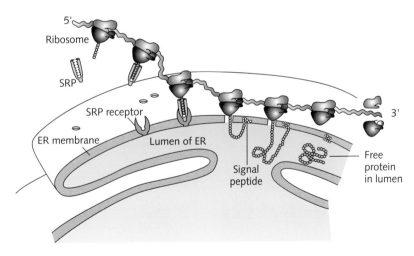

Fig. 2.14 Transport of newly synthesized proteins within the cell. The SRP is essential for transport of newly synthesized proteins into the ER. The SRP recognizes the signal sequence on a newly synthesized protein and binds to the SRP receptor in the ER membrane, allowing the growing polypeptide chain to be directed through the ER membrane. The signal sequence is cleaved off the protein chain releasing the newly synthesized protein into the ER (reproduced from Singer and Berg (1991)).

which inhibit DNA transcription or replication and mRNA translation at specific stages. For example, α-amanitin, an octapeptide isolated from a fungus, is a potent inhibitor of RNA polymerase II but only inhibits polymerase III transcription at very high concentrations (see Table 2.2). Rifamycin, isolated from *Streptomycetes*, or its synthetic analogue rifampicin, blocks transcription initiation in prokaryotes but not eukaryotes. Similarly, streptolydigins from *Streptomycetes* blocks prokaryotic but not eukaryotic transcription elongation, whereas actinomycin D, also isolated from *Streptomycetes*, intercalates between GC basepairs and inhibits transcription but not DNA replication.

There are also a number of specific protein translation inhibitors (see Table 2.2); specificity for prokaryotic but not eukaryotic translation inhibition gives rise to the successful use of such antibiotics to treat bacterial infections.

Mutation

It is clear that changes in nucleotides within the coding region of a gene can have drastic implications for the function of the encoded protein. Such mutations may take many forms. For instance, single base substitutions may cause the incorporation of inappropriate amino acids into the polypeptide chain or result in the generation of a stop codon—so-called **missense** and **nonsense** mutations, respectively. Both can have major effects on the function of the resulting protein. For instance, sickle

cell anaemia results from a mutation in the coding region of the β-globin gene in which the sixth amino acid from the amino-terminal end of the protein is changed from glutamine to valine. This results in aggregation of deoxygenated haemoglobin and deformation of the red blood cell. Similarly, small deletions or insertions of bases may have drastic effects on the resulting protein as they often shift the frame of translation — so-called **frame shift mutations**. Alternatively, large deletions or insertions in the genome may result in major rearrangements of genomic DNA. However, what is less obvious is that a mutation in the DNA sequence of *any* region of the gene which disrupts correct temporal or tissue-specific expression could have similar far-reaching effects. Consequently, mutations in the gene promoter might lead to changes in levels of expression; and even mutations within introns may affect the correct splicing of a transcript resulting in abnormal expression. Similarly, whilst not necessarily specific for any one protein, mutations in other genes encoding any of the components of the synthesis pathway (e.g. enzymes for protein glycosylation etc.) could result, generally, in abnormal protein synthesis.

In most situations mutations introduced into the genome are efficiently repaired during DNA replication (see p. 33), either by correcting the aberrant nucleotide directly or by **excision repair** in which the mutant bases are removed by enzymes and then replaced using the non-mutated DNA strand as the new template from which to make the correction. DNA polymerase itself has the ability to remove 3′ nucleotides on a growing DNA chain so that if nucleotides are misincorporated they can be removed and replaced by the DNA polymerase enzyme—so-called **proof reading**. However, such repair mechanisms are not foolproof. Indeed this is just as well because it must also be remembered that in some cases mutations may make the organism fitter or adapt better to the environment and, indeed, are essential for gene diversity and evolution. However, many mutations result in detrimental effects on the organism and it is these mutations which are the basis of many human genetic disorders and disease.

Table 2.2 Inhibitors of transcription and translation.

Inhibitor	Effects
Inhibitors acting on prokaryotes	
Tetracycline	Blocks binding of aminoacyl tRNA to the ribosome
Streptomycin	Causes miscoding during translation
Chloramphenicol	Blocks translation
Erythromycin	Blocks translation
Rifamycin	Prevents RNA synthesis
Inhibitors acting on prokaryotes and eukaryotes	
Puromycin	Causes premature release of polypeptides during translation
Actinomycin D	Binds DNA and prevents RNA synthesis
Inhibitors acting on eukaryotes	
Cycloheximide	Blocks translation
Anisomycin	Blocks translation
α-Amanitin	Binds RNA polymerase II and blocks transcription

Summary

Gene expression within a cell dictates the structure and function of that cell and, therefore, is critical for the correct growth and development of living organisms. All diseases with a genetic basis result from the incorrect expression of specific genes. Whilst these may result from incorrect temporal or tissue-specific expression, often disease is due to the expression of too high or too low a level of protein or due to expression of a protein which is aberrant in function. These aberrations result from mutation of the genetic code and may reflect mutation in any region of a gene. Mutations in coding regions more often than not result in non-functional proteins, whilst mutations in 5′ or 3′ regulatory regions of the gene may disrupt the correct transcriptional or translational control of the protein's expression.

Our understanding of disease, then, reflects a need to understand fully the structure and function of specific genes as well as how their expression is controlled in both the healthy and diseased state.

Further reading

Singer M. and Berg P. (1991) *Genes and Genomes*. Blackwell Scientific Publications, Oxford.

Stryer L. (1988) *Biochemistry*, 3rd edn. W.H. Freeman, San Francisco.

Watson J.D., Hopkins N.H., Roberts J.W., Steitz J.A. and Weiner A.M. (1987) *Molecular Biology of the Gene*, 4th edn. Benjamin Cummings, Menlo Park, California.

Chapter 3

Analysing human genes

Introduction

The explosion in molecular biological techniques over the last 15 years has helped enormously in our understanding of the molecular biology of human disease. In this chapter, rather than study a list of molecular techniques, we will work our way through a hypothetical analysis of a gene of interest. Such an analysis will require the isolation of the gene (cloning), determination of how many copies there exists in the genome, its chromosomal location and a detailed study of how that gene is regulated by analysing RNA and protein expression. It will become very clear that a complete understanding of gene structure, function and expression is essential for an understanding of the molecular basis of disease.

Cloning a gene for a purified protein

Consider a gene whose protein product is well defined and can be purified. It is now routinely possible to sequence this purified protein on an automated protein sequencer. From this the actual amino acid sequence of short pieces of the protein can be established. Any of these short protein sequences can then be compared to existing databases containing the protein sequences of all known proteins to determine if the protein is novel or is already known. If the protein sequence generated is novel and so far unknown, the protein sequence can be used to generate the corresponding RNA sequence of the mRNA encoding that protein by use of the known triplet codons for those amino acids (see Chapter 2). The DNA sequence can then be deduced from the RNA sequence. A short DNA sequence (**oligonucleotide**) can be synthesized very easily on an automatic DNA synthesizer

which is routinely capable of producing up to 100 base-pairs of synthetic DNA. Because of the redundancy of the triplet code (where one amino acid can be encoded by a number of codons), it is important to be aware that the short polypeptide sequence shown in Fig. 3.1 could be encoded by a number of slightly different DNA sequences. This can be compensated for by producing degenerate pools of oligonucleotides that take this redundancy into account. This involves predicting all possible variations around a particular DNA sequence that could encode the short polypeptide and then synthesizing a 'cocktail' of oligonucleotides. A single oligonucleotide or cocktail can easily be tagged with, for instance, radiolabel and then used directly as a **probe** to isolate the gene containing these DNA sequences by screening recombinant **complementary DNA (cDNA) libraries**.

cDNA libraries contain corresponding DNA sequences for all RNAs made in any cell or tissue of interest. They are made by making a cDNA to every RNA molecule in the cell by the use of the enzyme **reverse transcriptase**. This is done by first generating a single strand of cDNA, very often started off (**primed**) by large tracts of deoxythymidine (**poly(dT)**) which physically associates with (due to complementarity between A and T nucleotides) or **anneals** to the poly(A) tract at the 3′ end of the mRNA (the site of polyadenylation of the mRNA, see Chapter 2 and Fig. 3.2) due to DNA complementarity. Alternatively, priming can be carried out by large pools of random oligonucleotides (**random priming**) which will anneal all along the RNA molecule. This single-stranded cDNA is then used as a template to generate double-stranded cDNA by the use of DNA polymerase (see Chapter 2). These double-stranded cDNAs are then inserted into special **plasmid DNA**

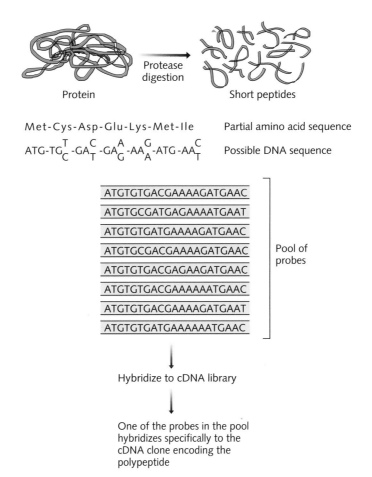

Fig. 3.1 Strategy for cloning a gene whose protein product can be isolated. Microsequencing of an unknown isolated protein can result in the amino acid sequence of small polypeptides within the protein. Based on the polypeptide sequence, small synthetic oligonucleotides can be synthesized which encode the corresponding amino acids of the polypeptide sequence. Because of redundancy in the genetic code some amino acids may be encoded by more than one triplet codon; therefore, mixtures of oligonucleotides representing all the possible combinations of DNA sequences that could encode the amino acid sequence of the polypeptide must be used as a probe. This pool of oligonucleotides is then used to screen either λ phage or plasmid cDNA libraries to isolate cDNA clones containing a complementary sequence to the probe.

sequences. Plasmids are small DNA molecules which can be introduced into bacteria by **DNA transformation** and replicated as circular DNA molecules to very high levels (Fig. 3.3). As only one recombinant plasmid can enter each bacterium, each individual cDNA is replicated in a single baterium and this permits the clonal propagation of a single cDNA—a cDNA clone, in a clone of bacteria. One sequence, one clone.

Plasmids are often based on naturally occurring circular DNAs which are found replicating in bacteria. They contain DNA sequences which permit high levels of plasmid replication in the bacterium (origins of replica-

tion). Plasmids used in molecular biology also contain a selectable marker, such as ampicillin resistance, so that any bacterium carrying a recombinant plasmid is transformed to ampicillin resistance. Consequently, bacteria carrying an individual cDNA in the form of ampicillin resistance plasmids can be cultured under ampicillin-selective conditions generating bacterial clones on agar plates which, in total, carry cDNAs representing every expressed RNA from a cell or tissue of interest—a so-called cDNA library.

The ability to insert DNA sequences of interest into plasmids comes about from our ability to cut DNA

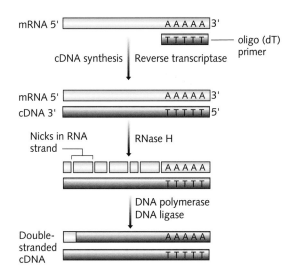

Fig. 3.2 cDNA synthesis of RNA molecules. mRNA molecules can be converted to a complementary single-stranded DNA molecule by the use of the enzyme reverse transcriptase. The reverse transcription reaction can be primed by synthetic deoxythymidine oligonucleotide or oligodT which anneals to the poly(A) tails of the mRNA. Reverse transcription of the mRNA molecule generates RNA–DNA hybrids which can be converted to double-stranded DNA molecules by the nicking of the RNA strand of the RNA–DNA hybrid with RNase H enzyme. The nicks then serve as primers for DNA synthesis by the enzyme DNA polymerase until all the RNA fragments are replaced with DNA and these short DNA fragments are then joined together by the enzyme DNA ligase.

DNA can be converted to a blunt end by the use of enzymes such as S1 nuclease which removes single-stranded DNA 'overhangs', or by **filling in** the overhangs using a subunit (**Klenow fragment**) of DNA polymerase (Fig. 3.5). Similarly, the joining (**ligation**) of synthetic double-stranded DNA sequences, termed **adaptors**, to one cohesive end of restricted DNA can turn one restriction enzyme site to another (Fig. 3.6).

The ability to transform bacteria with plasmid DNA is relatively inefficient, such that for 1 µg of plasmid DNA only about 10^5 transformed bacterial clones will be generated. As a human fibroblast cell may contain 10 000–30 000 mRNAs and a cDNA library needs to contain a cDNA for every RNA molecule in a cell, any cDNA library needs to contain between 100 000 and 200 000 clones in order to have a good probability that all mRNA species are included. Consequently, it is clear that generating enough bacterial clones by bacterial transformation to contain a complete cDNA library can be difficult. As a result, many cDNA libraries are not made in plasmids but in bacteriophage, such as lambda (λ), in which cDNAs are cloned into recombinant bacterial viruses. λ phage libraries contain cDNAs inserted by ligation into a λ phage genome (Fig. 3.7), itself a DNA molecule which has been engineered to contain known restriction enzyme sites. These recombinant λ clones can

sequences at specific sites (restrict) and then rejoin them (ligate) with any other DNA sequences by the use of DNA restriction enzymes and DNA ligase enzyme, respectively. **DNA restriction enzymes** recognize specific DNA sequences and cut the double-stranded DNA (Fig. 3.4a). These DNA ends can then be joined back together either to themselves or to other DNA sequences by the use of a DNA joining enzyme, **DNA ligase**.

Restriction enzymes generate two types of DNA ends, staggered (cohesive, sticky) or blunt (non-cohesive). Whilst blunt-ended DNA can be joined to any other blunt-ended DNA, DNA with cohesive ends can only be joined to DNA sequences with compatible cohesive ends (Fig. 3.4b). For instance, ends of DNA generated by restriction with the enzyme *Bam*HI can be joined to any other DNA ends generated by *Bam*HI or by the enzyme *Bgl*II, but not the enzyme *Eco*RI (Fig. 3.4b). However, it is relatively easy to convert one type of restriction enzyme site to another. For instance, any cohesive end of

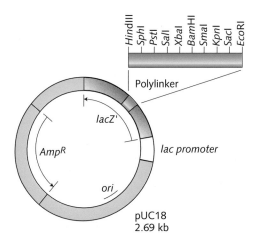

Fig. 3.3 Plasmids as vehicles for DNA and cDNA. pUC18, a typical plasmid vector, is about 2.69 kilobases in size and contains an origin of replication which permits the replication of the plasmid DNA to high copy number in bacteria, a drug resistance marker (ampicillin resistance) to allow selection of bacterial cells carrying the plasmid DNA, and sites to allow the insertion of a cDNA or genomic DNA sequence.

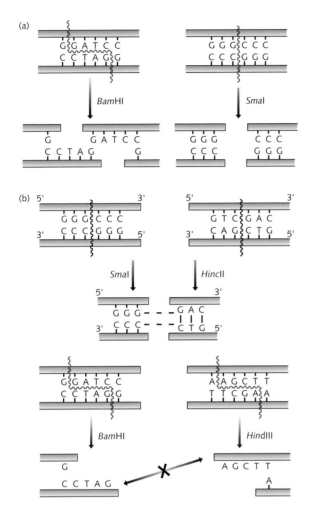

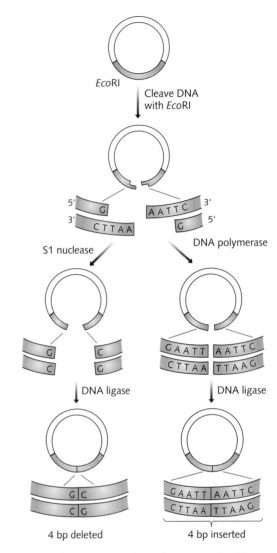

Fig. 3.4 (a) Restriction enzymes recognize defined DNA sequences. The restriction enzyme *Bam*HI recognizes and cuts a defined DNA sequence generating DNA ends that are sticky or cohesive. In contrast, the restriction enzyme *Sma*I cuts DNA leaving flush or blunt ends. (b) DNA ligase joins DNA ends. Blunt DNA ends can be joined to any other blunt DNA ends by the action of DNA ligase. In contrast, cohesive DNA ends can only be ligated to other compatible cohesive DNA ends. For instance DNA ends generated by the restriction enzyme *Bam*HI can be ligated to other *Bam*HI-generated DNA ends but not to DNA ends generated by the restriction enzyme *Hin*dIII. Ligation of cohesive DNA ends generated by restriction enzymes such as, for instance, *Bam*HI regenerates the *Bam*HI site, whereas ligation of cohesive ends generated by *Bam*HI and *Xho*I does not regenerate either enzyme site, even though these enzymes generate compatible cohesive ends.

Fig. 3.5 Cohesive DNA ends can be converted to blunt ends. Cohesive DNA ends generated by, for instance, the restriction enzyme *Eco*RI can be treated with S1 nuclease which removes DNA ends that are unpaired. Alternatively, DNA polymerase will extend recessed DNA ends also generating blunt-ended DNA. This allows ligation of the treated DNA ends to any other DNA with blunt ends. Note that ligation of *Eco*RI-generated cohesive ends that have been made blunt by S1 nuclease or DNA polymerase does not regenerate the original *Eco*RI site.

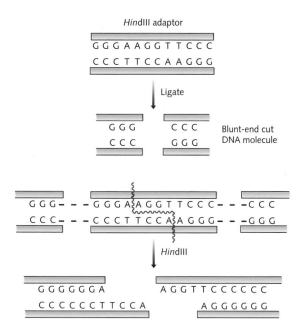

HindIII adaptor

GGGAAGGTTCCC
CCCTTCCAAGGG

Ligate

GGG   CCC   Blunt-end cut
CCC   GGG   DNA molecule

GGG– – –GGGAAGGTTCCC– – –CCC
CCC– – –CCCTTCCAAGGG– – –GGG

HindIII

GGGGGGA   AGGTTCCCCCC
CCCCCCTTCCA   AGGGGGG

Fig. 3.6 The compatability of DNA ends can be converted by adaptors. An alternative method of converting DNA ends of one type to DNA ends of another type is by the use of adaptors which are synthetic double-stranded oligonucleotides that are blunt-ended but contain a specific restriction enzyme site. Ligation of the adaptors to a blunt-ended DNA molecule followed by cutting with the appropriate restriction enzyme will generate new molecules with specific cohesive ends.

tor has some idea of a partial DNA sequence present in their gene of interest. In this case it is possible to screen cDNA libraries directly with this sequence. Such hybridization works because complementary DNA sequences will physically anneal together due to complementary basepairing (see Chapter 2). On many occasions the first cDNA clone isolated does not contain a full length cDNA due to, for instance, the reverse transcription reaction not proceeding all the way to the full 5′ end of the transcript on that RNA molecule. This may be due to loops or kinks in the RNA molecule physically blocking the progress of the reverse transcriptase enzyme. In this situation, the cDNA library can be continually rescreened with either the original probe or the short cDNA clones until the fullest length cDNA clone possible is isolated.

Whilst we have talked specifically about cDNA libraries in our example, it is also possible to generate

then be **packaged** into infectious virus particles which can then be used to infect a lawn of bacteria generating plaques (areas of the bacterial lawn which have been generated by infection and lysis of a single bacterium with a single recombinant λ phage) but at much higher frequencies than one is able to transform bacteria (up to 10^7 recombinant phage/μg of recombinant phage DNA). Clones of bacteria from plasmid libraries or plaques of phage from λ libraries can then be transferred to nitrocellulose filter papers (Fig. 3.7) by carefully placing the filter paper onto each Petri dish containing the bacterial clones or plaques. This allows easy manipulation of filter papers rather than Petri dishes of bacteria. These filters can then be incubated with a radiolabelled DNA probe and the phage plaques or bacterial clones which contain DNA sequences complementary to the probes can be detected. This allows the isolation of a plasmid or λ clone which contains the same cDNA sequence as the DNA probe sequence originally generated by, for instance, a partial protein sequence from a protein of interest. Alternatively, in many situations the investiga-

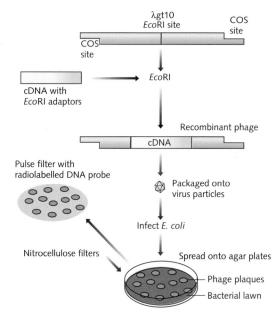

Fig. 3.7 Lambda phage as a vehicle for cloning DNA and cDNA. Bacteriophage λ is used extensively as a cloning vector for DNA. The left and right 'arms' of the phage encode phage structural genes and so are indispensible for phage replication. Sequences in the middle of the phage are dispensible and can be deleted to allow the insertion of specific DNA or cDNA. The ends of the λ phage also contain single-stranded cohesive DNA sequences, the COS sites, which are required for packaging the phage genome into the phage particle. The packaged phage are used to infect *Escherichia coli* and the infected cells form plaques on a bacterial lawn. The phage plaques can be transferred to nitrocellulose filters and the filters are probed with DNA or RNA probes.

genomic DNA libraries in which fragments of genomic DNA (generated by partial restriction enzyme digests or by random fragmentation of total genomic DNA), rather than cDNA, are cloned into λ phage. Plasmid genomic libraries are seldom used because the size of the DNA insert, restricted to about 10 kilobases, and the low frequency of bacterial transformation (about 10^5 clones/μg of plasmid DNA) would mean that an unmanageable number of plasmid clones and too large an amount of genomic DNA starting material would be required to cover an entire genome. In contrast, the frequency of infection with λ phage (10^7 clones/μg of recombinant phage DNA) and the ability to insert up to 30 kilobases of DNA into recombinant λ vectors allows a more manageable number of recombinant phage and much less genomic DNA starting material to cover an entire genome. Similarly, the use of **cosmids**, which are special plasmids that can also be packaged into λ phage, allows up to 50 kilobases of insert DNA to be cloned.

Another more recent development is the ability to clone and propagate extremely large pieces of genomic DNA, up to 150 kilobases in size, using yeast artificial chromosomes or **YACs** (Fig. 3.8). These vectors are based upon yeast chromosomal sequences which include a yeast autonomously replicating sequence (ARS), which is a yeast DNA sequence that allows replication of the DNA in yeast cells, as well as yeast centromeric (CEN) and telomeric sequences. These sequences help control copy number and stability of the synthetic chromosome. Such genomic libraries are invaluable for analysing gene sequences not expressed as RNA, i.e. introns, upstream promoter/regulatory regions of genes and other noncoding regions of DNA which will never be represented in cDNA libraries because cDNA clones, based on mRNA, will not include such sequences.

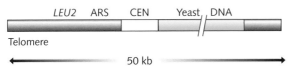

Fig. 3.8 Yeast artificial chromosomes. YACs contain a yeast chromosomal centromere (CEN) and two yeast chromosomal telomeres which allow this yeast vector to be stably replicated like linear yeast chromosomes. These vectors can accomodate several hundred basepairs of DNA.

Cloning a gene encoding a protein recognized by an antibody

So far we have considered a situation in which we have cloned a cDNA encoding a protein which can be purified. Obviously, this rationale cannot be carried out in many situations. Alternatively, access to an antibody, immunoglobulins that specifically recognize a protein of interest (see Chapter 10), can help directly in cloning of the cDNA expressing that protein. In this situation a cDNA library, in which cDNAs have been cloned into λ phage vectors in such a way that the proteins of interest are expressed at the protein level in infected bacteria (expression libraries), can then be screened directly with the antibody (Fig. 3.9). However, the ability to express cDNA in such recombinant phage requires special types of λ vectors. In these vectors, cDNAs are ligated to a coding region for the *Escherichia coli* β-galactosidase (*lacZ*) gene product such that the RNA expressed from them encodes a **fusion protein** containing *lacZ* and the protein of interest. In this situation the start of the *lacZ* mRNA provides correct initiation of translation for the cDNA, resulting in a protein starting with the amino acids for *lacZ* but then continuing with the amino acids encoded by mRNA encoding the protein of interest. Because amino acids are encoded by triplet codons, expression of a cDNA in such expression libraries requires that they are ligated into the *lacZ* portion of the cDNA in a way that translation through the *lacZ* region and into the region of the gene of interest are in the same phase of triplet codons (the same translation frame) as the starting *lacZ* coding region (Fig. 3.9). Consequently, such λ vectors have restriction enzyme sites engineered in all three potential translation frames (Fig. 3.10) to ensure that a cDNA will be ligated to the *lacZ* sequences in such a way to allow the fusion protein to be expressed. Such expression libraries can then be screened directly with an antibody to isolate the cDNA clone which expresses a specific protein recognized by the antibody.

Once cloned, a gene of interest can be analysed extensively for its structure, expression and function.

Sequencing the gene

One of the most important techniques available for the analysis of genes of interest is that of determining the precise order of nucleotides within the gene by **DNA sequencing**. Such DNA sequence analysis represents a first step in analysis of a gene of interest. With the help of DNA sequence analysis computer programs, sequence data can be used: (i) to determine all known restriction

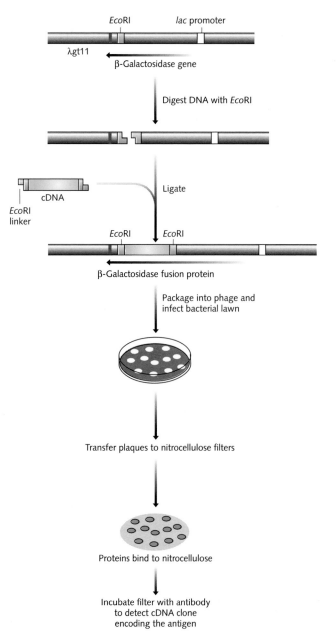

Fig. 3.9 Lambda vector for expression of cloned cDNAs. In the λ phage vector gt11, cDNAs are ligated into a site in the phage which encodes the *Escherichia coli lacZ* gene. If the cDNA is ligated into this region in the correct orientation, such that the reading frame of the cDNA is in phase with the reading frame of β-galactosidase, then a fusion protein is synthesized made up of β-galactosidase and the protein coded by the cDNA. Such expression libraries can then be screened with, for instance, an antibody to a gene of interest to isolate the phage clone expressing the cDNA encoding the protein recognized by that antibody.

enzyme sites within the gene; (ii) to predict the protein product encoded by the gene; (iii) to provide information about potential sites of introns in genomic DNA; and (iv) to give insights into the mechanisms by which the

expression of a gene is controlled, by analysing the 5′ non-coding region which may contain DNA sequences known to bind specific nuclear proteins that regulate transcription (transcription regulatory proteins or tran-

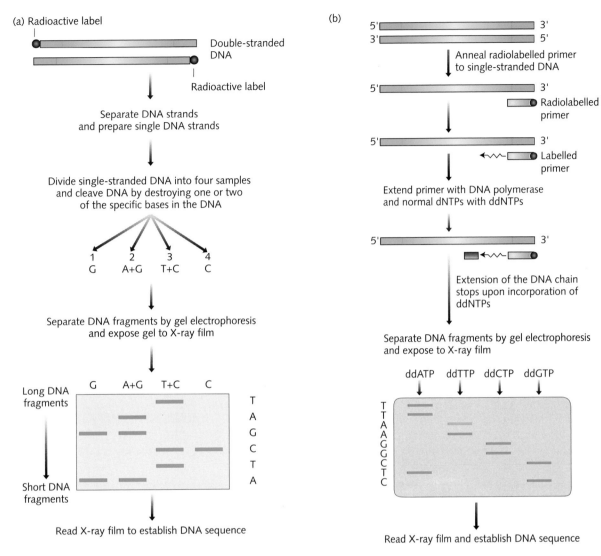

(a) Radioactive label

Double-stranded DNA

Radioactive label

Separate DNA strands and prepare single DNA strands

Divide single-stranded DNA into four samples and cleave DNA by destroying one or two of the specific bases in the DNA

| 1 | 2 | 3 | 4 |
| G | A+G | T+C | C |

Separate DNA fragments by gel electrophoresis and expose gel to X-ray film

Long DNA fragments

G　A+G　T+C　C

T
A
G
C
T
A

Short DNA fragments

Read X-ray film to establish DNA sequence

(b)

5' ———— 3'
3' ———— 5'

Anneal radiolabelled primer to single-stranded DNA

5' ———— 3'

Radiolabelled primer

5' ———— 3'

Labelled primer

Extend primer with DNA polymerase and normal dNTPs with ddNTPs

5' ———— 3'

Extension of the DNA chain stops upon incorporation of ddNTPs

Separate DNA fragments by gel electrophoresis and expose to X-ray film

ddATP　ddTTP　ddCTP　ddGTP

T
T
A
A
G
G
C
T
C

Read X-ray film and establish DNA sequence

Fig. 3.10 DNA sequencing. (a) Maxam and Gilbert **Chemical Degradation** sequencing is carried out by labelling one end of the DNA to be sequenced with [32]P. This labelled DNA is then divided into four samples and each is treated with a set of chemicals that degrades one or two of the four DNA bases in each sample (shown as G, A + G, T + C, C) in such a way that only a few sites in any one DNA molecule are degraded. This results in a set of DNA molecules of varying lengths. Each of the four samples is separated on an acrylamide gel side-by-side and the gel is exposed to X-ray film. The pattern of the labelled DNA fragments can then be used to determine the DNA sequence. (b) Sanger **Chain Termination** sequencing uses dideoxynucleotides which can be incorporated into growing DNA chains but which, once incorporated, prevent any further extension of that DNA chain. Such a sequencing reaction involves dividing the DNA sample to be sequenced into four and adding to each a radiolabelled oligonucleotide primer that is complementary to one end of the DNA strand to be sequenced. The primer is then extended with DNA polymerase in the presence of dNTPs but each of the four samples also contains one of the NTPs in the dideoxy form (shown as ddATP, ddTTP, ddCTP, ddGTP in the figure). Under the correct conditions, this generates a series of DNA molecules of varying lengths which can be separated on an acrylamide gel side-by-side and exposed to X-ray film. The pattern of the DNA bands can then be used to determine the DNA sequence.

scription factors) and confer upon the gene temporal or tissue-specific control (see Chapter 4). Two techniques for DNA sequencing were independently developed at about the same time, the **chain termination** method of Sanger

and Coulson and the **chemical degradation** method of Maxam and Gilbert (Fig. 3.10). Though very different techniques, they are both able to generate DNA sequences of several thousand bases in length, and have been improved and modified over the years to optimize resolution and minimize labour.

Gene location and copy number

It is relatively easy to determine how many copies (the copy number) of a gene of interest there are in a genome and the gene's chromosome location, which may have important implications for any genetic analysis of that gene.

Chromosome location can be determined by *in situ* hybridization to chromosome spreads. In this analysis a probe derived from the gene of interest, either radio-labelled or chemically tagged, is hybridized to specially prepared sections of chromosomes (see Chapter 6). The site of annealing of the probes to the chromosome sections will determine on which chromosome and where on that chromosome the gene is present.

The copy number of the gene in the genome can routinely be estimated using **Southern blot hybridization** (named after E. Southern, who first described this technique). In this assay, total genomic DNA is cut with known restriction enzymes and the genomic digest is separated on the basis of size by electrophoresis on agarose gels (Fig. 3.11). The DNA fragments are then transferred (**blotted**) onto nitrocellulose filter sheets and the filter hybridized to a radiolabelled probe to the gene of interest (Fig. 3.11). If a known number of copies of a plasmid containing the gene of interest is also included on the gel and the amount of total genomic DNA analysed is known, then the copy number of the gene within the genome can be quantified by comparing the intensity of radiolabelled probe binding to the genomic DNA and the known copy number samples. Also, much Southern blot analysis can be used to detect gene mutations if the mutation generates a new restriction enzyme site or removes a site normally present. This results in detectable changes in restriction enzyme fragments (so-called restriction fragment length polymorphisms (RFLPs)).

For many genes the ability to separate short DNA fragments (less than 20 kilobases) by conventional agarose gel electrophoresis is sufficient for their analysis by Southern blotting. However, some genes containing many introns may be spread over several thousand kilobases of genomic DNA. Separation of DNA fragments over about 20 kilobases in size on agarose gels is difficult using conventional electrophoresis and, therefore, such large genetic loci cannot be analysed by conventional agarose gel electrophoresis. **Pulsed field gel electrophoresis** (PFGE) allows the separation of very large fragments of genomic DNA (up to 5000 kilobases) by electrophore-

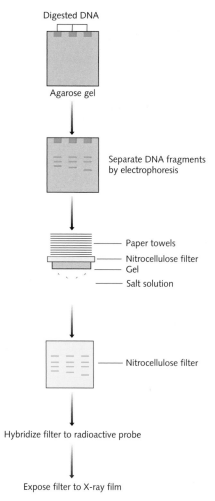

Digested DNA

Agarose gel

Separate DNA fragments by electrophoresis

Paper towels
Nitrocellulose filter
Gel
Salt solution

Nitrocellulose filter

Hybridize filter to radioactive probe

Expose filter to X-ray film

Fig. 3.11 Southern blot analysis of DNA. DNA digested with specific restriction enzymes can be fractionated on the basis of fragment size by electrophoresis in agarose gels. The DNA fragments in the gel can be transferred to a solid support such as nitrocellulose either electrophoretically or by transfer of solute up through the gel onto the nitrocellulose sheet. The filter can then be hybridized to a radioactive probe containing a DNA or RNA sequence of interest, the unbound probe washed off and the positions of the DNA fragments in the gel complementary to the probe can be localized by autoradiography on X-ray film.

sis on gels where, as well as current being applied from the top of the gel to the bottom, the electric current is also pulsed across the gel. These gels can then be blotted and analysed in the same way as standard agarose gels.

Alternatively, it is also possible to gain similar information by simply dotting DNA straight onto the nitro-cellulose filter sheets and probing these directly. However, such assays (known as **DNA dot** or **slot blots**) do not generate additional information, such as sizes of DNA fragments encompassing the gene of interest, which is intrinsic to size fractionation by gel electrophoresis prior to blotting.

Gene structure—does the gene contain introns?

A number of techniques can be used to determine if a gene of interest contains introns and, if so, their location within the gene. A full understanding of the relationship between the genomic DNA and its corresponding mRNA is essential to understand the many mechanisms by which expression of the gene may be controlled. Annealing of a genomic DNA sequence to RNA expressed from that DNA (single-stranded DNA and RNA will anneal as well if not better than single-stranded DNA molecules) will result in so-called **R-loops** (Fig. 3.12), in which the genomic sequences not present in the cDNA loop out of the annealed duplex. These structures can be seen in the electron microscope or can be digested away with single strand-specific nucleases such as S1 or mung bean nuclease, and separation of such digests by gel electrophoresis can determine the number of introns within a known segment of genomic DNA (Fig. 3.13). Precise definitions of the location of intron/exon boundaries can routinely be obtained by techniques such as **S1 nuclease mapping**, in which single

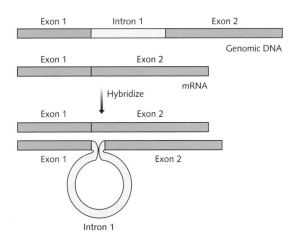

Fig. 3.12 R-loops to detect introns. The use of electron microscopy to look at the physical structure of mRNA–DNA hybrids can show the presence of introns in the DNA portion of the hybrid which loops out from the hybrid structure because there is no complementary sequence to the mRNA molecule.

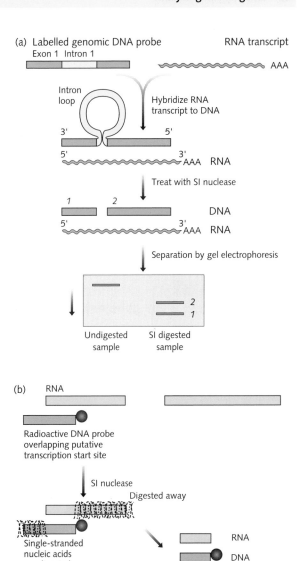

Fig. 3.13 S1 analysis of RNA. S1 mapping can be used to determine the start of an RNA transcript or the precise location of intron boundaries. A radioactively labelled genomic DNA probe can be hybridized to total cellular RNA. This forms an mRNA–DNA hybrid with DNA overhangs if the start of the RNA transcript lies within the DNA probe (a) or with R-loops if the DNA probe has intronic sequences (b). Treatment of the hybrids with S1 nuclease digests single-stranded loops or overhangs. Separation on agarose gels of the fragments of the DNA probe protected from digestion by S1 because of it annealing to complementary RNA in the hybrid can then determine the length and location of the intron sequence or the precise start of the RNA transcript.

strands of cloned fragments of genomic DNA which overlap potential intronic regions are annealed to total cellular RNA. Such DNA/RNA hybrids between complementary DNA and RNA molecules will contain single-stranded regions where any exonic sequences within the genomic DNA has no homologous RNA sequence to anneal to (Fig. 3.13). Digestion with S1 nuclease will remove all such single strands generating precise DNA/RNA hybrid molecules. By precisely sizing these double-stranded DNA/RNA hybrids, the site of the exon/intron boundary can be defined. A judicious choice of the genomic DNA sequence used for the mapping analysis can also generate information not only about intron/exon boundaries but the precise start and end of the transcript.

Where and when is the gene expressed?

Many diseases result from the inadequate or incorrect expression of specific genes. Consequently, an understanding of the exact site and level of expression of a gene of interest is often important in understanding the molecular basis of disease. A number of techniques are available to analyse the expression of a gene of interest, either at the RNA or protein level.

RNA can be analysed for the presence of specific sequences by **Northern blot** analysis, named somewhat tongue-in-cheek from Southern blot analysis. In this case total RNA or polyadenylated (poly(A+)) mRNA from cells or tissues of interest can be separated by size on agarose gels, blotted onto nitrocellulose filters and probed with a radiolabelled DNA sequence of interest to determine the presence of this specific RNA (Fig. 3.14). Analysis of specific cells or tissues over time courses of growth or differentiation can give information about tissue and temporal specificity of RNA expression. Similarly *in situ* hybridization, a technique involving the detection of RNA by probing for specific RNA species in specially prepared tissue sections by hybridization to known DNA probes, can also be used to establish levels of gene expression. A somewhat more sensitive system to detect specific RNA sequences, **RNase protection assay**, is based on S1 nuclease assays (Fig. 3.13a). In this assay, radiolabelled RNA complementary to an RNA of interest is hybridized to total cellular RNA. RNA species within the total cellular RNA complementary to the probe will hybridize to the radiolabelled RN probe and protect it from digestion with specific RNase enzymes. Protected species can then be visualized by separation on agarose or acrylamide gels

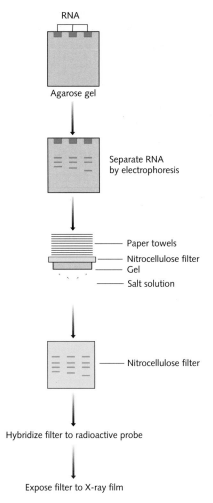

Fig. 3.14 Northern blot analysis of RNA. RNA can be size fractionated on agarose gels and transferred to nitrocellulose. The filter can then be probed with specific probes to detect the presence and size of RNA species of interest.

after detection on X-ray film by autoradiography. Because of the high specific activity of the radiolabelled RNA probes, this assay is much more sensitive than assays such as Northern blotting or S1 mapping to detect RNA species of interest

Expression at the protein level is most easily detected by antibodies to proteins of interest. Separation of proteins from specific cells or tissues by sodium dodecylsulphate–polyacrylamide gel electrophoresis (SDS-PAGE), which separates proteins on the basis of their size, followed by transfer onto nitrocellulose—so-called **Western blotting**—allows specific detection of a protein for which an antibody is available. Similarly *in situ* detection of proteins in specially prepared tissue sections can also be carried out with such antibodies.

What does the gene product do?

The primary amino acid sequence encoded by a gene of interest can sometimes help directly to determine protein function. Comparison of the novel protein sequence to all other known proteins in protein sequence databases will, obviously, immediately determine if the new protein sequence is of an already known protein. However, even if it is not, amino acid homologies between small regions (**protein domains**) of the novel protein and already defined proteins with known functions may give insight into what functions the novel protein may have. For instance, some specific enzyme activities are known to be defined by specific amino acid sequences within proteins (e.g. kinases). The presence of such a string of amino acids in any novel protein may indicate the relevant enzyme activity encoded by that protein.

In many situations, the ability to express a gene of interest either *in vivo* or *in vitro* can be immensely helpful in its analysis. It is possible to clone a cDNA of interest into special plasmids termed **expression vectors** which drive expression of the cDNA to RNA *in vitro* (Fig. 3.15a). This RNA, as well as being used for probes for RNA structure or *in situ* hybridization, can also be translated into protein in cell-free *in vitro* translation systems, such as reticulocyte lysates, to generate radio-labelled protein. Alternatively, plasmid vectors in which the cDNA of interest is expressed from bacterial promoters can be introduced and expressed at the protein level in bacteria (Fig. 3.15b). However it is important to be aware that, whilst the primary amino acid sequence of the bacterially expressed protein will be faithful to that encoded by the cDNA, any post-synthetic modifications such as protein glycosylation normally observed in the eukaryotically expressed protein will not be faithfully carried out in bacteria, as such signals for protein glyco-sylation are different between prokaryotic and eukaryotic cells. Also, such expression systems can only be used for cDNAs as neither *in vitro* transcription/translation systems nor bacteria will carry out RNA splicing reactions.

Such problems can be overcome by expressing the gene in eukaryotic cells. There are innumerable plasmid DNA vectors which have been developed to do this, many of which are based on expressing the gene from strong eukaryotic viral promoters (Fig. 3.16). As with bacterial transformation, it is possible to introduce

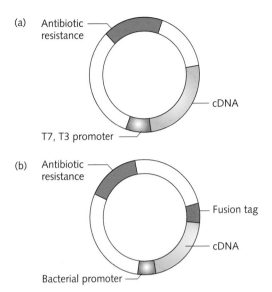

Fig. 3.15 (a) Plasmids that allow *in vitro* transcription and translation. Certain plasmids contain cloning sites downstream of bacteriophage promoters such as T7. This allows the transcription *in vitro* of the plasmid generating RNA of the cDNA coding region of interest. This RNA can also be translated *in vitro* using reticulocyte lysate extracts which contain ribosomes and all the other constituents to translate the RNA into protein. (b) Expression of fusion proteins in bacteria. High levels of proteins of interest can also be generated by expression of cDNAs in specialized bacterial expression vectors. In many cases these vectors permit the expresion of fusion proteins containing a protein of interest and a short amino acid 'tag', which allows the rapid purification of the recombinant protein from bacterial extracts by the use of specific antibodies to the 'tag'. Alternatively, the use of so-called 'HIS–tag' fusion in which the protein of interest is tagged with a string of histidine residues allows purification of this fusion protein on nickel columns, due to the high affinity of histidine for nickel.

plasmid DNA directly in cultured eukaryotic cells by **DNA transfection**. A number of transfection procedures are currently in use and all rely on techniques to enhance DNA uptake by the cell. These include presenting the DNA as a calcium phosphate precipitate or DEAE-dextran (a dextran sugar derivative that binds DNA) complex to the cell, stimulating uptake of DNA by breaching the cell membrane by electric currents (**electroporation**), or by fusing either bacterial protoplasts or artificial membrane vesicle (**liposomes**) containing plasmid DNA to cell membranes. Depending on whether the plasmid DNA also carries selectable markers (such as resistance to the translation inhibitor G418), cells can be

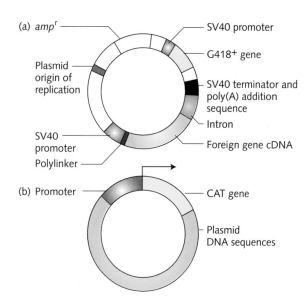

(a)
- amp^r
- Plasmid origin of replication
- SV40 promoter
- Polylinker
- SV40 promoter
- G418+ gene
- SV40 terminator and poly(A) addition sequence
- Intron
- Foreign gene cDNA

(b)
- Promoter
- CAT gene
- Plasmid DNA sequences

Fig. 3.16 Eukaryotic expression vectors. Expression vectors for high-level expression of genes in eukaryotic cells often contain different DNA domains from different sources that each function to optimize expression of the gene of interest. (a) Shown here is a vector in a plasmid backbone carrying antibiotic resistance and an *Escherichia coli* origin of replication in order to grow the plasmid efficiently in bacteria. The plasmid also contains a cloning site to insert DNA sequences of interest downstream of the simian virus 40 (SV40) promoter. This strong promoter, as well as a globin intron and an SV40 polyadenylation signal, all help confer high levels of expression of the insert in eukaryotic cells by maximizing transcription, RNA stability and transport. (b) Alternatively, other expression vectors can allow the analysis of gene promoter function. In these so-called reporter constructs, a gene promoter of interest is cloned upstream of a gene which is not usually expressed in eukaryotic cells and whose expression can be easily quantified. The example shown here is a reporter construct which expresses the chloramphenicol acetyl transferase (CAT) gene.

stably transfected. This means that the transfected cell continuously carries the transfected DNA due to continuous selection for drug resistance during culture of the transfected cells. Alternatively, cells can be **transiently transfected**, where no selection for maintenance of the transfected DNA is applied and the majority of cells that have not taken up the transfected DNA rapidly outgrow those that have. Generally, stably transfected cells carry the transfected DNA as large multimers (**concatamers**) of DNA which are predominantly integrated randomly into the cell genome by **non-homologous recombination** between transfected and genomic DNA. Plasmid DNA can also be microinjected directly into cell nuclei.

Obviously, it is difficult to carry out this technique on any large scale.

Alternatively, the ability to introduce genes of interest into a range of cell types by recombinant viral vectors, either retroviruses or DNA viruses, is currently under extensive use in potential gene therapy strategies (see Chapter 16), as this results in virutally every cell becoming infected with concomitant high levels of expression of the gene of interest. For instance, mammalian retroviruses are being extensively used to introduce and express potentially therapeutic genes in cells. Similarly, insect DNA viruses such as the polyhedrosis virus (baculovirus) that can infect *Spodoptera frugiperda* cells in culture are used extensively to express large amounts of gene product of interest.

Such ability to express cloned DNA at the protein level in prokaryotic or eukaryotic cells can allow direct analysis of protein function. The generation of DNA clones containing deletions or mutations in specific sites within the gene and their introduction back into cells as expression vectors permits an analysis of DNA sequences necessary for specific functions at the protein level. Similarly, isolated recombinant proteins can be analysed directly for biochemical function, used as immunogens to generate antibodies and, increasingly, used to ask specific questions about three-dimensional protein structure by biophysical analyses such as X-ray crystallography or nuclear magnetic resonance spectroscopy.

Many of the techniques for analysing gene function we have discussed so far have depended upon gene expression in bacteria or eukaryotic cell lines. However, the ability to introduce and express cloned genes in animals has extended our ability to analyse gene structure and function. Animals carrying recombinant DNA (**transgenic animals**) can be generated by microinjecting DNA directly into recently fertilized embryos. Alternatively, totipotent embryonal stem (ES) cell lines (undifferentiated cells capable of differentiating into all types of tissues) can be transfected with a gene of interest and these cells can be introduced into a developing embryo by micromanipulation (Fig. 3.17). After development, animals derived from such embryos often contain the foreign DNA in all cell types including their germ line and, hence, the foreign DNA is inherited from generation to generation. Such 'transgenics' have helped define control regions of genes necessary for their expression in the right tissue and at the right time of differentiation and development.

More recently, an elegant method based on transgenic animals has been used to ask about the function of specific genes *in vivo*. These **gene knockout** experiments rely

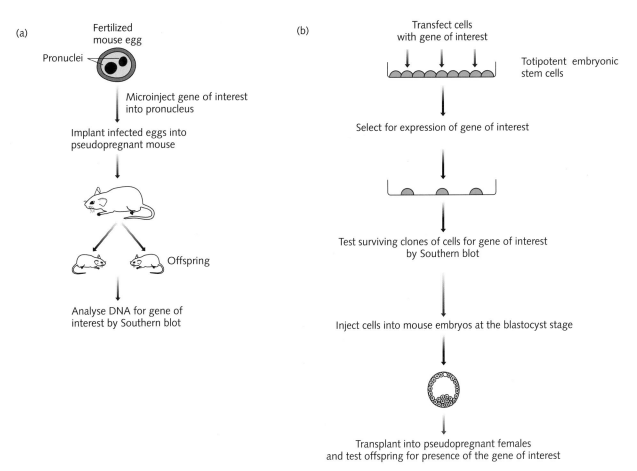

(a)

Fertilized mouse egg

Pronuclei

Microinject gene of interest into pronucleus

Implant infected eggs into pseudopregnant mouse

Offspring

Analyse DNA for gene of interest by Southern blot

(b)

Transfect cells with gene of interest

Totipotent embryonic stem cells

Select for expression of gene of interest

Test surviving clones of cells for gene of interest by Southern blot

Inject cells into mouse embryos at the blastocyst stage

Transplant into pseudopregnant females and test offspring for presence of the gene of interest

Fig. 3.17 Generation of transgenic mice. (a) DNA of interest can be introduced into fertilized mouse eggs by microinjection and transferred to pseudopregnant mice. After birth, offspring can be tested for insertion of the transgene by Southern blot or polymerase chain reaction (PCR)-based analyses. (b) Alternatively, DNA can be introduced into totipotent embryonal stem (ES) cell lines by stable transfection of a plasmid containing the gene of interest and a selectable marker, allowing cells expressing the DNA of interest to be selected for. Surviving cell clones can be tested by PCR or Southern blot analysis to confirm the presence of the transfected DNA and these cells are then injected into mouse embryos at the blastocyst stage. Embryos are then transplanted into pseudopregnant mothers and offspring analysed for the presence and expression of the gene of interest.

on the fact that on rare occasions transfection of cells with foreign DNA can result in the integration of the incoming DNA into genomic DNA of the same DNA sequence (**homologous recombination**). Consequently, use of specific DNA sequences for transfection carrying flanking sequences to a specific gene located in the cell genome (a so-called replacement vector) can result in homologous recombination between the target gene and the transfected DNA resulting in gene disruption (Fig. 3.18). Confirmation of this, and only this, specific recombination can be carried out by Southern blot analysis. This cell clone can then be introduced into a fertilized embryo resulting in a mutant transgenic animal unable to express a specific gene of interest. The resulting phenotype of the mutant can then give major insight into the function of that gene *in vivo*.

Does the protein interact with nucleic acids or other proteins?

It has become increasingly clear that many proteins exert important functions by interacting with other proteins or with nucleic acids. For instance, many transcription factors interact specifically with defined double-stranded DNA sequences (their DNA binding site) and also undergo defined protein–protein interac-

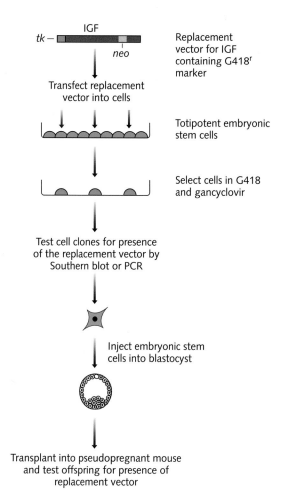

Fig. 3.18 Targeted gene disruption in transgenic mice. Specific genes can be 'knocked out' in transgenic mice by selection of ES cell transfectants that have specifically incorporated a replacement vector into the site of the wild-type mouse gene of interest. In the example shown, a replacement vector containing a cDNA encoding the enzyme thymidine kinase and a genomic DNA clone encoding the insulin-like growth factor (IGF) in which one of the exons was replaced with a gene conferring resistance to the drug G418 (*neo*), is transfected into ES cells. Expression of thymidine kinase (TK) will make cells susceptible to killing with gancyclovir, whilst expression of *neo* will make cells resistant to G418. Consequently, only cells that have homologously recombined the replacement vector with the genomic IGF gene will grow as these will contain the *neo* gene but not contain the *tk* gene which is lost during homologous recombination. This eliminates cells that have just incorporated the replacement vector randomly.

tions with other protein species for function (see Chapter 4).

A number of assays to determine if a protein of interest forms protein–protein interactions have been devised. *In vivo* assays such as co-immunoprecipitation rely on immunoprecipitations of, for instance, complex mixtures of radiolabelled proteins by a specific antibody to determine if any other protein species co-precipitates with the primary antibody–protein complex (Fig. 3.19).

Similarly, **Far-Western** blot analysis (like Western blot) relies on the ability to detect any protein–protein interaction between a protein probe and proteins on nitrocellulose filters after transfer from SDS-PAGE gels, but in this case the protein probe is not an antibody but a radiolabelled protein of interest.

Analysis of the ability of a protein of interest to bind DNA or RNA usually requires some idea of the DNA or RNA sequence that specifically interacts with that

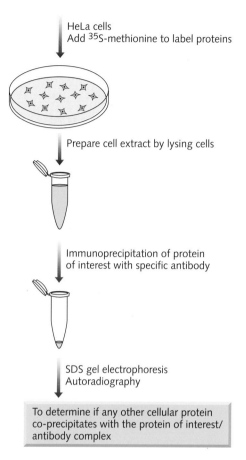

HeLa cells
Add ^{35}S-methionine to label proteins

Prepare cell extract by lysing cells

Immunoprecipitation of protein
of interest with specific antibody

SDS gel electrophoresis
Autoradiography

To determine if any other cellular protein
co-precipitates with the protein of interest/
antibody complex

Fig. 3.19 Double immunoprecipitation assays to analyse
protein–protein interactions. The ability of one protein to
interact specifically with another protein can be analysed easily
by immunoprecipitating one of the proteins with a specific
antibody and determining if this co-precipitates the other
protein of interest.

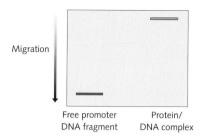

Migration

Free promoter
DNA fragment

Protein/
DNA complex

Fig. 3.20 Mobility shift assays to detect protein–DNA
interactions. If a radioactively labelled piece of double-
stranded DNA is mixed with a protein that is known to bind
specifically to that DNA sequence and the mixture is separated
by electrophoresis on non-denaturing acrylamide gels, the
mobility of the DNA probe is retarded or 'shifted' with respect
to the unbound DNA probe. This is because the large
DNA–protein complex migrates more slowly than the free
unbound probe. This type of analysis can also be used to ask if
a complex mixture of proteins such as a nuclear extract
contains DNA-binding proteins of specific interest.

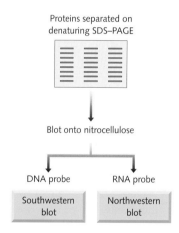

Proteins separated on
denaturing SDS–PAGE

Blot onto nitrocellulose

DNA probe   RNA probe

Southwestern
blot

Northwestern
blot

Fig. 3.21 Southwestern or Northwestern blots allow detection
of protein–DNA or protein–RNA interactions, respectively. As
well as mobility shift assays, it is possible to detect the specific
interaction of DNA with a protein using systems based on
Western blotting. In this type of assay, proteins of interest are
separated by denaturing polyacrylamide gel electrophoresis
(SDS-PAGE) and blotted onto nitrocellulose membranes.
These membranes can then be probed with radioactively
labelled DNA and any protein on the nitrocellulose membrane
that binds the DNA probe can be detected by autoradiography.
If the probe is RNA, then specific protein–RNA interactions
can also be detected and this has been termed Northwestern
blot analysis.

protein. If this is known, two major types of assay can
routinely be used to detect protein–nucleic acid interactions. **Mobility shift** assays rely on the observation
that protein–nucleic acids complexes migrate more
slowly upon gel electrophoresis compared to free
unbound nucleic acid probe (Fig. 3.20). Consequently, if
radiolabelled DNA or RNA probes are mixed with a
protein of interest and separated on acrylamide gels, a
specific interaction between that protein and DNA or
RNA probe can be detected by a shift in mobility of the
nucleic acid. Alternatively, yet other derivations of the
Western blot can be used to detect protein–nucleic acid
interactions. Proteins separated by SDS-PAGE and transferred to nitrocellulose filters can be probed with specific
radiolabelled double-stranded DNA or single-stranded

RNA to detect specific interactions with protein species.
These have been termed **Southwestern** blots for DNA
probing of protein filters or **Northwestern** for RNA
probing of protein filters (Fig. 3.21). Such assays have

helped enormously in our understanding of how transcription factors bind their target DNA sequences and specifically regulate gene expression.

The exact DNA sequence that interacts with a protein of interest can be determined by so-called **DNase I footprinting** assays. In this assay DNA sequences are radioactively labelled with ^{32}P. The radiolabelled DNA fragment is incubated with a purified protein of interest or, indeed, with a mixture of cellular proteins if the identity of the protein which binds that piece of DNA is not known. If the test protein binds to the labelled DNA probe, then the protein-bound DNA will be protected from digestion by the enzyme DNase I. Thus a 'naked' DNA molecule, not protected by a bound protein, will be cleaved by the DNase I between every adjacent nucleotide. DNase I cleavage of naked DNA will be visualized as a ladder of nucleotides on an acrylamide gel. If a protein is bound to a specific sequence of nucleotides within the labelled DNA fragment, the enzyme DNase I will be prevented from cleaving that sequence of nucleotides, and that portion of the sequence ladder will not be visualized. The missing portion of the sequence ladder looks like a window in the gel, and is called a footprint (Fig. 3.22).

Analysis of gene control regions

In many situations, once a gene of interest has been cloned, an analysis of its gene control regions, the so-called promoter/regulatory regions, will be essential for a full understanding for its function.

The control regions of a gene can be analysed by their introduction into cells by transfection attached to so-called **reporter** genes. In this situation, gene promoter/regulatory regions can be linked to a marker gene encoding, for instance, the chloramphenicol acetyl transferase (CAT) gene. This gene encodes an enzyme that acetylates chloramphenicol and is not found in eukaryotic cells. CAT activity can easily be measured in cell extracts and the levels reflect the activity of the promoter sequences attached to it—that is the CAT activity reports the promoter strength used in the reporter vector (Fig. 3.23).

Such DNA transfection assays of the putative gene control regions in reporter vectors will help define the DNA sequences containing all the gene's promoter/regulatory region. Similarly, such analyses can also be carried out *in vitro*. For instance, promoter/regulatory regions can be added to cell nuclear extracts and are capable of initiating mRNA synthesis which can be measured. Such *in vitro* **transcription** assays can be used to measure promoter activity and can also be used to analyse the effect

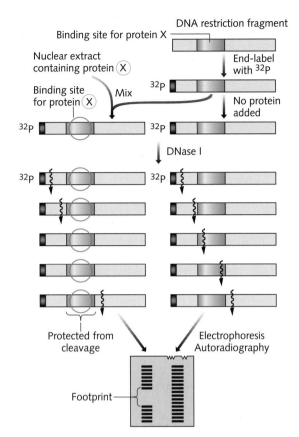

Fig. 3.22 DNase I footprinting identifies specific DNA sequences that interact with proteins. In DNase I footprinting analysis, a DNA fragment that is known to bind specifically to a protein (X) is radioactively labelled at one end of the DNA fragment. The DNA probe is then incubated with protein X or a mixture of proteins containing protein X and the mixture is briefly treated with DNase I so that the probe DNA is randomly cut once on average. If no protein is bound to the DNA probe the DNase I digestion generates a ladder of probe DNA subfragments on polyacrylamide gel electrophoresis. If, however, the probe is bound by a protein, this region of the DNA cannot be cut by the DNase I and shows up as a gap on the gel ladder of DNA subfragments. The position of the gap in the DNA ladder—the so-called footprint or protected area— corresponds to the specific DNA sequence protected by the protein.

of recombinant proteins on transcription. For instance, the effect of a transcriptional activator or repressor (see Chapter 4) on a promoter can be assayed by adding the pure protein to an *in vitro* transcription assay containing that promoter.

The use of mobility shift assays, Southwestern blotting and DNase I footprinting assays will all help define cellular protein factors that might interact with a pro-

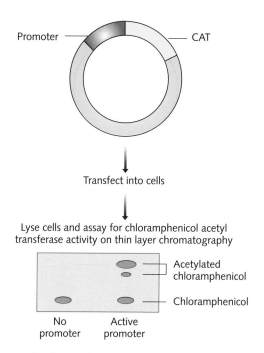

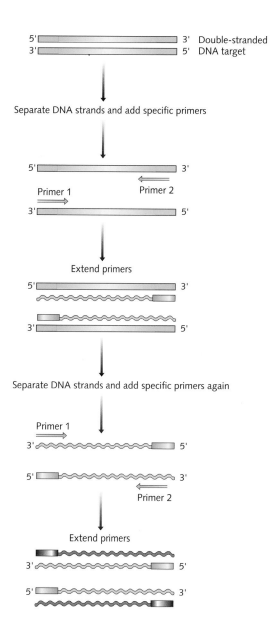

Fig. 3.23 The choramphenicol acetyl transferase (CAT) reporter assay. The strength of a gene promoter can be analysed by transfection of promoter reporter constructs. Transfection of CAT reporter vectors into eukaryotic cells results in the expression of the CAT gene which can be easily assayed by measuring the conversion of ^{14}C-chloramphenicol to acetylated chloramphenicol in the presence of transfected cell extracts. If these assays are then analysed by ascending thin layer chromatography the amount of acetylated chloramphenicol can be measured by autoradiography. Acetylated chloramphenicol products migrate faster up the chromatogram.

Fig. 3.24 The polymerase chain reaction (PCR). Any double-stranded DNA molecule can be amplified by the use of specific primers to the two DNA strands and a thermostable DNA polymerase enzyme. In the PCR, the two strands of a DNA target are separated by heating and the DNA is cooled in the presence of oligonucleotide primers complementary to each DNA strand at either end of the region of the DNA to be amplified. These prime new DNA strand synthesis from the target DNA template using a thermostable polymerase such as *Taq* polymerase (isolated from *Thermophilus aquaticus*, hence the name *Taq*). New DNA synthesis will be limited to the region of DNA bounded by the two primers. If the reaction is heated again, the original template DNA strands and the newly synthesized DNA strands are again denatured, primers now bind to both newly synthesized and original template DNA strands, and DNA synthesis proceeds again. By repeating this cycle, a single copy of target DNA can be exponentially amplified.

moter/regulatory region of interest and control its expression.

Polymerase chain reaction—a wide-ranging technique in molecular biology

The polymerase chain reaction allows the massive amplification of specific DNA sequences and has become a powerful aid to the molecular biologist. The reaction relies on the annealing of two short primers each complementary to flanking DNA sequence of the region of DNA to be amplified (Fig. 3.24). These primers are then

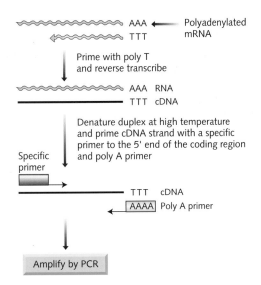

Fig. 3.25 Cloning by PCR. Total cellular RNA can be reverse transcribed using a poly(dT) primer. If the amino acid sequence of the gene of interest is known, specific primers complementary to the 5′ end of the coding region can be used together with a poly(dA) primer to amplify the gene of interest specifically by PCR.

acid sequence encoded by the 5′ end of the gene is known. If reverse transcription of RNA is carried out using poly(dT) priming, then carrying out PCR using a 5′ oligonucleotide primer complementary to the DNA sequence encoding the known amino acid sequence and a poly(dT) 3′ primer will result in the amplification of the cDNA of interest directly (Fig. 3.25). No cDNA library screening is required.

PCR can also be used to change the precise sequence of an amplified target to any sequence of choice. For instance, if the 5′ ends of the PCR primers are made to contain restriction enzyme sites, then the final PCR product will be flanked by these sites (Fig. 3.26) which can help enormously in their subsequent cloning and manipulation.

PCR techniques can also be used efficiently to screen for mutations in genes of interest. For instance, the choice of oligonucleotide primers can allow specific amplification of normal but not mutant DNA sequences (the so-called amplification refractory mutation system—ARMS).

extended with a special thermostable DNA polymerase enzyme (*Taq* polymerase). The new double-stranded DNA molecule (**DNA duplex**), consisting of one template strand and one extended strand, is then denatured under high temperature. The primers are then allowed to anneal again and are once more extended by the *Taq* DNA polymerase. This series of denaturation/annealing/extension is carried out in multiple cycles resulting in a logarithmic amplification of the target DNA sequence (Fig. 3.24). Similarly, if reverse transcription (RT) of RNA is first carried out, then the resulting single-stranded cDNA can also be used as starting material from which to amplify any specific RNA sequences of choice, by so-called **RT-PCR**.

This ability to amplify a target DNA sequence has found many applications in clinical molecular biology. Perhaps its primary uses have been in detecting rare DNAs or RNAs such as viral or bacterial nucleic acids in clinical samples (see Chapter 12), and for detection of mutations in known genetic disorders (see Chapter 6). However, it is increasingly being used in a variety of molecular cloning techniques and for analysis of gene expression.

In some situations there is no need to screen cDNA libraries to isolate a cDNA clone of interest. For instance, consider a gene of interest for which the amino

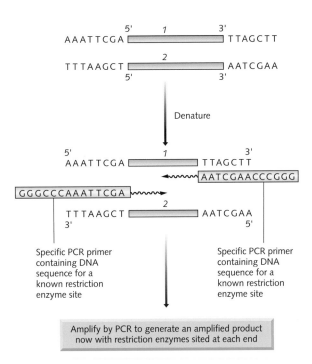

Fig. 3.26 Modifying DNA ends by PCR. If PCR primers are synthesized so that they contain known restriction enzyme sites, then the target DNA that is amplified will contain these restriction enzyme sites at their ends.

More recently, the ability to carry out PCR analysis *in situ* on specially prepared sections has permitted the localization of specific viral nucleic acids present in samples at too low a level for detection by routine *in situ* hybridization and, in the future, will help enormously in localizing specific rare RNA or DNA sequences.

Further reading

Sambrook J., Fritsch E.F. and Maniatis T. (1989) *Molecular Cloning*, 2nd edn. Cold Spring Harbor Laboratory Press, New York.

Watson J.D., Gilman M., Witowski J. and Zoller M. (1992) *Recombinant DNA*, 2nd edn. W.H. Freeman, San Francisco.

Chapter

4 Transcriptional control of human gene expression

Introduction

Aberrant expression of genes can have far-reaching consequences. The expression of too much or too little of a gene product or expression of a gene product at the wrong time or in the wrong place can all result in the manifestation of disease. Consequently, an understanding of the control of cellular gene expression can only help in our understanding of the molecular basis of many human diseases.

Gene expression dictates the cell phenotype

The amount of a specific cellular protein can vary over 100 million-fold between different cell types in human tissues. For instance, in adult human reticulocytes, 95% of the polypeptide chains synthesized are α- or β-globin, whereas in the somatotrophs of the anterior pituitary up to 30% of the protein made is growth hormone. In contrast, neither globin nor growth hormone is detectable in adult hepatocytes. A hypothetical explanation for the differences between cells in their levels of proteins is that genes encoding specific proteins are present in certain cell types but not others. However, it is clear that this is not the case because, except for a few certain cell types, most cells contain identical complements of DNA—that is they have the same genotype. It is differences in the levels of expression of genes within the cell which determines cell type—the cellular phenotype. The phenotypic differences between cell types thus

requires that the same cellular DNA is used uniquely in each of the tissue types. Not only is selective expression of genes a determinant of cellular differentiation, it is also required for living cells to respond to changes in their environment. Thus, the control of gene expression is required for cellular differentiation and maintenance of cell viability in diverse environments.

When a polypeptide such as β-globin is measurable, it is said that 'the gene encoding for β-globin is expressed'. The first step in gene expression is the process of transcription, which results in the production of RNA on a DNA template. The newly synthesized RNA may be a messenger RNA (mRNA) (whose protein product will require translation), or it may be a small nuclear RNA (snRNA) needed for splicing, or ribosomal RNA (rRNA), or transfer RNA (tRNA), required for translation of mRNAs. But it has become clear that levels of expression of specific genes can be controlled at many stages, either directly at the level of their transcription (transcriptional control), at the level of splicing (post-transcriptional control) or, as with some mRNAs, at the level of their translation (translational control). Whilst there are examples of control of gene expression at each of these levels, by far the most common mechanism of control is at the level of transcription.

Of the estimated 100 000 human genes, the transcription of many is restricted to cells of a specific tissue lineage, to a specific time in the development of a tissue, or in response to a specific environmental inducing factor such as a hormone. In contrast, other genes are transcribed constitutively in all tissues and are called 'housekeeping genes'. Tissue-, time- or induction-specific gene transcription cannot, therefore, be explained on the basis of changes in the genotype, but on mechanisms that control gene expression from identical genomes. It is now becoming clear that the regulation of gene expression can be explained by a hierarchical control of transcription at the level of the structure of the chromosome (so-called **chromatin structure**) and by combinatorial interactions between a limited number of cell-specific transcriptional regulatory proteins and RNA polymerase (the enzyme required for the synthesis of RNA).

Whilst the transcriptional regulation of a specific gene in one specific organism will, or course, always be a special case, the study of transcriptional regulation in viruses, prokaryotes, and eukaryotes reveals many common mechanisms because the process is governed by the rules of chemistry and thermodynamics. In this chapter, we will look at the mechanisms that control cellular gene expression using the regulation of β-globin expression as an example. Similar mechanisms will operate in the control of a number of other cellular and viral genes that we will study in later chapters.

Cellular proteins regulate transcription

The initial step of RNA synthesis for all three RNA polymerases is the localization of RNA polymerase to a sequence of double-stranded DNA at the so-called promoter of the gene that is to be transcribed. The promoter sequence defines the site of initiation of mRNA transcription (Fig. 4.1). For rRNA genes transcribed by RNA polymerase I, this is located at their 5′ end. Similarly, genes transcribed by RNA polymerase II also contain promoter sequences usually at their 5′ end which often, but not always, contain a DNA sequence resembling the DNA sequence TATA about 30 basepairs upstream from the start of transcription—the **TATA motif**. RNA polymerase III-transcribed genes may also have upstream promoter elements containing a TATA element (e.g. snRNA genes) or may have TATA-less promoters internal to the coding region (e.g. tRNA genes).

Unlike bacterial RNA polymerases, eukaryotic RNA polymerases do not contact the promoter DNA directly but are recruited to the promoter by complexes of proteins specific for each RNA polymerase (Fig. 4.1). These complexes have been termed SL1 for RNA polymerase I, TFIID for RNA polymerase II and TFIIIB for RNA polymerase III. In the case of TATA-bearing promoters transcribed by RNA polymerase II, TFIID binds directly to TATA elements via direct binding of a component of TFIID known as **TATA binding protein** or TBP which is known to be a universal component of all three

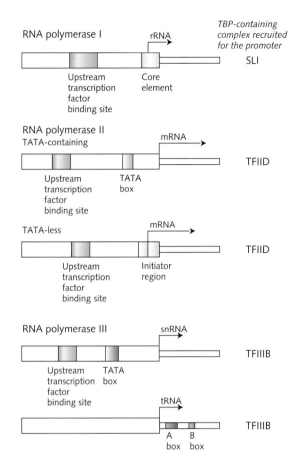

Fig. 4.1 Typical gene promoter elements important for transcription by the three RNA polymerases, RNA polymerase I, II and III. RNA polymerase I-dependent promoters contain a core element spanning the site of initiation of RNA trancription and an upstream control element that is believed to activate transcription from the core region by binding the cellular transcription factor UBF. RNA polymerase II-dependent promoters often contain a TATA element which acts as a basic promoter element as well as upstream elements that bind specific cellular transcription factors. Some RNA polymerase II-dependent promoters are TATA-less but contain an alternative basic promoter element called the initiator region. RNA polymerase III-dependent promoters which control transcription of tRNA genes contain promoter elements that reside within the coding region of the gene, often referred to as the A and B box. Alternatively, small nuclear RNAs (snRNAs) which also depend on RNA polymerase III for their transcription do contain a TATA element as well as upstream elements. The ubiquitous TATA binding protein (TBP) is required for activity from promoters driven by all three RNA polymerases and is recruited to the promoter in the form of the SL1, TFIID or TFIIIB complex for RNA polymerase I-, II- and III-dependent promoters, respectively.

polymerase-specific complexes (Fig. 4.1). For RNA polymerase II promoters that have no TATA elements, TFIID is recruited to the promoter DNA at so-called initiator elements probably via direct interaction between the initiator DNA element and another component of TFIID known as TAF 150 (Fig. 4.1). In the case of RNA polymerase II promoters, the TFIID complex then acts as a site where other protein cofactors such as TFIIA and TFIIB are recruited to the promoter and help stabilize the interaction between TFIID and DNA. This stable promoter–protein complex then acts to recruit RNA polymerase along with other **general transcription factors** (GTFs) to allow transcription (Fig. 4.2), and it is these DNA–protein complexes containing the ubiquitous general transcription factors and RNA polymerases, the

so-called **basal transcription complex**, which act as targets for transcriptional activation or repression by tissue-specific transcription regulatory proteins. These tissue-specific transcription factors also bind specifically to other DNA sequences in the control regions of genes and it is their control of the basal transcription complex which results in regulated tissue-specific gene expression. The ability of general and tissue-specific transcription factors to interact directly with DNA is fundamental to such control of gene transcription.

Transcription factors contain different functions

Tissue-specific transcriptional regulatory proteins bind to specific promoter/regulatory regions of genes and regulate levels of transcription from the basal transcription complex. Aside from their DNA binding region or domain, transcriptional regulatory proteins may have domains for reversible, non-covalent protein–protein interaction sometimes termed **dimerization domains**. Interactions between one specific protein via a similar dimerization domain on another protein is a prerequisite for binding of some transcription regulatory proteins to DNA. Therefore the binding of transcription factors to DNA is often co-operative, that is the presence of one protein can change the affinity of other proteins for binding to DNA.

Whilst many transcription factor dimers contain two of the same protein species (**homodimers**), others are formed between two non-identical proteins (**heterodimers**) (Fig. 4.3). Consequently, different transcription factor homodimers and heterodimers may recognize the same or related DNA sequences and this allows the generation of combinatorial diversity in the regulation of transcription. For instance, the DNA sequence TGAGTCA is a DNA sequence recognized by a family of transcription regulators called activator protein-1 (AP-1) proteins (Fig. 4.4). This DNA motif is found in the promoter elements of many genes, both tissue-specific and non-specific. The AP-1 group of factors consists of heterodimeric protein complexes encoded by the cellular *fos* (c-*fos*) and cellular *jun* (c-*jun*) gene families and these proteins need to form dimers in order to bind to DNA (Fig. 4.4a).

Like other transcription regulators, the AP-1 proteins are DNA binding proteins which have different domains for different functions. One domain of an AP-1 protein is the dimerization domain, which mediates dimer formation through a structure called the leucine zipper. This region of the protein contains amino acids that form a helical structure or coil, such that one side of the protein structure consists of hydrophilic amino acids while the

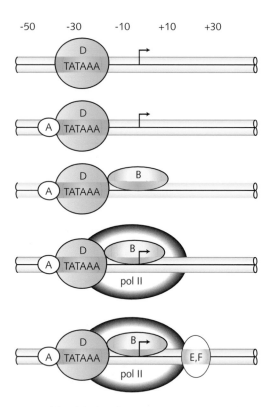

Fig. 4.2 Assembly of the basal transcription on a typical RNA polymerase II-responsive promoter involves a sequential recruitment of general transcription factors. The first general transcription factor to bind to the promoter is TFIID which directly contacts the TATA box of the promoter DNA via the TBP component. If the promoter contains no TATA box, it is likely that TFIID contacts the promoter DNA at the initiator region of the promoter via one of the other TAFs in TFIID, probably TAF150. Once TFIID has bound, the other GTFs bind sequentially, finally resulting in the recruitment of RNA polymerase and its associated factors (reproduced from Singer and Berg (1991)).

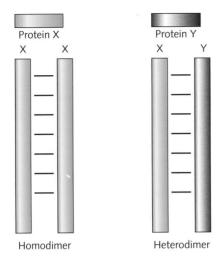

Fig. 4.3 Transcription factor function often requires protein dimers containing identical (homodimer) or different (heterodimer) partners.

domain of AP-1 proteins is also found in many other transcriptional activating proteins, but other activation domains in other transcriptional regulatory proteins may be proline rich or may have no obvious pattern of amino acids; how these domains of transcriptional regulatory factors increase the activity of RNA polymerase II is the subject of intensive study but it is believed that many contact the basal transcription complex by direct interaction with TFIID, and increase the speed at which

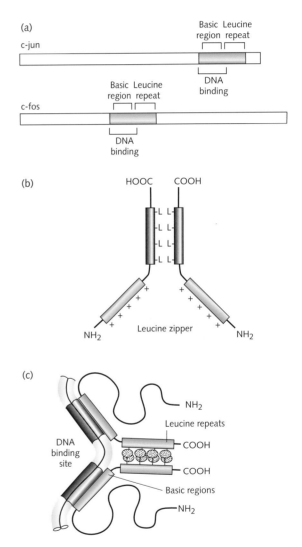

Fig. 4.4 (a) The cellular transcription factor AP-1 consists of a heterodimer of the Fos and Jun proteins. These proteins dimerize by interaction of their leucine zipper regions (b) and contact DNA via their basic DNA binding domain (c). Whilst Fos and Jun heterodimers bind the consensus AP-1 site DNA sequence TGACGTCA tightly, homodimers of Fos do not bind DNA at all (reproduced from Singer and Berg (1991)).

other side has hydrophobic amino acids. Every seventh amino acid in the helical structure is the amino acid leucine; leucine is a hydrophobic amino acid so all the leucines are found on the hydrophobic side of the coil. The hydrophobic side of the coil can engage in non-covalent bonding with a similar hydrophobic coil containing a leucine at seven amino acid intervals. Protein dimers are formed by the interdigitation of these hydrophobic coils which can be described as a (leucine) zipper or a coiled coil (Fig. 4.4b).

The coiled coil formed between the two monomers permits the DNA binding domain within each protein monomer to interact with its binding site within DNA. The DNA binding domain of each monomer is also a helical structure consisting of many basic amino acids. The positively charged helix of the DNA binding domain of each member of the dimer forms hydrogen bonds with the sequence TGA in the TGAGTCA element. Since the sequence TGA is found on both strands of the DNA duplex (as the sequence TGACTCA has dyad symmetry and the complementary sequence to TGACTCA is also TGACTCA), the dimer actually contacts both strands of the DNA duplex and grasps the DNA as if in a scissors grip (Fig. 4.4a). The leucine zipper domain and the DNA binding domain of AP-1 proteins are necessary but not sufficient for increased transcriptional activity. Yet another domain within each monomer, the so-called **transcriptional activation domain** (Fig. 4.5), rich in acidic amino acids, is required for increasing the transcriptional activity of a promoter. The acidic activation

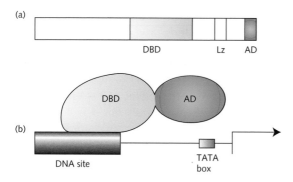

Fig. 4.5 As well as protein domains which mediate DNA binding (the DNA binding domains (DBD)) and protein dimerization (e.g. the leucine zipper), transcription factors also contain domains which are responsible for transcriptional activation (activation domains (AD)). Often these activation domains contain stretches of acidic amino acids (acidic activation domains) or proline-rich regions and these are believed to mediate transcriptional activation via direct interactions with the basal transcription complex. Many transcription factors contact TBP or TFIIB directly and others have been shown to interact specifically with one or other of the TAFs. Transcriptional activation may involve an increase in recruitment of the GTFs to the promoter by such interactions.

a functional basal transcription complex is formed (Fig. 4.5).

There are at least three proteins in the c-*jun* family and three in the c-*fos* gene family; this allows for the generation of various AP-1 heterodimers, each of which may have different levels of transcriptional activation. In addition, it has been shown that c-Jun can form heterodimers with proteins of other transcriptional activating proteins such as steroid hormone receptors, which, like other transcriptional activating proteins, are also multidomain proteins. Hormone receptors may also contain a dimerization domain, a DNA binding domain and a transcriptional activation domain as well as a binding domain for the hormone.

Growth factors and other agents can activate transcription

Cells that are not actively growing and dividing because of growth factor starvation express the Jun and Fos proteins at a low level. Within 15 minutes of the addition of growth factors to the medium, there is an increase in the amount of c-*fos* and c-*jun* mRNA followed by a burst of synthesis of these transcription factors.

As well as an increase in the amount of Jun and Fos proteins, there are changes in the phosphorylation of

some of the amino acids within Jun/Fos proteins. There is decreased phosphorylation of the DNA binding domain of the Jun protein. Since phosphorylation of an amino acid changes its charge to negative, decrease in the phosphorylation of the DNA binding domain would increase the net positive charge of the DNA binding domain. Increase in the net positive charge of the DNA binding domain could increase the interaction of the DNA binding domain with the net negatively charged phosphodiester backbone of the DNA duplex. There is increased phosphorylation of amino acids in other domains of c-*jun* that could lead to an increase in the ability of the Jun/Fos heterodimer to activate transcription following binding to the DNA duplex.

The increased amount and activity of AP-1 proteins in growth factor-stimulated cells likely leads to activation of many genes that contain AP-1 binding sites. Some of the protein products of the genes activated by binding of AP-1 proteins to transcriptional regulatory sequences are required to maintain replication through the cell cycle. For this reason Fos/Jun dimers, i.e. AP-1 factors, have been called early response genes or competency genes because they control the entry of the cell into a cycle of growth and division.

However, it is becoming increasingly clear that other mechanisms besides the simple presence or absence of tissue-specific transcription factors also play an important role in the regulation of gene expression, and involve the higher order structure of chromatin.

Chromatin and transcription

Chromatinization of a cell's genomic DNA by interaction with histones permits a metre of DNA to be compacted within the 10 μm diameter of the cell's nucleus. Using special stains, chromatin in the nucleus of a cell can be seen by light microscopy. Some chromatin, called heterochromatin, appears to be darkly stained and compact, while the less densely stained chromatin is more dispersed and called euchromatin. Heterochromatin corresponds to transcriptionally inactive DNA, while euchromatin is transcriptionally active. Transcriptionally inactive heterochromatin is compacted so tightly that RNA polymerase cannot easily access the DNA. In contrast, there are regions of DNA within euchromatin that are quite accessible to transcriptional regulatory factors and RNA polymerase.

Since there are large regions of chromatin that are inaccessible to transcription factors, even the presence of the correct combination of transcription factors that should recruit RNA polymerase to that promoter does not guarantee that transcription will be initiated at the promoter. If the promoter is in a region of closed chromatin, the transcription factors and RNA polymerase will not have access to the promoter. Therefore, chromatin structure regulates the accessibility of the DNA to these transcription factors and so represents an important regulatory step in the process of tissue-specific transcription. How chromatin switches from inactive to active chromatin is not known at present, and is the subject of much experimentation. Some experiments using chromatin from viruses have helped shed some light on chromatin structure. For instance, active chromatin, along a short stretch of nucleosomes, has been visualized by electron microscopy in some experimental systems. SV40 (simian virus 40) is a small, about 6000 basepairs, double-stranded DNA virus that infects monkey cells. Following entry into the cell nucleus, the viral genome is chromatinized by histones. About 200 basepairs of the SV40 virus contain the DNA sequences that serve as the promoter for viral transcription as well as the origin of replication for viral DNA replication. This 200 basepairs region of the virus appears to be devoid of nucleosomes, so that the DNA is 'naked' and freely accessible to transcription and replication factors. However, other experimental systems suggest that complete removal of histones from a DNA template is not needed for transcription to occur.

Unfortunately, it is not possible to identify regions of active chromatin in a long sequence of chromatinized DNA such as a human chromosome by, for instance, electron microscopy. However, as active euchromatin is open to access by transcription factors and RNA polymerase, these regions of euchromatin are also accessible to enzymes that can probe chromatin structure. When chromatinized DNA within a cell's nucleus is exposed to the enzyme DNase I, adjacent phosphodiester bonds in the DNA chain are cleaved. About 10% of the cell's DNA is easily cut into nucleotides by this enzyme; the remaining 90% remains uncut.

After the nuclei of erythroblasts that express the globin gene are exposed to DNase I, the region of the genome encoding globin is preferentially digested to nucleotide bases. In contrast, the region of the genome encoding albumin, which is not expressed in erythroblasts, is protected from DNase I cleavage. Therefore active euchromatin globin gene DNA is preferentially digested into nucleotides and is said to have increased **DNase I sensitivity** in comparison to the inactive heterochromatin albumin gene DNA.

Discovery of the relative 'openness' of the chromatin of the transcribed globin genes in erythroid cells, in comparison to the non-transcribed albumin gene, was a starting point for investigation of the erythroid-specific transcription of the globin genes.

Regulation of human globin gene expression

The human β-like globin gene domain, located on the short arm of chromosome 11, has five linked transcriptionally active genes that are expressed in a developmentally specific manner and transcribed by RNA polymerase II. These genes are arranged over a distance of 45 kb and are ordered along the chromosomal DNA in the same order as their temporal activation (Fig. 4.6). The most 5′ gene is the ε-globin gene; this gene is expressed very early in embryonic life by erythroblasts, in the yolk sac. Transcription of this gene is extinguished by about 8 weeks of gestation. The site of globin gene transcription then moves to the fetal liver where the two fetal γ genes are expressed until about 36 weeks of gestation. The site of globin gene transcription then moves again to its final tissue location—the bone marrow. Fetal globin gene expression is extinguished, and adult globin gene expression, which starts at about 8 weeks, increases to high levels. Adult globin gene expression within the β-like domain primarily involves β-globin with a small amount of δ-globin.

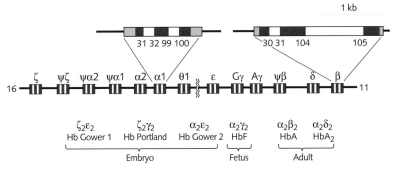

Fig. 4.6 In humans, the β-globin gene cluster containing the β-, γ- and δ-globin genes is found on chromosome 11, with genes arranged in their order of expression. The α- and ζ-globin genes are clustered on chromosome 16.

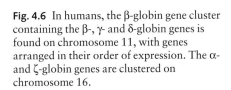

The human α-globin gene domain is located on chromosome 16. The embryonic ζ-globin gene is expressed in the yolk sac, while the adult α-globin gene is expressed in fetal liver and bone marrow. For the α-like globin genes there is only a single embryonic to adult switch, with no fetal intermediate. To assemble a functional haemoglobin molecule, a dimer of β-like globin chains must join with a dimer of α-like globin chains to form the heteromeric tetramer.

The thalassaemic phenotype
(see Plate 5, facing p. 214)

Since all functional human haemoglobins are tetrameric proteins consisting of two α-like and two β-like polypeptide chains (Fig. 4.7), decreased synthesis of either globin chain leads to reduction in the amount of haemoglobin per erythrocyte. Decreased production of α- or β-globin polypeptide is characteristic of the thalassaemias. There are many thalassaemic genotypes that produce the easily recognized thalassaemic phenotype: erythrocytes that are small (microcytic) and not well haemoglobinized (hypochromic). The hypochromic and microcytic phenotype is not unique to thalassaemia, iron deficiency and other defects of haemoglobin synthesis also cause it. The application of recombinant DNA technology to the identification of the mutant genotypes which decrease the production of β-globin chains has shed light on the study of chromatin structure and transcription within the β-globin gene domain. Studies have led to the identi-

fication of *cis*-acting DNA sequences (DNA sequences physically linked in close proximity) and *trans*-acting transcriptional regulatory proteins (essentially diffusible factors) that regulate expression of globin molecules in erythroid cells.

All the globin genes have three exons separated by two intervening intronic sequences that are spliced out from the heterogeneous nuclear RNA transcript (Fig. 4.6). Many of the genetic mutations that cause so-called β_0-thalassaemia, where no globin chains are produced, are mutations in a single nucleotide within the gene that either prevent splicing of an intron or result in the generation of a translational stop codon. Another group of β_0-thalassaemia mutations, the frame shift mutations, are caused by the addition or deletion of nucleotides within the β-globin gene. This results in an mRNA that when translated produces a non-functional protein. Mutations within the β-globin gene itself, leading to sequence changes in the transcribed mRNA, do not (in almost all cases) cause a change in the rate of transcription, because these mutations do not involve the promoter of the β-globin gene which is the site of transcriptional initiation.

Regulatory sequences in the β-globin promoter

Each of the five linked globin genes within the β-globin gene domain has its own promoter element located 5′ to the DNA sequence encoding the globin chain. Mutations within the promoter sequence define another class of nucleotide changes that cause the β_+-thalassaemic phenotype. In contrast to β_0-thalassaemia, in which no globin chains are produced, the β_+-thalassaemic phenotype is due to point mutations which result in a decrease in the rate of β-globin mRNA transcription. These mutations also define *cis*-acting DNA sequences in the promoter that bind transcriptional regulatory proteins which control β-globin gene transcription. Such point mutations causing the β-thalassaemic phenotype are found in the TATA motif located at bases −31 to −27 with respect to the site of initiation of transcription and decrease the formation of the basal transcription complex, and also produce variability in the start site of transcription.

Point mutations in overlapping CCAAT and CACCC DNA motifs located at −90 to −84 (Fig. 4.8) also cause the β_+-thalassaemic phenotype. The CCAAT sequence motif is bound by many transcriptional factors of the NF1/CTF family of transcription regulatory proteins which act as transcriptional activators. The CACCC sequence is also bound by many proteins including the transcriptional regulatory protein Sp1 and erythroid

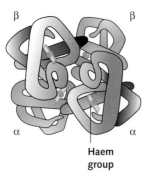

Haem group

Fig. 4.7 All the human globins have a tetrameric structure: adult and fetal globins contain two α chains combined with two β chains in haemoglobin A (α2β2), two δ chains in haemoglobin A2 (α2δ2) or two γ chains in haemoglobin F (α2γ2). Two forms of γ chains exist, Gγ and Aγ, depending on the presence of an alanine or glutamine amino acid at position 136 in the amino acid. In the embryo, the two ζ chains combine with two ε or two γ chains to generate Gower (ζ2ε2) or Portland haemoglobin (ζ2ε2) and two α chains combine with two ε chains to form the Gower2 haemoglobin.

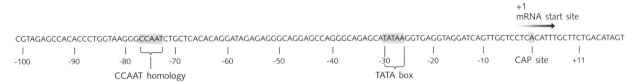

Fig. 4.8 The human β-globin promoter is a typical RNA polymerase II-dependent promoter containing a TATA motif, a CCAAT box homology and GC-rich sites that bind the cellular transcription factor Sp1 and EKLF.

Kruppel-like factor (EKLF). Mutations that decrease binding of the EKLF protein, which is a positive regulator of adult β-globin gene transcription, also decrease mRNA production. In contrast, some forms of hereditary persistence of fetal haemolobin (HPFH) may be due to point mutations at an Sp1 binding site in the γ-globin promoter that increase the affinity of the binding site for Sp1.

The TATA, CCAAT and CACC sequence motifs are found not only in the promoter sequences of the globin genes elements but in the promoters of many tissue-specific and housekeeping genes. Erythroid cells may have tissue-specific versions of proteins that bind to these motifs, such as EKLF to the CACC sequence. It is also likely that ubiquitous transcriptional regulatory factors bind to globin promoters in conjunction with erythroid-specific factors.

Additional *cis*-acting transcriptional regulatory sequences within the human β-globin gene promoter have been defined by identification of highly conserved nucleotide sequences shared between the promoters of β-globin genes of many mammalian species. A sequence containing the tetranucleotide GATA is found in virtually all globin promoters in species such as chicken, mouse and humans. This sequence has been shown to bind a transcription factor called GATA-1 (also known as Eryf1 or GF-1). GATA-1 is an erythroid-specific factor, related to other GATA binding factors. Binding sites for GATA-1 are also found in the promoters of some of the genes that encode enzymes of the haem synthetic pathway as well as the promoter of the erythropoietin receptor gene. It is possible that the GATA-1 transcription factor controls the transcripion of a battery of erythroid-specific genes. (GATA-1 is discussed in more detail on p. 70.)

In addition to these well-defined sequences within the β-globin promoter, there are likely to be specific sequences within each of the β-like globin promoters that bind factors involved in the positive regulation of specific stages of transcription, i.e. embryonic or fetal or adult. Since there is also stage-specific shut-off of globin gene transcription it is also likely that there are binding sites for proteins which regulate transcription negatively at the globin promoters. A binding site for a protein that may extinguish ε-globin gene transcription has been located in the ε-globin promoter.

The β-globin promoter element linked to the β-globin gene has been found, in transgenic mice, to contain all the nucleotide sequence information required for erythroid-specific transcription. Therefore within the promoter element of each of the globin genes within the β-globin gene domain there are many *cis*-acting regulatory sequences that can be bound by a large number of cellular transcription factors. It is likely that occupancy of all of the transcriptional regulatory sites within the promoter as well as β-globin intragenic sequences is required for erythroid-specific transcription.

Not all β-thalassaemias are caused by point mutations within or near the β-globin gene. This finding indicates that additional *cis*-acting sequences are required for the high level of erythroid-specific expression of globin genes.

Promoter sequence deletions result in the γ/δ/β-thalassaemias

One particularly informative group of thalassaemias is the γ/δ/β-thalassaemias. As a result of decreased production of β-globin polypeptide chains, individuals who have γ/δ/β-thalassaemia have hypochromic microcytic erythrocytes. A simple explanation for the decreased production of β-globin polypeptide is that the gene is deleted on at least one of the two chromosomes 11. This would result in a decreased β-globin mRNA and reduced quantities of translation product.

Analysis of the structure of the β-globin gene domains of individuals with γ/δ/β-thalassaemia has shown deletions, but not of either of the two β-globin genes. Within one of the two chromosomes 11, a large deletion leaves the adult β-globin gene intact, while removing about 100 000 basepairs of DNA upstream (5′) to β-globin. The extent of this deletion varies from individual to individual. In some there is a deletion of about 100 000 base-pairs of DNA ending as close as 2.5 kb 5′ to the β-globin gene, removing all other β-like globin genes. In others, a large deletion leaves intact all the β-like globin genes but removes DNA ending about 10 kb 5′ to the ε-globin gene or about 55 kb 5′ to the β-globin gene. All affected individuals have a genotype containing two intact β-globin genes while their phenotype suggests that only one β-globin gene is expressed.

An explanation for the absence of mRNA transcripts from the β-globin gene on the chromosome 11 having the deletion mutation, is that there are additional point mutations within the linked β-globin gene causing the thalassaemic phenotype. The β-globin gene from the deleted chromosome is easily distinguished from the β-globin gene on the intact chromosome because the genomic restriction maps are different; this allows cloning of the β-globin allele from the deleted chromosome. When inserted into transcriptionally active, non-erythroid cells this cloned β-globin allele is transcribed at the same (low) rate as cloned β-globin alleles from intact chromosomes 11. This indicates that the absence of transcription from the β-globin allele on the deleted chromosome is not caused by additional inactivating point mutations within the β-globin gene or its promoter sequences.

Another possible explanation for the lack of expression of the β-globin gene allele from the deleted chromosome is that the deleted DNA sequence encodes for a protein required for β-globin gene expression. A more formal statement is that a sequence coding for a *trans*-acting transcriptional regulatory protein factor required for β-globin transcription is deleted. However, since the other chromosome 11 has no deletion, at least one gene for the putative *trans*-acting factor would remain, ensuring a 50% of normal level of the factor. Assuming that 50% of the level of this putative *trans*-acting factor is sufficient to permit transcription of both β-globin genes, we must conclude that the deleted sequence does not encode for a transcriptional regulatory protein. Rather the missing DNA sequence is required to be covalently linked, and must be in *cis*, to the β-globin gene for this gene to be expressed. To locate specific DNA sequences that are deleted in γ/δ/β-thalassaemia and regulate transcription of the β-globin gene cluster, the chromatin structure of the intact β-globin domain was examined.

Tissue-specific globin gene expression

To determine the chromatin structure of the human β-globin gene domain, it is necessary to have uniform populations of cells that express β-like globin genes.

Fortunately, there are human cells that have become immortal and transformed, as a result of oncogene (see Chapter 8) activation, and can be grown in tissue culture. These cell lines are often derived from human tumour tissues but retain some normal characteristics. The cell line K562 was derived from the blood cells of a patient with the blast crisis of chronic myelogenous leukaemia (CML). In tissue culture, K562 cells produce the embryonic haemoglobins Gower I and II and the fetal haemoglobin F; no adult haemoglobin A is synthesized because the adult β-gene is not transcribed. K562 cells, the progeny of human bone marrow cells, can be used as a model for the transcription of erythroid-specific genes. The leukaemic cell line HL60 does not transcribe any of the globin genes and can be used as a model for non-erythroid gene expression.

Since genes within the β-globin gene domain of K562 cells are transcribed, while those of HL60 cells are not, DNase I will preferentially cleave the β-globin gene DNA domain of K562 cells (Fig. 4.9a). If the hypothesis that some chromatin sequences are easily accessible to transcription factors is true, then identification of specific sequences of DNA within K562's β-globin gene domain that are cleaved by DNase I should also localize regulatory DNA sequences required for transcription of the β-globin gene.

ε-Globin chromatin structure is erythroid specific

Such mapping of the chromatin structure of the β-globin gene domain in K562 cells by DNase I revealed that there were four regions of hypersensitivity upstream (5′) of the embryonic ε-globin gene (Fig. 4.9b). These hypersensitive sites (HS) are called 5′HS1, 5′HS2, 5′HS3 and 5′HS4; 5′HS1 is closest to the promoter of the ε-globin gene, and 5′HS4 is the furthest away. These hypersensitive chromatin sites were located far from the promoter of the ε-globin gene and more than 50 000 basepairs from the β-globin gene promoter. As expected, the non-erythroid cell line HL60 did not have these hypersensitive sites. When adult human bone marrow containing erythroid precursor cells was tested, hypersensitive sites upstream to ε-globin were also detected. This result confirmed that open regions of chromatin were found far upstream of the β-globin gene cluster in cells of erythroid lineage only. Furthermore these erythroid-specific hypersensitive sites were detected at all developmental stages of globin gene expression; embryonic ε-globin in K562 cells, adult β-globin in bone marrow cells.

The deleted region of DNA common to all forms of γ/δ/β-thalassaemia is the region of the DNase hypersensitive sites far upstream of the human ε-globin gene.

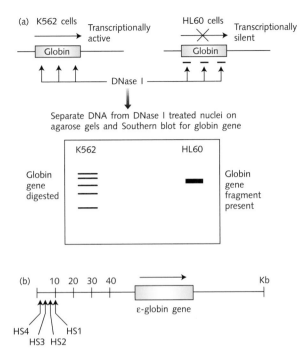

Fig. 4.9 DNase I-sensitive sites of the β-globin promoter. Genes which are actively transcribed contain a more open chromatin configuration and are therefore more susceptible to digestion with enzymes such as DNase I. Consequently, DNase I treatment of cell lines that express β-globin will result in digestion of the β-globin coding region compared with cell lines in which β-globin genes are not transcribed (a). Similarly, promoter regions that have an open chromatin structure are also hypersensitive to DNase I digestion (b).

Determination of the chromatin structure of the β-globin gene cluster indicated that sequences readily accessible to transcription factors are located far 5′ of the human ε-globin gene. The experimental evidence strongly suggested that this region of DNA contained far upstream *cis*-acting sequences required for transcription within the β-globin gene domain, and helped define another DNA element besides the promoter which is essential for the high-level expression of a number of cellular and viral genes — the so-called **enhancer**. Enhancers are DNA sequences that have been defined in DNA transfection assays to increase the expression of genes that they are linked to. In contrast to promoters which only function close (some 30 basepairs) to the site of initiation of RNA transcription, enhancers increase transcription from promoters independent of their orientation or site of location. Consequently, an enhancer can still activate promoters even if located many kilobases away or on the complementary strand of DNA to the promoter in ques-

tion. Such was the case for the 5′ HS sites of the ε-globin gene defined above.

DNase I hypersensitive sites correspond to regions of chromatin that are accessible to transcription factors. The formation of a DNase I hypersensitive site at the 5′ end of a gene in the promoter region or at a distance from a gene is one of the initial steps in the process of transcription. DNase I hypersensitive sites probably form before the localization of an RNA polymerase II-containing transcription complex at the promoter. Therefore, DNase I hypersensitive sites are necessary, but not sufficient, to initiate transcription.

Though we can identify regions of chromatin that are accessible to transcription factors using DNase I, it is still not clear how regions of chromatin become accessible to transcription factors. Furthermore, DNase I hypersensitive sites at specific gene locations are passed on to daughter cells as cells divide. It is probable that the chromatin structure of DNA is altered during the process of DNA replication such that regions of DNA that should be transcriptionally active in a certain cell are maintained in open chromatin conformation as the cell replicates. This hypothesis will be discussed later.

The locus control region for β-globin expression

The DNase hypersensitive sites upstream of ε-globin contain powerful transcriptional enhancer elements which may also confer a degree of position independence to genes when they are stably integrated into mouse chromatin. For instance, when a gene and its control elements are introduced and stably integrated into the chromosomes of a transgenic mouse, that gene is transcribed to a variable extent, depending on the position of integration of the gene in each particular transgenic mouse. If the gene integrates into an active accessible chromatin position, it is expressed at higher levels than at other positions. This variability in transcription activity is termed the position effect. When the human β-globin gene is linked in *cis* to the hypersensitive sites and used to create a transgenic mouse, the hypersensitive sites protect the β-globin gene from such position effects. Regardless of the mouse chromosome into which the human β-globin gene integrates, the level of human β-globin gene expression remains the same. The hypersensitive sites upstream of ε-globin appear to be dominant over position in their effects on transcription. Because of this, the hypersensitive sites have been termed the locus control region (LCR) for β-globin gene expression in humans.

The experiments described above indicate that an enhancer element and a promoter element, as well as accessibility of these elements to erythroid-specific transcription factors, are needed to achieve physiological rates of erythroid-specific transcription of any of the genes within the β-globin gene domain.

The LCR contains transcriptional enhancer elements, that also confer some position-independent expression onto linked genes. As we shall see, the LCR contains many binding sites for transcriptional regulatory proteins, but how these proteins initiate transcription at promoters located many kilobases away is still unclear.

The LCR for α-globin expression

DNA sequences that serve as position-independent transcriptional enhancers are not unique to the human β-globin gene cluster; the human α-globin gene domain also has a LCR far upstream of the α-globin genes. These LCRs are not unique to the human globin gene domains, animals as distant as the mouse and goat also have them. Comparison of the nucleotide sequences between mouse, goat and human shows that there are runs of nucleotides that are virtually identical between the species. Conservation of the nucleotide sequence of *cis*-acting regulatory sequences between species is highly suggestive that conserved DNA sequences serve to bind *trans*-acting regulatory proteins that have also been highly conserved during evolution.

Silencer elements of the β-globin gene

Transcription of the embryonic ε-globin gene is turned off by about 10 weeks of fetal gestation. Investigation of the promoter of this gene has revealed the sequence motifs noted above — TATAA, CCAAT, CCACC and GATA binding sites. When DNA containing the ε-globin promoter and additional sequences 5' to the known protein binding sites was analysed for the ability to control gene expression in erythroid and non-erythroid cell lines by transfection assays, a sequence between −177 and −392 was shown to repress promoter activity. This finding suggests that there is a negative regulatory element, that when removed allows increased transcription. Furthermore, this element repressed promoter activity regardless of its position or orientation with respect to the promoter. Thus, this sequence decreases transcription in a position- and orientation-independent manner. Sequences which act in this way are called **transcriptional silencer elements**. Transcriptional silencer elements bind proteins that act negatively to regulate the activity of transcription.

Hypersensitive sites bind transcriptional regulatory proteins

DNase footprinting has helped identify transcriptional regulatory factors that bind at enhancers, silencer or promoters.

When the 5'HS2 DNA sequence is analysed by DNase I footprinting using nuclear factors isolated from erythroid or non-erythroid cell lines, a large number of protected DNA regions are detected, indicating the binding of a number of transcriptional regulatory proteins to this region of DNA. The DNA sequences of these protected regions have been compared to DNA sequences that are known to serve as binding sites for transcription factors. One of the protected DNA sequences in the 5'HS2 region is the sequence GGGGTGGGGG, and this sequence is protected regardless of whether a nuclear extract from the erythroid cell line K562 or a non-erythroid extract from HL60 or HeLa cells is used.

Fractionation and analysis of the numerous proteins found in these nuclear extracts that bind to this DNA sequence show that at least one of them was the transcription regulatory protein SP1. This transcriptional regulatory factor is found in all cells and belongs to a family of transcription factors called zinc finger proteins. Zinc finger proteins contain zinc ions that serve to co-ordinate amino acids into a finger-like structure that can reach into the major groove of the DNA helix and contact the nucleotides to form a non-covalent bond. Although Sp1 binds to 5'HS2, as well as to globin gene promoters, this protein is probably not responsible for the erythroid-specific activity of 5'HS2 as it is ubiquitously expressed and found in many if not all cells.

GATA-1 is an erythroid-specific transcription factor

Binding sites within 5'HS2 for the erythroid-specific transcription factor GATA-1 are also detected by DNA binding assays. Therefore this erythroid-specific enhancer as well as erythroid promoter elements appears to bind GATA-1. The presence of binding sites for this transcription factor in the regulatory elements for many erythroid lineage-specific genes suggests that the GATA-1 transcription factor may be a major control protein, regulating transcription of erythroid-specific genes by acting as a master switch to turn on a battery of erythroid-specific genes. If this hypothesis is true then loss of the GATA-1 protein from cells should decrease the general expression of erythroid-specific genes. Since the gene encoding for GATA-1 is found on the X-chromosome, there is only one copy of this gene in males. It was, therefore, possible to disrupt this single copy gene specifically in cells of male transgenic mice.

Embryonic stem cells containing a GATA-1 gene disruption resulted in mice with little development of circulating erythrocytes, indicating that the transcription factor GATA-1 is required for erythroid differentiation. An explanation for this appears to be that there is a single GATA-1 binding site in the promoter of the gene encoding the erythropoietin (EPO) receptor. If GATA-1 cannot bind to the promoter then the transcription of the EPO receptor gene is insufficient to permit the EPO-mediated proliferation of cells derived from the most immature pool of erythroid stem cells. Since GATA-1 binding sites are found in other erythroid-specific genes, even if the number of erythroid progeny cells did not decrease, phenotypic expression would not have been recognizable because the globin genes and other erythroid-specific genes such as those encoding the enzymes of haem biosynthesis would be transcriptionally inactive.

The erythroid enhancer binds many proteins

The sequence within 5′HS2 that has been shown to be required for its regulatory activity binds factors from erythroid and non-erythroid nuclear extracts alike. The core nucleotide sequence of this 5′HS2 region is GCTGAGTCATGATGAGTCATG and binds many nuclear proteins as defined by electrophoretic mobility shift assays (see Chapter 3) with erythroid nuclear extracts.

The core sequence contains a tandem repeat of the heptameric sequence TGAGTCA which binds the AP-1 family of transcription regulatory proteins. The 5′ nucleotides of each heptamer are spaced 10 basepairs apart, just the distance of one full turn of the double helix. This suggests that the AP-1 factors that bind to each heptamer will be on the same side of the helix and able to interact co-operatively. How binding of AP-1 factors to recognition sites within the LCR activates the β-globin gene domain is not known at present.

Haemin inducibility of the erythroid enhancer

The core sequence element of the 5′HS2 enhancer binds additional factors beyond the many possible combinations of heterodimers that recognize AP-1 binding sites. The core sequence of 5′HS2 also contains the sequence GCTGAGTCA. When the 5′ G of this sequence is mutated, and this mutant oligonucleotide is used in DNA binding assays with erythroid nuclear extracts, the mutant oligonucleotide generates one less band than the

non-mutated oligonucleotide. Since the mutant oligonucleotide still contains an AP-1 binding site the additional band formed with the wild-type oligonucleotide must be generated by a protein other than AP-1.

To date, this protein has not yet been definitively identified; candidates include NF-E2 and its family members. This protein/s appears to be relevant to erythroid transcription because it appears essential for haemin-induced promoter activation in DNA transfection assays. Consequently, at least one of the proteins that binds to the core element of 5′HS2 confers haemin inducibility upon the LCR.

Regulation of the transcriptional activity of 5′HS2 by haem could serve a useful purpose in erythroid cells. Without sufficient haem in an erythroid cell to form haemoglobin, the transcription of globin mRNA and synthesis of globin chains would be useless. Therefore the requirement for haemin to increase the transcriptional activity of the β-globin gene domain (as well as α-globin since the α-globin LCR has a similar binding sequence) ensures that globin chains will be produced when there is the capacity to form functional haemoglobin.

Transcriptional activation—the interaction of erythroid enhancers and promoters

All the experimental evidence so far indicates that sequences far upstream of the human ε-globin gene are required for high-level erythroid-specific transcription within the β-globin gene domain. Investigation of the proteins that bind to sequences within the 5′HS2 enhancer indicates that many proteins can bind to this enhancer. Similarly, the promoters of the globin genes also contain many of the same transcription factor binding sites as the enhancer.

Transcription initiation at promoters of genes for mRNAs requires that RNA polymerase II be recruited to the promoter. For general transcription factors such as TFIID, it is readily understandable how the binding of these proteins close to the site of action of RNA polymerase may help recruit and increase the formation of a functional transcriptional complex. It is more difficult to understand how a protein binding at the 5′HS2 enhancer can activate transcription by RNA polymerase II from the TATA box of the β-globin gene promoter when this TATA box is thousands of basepairs away from 5′HS2.

One hypothesis is that enhancer elements can loop to promoter elements (Fig. 4.10), allowing proteins that bind at the enhancer to contact proteins that bind at the promoter forming a complex of proteins that

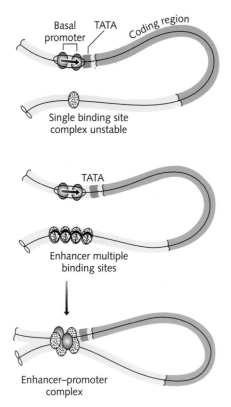

Fig. 4.10 The mechanism by which enhancers, which can act in a position- or orientation-independent manner, activate transcription is not well understood. One model suggests that the chromatin between the enhancer and the promoter region loops out to allow direct interaction between enhancer-bound proteins and the general transcription factors of the basal transcription complex (reproduced from Singer and Berg (1991)).

increase the recruitment of RNA polymerase II to the TATA box.

At present this result may be considered as a model for the study of eukaryotic enhancer elements which also bind transcriptional regulatory proteins and act at a great distance from the promoter. Recently, *in vitro* systems for the study of eukaryotic transcription have yielded insight into how histones, DNA, RNA polymerase III and transcriptional regulatory proteins may interact to specifically increase transcription of genes.

Nucleosomes inhibit transcription *in vitro*

It is possible to analyse transcriptional activation of specific promoters by specific transcriptional regulatory proteins *in vitro* using *in vitro* transcription assays. Such assays have shown that if all the components of the tran-

scriptional initiation complex are added to promoter elements that have been chromatinized by histones, so that the template has nucleosome structure, the level of transcription of chromatinized templates is reduced by two orders of magnitude compared to naked promoters. This indicates that nucleosomes may serve to inhibit the transcription of promoters. If a transcriptional activator protein is added to the *in vitro* transcription reaction after the assembly of the nucleosome structure, the rate of transcription is not increased. However, if a transcriptional activator protein is added at the same time as histones required for nucleosome assembly on the DNA template and prior to the addition of the RNA polymerase II initiation complex, the rate of transcription is now increased about 30 times compared with chromatinized templates formed in the absence of transcriptional activator proteins. An interpretation of this finding is that transcriptional activator proteins compete with histones for access to DNA. The competition with histones would disrupt the formation of nucleosomes, exposing regions of DNA and thereby increasing access of the components of the transcriptional initiation complex to the promoter. Therefore one role of some types of transcriptional activator proteins could be to prevent the inhibition of transcription produced by the assembly of nucleosomes, whilst others may directly interact with the transcriptional initiation complex to increase the rate of formation of the open complex.

It is apparent from all the experimental data discussed above that the regulation of globin gene transcription is very complex owing to its combinatorial diversity. It is likely that the initial step in activation of transcription within the β-globin gene domain is the binding of transcriptional regulatory proteins to the LCR. This statement implies that the chromatin structure of the LCR is not so tightly closed that it is inaccessible to some regulatory proteins. When erythroid cells undergo DNA replication and mitotic division, the chromatin structure is altered to permit DNA replication by the DNA polymerase complex. It may be that in the time immediately following DNA replication, transcription factors can bind, thus sustaining the replication-induced alteration of chromatin structure. The linkage between replication and transcription is no longer speculative: there is experimental evidence that the portion of the genome that replicates early in cell division contains the genes that are transcriptionally active.

Transcription and cell division

Experiments have shown that the globin gene domain

DNA replicates early in the S phase of erythroid cells. In contrast, in non-erythroid cells in which there is no transcription of globin genes, the globin gene DNA is replicated later.

When a mouse erythroleukaemia cell line is engineered to contain a human β-globin gene domain that has a deletion of the LCR (similar to a deletion found in a type of γ/δ/β-thalassaemia) for β-globin expression, the human β-globin gene is not expressed; this gene is replicated later in S phase. However, when the cell line contains a human β-globin gene domain with an intact LCR, permitting expression of the gene, the β-globin gene DNA is in the early replicating pool of DNA.

These experiments confirm that there is a linkage between DNA replication and gene transcription. In addition, the LCR for the β-globin gene domain appears to be required for the early replication of the DNA of the globin gene domain as well as the transcription of the domain's genes into mRNA. Perhaps the DNA in the early replicating pool has greater access to the limited amount of transcription factors. If this is so, then a valid hypothesis to explain the inheritance of DNase I hypersensitive sites could be that shortly after DNA replication transcription factors can bind to their sites in DNA, and binding of transcription factors to DNA alters nucleosome structure, producing DNase I hypersensitivity. As a corollary to this hypothesis, after the pool of transcription factors is exhausted, the DNA that replicates too late to bind to transcription factors would not sustain the necessary alteration in chromatin structure required for transcription. The late replicating DNA would be in the closed heterochromatin conformation. Just how the cell decides whether a chromosome will replicate early or late is not presently understood. How the cell maintains DNA in a closed conformation inaccessible to transcription factors will be discussed later.

Transcription factors regulate chromatin structure

Though many of the proteins that bind to 5'HS2 are found in all tissues, some regulatory proteins such as GATA-1 and NF-E2 are restricted in their distribution. Furthermore, since many of the proteins that bind to 5'HS2 bind as heterodimers, it is possible that in erythroid cells the heterodimers consist of a ubiquitous regulatory protein as well as one that is erythroid specific. It is also possible that once a DNA binding site is occupied by a transcriptional regulatory protein, that protein preferentially interacts with a subset of transcriptional regulatory proteins, permitting those proteins to bind to other regulatory sites, thereby excluding the binding of other proteins.

As regulatory proteins bind to the LCR, perhaps the chromatin structure of the LCR is perturbed so that nucleosome formation is altered. In some way this change in the chromatin structure in the LCR may also alter the chromatin structure at the promoters of the globin genes, allowing the binding of other regulatory proteins to the promoter of a globin gene. Some of the transcriptional regulatory proteins that bind to globin promoters are limited in their tissue distribution, or may only bind to a globin promoter if transcriptional regulatory proteins are binding to the LCR. The nucleosome structure of the promoter is altered further, allowing formation of an RNA polymerase II transcriptional initiation complex. Perhaps some of the proteins binding at the LCR loop to proteins bound at the promoter causing a conformational change in the transcriptional initiation complex, allowing the formation of an open complex and the production of globin mRNA.

Stage-specific expression of the β-like globin genes

What accounts for the stage-specific expression of the β-like globin genes? Experiments in transgenic mice have demonstrated that the promoter and intergenic sequences contain sufficient binding sites for transcription factors to allow erythroid-specific gene expression. It is quite likely then that there are stage-specific transcription factors that activate or possibly repress transcription of the individual globin gene promoters. As noted above, within the embryonic ε-globin gene promoter, there is a binding site for a silencer of ε-globin gene expression. Perhaps at the stage of fetal globin gene expression in the fetal liver, a transcriptional silencer protein binds to the ε-globin promoter shutting off ε-globin expression. At the same time a fetal specific transcription factor binds to the two γ-globin gene promoters and increases the rate of transcription.

It is also possible that there is a change in the interaction between the LCR and globin gene promoters. Perhaps when the silencer of ε-globin gene transcription binds to the ε-globin promoter it disrupts a loop formed between the LCR and the ε-globin promoter. Now the LCR could be free to loop to the γ-promoters and increase the rate of transcription of the fetal globin genes. Finally, in the adult stage of globin expression in the bone marrow there is a factor that binds to the β-globin promoter and causes the LCR to loop to the β-globin promoter to increase the rate of adult globin gene transcription. Though speculative, it is very likely that these types of mechanisms play a major role in the tissue- and temporal-specific control of β-globin gene expression.

Heterochromatin may contain methylated DNA

What accounts for the maintenance of large regions of non-transcribed DNase I-resistant chromatin? It has been shown that DNA that is transcriptionally inactive contains increased amounts of methylated cytosine nucleotides. Methylated cytosines usually are found in the dinucleotide sequence 5′CpG3′; the complementary strand would read 5′GpC3′, so both strands of the duplex could be methylated. At replication the daughter DNA molecules would each contain one strand that contained a methylated cytosine. It is possible that there is a methylase enzyme which recognizes the sequence 5′methyl-CpG3′ and methylates the cytosine residue on the complementary strand. This may explain how the methylation state of CpG dinucleotides is inherited.

Upstream of many transcribed genes are sequences that contain about 60% CpG dinucleotides. This high percentage of CpG dinucleotides is much greater than the average, which is about 20% in a random sequence of human DNA. These CpG-rich islands are hypomethylated in transcribed genes, and are heavily methylated if the gene is not transcribed. Recently, a protein has been found that binds specifically to methylated CpG dinucleotides. Binding of this protein to DNA prevents the binding of the activating factors, thus inhibiting transcription.

Summary of transcriptional regulation

Transcription in nucleated cells requires the multisubunit enzymes RNA polymerase I, II and III, to recognize and initiate transcription from genes at their promoter elements. The RNA polymerases do not directly bind to promoters for transcription. Instead a group of general transcription factors bind to promoter elements and recruit RNA polymerase to the promoter, forming a basal transcription complex. In order to activate basal transcription, transcriptional activator proteins must bind to sites near to the promoter or distant to the promoter at enhancer elements and form an open complex, which melts the DNA duplex exposing the DNA template strand for mRNA synthesis. In many cases, activated transcription by a transcription regulatory protein involves the direct interaction between the DNA-bound transcription factor and the basal transcription complex. Some proteins that are transcriptional activators are

found in all cells while other activators are limited in their tissue distribution. To achieve full transcriptional activation it is also likely that multiple transcriptional regulators must bind to enhancer elements and promoters. However, the presence of the required transcription factors within the nucleus is not sufficient to ensure that a gene is transcribed.

Because the DNA of eukaryotic organisms is organized into chromatin by histone proteins, access by transcription factors and RNA polymerases to some regions of chromatin is prevented and, therefore, these regions of DNA cannot be transcribed. In contrast, open chromatin is accessible to transcription factors. The formation of open regions of chromatin may occur shortly after DNA replication when transcription factors can bind and alter nucleosome structure, allowing the formation of a transcription initiation complex at the promoter.

Regulatory elements that act at a distance such as enhancer elements probably alter the structure of chromatin over a long distance. It is possible that enhancer elements may loop to promoter elements over great distances to increase the recruitment of RNA polymerases at the promoter and to change the closed transcription complex into an open one.

The rate of transcription of the thousands of tissue-specific genes is regulated by a limited number of transcription factors, as well as the state of accessibility of the promoter to the transcription factors. The transcription of a gene requires the presence of the correct combination of transcription factors binding to promoter and enhancers. The occupancy of some of the transcriptionl regulatory sites may facilitate the binding of additional transcriptional regulators, and if the appropriate combination of regulatory factors does not bind, transcription of that gene is not activated.

Transcription can also be repressed. One mechanism may be methylation of cytosine residues with the binding of a protein that inhibits binding of transcriptional activator proteins. Methylation of a sufficient number of cytosines in the promoter or enhancer of a gene may lead to a closed chromatin conformation, and this closed chromatin conformation can be inherited so helping to define the phenotype of a cell. Some transcription factors may themselves be negative regulators of the basal transcription complex. By binding to DNA sequences near the promoter they may destabilize the basal transcription complex or prevent its formation directly. Alternatively, some negative regulators may bind to positive transcription factors either preventing their correct localization (e.g. the IκB factor prevents the nuclear localization of the NFκB transcription factor) or act by sequestering these positive factors away from their DNA

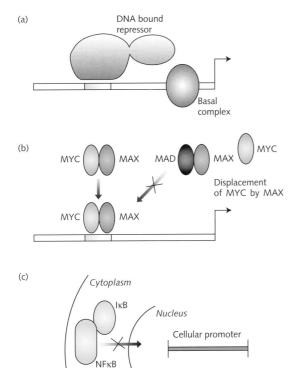

Fig. 4.11 Transcriptional activation plays a major role in ensuring the tissue- and temporal-specific expression of genes. However, it is becoming increasingly clear that transcriptional repression also plays a major role in such control. Repressors may act directly by binding to DNA sequences close to the promoter, destabilizing or preventing basal transcription complex formation (a). Alternatively, some transcriptional repressors may bind to other factors, preventing them from dimerizing with a specific partner which would be required for the formation of an active heterodimer. Such a mechanism occurs with the transcription factor MYC. For MYC to function as an activator, it must dimerize with another protein called MAX. Functional MYC–MAX heterodimers are, however, prevented from forming by another protein called MAD which binds MAX and prevents MAX from pairing with the MYC protein (b). A similar phenomenon occurs with the cellular transcription factor NFκB. When associated with the inhibitory protein IκB, NFκB is prevented from entering the nucleus. Mitogens and other stimuli can cause dissociation of the IκB/NFκB complex, releasing NFκB which can then enter the nucleus and act as a DNA binding transcription factor.

binding sites (Fig. 4.11). For instance the transcription factor **MYC**, a member of the so-called helix-loop-helix (HLH) family of transcription regulatory proteins, dimerizes with another cellular protein termed **MAX** to form a functional transcriptional activator. However, the **MAD** protein can bind MAX, preventing the formation of the functional MYC–MAX complex. This indirect mechanism of negative regulation has been termed **squelching**.

Transcriptional control and insights towards gene therapy

The disease sickle cell anaemia is caused by the presence of two mutant haemoglobin alleles (*HbS* alleles), transcription of which results in the production of HbS protein in the erythrocyte. Conditions that cause localized hypoxia or acidosis such as exercise or infection produce increased amounts of deoxyHbS. DeoxyHbS polymerizes and causes the erythrocyte to change from its usual biconcave shape into a sickle shape (Plate 6, facing p. 214). The sickled erythrocyte is not deformable, and cannot pass through the microcirculation. This results in localized ischaemia and necrosis of bone, spleen and kidney. Erythrocytes that contain one copy of the *HbS* gene and one copy of the wild-type haemoglobin (HbA) gene do not sickle unless subjected to extreme hypoxia. Individuals heterozygous for the *HbS* gene are not anaemic nor do they suffer the catastrophic manifestations of sickle cell anaemia. Therefore if an erythrocyte contains 50% HbA it will be protected from sickling. If it were possible to introduce a functional *HbA* gene into erythroid precursor cells, the bone marrow stem cells, of an individual homozygous for the *HbS* gene that person would no longer suffer from sickle cell anaemia.

However, at present there is one critical problem to be solved before we can produce HbA within the erythrocytes of individuals homozygous for the *HbS* gene. The problem is not what *cis*-acting sequences are required to get high-level erythroid-specific transcription of the β-globin gene, rather it is how to target all the sequences required for high-level β-globin gene expression into bone marrow stem cells. Regardless of the method used, our understanding of the process of transcription within the β-globin gene domain contains the recipe for the recombinant β-globin construct needed. To ensure a high level of β-globin gene expression, there is a requirement for the interaction of the β-globin gene LCR, the promoter of the β-globin gene, and of course the β-globin gene itself. The LCR for β-globin gene expression consists of the four DNase I hypersensitive sites upstream of the embryonic ε-globin gene. In the genome, the LCR spans 12 kb of DNA, but smaller recombinant versions of the LCR have been made. These recombinant versions contain portions of each of the DNase I hypersensitive sites including the sequences within 5′HS2 which contain the powerful erythroid-specific enhancer. We therefore now have the knowledge needed to generate recombinant constructs that contain all the *cis*-acting DNA sequences required for high-level, position-independent, erythroid-specific β-globin gene transcription. We can insert exogenous DNA sequences into cells by the process of transfection or electroporation, but the efficiency of insertion is low and the rate of cell loss is high. Since the frequency of stem cells within the nucleated cell population of the bone marrow is low, perhaps 1 in 10 000, we need to have a highly efficient method for inserting the functional recombinant β-globin construct into erythropoietic tissue.

The methods that are under consideration now include the isolation of pure populations of bone marrow stem cells that can be used as targets into which to introduce clone genes, and the use of recombinant viruses to infect bone marrow stem cells to high efficiencies (see Chapter 16).

It is likely that within the not too distant future we shall hear of the introduction of such a construct into bone marrow cells of an individual with sickle cell anaemia resulting in a cure. This will represent the practical consequence of our understanding of the regulation of transcription in eukaryotic cells and its role in the development and differentiation of the tissues.

Further reading

Singer M. and Berg P. (1991) *Genes and Genomes*. Blackwell Scientific Publications, Oxford.

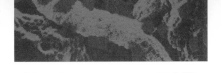

Chapter 5 Principles of medical genetics

Introduction

This chapter introduces:
- the human karyotype and the basis of chromosomal disorders;
- Mendelian principles as reflected in the inheritance of human diseases;
- pedigree analysis and investigation of genetic linkage in man—lod scores;
- non-Mendelian genetics, including mitochondrial disorders (matrilineal inheritance);
- genes in populations: distribution, selection, drift, inbreeding, polymorphism;
- human linkage disequilibrium.

Medical genetics encompasses the study of **human variation** and **heredity** (human genetics) and its application to medical practice. Heredity represents the transmission of information required for the formation and regulation of proteins. The primary structure of all proteins is encoded in DNA, most of which is packaged into chromosomes within the nucleus; a minute, independent genome in the mitochondria codes for components that participate in intramitochondrial protein synthesis and 13 polypeptide constituents of the enzymes that transfer electrons in the respiratory chain. The practical questions that surround much of the practice of human genetics are concerned with transmission of heritable traits. Scientific study of human variation largely depends on analysis of the outcome of matings of individuals with scientific study of definable differences, but lack of controlled experiment and small families limit the applicability of the classical approach to genetics. As Morgan stated, humans are poor breeders and their family pedigrees are too meagre to furnish good material for analysis. However, studies in many other organisms provide the foundation for interpretative studies in humans. Medical genetics additionally deals with the application of these principles to the investigation and management of human disease. In this chapter, the analytical principles that underlie transmission of disease traits in humans are presented as the basis for the deeper understanding of human genetics which now, thanks to the development of analytical methods in molecular biology, has wide social, ethical and therapeutic implications.

Chromosomal basis of inheritance

Every cell nucleus contains a set of **chromosomes** (Greek: *chromos* = coloured, *soma* = body) which are named from their ability to take up certain stains. Each chromosome consists of a single molecule of DNA (deoxyribonucleic acid) together with associated acidic and basic proteins. Between cell divisions (**interphase**) the chromosomes are fully extended and are not individually distinguishable within the nucleus. During cell division each DNA molecule becomes coiled and condensed and the individual chromosomes can then be seen with the light microscope.

Most cells contain 46 chromosomes (the diploid number) which can be arranged into 22 pairs of **autosomes**, which are alike in males and females, and a pair of **sex chromosomes**: XX in a female and XY in a male (Fig. 5.1). In some tissues, such as the liver, the cellular complement of chromosomes is increased by duplication, e.g. tetraploidy, hexaploidy and so on. Each chromosome has a narrow waist called the **centromere** which has a constant position for a given chromosome. The centromere divides each chromosome into short and long arms which are labelled p (French: *petit*) and q, respectively; the tip of each arm is called the **telomere**. Chromosomes 13–15, 21 and 22 have ribosomal genes located in their short arms and during cell division these regions often do not condense, as a result of their involvement in the organization of nucleoli. Thus the ends of their short arms appear as 'satellites' separated from the rest of chromosome arm by narrow stalks, known as secondary constrictions. There is interindividual variation in the number of copies of these ribosomal

(a)

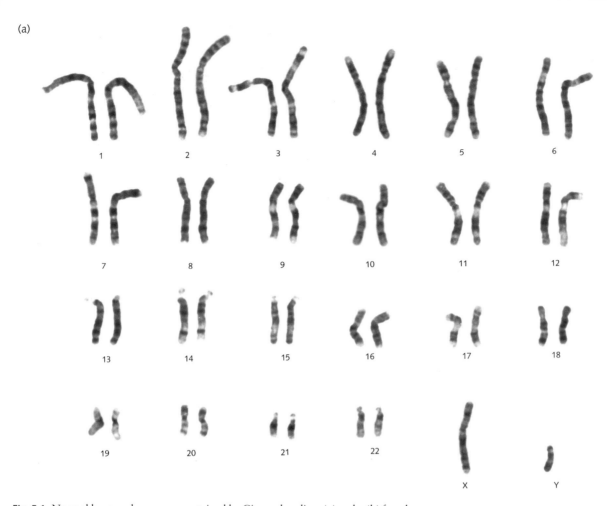

Fig. 5.1 Normal human chromosomes stained by Giemsa banding: (a) male; (b) female.

genes and hence in the length of the short arms of these chromosomes. This variation has no clinical significance and resembles other common chromosomal variants or heteromorphisms that involve the number of copies of repetitive DNA. These include the size of the long arm of the Y-chromosome and the sizes of centromeric heterochromatin of chromosomes 1, 9 and 16.

At **mitosis** each chromosome replicates to form a pair of sister chromatids which are held together at the centromere. Exchange of material by crossing over (sister chromatid exchanges, SCEs) can occur during this process but as each sister chromatid is identical, no clinical consequence results and at the end of cell division, each daughter cell has an identical set of 46 chromosomes (Fig. 5.2a).

The chromosomal complement (or **karyotype**) may be described using a shorthand system of symbols and in general this has the order: total number of chromosomes, sex chromosomes and description of any abnormality. Thus a normal female is 46,XX and a normal male is 46,XY. Table 5.1 lists the other commonly used symbols. For routine karyotyping Giemsa banding (G-banding) is usually preferred. This produces 300–400 alternating light and dark bands which are characteristic for each chromosomal pair and which reflect differential chromosomal condensation. A standardized numbering system is used for these bands and this permits accurate description of structural chromosomal abnormalities.

In contrast to mitosis, reductive cell division, or **meiosis**, results in cells with a half set (haploid number) of 23 chromosomes. Meiosis is confined to gonadal cells involved in gametogenesis. It consists of two successive divisions in which the DNA replicates only once—before

(b)

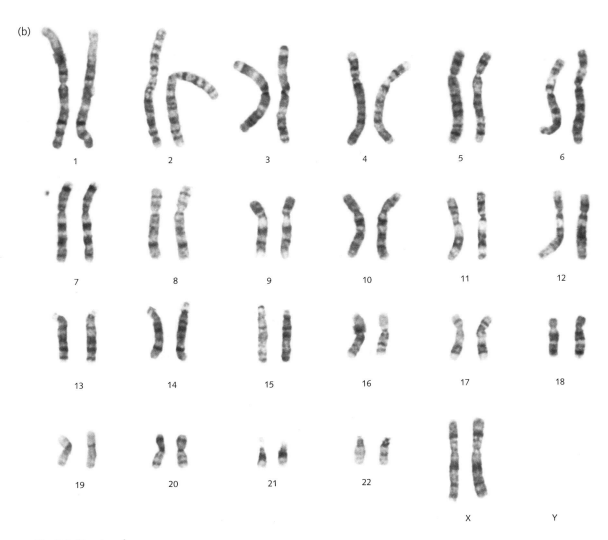

Fig. 5.1 *Continued.*

the first division (Fig. 5.2b). Each mature egg thus normally contains one of each pair of autosomes and the X- or the Y-chromosome. At fertilization the diploid number is restored and in consequence half of each individual's autosomes are derived from each parent, and a female has an X from each parent whereas a male has a maternal X and a paternal Y sex chromosome. Exchanges of material by crossing over routinely occur during the first meiotic division. The locations of these crossovers can be identified as points of contact or chiasmata when the chromosomal pairs separate at diplotene (Fig. 5.2b). The chromosomes which have exchanged

material are called **recombinants** and, in contrast to the sister chromatid exchanges, differ from the non-recombinant originals. On average, there are about 52 crossovers per human male meiosis with at least one chiasma per chromosome arm (with the exception of the short arms of chromosomes 13–15, 18, 21 and 22). Hence few chromosomes are inherited intact from a parent and co-segregation or linkage of genes on a chromosome will only be observed if they are physically close (see 'Recombination and linkage', p. 86). The sex chromosomes in the male are an exception and crossing over is confined to the distal parts of the short arms of the X

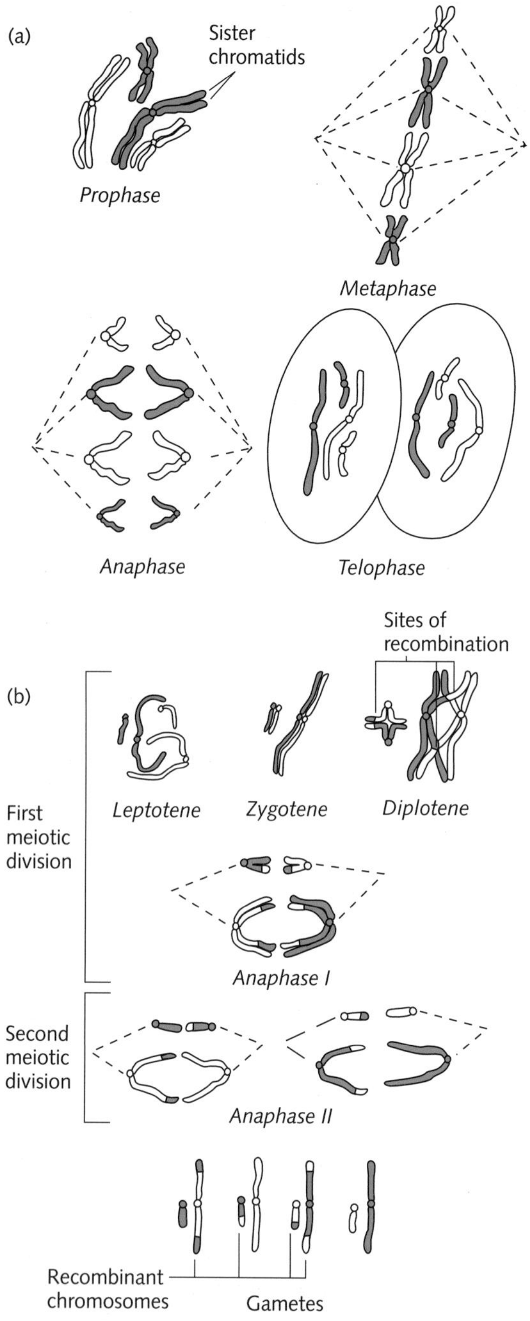

Fig. 5.2 Diagrams of (a) mitosis and (b) meiosis. Only two chromosome pairs are shown; the chromosomes from one parent are in outline, those from the other are in blue.

and the Y, with the remainder of each chromosome being transmitted intact to offspring.

Lyonization and imprinting

Lyonization is the name given to the process of inactivation of one member of the pair of X-chromosomes in every female cell (after Mary Lyon, a British geneticist). It occurs in all somatic cells (but not germ cells) of the female embryo on the sixteenth day after fertilization, when it comprises about 5000 cells. For any somatic cell the choice as to whether the paternal X or the maternal X is inactivated is random but thereafter it is fixed for all descendants of that cell. The X chromosome inactivation centre lies in the proximal part of Xq and the inactive X is not transcribed, with the exception of a cluster of genes close to the tip of Xp and a few other genes on Xp and Xq. Hence for most genes on the X-chromosome, the level of protein expression is similar to that in the male where the single X always remains active. Thus normal females are **mosaics** with a mixture of cells some of which have an active paternal X-chromosome and some with an active maternal X-chromosome. Because of the intrinsic randomness of the inactivation process, the relative proportions vary from female to female (even in identical twins). This accounts for the variable expression of X-linked recessive traits in heterozygous females, who may be symptomatic if most cells are utilizing the

Table 5.1 Symbols used for karotypic description.

p	Short arm
q	Long arm
pter	Tip of short arm
qter	Tip of long arm
cen	Centromere
h	Heteromorphism
del	Deletion
der	Derivative of a chromosome rearrangement
dic	Dicentric
dup	Duplication
i	Isochromosome
ins	Insertion
inv	Inversion
mat	Maternal origin
pat	Paternal origin
r	Ring chromosome
t	Translocation
/	Mosaicism
+/−	Before a chromosome number indicates gain or loss of that whole chromosome
+/−	After a chromosome number indicates gain or loss of part of that chromosome

defective gene on the X-chromosome (see 'X-linked recessive inheritance', p. 85).

In contrast, all autosomes remain active in males and females. However, it is now apparent that normal autosomal function requires not only the normal number of autosomes but also paternal and maternal contributions for many autosomal pairs. For example, if a conception results from a double paternal contribution to give 46,XX then, despite the superficially normal karyotype, no fetus develops and the placenta is grossly abnormal with hydatidiform changes. Similarly the parental origin of certain chromosomal deletions profoundly influences the clinical appearance (with for example, paternally derived deletions of proximal 15q resulting in Prader–Willi syndrome and comparable maternally derived deletions resulting in the phenotypically distinct Angelman syndrome). Experimental studies in mice suggest that not all regions of a chromosome are susceptible to such **parental imprinting** but at present the reason for this phenomenon and its molecular basis is not fully understood.

Chromosomal disorders

Chromosomal disorders by definition are characterized by abnormalities of chromosomal number or structure that can be seen by light microscopy. They may involve either the sex chromosomes or the autosomes and may occur either as a result of germ cell mutation in the parent or a more distant ancestor or as a result of somatic mutation in which only a proportion of cells will be affected (mosaicism). Over 600 different chromosome abnormalities have already been described which collectively affect seven per 1000 live births. The frequency is estimated to be 10-fold higher at conception but the majority are lost as a result of spontaneous abortion.

A chromosome number which is an exact multiple of the haploid number (23) and which exceeds the diploid number (46) is called **polyploidy** and one which is not an exact multiple is called **aneuploidy**. Aneuploidy usually arises from failure of segregation (non-disjunction) of paired chromosomes at one of the meiotic cell divisions and so results in cells with either an extra copy of a chromosome (trisomy) or with a missing copy of a chromosome (monosomy). The cause of meiotic non-disjunction is not known but it occurs at increased frequency with increasing maternal age, in the setting of maternal hypothyroidism and possibly after irradiation or as a familial tendency.

Table 5.2 shows examples of common numerical chromosomal aberrations. In general aneuploidy has less

Table 5.2 Examples of numerical chromosomal aberrations.

Chromosomal disorder	Karyotype	Frequency in live births
Trisomy 21	47,XY,+21 or 47,XX,+21	One in 700
Trisomy 18	47,XY,+18 or 47,XX,+18	One in 3000
Klinefelter's syndrome	47,XXY	One in 1000 males
Turner's syndrome	45,X or variants	One in 2500 females
Triple X	47,XXX	One in 1000 females
XYY syndrome	47,XYY	One in 1000 males
Triploidy	69,XXY or 69,XXX or 69,XYY	Rare in live births

serious phenotypic consequences when it involves the sex chromosomes than when it affects the autosomes, and whilst monosomy X is seen in live births (Turner's syndrome) autosomal monosomy usually results in early spontaneous abortion. Autosomal trisomies also tend to be miscarried; the surviving infants show mental disability and multiple congenital malformations. A complete extra set of chromosomes will raise the total number to 69 (triploidy). This usually arises from fertilization by two sperm or from failure or one of the maturation divisions of the egg or the sperm so that fertilization occurs with a diploid gamete. Triploid pregnancies usually miscarry in early pregnancy.

Structural aberrations all result from chromosomal breakage. When a chromosome breaks two unstable 'sticky' ends are produced. Generally, repair mechanisms rejoin these two ends without delay. However, if more than one break has occurred, then as the repair mechanisms cannot distinguish one sticky end from another, there is the possibility of rejoining the wrong ends. The spontaneous rate of chromosomal breakage may be markedly increased by exposure to ionizing radiation or mutagenic chemicals and is also increased in some rare inherited conditions. Chromosomal breakages are not randomly distributed and overall (see below) the spontaneous rate of translocation is one in 1000 gametes (which is about 100 times greater than the mutation rate at individual gene loci).

Several different types of structural aberration are recognized (Table 5.3). A **translocation** is the transfer of chromosomal material between chromosomes; the

Table 5.3 Examples of structural chromosomal aberrations.

Karyotype	Comment
46,XY,t(5;10)(p13;q25)	Balanced reciprocal translocation involving the short arm of chromosome 5 and the long arm of chromosome 10 (with breakpoints at bands 13 and 25 respectively)
45,XX,t(13;14)(p11;q11)	Centric fusion translocation of chromosomes 13 and 14
46,XY,del(5)(p25)	Short arm deletion of chromosome 5 (cri du chat syndrome)
46,X(Xq)	Isochromosome of Xq
46,XX,dup (2)(p13p22)	Partial duplication of the short arm of chromosome 2 (p13 to p22)
46,XY,r(3)(p26→q29)	Ring chromosome 3
46,XY,inv(11)(p15q14)	Pericentric inversion of chromsome 11

process requires breakages of both chromosomes with repair in an abnormal arrangement. This exchange usually results in no net loss or gain of DNA and in that case the individual will be clinically normal (**balanced translocation carrier**). The medical significance is for future generations because a balanced translocation carrier is at high risk of producing chromosomally unbalanced offspring.

Deletions usually arise from the loss of a portion of the chromosome between two break points or as a result of a parental translocation. As the smallest visible loss from a chromosome is about 4000 kb of DNA, individuals with visible deletions are rendered monosomic for many contiguous genes. Thus with autosomal deletions, mental disability and multiple malformations are usual. Small deletions close to and beyond the limit of light microscopy (microdeletions) are still clinically important and can be demonstrated by failure of hybridization of DNA probes to the deleted area. Deletions may also result from unequal crossing over at meiosis in which case the other chromosome has a duplicated segment (Fig. 5.3). Duplications may also result from a parental translocation and are in general less harmful than deletions. Indeed, tiny duplications at a molecular level (repeats) may play an important role in permitting gene diversification during evolution.

Inversions arise from two chromosomal breaks with inversion through 180° of the segment between the breaks. If both breaks are in a single arm so that the centromere is not included then it is called a **paracentric**

inversion, whereas if the centromere is included in the inverted segment it is a **pericentric** inversion. Generally this change in gene order does not produce clinical abnormality in the individual that harbours it but there is an increased risk of chromosomally unbalanced offspring.

Mendelian inheritance

Mendel's laws

Before Mendel, parental characteristics were believed to blend in the offspring. Whilst this was plausible for continuous traits such as height or skin colour that turn out to be controlled at many separate gene loci, it was clearly difficult to account for the family patterns of discontinuous traits such as haemophilia or muscular dystrophy. Mendel studied clearly defined pairs of contrasting characters in pea breeding experiments and concluded that inheritance of these characteristics (traits) must be particulate with pairs of hereditary elements (now called genes with alternative forms called alleles) which segregated at meiosis: one gene of a pair to one gamete and one to another gamete (**Mendel's first law**). If two characteristics were considered there was no tendency in his experiments for the genes arising from one parent to stay together. In other words members of different gene pairs assort to gametes independently of one another (**Mendel's second law**). The characteristics studied by Mendel were by chance determined by genes on different chromosomes. In contrast if gene pairs are considered which are close together or linked on the same chromosome then Mendel's second law is apparently violated and independent assortment will not be seen (see 'Recombination and linkage', p. 86).

Pedigree analysis

A family tree or pedigree is a particularly useful way of

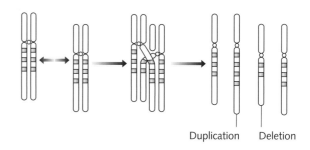

Duplication   Deletion

Fig. 5.3 Diagram to show results of unequal crossing over.

recording genetic information. A standardized set of symbols is used (Fig. 5.4). The male line is conventionally placed on the left and all members of the same generation are placed on the same horizontal level. Roman numerals are used for each generation, starting with the earliest, and arabic numerals are used to indicate each individual within a generation (numbering from the left). The offspring of each set of parents are given in birth order with the eldest on the left.

Autosomal dominant inheritance

In autosomal dominant disorders the condition is produced by a mutation of one member of an autosomal gene pair. The affected person thus has one normal gene and one mutant gene and is said to be **heterozygous** at this gene location (or locus). The affected person must pass on one copy of each chromosome pair and hence of each gene pair and thus the offspring are equally likely to be affected as to be unaffected (a one in two or 50% risk to the offspring). As indicated in Fig. 5.5 these autosomal dominant traits tend to show a vertical type of pedigree pattern with approximately equal numbers of males and females affected.

So far 4458 human autosomal dominant traits have been described which collectively affect about one in 100 live births (Table 5.4). In general they tend to be of later onset/less severe than recessive traits and, whereas recessive traits usually involve defective enzymes, dominant traits often result from mutations in proteins that function as receptors or ligands or are involved in the maintenance of cellular or tissue integrity.

Many dominant traits show **variable expression**. This implies that affected individuals in the same family vary in their clinical severity. For some conditions (e.g. Huntington's disease and myotonic dystrophy) this reflects mutational instability with variably sized length mutations in different members of the same family, but in other conditions the basis for this and the occasional occurrence of **non-penetrance** where a clinically normal individual carries and transmits the mutant gene for an autosomal dominant condition (e.g. individual III2 in Fig. 5.5) is not understood. For some autosomal dominant traits there is a sex influence on expression (e.g. male pattern baldness), which in an extreme form results in only males affected and a pattern of inheritance resembling that of X-linked recessive inheritance (sex-limited expression). Variable expression and non-penetrance are important considerations when counselling family members at risk. Another pitfall for the geneticist is **gonadal mosaicism** where the mutation is confined to the gonad of one parent. In this situation the parents of an affected child are clinically normal but whereas a new mutation in the child would carry a very low recurrence risk for brothers and sisters, the recurrence risk for gonadal mosaics may be as high as 50%.

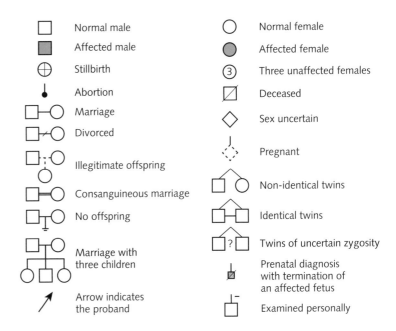

Fig. 5.4 Symbols used in pedigree construction.

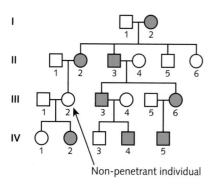

Non-penetrant individual

Fig. 5.5 Pedigree showing autosomal dominant inheritance.

Furthermore, when counselling any family the possibility of genetic mimics or **phenocopies** needs to be considered. Phenocopies arise when mutations at different loci produce a similar clinical appearance (**genetic heterogeneity**). This heterogeneity emphasizes the need for a precise diagnosis in the index case, if possible with biochemical and molecular analysis of the condition in order to avoid errors in counselling.

Autosomal recessive inheritance

Unlike autosomal dominant disorders where heterozygotes manifest the condition, in autosomal recessive disorders the affected person has mutations in both members of a gene pair (**homozygous** at the locus). Usually the parents are unaffected yet each harbours one defective gene and is thus a heterozygote, and, in completely recessive traits, is an asymptomatic gene carrier. For two heterozygous parents the chance of further affected children is the chance of each handing on the mutant gene, or one-half multiplied, i.e. an average risk of one in four or 25% with each successive pregnancy. The risk of homozygosity in other family members is low and thus the pedigree shows horizontal transmission of disease, with brothers and sisters affected but usually no other history of disease in the family (Fig. 5.6).

Many autosomal recessive traits concern enzyme proteins which are usually present in excess over that required of the normal activity so that a reduction to 50% of the normal activity in the heterozygote does not result in disease. Homozygotes have little or no enzyme activity and are affected. The chance of having a child with an autosomal recessive trait is greatly increased if the parents are blood relatives (**consanguineous**): here the affected individuals inherit two mutant genes that are identical by descent from an ancestor common to both parents. So far 1730 autosomal recessive traits have been

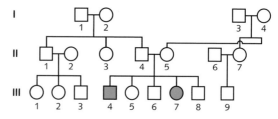

Fig. 5.6 Pedigree showing autosomal recessive inheritance.

Table 5.4 Examples of common autosomal dominant disorders.

Condition	Frequency in 1000 births	Gene locus	Gene cloned
Dominant otosclerosis	3	?	–
Familial hypercholesterolaemia	2	19	+
Adult polycystic kidney disease	1	16p,4	+,–
Multiple exostoses	0.5	19,11,8	–,+,+
Huntington's disease	0.5	4pter	+
Neurofibromatosis type I	0.4	17	+
Myotonic dystrophy	0.2	19	+
Tuberous sclerosis	0.1	16p,9q	+,–
Polyposis coli	0.1	5q	+
Dominant blindness	0.1	Several	Some
Dominant congenital deafness	0.1	Several	–
Other	2.0		

Total 10/1000 (4458 traits)

described which collectively affect two per 1000 live births (Table 5.5).

X-linked recessive inheritance

The uneven distribution of sex chromosomes results in a characteristic pattern of inheritance for mutations of genes on the X-chromosome. Males have only a single X-chromosome, i.e. they are **hemizygous** and thus are affected if the sex chromosome they inherit harbours a defective gene. Females have two X-chromosomes and thus may compensate for a mutant gene on one X-chromosome (carriers, heterozygotes). A maternal carrier for an X-linked disorder transmits the mutant gene on average to one-half of her sons and to one-half of her daughters. If the affected male survives to reproduce then he transmits his X-chromosome, and hence the mutant gene to all his daughters, who will be heterozygous carriers. His sons all receive his Y-chromosome and thus cannot be affected (Fig. 5.7).

X-linked recessive traits tend to show consistent male severity within a family. Female carriers are usually clinically normal but may be affected (usually mildly) because of non-random inactivation of their X-chromosomes (see 'Lyonization and imprinting', p. 80). So far 412 human X-linked recessive traits have been described which collectively affect 82 in 1000 males (with 80 in 1000 of this total due to red–green colour blindness). Some of the more common and important of these traits are shown in Table 5.6.

X-linked dominant inheritance

So far very few X-linked dominant traits have been

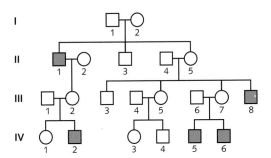

Fig. 5.7 Pedigree showing X-linked recessive inheritance.

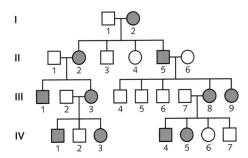

Fig. 5.8 Pedigree showing X-linked dominant inheritance.

described, and with the exception of the Xg blood group most of these are rare (e.g. vitamin D-resistant rickets). Males and females are affected, with a uniformly severe disease in males but a variable picture in heterozygous females as a result of random X-inactivation. Superficially the family tree resembles that of an autosomal dominant trait but key differences are the lack of male-to-male transmission and the transmission of disease from a male to all his daughters (Fig. 5.8). In some X-linked dominant conditions (e.g. incontinentia pigmenti and focal dermal hypoplasia) the affected males are believed to be so severely affected that spontaneous abortion is usual and hence only affected females are observed.

Autosomal and X-linked co-dominant inheritance

The phenomenon of co-dominant inheritance results from the ability to distinguish the effects and follow the inheritance of more than one allelic form of a gene within a family. Thus heterozygotes can be readily distinguished from homozygotes for either allele. This type of inheritance applies to many traits including blood

Table 5.5 Examples of common autosomal recessive disorders.

Condition	Frequency in 1000 births	Gene locus	Gene cloned
Haemochromatosis	3	6p	+
Cystic fibrosis	0.5	7q	+
Recessive mental retardation	0.5	Several	Some
Congenital deafness	0.2	Several	
Phenylketonuria	0.1	12q	+
Spinal muscular atrophy	0.1	5q	+
Recessive blindness	0.1	Several	Some
Others	0.5		

Total 5/1000 (1730 traits)

Table 5.6 Examples of common X-linked recessive disorders.

Condition	UK frequency in 10 000 males	Gene locus	Gene cloned
Red–green colour blindness	800	Xq28	+
Fragile X-associated mental retardation	5	Xq27.3	+
Duchenne muscular dystrophy	3	Xp21	+
Becker muscular dystrophy	0.5	Xp21	+*
Haemophilia A	2	Xq28	+
Haemophilia B	0.3	Xq27	+
X-linked ichthyosis	2	Xp22	+
Others	2.2		

Total 820/10 000 males (412 traits)

* Duchenne and Becker muscular dystrophy are allelic

groups (ABO, MNS, rhesus), red cell enzymes (acid phosphatase, adenylate kinase), cell surface antigens (HLA) and restriction fragment length polymorphisms (RFLPs, Chapter 3).

Figure 5.9a shows the inheritance of an autosomal RFLP with allelic fragments of 1 and 2 kb in size. Each parent is heterozygous (1 kb, 2 kb) as are two children, and one child is homozygous for each allelic fragment. Figure 5.9b shows the inheritance of an X-linked RFLP with allelic fragments of 3 and 4 kb in size. The mother is heterozygous (3 kb, 4 kb) whereas her husband with a single X-chromosome is hemizygous (3 kb). Each child receives one or other of their mother's fragments and in addition each daughter receives the paternal fragment. Many RFLPs and other co-dominant traits have rare allele frequencies of more than 2% and are thus examples of **genetic polymorphisms** (see 'Population genetics', p. 90) and as such are useful in linkage studies (see below).

Recombination and linkage

Two genes are said to be **linked** if they are close together on the same chromosome. In this situation the alleles at these two loci tend to pass together rather than independently into each gamete. Thus disturbance of the phenomenon of independent assortment (Mendel's second law) is an important clue that two genes are linked. If the chromosomal location of one of the genes is known, then by inference the other can be mapped to that region of the chromosome. Thus in seeking to find linkage, two loci are considered, one for the single gene disorder or trait in question and another for the marker.

If the disease and marker loci are on separate chromosomes then independent assortment will occur and the disease and marker should be found as often together as apart in the gametes and hence in the offspring (Fig. 5.10a). If, however, the disease and marker loci are close together on the same chromosome then independent assortment will not occur and the disease and marker will occur together in each child unless by chance they are separated by a crossover at meiosis (Fig. 5.10b). As the distance between the disease and marker loci increases, so the opportunity for recombination in the interval increases and the percentage of recombinants increases (Fig. 5.10c). If the disease and marker loci are far apart on the same chromosome, a crossover between the loci is very likely: the disease and marker traits will occur separately in each recombinant but together in the non-recombinants (Fig. 5.10d). So for a distant marker trait the number of recombinants will approximate to

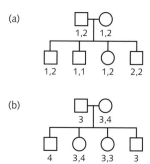

Fig. 5.9 Families showing inheritance of restriction fragment length polymorphisms: (a) autosomal with allelic fragments of sizes 1 and 2 kb; (b) X-linked with allelic fragments of sizes 3 and 4 kb.

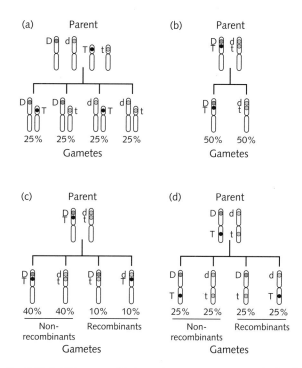

Fig. 5.10 (a) Diagram of independent assortment at meiosis of the disease locus (disease allele D and normal allele d) and the marker locus (alleles T and t) on different chromsomes. (b) Absence of independent assortment at meiosis for disease and marker loci very close together on the same chromosome (tight linkage). (c) Disease and marker loci nearby on the same chromosome showing linkage. The recombination fraction is 20%. (d) Disease and marker loci far apart on the same chromosome mimic independent assortment and linkage cannot be detected. The recombination fraction is 50%.

the number of non-recombinants and the **recombination fraction** (number of recombinants divided by the total number of offspring) will be 0.5 or 50% which mimics independent assortment. As the distance between the marker and disease loci decreases, the chance of crossing

over diminishes, the number of recombinants becomes fewer, the recombination fraction is reduced, and the disturbance of independent assortment increases (Table 5.7). Thus the recombination fraction varies from 0% (tight linkage) to 50% (equivalent to independent assortment).

Linkage is demonstrated or excluded by identifying suitable families which are segregating for the condition in question and for a variety of test markers. Thus, for example, the affected man in the second generation of family A (Fig. 5.11) has received the mutant allele for an autosomal dominant trait together with the marker allele T from his father. Similarly he has received the normal allele and marker allele t from his mother. If these two loci are on the same chromosome then it follows that he must have one chromosome that carries the disease allele together with T, while the other chromosome of the pair carries the normal allele and t. Hence the arrangement of the disease and marker alleles (the **phase**) can be deduced with certainty in this individual. If the loci are linked, it should be apparent in the next generation as a tendency for the disease allele to segregate with marker T and the normal allele to segregate with marker t, and this is what is observed since all four affected offspring inherit T from their father (and t from their mother) while the five unaffected offspring inherit t from their father (and t from their mother).

If the loci are not linked, the probability of such a striking departure from independent assortment occurring by chance is the same as the probability of correctly calling heads or tails for nine consecutive tosses of a coin, that is $(0.5)^9$ or 0.002. However, if these two loci are linked with a recombination fraction of, say, 0.1 (10%) the probability of the disease segregating with T or the normal allele segregating with t is 0.9 for each child and the probability of not observing a single recombinant event in all nine children in $(0.9)^9$ or 0.4. It follows that linkage at 10% recombination is a more likely explana-

Table 5.7 Comparison of linked and unlinked loci.

	Situation of the two loci			
	Same chromosome			Different chromosomes
	Very close	Nearby	Far apart	
Frequency of crossing over between the two loci	Rare	Some	Frequent	—
Independent assortment	Little or none	Some	Normal	Normal
Linkage	Present	Present	Absent	Absent
Number of recombinants	Few or none	Some	50%	50%
Recombination fraction	0%	0–49%	50%	50%

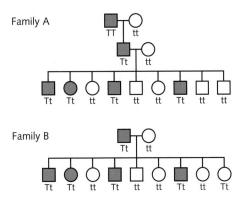

Fig. 5.11 Pedigrees of two families showing linkage between an autosomal dominant condition and a marker trait (alleles T and t).

tion for the family than no linkage: 200 times more likely to be exact (0.4/0.002 = 200). Similarly for a recombination fraction of zero (0%) we would not expect any recombination and the probability of observing this family would be $(1.0)^9$ or 1.0. This is 500 times more likely than no linkage (1.0/0.002 = 500). To proceed with the analysis, the logarithms of these probability ratios are calculated and referred to as **lod (logarithms of odds) scores**. For family A at a recombination fraction of 10% the lod score is therefore $\log_{10} 200 = 2.3$ and at a recombination fraction of zero the lod score is $\log_{10} 500 = 2.7$. In practice, proof that two loci are linked usually requires that data from several families are combined mathematically; before this can be done, lod scores must be calculated in the same way for all possible values of the recombination fraction, as shown in Table 5.8.

Suppose a second family, resembling the first but with only two generations (family B, Fig. 5.11), is studied. All four affected children have inherited T from their father (and t from their mother) and four of the five healthy children have inherited t from their father (and t from their mother). As in family A, this signifies a disturbance of independent assortment and suggests linkage between the disease and marker loci, marker T segregating with the disease allele as in family A. If this were the case, the youngest child would represent a recombination since she has inherited marker T from her father but not the disease allele with it. The alternative explanation is that marker T did not segregate with the disease allele but with the corresponding normal gene, in which case the youngest child is a non-recombinant and all her brothers and sisters represent recombinations. This is a less likely possibility but it cannot be excluded, because without information about the grandparents the relationship

between the disease and marker alleles in the father cannot be determined. In other words, the phase of the putative linkage is unknown. Calculation of the lod scores for such a family is more complicated since the two possible phases must be taken into account. Whichever phase is considered in this pedigree, at least one recombination between disease and marker loci must have taken place, so that the possibility of close linkage, with a recombination fraction of zero, is excluded.

To combine the data from these two families, the lod scores at each recombination fraction are simply added together (Table 5.8). The maximum value of the lod score then corresponds to the most likely value for the recombination fraction between the two loci. In this example the maximum lod score is 3.3 at 10% recombination. The ease with which data from phase-known and phase-unknown families can be summated in this way is the reason why the use of lod scores has become almost universal for the analysis of linkage data.

The maximum value of the lod score gives a measure of the statistical significance of the result. A value greater than 3 is usually accepted as demonstrating that linkage is present and in most situations it roughly corresponds to the 5% level of significance used in conventional statistical tests. Conversely if lod scores below −2 are obtained, this indicates that linkage has been excluded at the corresponding values of the recombination fraction.

For three-generation phase-known families represented in family A and two-generation phase-unknown families like family B the lod scores can be calculated directly or obtained from tables. Computer programs are available to deal with more complex or extensive predigrees and for analysis of data involving more than two linked loci.

The relationship between recombination fraction and the actual physical distance between loci depends upon several factors. A recombination fraction of 0.1 (10%)

Table 5.8 Lod scores at values of the recombination fraction from 0% to 40% for the two families shown in Fig. 5.11 (the data are combined by adding together lod scores at each value of the recombination fraction).

	Recombination fraction				
	0%	10%	20%	30%	40%
Family A	2.7	2.3	1.8	1.3	0.7
Family B	−∞	1.0	0.9	0.6	0.3
Both families	−∞	3.3	2.7	1.9	1.0

corresponds by definition to a map distance of 10 centimorgans (100 centimorgans = 1 Morgan; after the American geneticist T.H. Morgan (1866–1945)) but with increasing distance apart, the apparent recombination fraction falls due to the occurrence of double crossovers. Furthermore, crossovers for autosomes are more frequent in females than males. The frequency of crossing over also varies in different parts of the chromosome and seems to be greater at the ends of the chromosomes compared with closer to the centromeres. The total length of the haploid genome is estimated to be 3000 centimorgans, and as the DNA therein has 3×10^9 basepairs, 1 centimorgan is roughly equivalent to 1 megabase (Mb) of DNA. In practice it is difficult to detect linkage for loci more than 25 centimorgans apart, and beyond 50 centimorgans the frequency of multiple crossovers mimics the occurrence of independent assortment.

Non-Mendelian inheritance

Multifactorial/polygenic inheritance

Multifactorial disorders are defined as those that require the interaction of environmental and genetic factors to become manifest. Generally, several genetic loci are considered to participate, although for most of these disorders the nature of these loci is currently unknown. In contrast to monogenic and mitochondrial inheritance, the pedigree pattern is not diagnostic in multifactorial disorders. Generally only a single individual is affected in the family, and only an examination of many families will demonstrate the increased incidence of the condition in close relatives compared with the general population. These observed (or empiric) risks in family studies cannot be quantified rationally but are widely used for genetic counselling for these conditions.

Twin studies may provide a powerful means to detect multifactorial inheritance. The frequency that both twins are affected (**concordant**) is compared for identical (i.e. all genes in common) and non-identical twins (i.e. 50% of autosomal genes in common). Table 5.9 compares the findings for different genetic and non-genetic conditions. Characteristically in multifactorial traits the degree of concordance in identical twins exceeds that seen in the non-identical twins but is less than 100% as a result of inequalities in the environmental contribution. These twin and family studies help to confirm the existence of genetic contributions to disease but do not provide information about the number or the nature of the involved genes. Possible approaches to analysis of polygenic disorders are considered in more detail in Chapter 7.

Table 5.9 Concordance rates in twins.

Disorder	Concordance	
	Identical	Non-identical
Single gene	100%	As sibs
Chromosomal	100%	As sibs
Multifactorial	<100% but > sibs	As sibs
Somatic cell genetic	As sibs*	As sibs*
Non-genetic	As sibs*	As sibs*

* Sib risk in these conditions would equal the general population frequency

Somatic cell genetic disorders

When a mutation is present in the fertilized egg it will be transmitted to all its daughter cells. If, however, a mutation arises after the first cell division then this mutation will only be found in a proportion of cells and the individual is **mosaic** (two or more different genetic constitutions in one individual). The mutation may be confined to gonadal cells (gonadal or germline mosaic) or to somatic cells (somatic mosaic) or occur in a proportion of both. Irrespective of the distribution of the initial mutation within the individual, there would be no preceding family history. If the mutation is confined to somatic tissues there would be no increased risk to offspring but in gonadal mosaics the risk of transmission of the mutation can be as high as 50%. Cancer provides many examples of somatic cell genetic disorders (Chapter 9) and it is suspected that other common problems such as autoimmune disorders and ageing might have their basis, at least in part, in alterations of DNA in somatic cells.

Mitochondrial disorders

Human mitochondria each have about ten small, circular 'chromosomes' which contain, in their 16 596 basepairs, genes for 22 transfer RNAs and two types of ribosomal RNA required for mitochondrial protein synthesis, in addition to 13 peptides which are subunits of various enzyme complexes involved in electron transfer reactions of oxidative phosphorylation. Diseases due to mutations in these chromosomes show a characteristic pattern of inheritance as the egg not the sperm is the source of the zygote's mitochondria. Hence an affected mother will transmit the condition to all of her children whereas an affected man does not have affected offspring (maternal inheritance, Fig. 5.12).

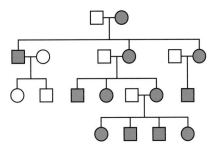

Fig. 5.12 Pedigree showing matrilineal inheritance.

The situation is often complicated by the fact that the mutation is only present in a proportion of an individual's mitochondrial DNA (**heteroplasmy**). This contributes to the range of phenotypic variability seen within affected families. For example, in families with myoclonic epilepsy and ragged red fibres on muscle biopsy (MERRF) carriers of only a small proportion of mutant mitochondria may be asymptomatic, whereas at the other extreme, if a threshold is exceeded, a severe encephalopathic picture (Leigh's disease) is seen. Mitochondrial molecular pathology includes point mutations, partial deletions and partial duplications and the phenotype depends not only upon the nature and site of the molecular lesion but also, as indicated earlier, upon the proportion of mitochondria in each tissue that is affected.

Population genetics

Population genetics is the study of gene distribution in populations and of how the frequencies of genes are maintained or changed.

Hardy–Weinberg equilibrium

Hardy and Weinberg were able to show mathematically (see 'Further reading', p. 93 for details) that, in a randomly mating population in the absence of selection, the relative frequencies of different alleles tend to be constant and may be described by a simple equation. Thus for an autosomal recessive trait due to homozygosity of a mutant allele which has a frequency q (normal allele A with a frequency p), if these are the only alleles at the locus, the sum of p and q must be 100% or 1. Similarly, the sum of the frequencies of the normal homozygote (AA, frequency $p \times p$ or p^2), the heterozygote (Aa, frequency $2 \times p \times q$ or $2pq$) and the affected homozygote (aa, frequency $q \times q$ or q^2) must be 100% or 1 ($p^2 + 2pq + q^2 = 1$).

Comparison of these calculated values with observed allele frequencies at a given locus provides evidence that these frequencies are consistent with the Hardy–Weinberg equilibrium. Under these circumstances the formula can be used to predict the frequencies of heterozygotes in the population at large when counselling for autosomal recessive conditions. For example, if an autosomal recessive disease has a frequency (q^2) of one in 10 000 (phenylketonuria occurs at about this frequency in most European populations) then q is the square root of this figure, i.e. one in 100; p approximates to 1 ($p = 1 - q$) and thus the heterozygote frequency is one in 50 ($2pq = 2 \times 1/100 = 1/50$). These considerations show how, even for apparently rare disorders, mutant genes may approach polymorphic (>1%) frequency in the population and heterozygous individuals who are asymptomatic carriers of recessive disease are similarly frequent. For cystic fibrosis, with a disease frequency of about one in 2000, heterozygous carriers would be predicted to occur with a frequency of one in 23. Such a high frequency immediately poses questions as to how an apparently deleterious gene has become so prevalent. This raises the possibility that evolutionary forces have operated to apply selective pressure in favour of heterozygotes (or homozygotes) for mutant genes that cause the more common inherited disorders (see below).

Several factors may distort the gene frequencies in a population and lead to either an increase or a decrease in allele frequencies from one generation to the next.

Selection

Selection may greatly influence the distribution of genes in a population. It may operate to reduce (**negative selection**) or increase (**positive selection**) a particular trait and hence its genetic distribution. In practice, selection acts at the level of individuals by favouring or hindering reproduction and hence the propagation of that individual's genes. Any increase in the ability of the affected person to reproduce (the **biological fitness** or f), for example as a result of therapy, will increase the frequency of the mutant allele. This change would produce a rapid increase in the number of affected people for an autosomal dominant trait (birth frequency at equilibrium = $2\mu(1 - f)$ where μ is the mutation rate and f is the biological fitness which ranges from 0 to 1). The increase would be of intermediate frequency for an X-linked recessive trait (birth frequency at equilibrium = $3\mu(1 - f)$) and extremely slow for an autosomal recessive trait (birth frequency at equilibrium = $\mu(1 - f)$). Thus for example if the biological fitness for a lethal autosomal dominant condition was restored from 0% to 100% the gene frequency would double in a generation and continue to increase at a similar pace until equilibrium was achieved (see above formula). With complete negative selection ($f = 0$) the gene frequency for an autosomal dominant condition would settle to 2μ.

For an autosomal recessive trait, selection against the recessive homozygote is much less powerful since most people in the population with the gene are heterozygous carriers. Restoration of the homozygote's biological fitness from 0% to 100% would only double the gene frequency after 50 generations if the initial disease frequency was one in 15 000. If less frequent then the increase would be even slower. A reduction in homozygote biological fitness would result in a similar slow change in gene frequencies. For an X-linked recessive trait of comparable frequency the situation is intermediate between that seen for autosomal dominant and recessive traits and an increase of biological fitness from 0% to 100% would double the incidence at birth in about four generations.

Selection may also operate on the recessive heterozygote as exemplified by sickle cell disease. Affected homozygotes in most parts of the world have an extremely low biological fitness and in view of this and the average mutation rate for a gene locus of 10 mutations per million gametes, the predicted birth frequency might be expected to approach one in 100 000 (see earlier formula). In certain areas such as equatorial Africa, however, the frequency at birth may exceed one in 40. Clearly the homozygote who dies without reproducing cannot have a selective advantage, and so the advantage must lie with the heterozygote. This state of affairs is referred to as a **balanced polymorphism**. The areas where sickle cell disease is most prevalent correspond geographically with the distribution of *Plasmodium falciparum* malaria. This clue led to the discovery that in the heterozygote the red cells parasitized by *P. falciparum* undergo sickling and are destroyed in the spleen. The sickle cell disease heterozygote thus more readily overcomes malarial infection than the normal homozygote and possesses a reproductive advantage. Increased biological fitness in comparison with normal homozygotes leads to a relatively rapid change in gene frequencies, but clearly the selective advantage no longer operates in regions where malaria has been eradicated. This may in part explain why sickle cell gene frequency appears to have fallen from about one in three to one in ten in the descendants of Africans who were transported to North America some ten generations ago.

In this connection, sickle cell anaemia is an unusual disorder. For most recessive diseases where the gene frequency exceeds 1%, no clear explanation beyond speculation has been apparent. Given that the selective forces may have been indirect or operated early in the evolution of the population group in question, this is perhaps not surprising. It also makes experimental testing of any notional advantage conferred on individuals that harbour the given trait very difficult. In cystic fibrosis, it has been suggested recently that the heterozygotes who carry one copy of a gene that leads to abnormal chloride transport in the intestine have relative resistance to microbial gut infections, and even cholera. Since enteric illnesses are a common cause of infant deaths, especially in poor communities, this hypothesis is superficially plausible. However, there are formidable obstacles to testing the theory in living populations currently at risk from fatal enteric illnesses.

Small populations

For religious, geographical or other reasons, a small group of individuals may become genetically isolated from the rest of the population. This may provide another explanation for the existence of mutant alleles of human genes at a high frequency in certain populations. The founder members of the group may harbour mutant alleles that are responsible for some autosomal traits (recessive or late-onset dominant) and so within this population these genes would exist at a higher frequency than within the general population (e.g. variegate porphyria in Afrikaners, congenital adrenal hyperplasia in Yupik Eskimos and congenital nephrotic syndrome in Finns). With only a small number of individuals in a breeding population the actual frequencies of alleles vary widely from one generation to the next (**random genetic drift**). By chance one allele may fail to be passed on to the next generation and so disappear (extinction) leaving only the alternative allele at that locus (fixation).

Other factors

As indicated by the formulae in 'Selection', any change in the mutation rate at a given locus would influence gene frequencies. Consanguinity (marriage between blood relatives) in a population influences gene frequencies by increasing the prevalence of carriers for certain traits. However, at the same time, by promoting homozygosity for autosomal recessive traits there will be the loss of two mutant alleles for each affected homozygote that fails to reproduce. A further influence on gene frequencies in the population is **migration**. The best example of this is the gradual fall in frequency of the ABO blood group allele B in populations as one moves westward from Asia through Europe. The frequency of B in eastern Asia is 0.3, but in western Europe it is only 0.06. This would suggest that the B allele originally arose in eastern Asia and has subsequently spread as a result of large scale population migration.

Genetic polymorphisms

A genetic polymorphism is defined as the occurrence together in the same population of two or more discontinuous traits (genetically determined characteristics) at a frequency where the most rare could not be maintained by recurrent mutation alone. In general, if one in 50 or more of the general population has the rare allele, the condition is considered to be polymorphic. Table 5.10 lists some examples of human polymorphisms. Biochemical studies in the past suggested that up to 7% of proteins were polymorphic, but this was suspected to be an underestimate since only about one-third of proteins with altered amino acid sequence have a detectable change in electrophoretic mobility. More recently, DNA sequencing has revealed that most, if not all, genes are polymorphic. These DNA variants may result in no alteration to the protein product (if they affect intron sequences or if they are synonymous and encode the same amino acid) or may produce an altered protein product which may or may not have altered function and/or electrophoretic mobility.

DNA variants arise by mutation and if they result in an advantageous phenotype or are closely linked to another gene which causes an advantageous phenotype (see 'Linkage disequilibrium', across) then natural selection will result in an increased frequency of the DNA variant (and the trait). Thus, for example, there is evidence that one of the original point mutations of the β-globin gene to the mutant form which occurs in sickle cell disease occurred on an ancestral chromosome 11

Table 5.10 Examples of human polymorphic traits.

Chromosomal: length of Yq, size of centromeric heterochromatin
Blood groups: ABO, MNS, Rh
Cell surface antigens: HLA
Red cell enzymes: adenylate kinase, phosphoglucomutase
Serum proteins: haptoglobins
DNA: site polymorphisms, e.g. restriction fragment length polymorphisms; length polymorphisms, e.g. microsatellites and minisatellites

bearing the less frequent allele for the linked RFLP identified by *Hpa*I. As the sickle β-globin gene increased in frequency by selection, so too did the linked *Hpa*I RFLP on this ancestral chromosome.

Many common DNA variants, however, do not produce altered proteins or if they do there appears to be no obvious selective advantage or disadvantage nor is there usually evidence of a selective pressure on a neighbouring gene. The high frequency may reflect random genetic drift or it may also reflect the consequences of a small or now obsolete selective pressure.

Linkage disequilibrium

Alleles at closely linked loci (recombination fraction less than 0.5%) usually show the phenomenon of **linkage disequilibrium**. As indicated in Fig. 5.13, for such a pair of loci four allelic combinations or **haplotypes** are possible (AC, AD, BC and BD) and at equilibrium the frequency of each will equal the product of the individual allele frequencies. However, when for example the normal allele A mutated to B in this instance the neighbouring allele was C (i.e. B arose on a C background). For B to occur on the same chromosome as D, a crossover must occur and the frequency of such crossing over depends on the physical distance between the two loci. Eventually, with sufficient crossovers, an equilibrium will be reached, but in the meantime linkage disequilibrium exists. This situation is exacerbated if natural selection acts on a trait determined by one of these alleles. If, for example, B is advantageous then B (and its associated C) will rapidly increase in frequency within the population and linkage disequilibrium will be pronounced (i.e. the excess of B with C compared with the frequency of B with D). In the absence of disturbing effects such as natural selection, linkage disequilibrium (or gametic association) declines eventually to zero at a rate $(1-r)^n$ where n is the number of generations and r is the recombination fraction.

Linkage disequilibrium is important in medical genetics as a means of identifying disease-causing genes, as a guide to the underlying molecular pathology and for the identification of the origin and spread of mutations. The major histocompatibility complex (MHC; Chapter 10) provides many examples of diseases where the first clue to the genetic susceptibility was given by the identification of an association with a neighbouring gene in linkage disequilibrium. The autosomal recessive nature of the common adult disorder hereditary haemochromatosis (frequency of homozygotes approximately one in 400) was established after studies of pedigrees confirmed genetic linkage to the HLA Class I loci. Earlier

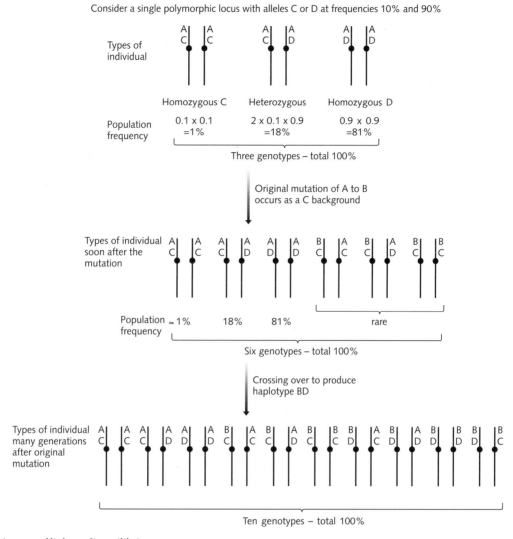

Fig. 5.13 Diagram of linkage disequilibrium.

studies had shown marked allelic association of the disease with the HLA-A3 antigen and an extensive region of DNA distal to the MHC cluster on chromosome 6 demonstrates marked linkage disequilibrium with the haemochromatosis gene.

The context of DNA polymorphisms in relation to a mutation often remains substantially unchanged for many generations and thus the occurrence of a given pattern of polymorphisms can be a clue to the presence of a particular mutation that is responsible for disease. Studies of this nature suggest that the sickle cell trait arose independently by several mutational events and spread subsequently as a result of selection. In contrast,

in phenylketonuria, due to defects in the enzyme phenylalanine hydroxylase, multiple mutations have occurred, each in association with distinct haplotypes that are recognizable as restriction fragment length DNA polymorphisms.

Further reading

Connor J.M. and Ferguson-Smith M.A. (1997) *Essential Medical Genetics*, 5th edn. Blackwell Science, Oxford.

Harper P.S. (1993) *Practical Genetic Counselling*, 4th edn. Butterworth-Heinemann, Oxford.

Mueller R. and Young I.D. (1995) *Emery's Elements of*

Medical Genetics, 6th edn. Churchill-Livingstone, Edinburgh.

Rimoin D.L., Connor J.M. and Pyeritz R.E. (1996) *Emery and Rimoin's Principles and Practice of Medical Genetics*, 3rd

edn. Churchill-Livingstone, New York.

Young I.D. (1991) *Introduction to Risk Calculation in Genetic Counselling*. Oxford University Press, Oxford.

Chapter **Monogenic disorders**

Introduction

This chapter:
- outlines approaches to the detection of loci that predispose to the development of inherited disorders, including some developmental conditions;
- indicates the advantages that result from the identification of disease genes;
- shows how the coordinated development of genome projects will improve the functional understanding of gene pathology.

Several thousand phenotypes have so far been attributed to distinct loci in the human genome; a similar number are additionally recognized as probably due to defects in single genes. These clinical phenotypes show dominant, recessive or sex-linked inheritance patterns and affected pedigrees clearly illustrate the Mendelian principles of allelic segregation and independent assortment (see Chapter 5). To date, genes for several hundred of the monogenic disorders have been isolated. The identification of mutant gene loci for disabling diseases such as cystic fibrosis and Duchenne muscular dystrophy (DMD) brings with it not only improvements in genetic counselling but the possibility of correction of the mutant phenotype after conception. Advances in the study of genetic diseases have attracted wide public attention — justifiably so, because the prospects for disease detection and definitive treatment have never been better. This chapter outlines how these advances have been achieved and illustrates why elucidation of single gene disorders provides the most conspicuous proof of the value of molecular biology to the study of human disease.

History of human genetics

The complementary nature of the strands of the DNA helix recognized by Watson and Crick provides a means for faithfully reproducing any change in its coding sequence. This strict order of **complementary base-pairing** represents the physical basis for fidelity of replication of the hereditary material and for fixation of its variants. In the transmission of this information by sexual reproduction in living organisms reside the essential but apparently conflicting characteristics of **invariance** and **diversity**. The origin of genetic diversity in humans is in the interplay of mutations and repair in germline DNA; it is modified by **natural selection** which may discriminate against, or favour the **fixation** of, novel mutations. Thus genetic variation provides the substrate for Darwinian evolution. Alternatively, variant genes may persist in a population because their effects are essentially neutral. Inherited diseases thus represent one extreme of the spectrum of **human genetic diversity**.

Until the emergence of molecular genetics, the study of function and heredity depended on the occurrence of natural mutants and, later, the experimental use of mutagenesis — especially in microbial genetics. Molecular genetics enables the function of genes to be explored directly in terms of their protein products because of our knowledge of the genetic code. Human molecular genetics allows these two approaches to act synergistically and reciprocally in our endeavour to understand the basis of inherited diseases as a step towards their early recognition and treatment (Fig. 6.1).

Human molecular genetics

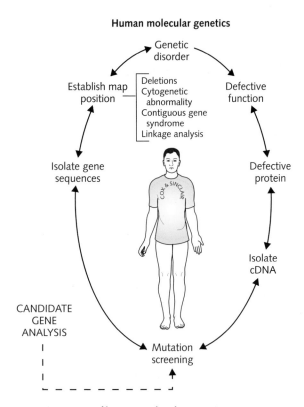

Fig. 6.1 Summary of human molecular genetics.

Inborn errors of metabolism

The application of these ideas to hereditary diseases can be traced in part to the work of the physician Archibald Garrod (1857–1936) who, while investigating congenital disorders of metabolism, demonstrated the link between heritable characters and defects in defined chemical reactions carried out in the tissues of the body. He proposed that defects in enzymes ('ferments') with specific actions on certain substrates were responsible for the disordered metabolism. This relationship was further clarified in 1908 by Garrod's observation that patients with these rare disorders, e.g. alkaptonuria, were more often than not the offspring of consanguineous marriages. Garrod's associate, the pioneering geneticist Bateson, suggested that the disorders were thus likely to result from the inheritance of two copies of a recessive Mendelian character that were identical by descent from a common parental ancestor. The full implications of Garrod's concept of '**inborn errors of metabolism**' were overlooked at the time but his notion was the antecedent of research into the genetics of eye colour determination in the fruit fly, *Drosophila*, and later work with auxotrophic mutants of the bread

mould, *Neurospora*, that led to the annunciation by Beadle and Tatum of the '**one gene–one enzyme**' (later 'one gene–one polypeptide') principle.

Chromosomes and genetic linkage

Recognition of the influence of physical proximity of genes on the inheritance of multiple characters has its origins in the rediscovery in 1900 of Mendel's experiments with garden peas. Mendel ensured that the seeds used in his experiments bred true for the seven pairs of contrasting characteristics he examined. In the progeny of crosses between defined parental types, each pair of characters **assorted independently** from the others. When Mendel's work was discovered and repeated in other plants, certain anomalies were noted. Bateson and Punnett in 1908 studied flower colour and pollen structure in the sweet pea: in the second filial generation of these experiments, although the expected ratio of 3 : 1 for long to round pollen was found to hold for white flowers, widely discordant ratios of pollen types were observed when sweet peas with purple or red flowers were studied. Thus the character of the pollen was linked or 'coupled' partially to flower colour. Similar observations with three sex-linked traits in *Drosophila* were made by T.H. Morgan, who found that the proportion of flies showing **recombination** between the parental characters was significantly lower than expected, indicating non-random assortment. This distribution of **segregation**, or **genetic linkage**, was explained by the discovery that genetic material is organized into a limited number of discrete units, or chromosomes. As a result of his sophisticated back-cross experiments in *Drosophila*, Morgan realized that genes and chromosomes showed parallel behaviour that provides a mechanistic explanation for linked inheritance of certain characteristics.

In 1902 Sutton observed the mechanics of chromosome separation at meiosis and concluded that this would allow numerous random combinations of parental chromosomes to pass to the germ cells. Ultimately de Vries and Morgan realized that if independent assortment of characters located on those same chromosomes were to occur, then this would require crossing over of short homologous regions of chromosomes that were paired at meiosis. This crossing over they referred to as **recombination**. Morgan also concluded that if characters were juxtaposed on the same chromosome then they would tend to **co-segregate** during gamete formation and thus show the phenomenon of genetic linkage. Should the regions bearing the characters be physically distant, then their transmission to the germ cells and offspring would more closely approach random segregation (50% recombination fraction). By determining the **recombination frequency** for multiple linked genes in three point back-cross experiments between heterozygous and homozygous parents, Morgan and his associates measured the relative levels of linkage between the different loci and in this way constructed a genetic linkage map for *Drosophila*. Low frequencies of recombination indicate close physical linkage of genes, whereas large recombination fractions show that the genes are widely separated on the chromosome (see Chapter 5).

It is noteworthy that the seven characters originally studied by Mendel in the garden pea show no linkage, although two of these traits are determined by genes on chromosome 1 and 3 by genes on chromosome 4. Thus four pairs of genes each share a chromosome — a property known as **synteny**. Three of these pairs of genes are found at distantly separated loci on their respective chromosomes and show approximately 50% recombination that precludes detection of linkage, even after numerous crosses.

Morbid anatomy of the human genome

As shown in Chapter 5 and described below, the concept of genetic linkage is fundamental to the isolation of many disease loci caused by lesions in single genes. This approach has proved productive in the study of monogenic (single gene) disorders beyond the analysis of disorders of metabolism, and their ultimate characterization has resulted in impressive leaps in our knowledge. The ability of physicians, medical scientists and clinical geneticists to retrieve and use burgeoning information about the functional anatomy of the human genome has been enhanced by the pioneering work of Victor McKusick to establish the, now on-line, clinical register of **Mendelian inheritance in man** (OMIM). McKusick's catalogue is continually updated and stored centrally in the Welch Medical Library at Johns Hopkins University, Baltimore, as part of the Genome Data Base. The on-line version of OMIM now carries about 6000 entries concerning human inherited disorders and is periodically downloaded to international reference centres and local networks for access by individual laboratories.

The Human Genome Project

In the mid-1980s discussion on the feasibility of characterizing the entire human genome at the nucleotide level began in earnest. Widespread enthusiasm for this ambitious endeavour resulted in the initiation of an international programme, the Human Genome Project (HGP), in 1990. Consisting of a number of individual genome projects established worldwide, the goals of this concerted action were several-fold: to obtain the 3000 megabases (Mb) of human DNA sequence, localize the 50 000 or so genes and construct detailed physical and genetic maps. Although the project had the scale and flavour of a space race and excited much scepticism, it is now well under way with some of its aims already realized. This has mainly been due to the factory-scale approaches employed by centres such as the **Centre d'Etude du Polymorphisme Humain** (CEPH) and the company **Généthon** in France, the **Institute for Genome Resources** (TIGR), the Whitehead Institute/MIT Centre for Genome Research and Washington University in the USA, as well as the international collaboration of hundreds of laboratories. Integration and accessibility of data has been greatly enhanced by the development of worldwide web protocols and the influence of the international body HUGO. Coupled with the establishment of local centres, such as the HGMP resource centre in the UK, that can provide many of the reagents and technology emerging from large-scale genome analysis, these public databases allow individual scientists to use HGP information to accelerate their own disease gene hunt.

To mark the fifth birthday of its inception, reviews on the HGP's progress at the end of 1995 were glowing with optimism (see 'Further reading', p. 127). In 1994 the efforts of over 100 laboratories resulted in the publication of the first complete **linkage map** of the human genome. Co-ordinated by CEPH and Généthon the map contains 5926 loci covering 4000 centimorgans (cM) representing an average marker density of 0.7 cM. Parallel physical mapping strategies have resulted in an STS-based radiation hybrid map with a marker sequence every 199 kb on average and contiguous sections of cloned sequences representing about 70% of the whole genome (see later sections for an explanation of some of the technology). None of these maps represents perfect resources for ultimate base-by-base characterization of the genome, but they provide an excellent start as well as valuable frameworks for expediting disease gene isolation. Further refinement of maps and improved technology will be required but the HGP is well on its way to obtaining a complete genome sequence soon after the turn of the century.

A further aspect of the evolving HGP that will accelerate the identification of disease genes is the development of large databases of partial sequences of cDNA clones from a variety of tissue sources. Literally hundreds of thousands of these expressed sequence tags (ESTs) are being generated by private companies and academic institutions. Although each 'tag' only contains part of a gene sequence, the accumulated data to date have confirmed previous estimates of human gene number (~100 000) as well as the recognition of gene families. The value of these sequences will be fully realized when they are placed on the evolving physical map to provide candidates for chromosomally localized disease loci.

Despite these achievements, the challenge to identify all human disease genes remains daunting. Whilst the availability of the entire human sequence will undoubtedly accelerate progress, much investigation will be needed to marry individual phenotypes with their respective genes and to unravel the biological messages encoded in the sequence blueprint of DNA.

Aims and utility of gene isolation

Given the size of the human genome (approximately 3×10^9 basepairs), with a genetic map length of 30 Morgans, mapping an unknown locus by linkage to defined markers followed by complete sequence characterization of the disease gene remains a formidable task. This task is justified because of the potential to alleviate suffering in families affected by serious inherited diseases and for the scientific revelations that emerge. Having isolated genes responsible for human disorders there is a need to ensure that the potential use of the resulting information is fully realized. As a result of the development of rapid sequencing methods and DNA amplification techniques based on the **polymerase chain reaction** (PCR), it is now possible to diagnose many genetic diseases directly by molecular analysis of small samples of DNA obtained non-invasively from affected individuals and putative carriers. The methods also improve existing techniques for antenatal diagnosis in mothers carrying a fetus at risk.

Table 6.1 Utility of isolating genes responsible for hereditary disease.

- Facilitates the detection of mutations responsible for disease and aids diagnosis and identification of disease carriers
- Nature of the gene product may lead to better understanding of the pathological or biochemical lesion and identify novel targets for therapy
- Characterization of the effects of naturally occurring mutations may allow more refined analysis of the molecular function of the gene product itself
- Identification of the disease locus is essential for the development of somatic gene therapy or for the production of recombinant proteins for therapeutic use

The utility of isolating genes responsible for hereditary disorders in humans needs little emphasis but some of the fruits that may be harvested from this rich source of molecular information about the human genome are set out in Table 6.1.

Isolation of disease loci via the protein product—functional cloning

Dissecting the pathology of a given hereditary disease necessarily involves identification of the faulty gene and understanding the nature of its protein product. In some cases where an underlying protein deficiency has been identified this information can be used to trace the mutated gene. Where the relevant protein is expressed in an obtainable tissue in sufficient quantity, protein purification, digestion and sequencing techniques can be used to obtain stretches of amino acid sequence corresponding to unique sections of the polypeptide. This sequence can be converted into nucleic acid sequence by reference to the genetic code and hence a short unique section of the gene can be identified.

This DNA sequence can be artificially synthesized, labelled with radioactive phosphorus and used to screen by hybridization a cDNA library that represents the genes expressed in a relevant tissue. This 'protein to gene' strategy is illustrated in Chapter 1 on haemophilia A and described in Chapter 2. Numerous other examples of this approach include the identification of genes for many inborn errors of metabolism such as phenylketonuria (phenylalanine hydroxylase), hereditary fructose intolerance (aldolase B) and Lesch–Nyhan disease (hypoxanthine–guanine phosphoribosyl transferase) as well as the haemoglobinopathies (including the thalassaemia syndromes). In fact, the precise cause of the first 'molecular disease', sickle cell anaemia (Plate 6, facing p. 214), was inferred from the primary discovery of Vernon Ingram in 1956 that human sickle haemoglobin differs from normal adult haemoglobin by the replacement of a single amino acid at the sixth position in the β-globin chain. The mutation ($Hb\beta glu^6 \rightarrow val$) results from an A $\rightarrow$ T transversion in the second nucleotide of the sixth codon in the β-globin gene.

In other cases, 'educated guesses' as to the nature of the defective protein can lead to identification of a mutant gene. This process is illustrated by the recent identification of *ZAP70* as the gene underlying development of one form of severe combined immunodeficiency (SCID). T-lymphocytes from patients with this disease were found to be unable to trigger a cascade of cytoplasmic tyrosine kinase reactions required for activation. ZAP70 was one of several T-cell-specific kinases known to participate in T-cell activation and the *ZAP70* gene was duly tested as a candidate disease locus.

Positional cloning and candidate genes

Isolation of a disease locus when the protein product is unknown

Where there are no indications as to the nature of the underlying biochemical defect in a single gene disorder, isolation of the mutated gene and subsequent characterization of its protein product offers the means for progress. This approach to understanding hereditary disorders has been called 'reverse genetics' or, more appropriately, '**positional cloning**'. The reason the latter term best describes the process is that isolation of an unknown disease gene relies heavily on initially identifying the position of the gene in a single subchromosomal region within the whole human genome. The scale of this task is illustrated by the following. The haploid human genome (one-half of the cellular diploid complement of homologous chromosomes) consists of 3×10^9 **basepairs** or 3×10^6 kilobase (kb) pairs. A single gene, on average, occupies only about 40 kb and could therefore be in any one of about **100 000 sites**. This is equivalent to searching the telephone directory for a single name with the added difficulty of not knowing how the name is spelt. Fortunately, classical genetics, cytogenetics and molecular biology in combination have provided us with methods to track down and recognize genes for hereditary diseases.

As we describe below, in general the location of a gene is first broadly determined to a region of about 10 000 kb, either by the detection of cytogenetic rearrangements associated with the disease, or the application of genetic linkage analysis in extended pedigrees. This region is then dissected using the tools of molecular genetics to provide closely linked DNA probes and potential 'candidate' disease genes from the region. Finally, individual genes from the relevant region are sequenced and screened to determine whether they do indeed contain mutations in individuals with the disease under study. It must be emphasized that positional cloning is not a single strategy but a form of detective work that involves concurrent application of many different techniques. Different approaches are often adopted by each set of investigators for the isolation of a given disease gene. The rapid evolution of the HGP with its attendant centralized resources means that increasingly the laborious task of positional cloning can be short-circuited to a 'candidate gene approach'. Once the approximate position of a disease locus has been defined

the relevant region can be surveyed for potential candidates by referring to the emerging maps of expressed sequences. Ultimately, the complete sequence will allow very rapid progression to candidate genes. The remainder of this chapter will first describe the tools of the gene mappers' trade and then use examples to illustrate how they are employed. Many of these have been used on a grand scale as part of the HGP. Figure 6.2 depicts the whole 'top-down' approach to gene isolation and should be used as a reference throughout the chapter.

X-linked disorders

Disease genes on the human X-chromosome can be recognized by their patterns of inheritance. X-linked recessive genes will give rise to the disease only in male children of asymptomatic carrier mothers as described in

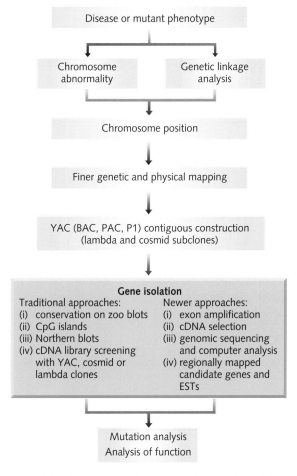

Fig. 6.2 'Top-down' approach to gene isolation (adapted from Monaco (1994) with permission).

Chapter 1. Haemophilia provides the best-known example of such a gene in humans (see Chapter 1). Dominant X-linked disorders are usually more severe in males, sometimes with the result that only female cases are observed. Recognition of X-linked inheritance facilitates gene isolation because the search is narrowed down to only 5% of the haploid genome. For this reason many more disease loci have been assigned to the X-chromosome than to any single autosome, although many of the X-linked disorders are very rare. By the same token it is not surprising that the first disease genes mapped to a particular chromosome were X-linked and include the genes for haemophilia A and B and colour blindness.

Cytogenetic clues to gene location

Valuable pointers to the location of a disease gene may result from the observation of cytogenetic rearrangements in affected individuals. These may take the form of translocations, large deletions or duplications and may affect one or more genes. Translocations have been particularly useful in the case of X-linked diseases where their effects are more apparent because of the effects of Lyonization in females. Where balanced translocations involve the X-chromosome in females, the normal unadulterated X is usually inactivated early in embryogenesis. This preserves a normal complement of expressed genes from the chromosomes involved in the exchange, with the exception of any gene disrupted by the translocation event. Female carriers of a translocation interrupting the gene for an X-linked recessive disorder will manifest the disease because their normal healthy gene copy is inactivated in all cells. Karyotypic analysis of women expressing X-linked recessive disorders is therefore an excellent means to localize a disease gene to a specific subchromosomal site. Two examples where identification of such female cases has been instrumental in the isolation of the disease locus are DMD and Menkes' disease — a rare disorder of metal transport associated with arterial fragility and skin and hair abnormalities, due to tissue copper deficiency.

Large deletions that are readily detected by karyotyping have also provided excellent clues to the site of a disease gene. Often these large deletions affect more than one gene and may result in a complex phenotype with multiple defects in a single individual. These are called **contiguous gene syndromes** and, again, are more commonly noted on the X-chromosome because of hemizygosity of X-linked genes in males. Examples of contiguous gene syndromes are listed in Table 6.2.

Where one component of a contiguous gene syndrome

Table 6.2 Contiguous gene syndromes.

Clustered phenotypes	Chromosomal location of deletion	Disease loci cloned	Gene function
Wilms' tumour	11p13	WT1	Tumour supressor
Aniridia		PAX6	Homeotic gene
Genital abnormalities		WT1	
Mental retardation		?	
Duchenne dystrophy	Xp21	Dystrophin	Muscle protein
Glycerol kinase deficiency		GK	Kinase
Chronic granulomatous disease		b-245	Cytochrome subunit
Retinitis pigmentosa		?	?
Adrenal hypoplasia		DAX-1	Putative nuclear hormone receptor
McLeod syndrome		XK	Putative membrane transporter
Mental retardation		?	?
Kallmann syndrome	Xp22	KAL	Neuronal guidance
X-linked ichthyosis		ARSC (STS)	Arylsulphatase C (steroid sulphatase)
Mental retardation		?	?
Chondrodysplasia		ARSE (CDPX)	Arylsuphatase E

can be related to a previously identified disease gene, the chromosomal rearrangement can lead rapidly to identification of the neighbouring genes. For example, large deletions of a region of Xp22 were identified in a few males with X-linked icthyosis as well as Kallmann syndrome and mental retardation. Kallmann syndrome is a developmental disorder of neuronal cell migration that results in anosmia and hypogonadism in males. X-linked ichthyosis is due to deficiency of the gene encoding steroid sulphatase (STS) and these males were deleted for this locus and a large amount of flanking DNA. A large series of overlapping deletions, some cytogenetically detectable and some submicroscopic, in individuals with and without Kallmann syndrome and STS deficiency were then used to define a region of DNA harbouring the Kallmann gene. Ultimately, this region was examined in detail and a gene was identified that is either deleted or mutated in individuals with Kallmann syndrome. The Kallmann syndrome gene product is a secreted protein involved in establishing and maintaining the olfactory bulb as well as dictating the migratory pathway of neurones destined to become the gonadotrophin-releasing hormone (GnRH) cells of the hypothalamus.

In a similar manner, characterization of deletions giving rise to the complex WAGR phenotype (Wilms' tumour, aniridia, genital abnormalities, mental retardation) has been used to identify genes involved in the development of aniridia (absent iris). Large deletions of the particular region of the short arm of the X-chromosome designated Xp21 not only assisted in the cloning of the DMD (Duchenne muscular dystrophy) gene but also served to localize the genes for three other X-linked diseases which have since been cloned (those for chronic granulomatous disease, glycerol kinase deficiency and adrenal hypoplasia).

A singular example of a chromosomal rearrangement acting as a cytogenetic signpost for the position of a disease gene is that of the fragile X or Martin–Bell syndrome (Box 6.1). This is a common hereditary disorder, predominantly but not exclusively affecting males and accounting for up to 50% of males with mental retardation. Affected males have characteristic facies and enlarged (oedematous) testes and expression of the disease is associated with fragility of a section of the long arm of the X-chromosome (Xq27.3) when fibroblasts obtained from affected individuals are cultured in folate-deficient medium. The inheritance of fragile X does not conform to any classical pattern, a fact which puzzled researchers until the gene was cloned. The existence of the fragile site focused the search for the gene on Xq27, a strategy which was rewarded in 1991 by the isolation of a candidate gene (*FMR1*) from this area of the X-

---

Fragile X or Martin–Bell syndrome

Frequency

Approximately one in 2000 males.

Characteristics

Large ears, prominent jaw, high-pitched speech, large (oedematous) testes, seizures in 10%. Moderate to severe retardation. Patients may survive to advanced old age.

Transmission

X-linked (Xq27.3).

Molecular defect

Expansion of trinucleotide repeat sequences in the *FMR1* gene.
   Condition demonstrates anticipation in affected families due to 'pre-mutation' expansion at meiosis.

Treatment

Symptomatic only; variable expression renders many affected males capable of active community life.

Box 6.1

---

chromosome. The gene is associated with an unusually unstable region of DNA consisting of a large number of tandem repeats of the trinucleotide sequence CGG. Expansion of this region in affected individuals gives rise to the unusual cytogenetic observations and the neurological phenotype. This and other examples of expanded repeats in human disease are discussed on p. 120.

Genetic linkage analysis

Although cytogenetic clues may provide an invaluable route to gene localization, they are the exception rather than the rule. The most generally applicable technique for localizing the genes for monogenic disorders is genetic linkage analysis. The fundamental principles of linkage are described in Chapter 5 and discussion here will focus on its application to the isolation of specific disease genes. By the same token, special procedures have been developed to isolate DNA sequences related to disease loci. These depend on an understanding of the techniques outlined in Chapter 5 and are discussed here in relation to human genetics.

Accurate positioning of a disease locus depends on the existence of a good genetic map of the human genome, that is, a large array of polymorphic DNA markers whose relative positions are known. The greater the number of markers and the more 'connected' the map is, the more likely it is that a given disease locus can be positioned within it. The success of any linkage study also relies on the nature of the polymorphisms used to develop the map, the most useful being those that can have a large number of alleles, i.e. variable number tandem repeats (VNTR) or microsatellite repeats. These maps have only very recently become available as part of the HGP.

In theory, analysing the segregation of these markers throughout disease pedigrees allows localization of any disease gene to within a distance of 5–10 cM or, approximately, 5000–10 000 kb. This then sets the stage for the directed isolation of additional polymorphic sequences within the relevant region and finer genetic mapping. Depending on the frequency of the disease and its mode of inheritance, it is often possible to narrow down the position of a disease to within 1 cM, which approximates to a physical distance of about 1000 kb. This is because of the need to obtain affected pedigrees of appropriate size and structure for linkage analysis. Before the development of comprehensive maps, localizing a disease gene by genetic analysis was a slow and painful business; a certain degree of luck was needed to ensure that the disease locus would lie within mapping distance of an available polymorphic probe. The mapping of the locus for cystic fibrosis, which will be discussed later, provides a good illustration of this principle. A fine example of rapid localization by linkage is the mapping of the gene for a disease of premature ageing or progeria called Werner's syndrome: 500 polymorphic loci were used to position the gene for this rare autosomal dominant disorder to a small region of chromosome 8.

The form of linkage analysis used to map a gene will depend on the mode of inheritance, the mortality associated with it and its frequency. Where large pedigrees with several affected individuals are available, family linkage studies are appropriate. Where these are limited, proband-based linkage disequilibrium or sib pair studies can be used. Linkage disequilibrium relies on the fact that for some monogenic disorders (e.g. cystic fibrosis, sickle cell anaemia) a single mutation is responsible for most cases. A founder effect accounts for the high frequency of a specific mutation: in a particular population all the disease alleles originate from an individual harbouring a single mutated chromosome. The original chromosome may be identified by the presence of particular allelic forms of closely linked genetic markers that associate specifically with the disease locus—a prop-

erty known as linkage disequilibrium. If a genetic map is sufficiently dense, this property can conceivably be used to identify the position of the disease locus. To date linkage disequilibrium has been used primarily to narrow down the interval containing a disease locus when a rough location has already been established.

Sib pair analysis is a powerful method that compares the inheritance of the alleles of a series of polymorphisms between affected members of the same sibship. If a given polymorphism lies close to the disease gene then affected siblings would be expected to have inherited the same marker allele significantly more than 50% of the time when a large series of sibs are examined. Sib pair methods have the advantage that they do not rely on a single disease-causing mutation and may avoid some of the diagnostic problems presented by late-onset diseases such as Huntington's chorea or familial Alzheimer's disease. Furthermore, sib pair methods provide an inbuilt control for the confounding effects of environmental factors (e.g. nutrition) or other genes that influence expression of the mutant allele predisposing to disease because only affected individuals are considered. However, sib pair studies may involve the examination of hundreds of individuals in families affected by a given disorder. Recently the introduction of automated scanning procedures, usually based on the polymerase chain reaction, to analyse the size of marker alleles at multiple polymorphic loci distributed throughout the genome, has greatly assisted in the conduct of such studies (Plate 7, facing p. 214).

The positions of even very rare autosomal recessive loci can be determined by the technique of 'homozygosity mapping'. This form of linkage analysis exploits the existence of consanguineous marriages that result in affected cases. Such cases are likely to have inherited an identical chromosomal fragment housing the same mutated gene from both parents, due to their relatedness. They thus become homozygous at all loci closely flanking the disease gene. A genome-wide search for regions of homozygosity in the affected progeny of only a few such marriages may be sufficient to provide statistical evidence for linkage to a disease locus.

Narrowing down the interval

With the combined use of cytogenetic and linkage analyses, a disease locus may be initially mapped to a region spanning approximately 10 000 kb of DNA. Clearly, this is too large an interval to search kilobase by kilobase and a degree of refinement will be needed to allow cloning of the gene. This will involve the construction of a physical map across the region and an essential first step in this process is the isolation of additional DNA sequences or probes. These are then used as reagents for developing polymorphic markers for further linkage analysis (including disequilibrium studies), as probes for creating a large-scale restriction site map of the region and, finally, for the isolation of large ordered sections of cloned DNA (**contigs**) which can be searched directly for **candidate genes**.

Isolation of DNA from the region

Many techniques have emerged that allow small sections of DNA (DNA probes or markers) from specific regions of the genome to be cloned: individual chromosomes can be selectively sorted using a fluorescence activated cell sorter (FACS) and used to create libraries of short (approx. 20 kb) DNA sequences enriched for the region of interest; individual chromosome bands can be dissected out by microdissection or laser technology and used to provide a battery of even smaller fragments (approx. 500 basepairs); and finally, somatic cell hybrids containing fragmented or whole human chromosomes in a rodent cell background can be used to provide libraries from which the human sequences can be readily identified. DNA fragments provided by any or all of these means can be used as anchor points in a developing physical and genetic map.

In general the map will develop along several complementary lines. Small fragments can be ordered relative to each other using somatic cell hybrids as well as pulsed field gel electrophoresis and used to isolate larger sections of DNA that, in turn, must be characterized by restriction mapping and sorted into overlapping contigs. The next two sections describe the mapping techniques that can be employed and some of their limitations.

Ordering small fragments of DNA

Sequence tagged sites

The advent of the PCR has brought with it the possibility of ordering small sections of DNA within the genome through limited knowledge of their DNA sequences. A short stretch (a few hundred basepairs) of DNA sequence is obtained and short oligonucleotide primers are generated that allow PCR amplification of a unique representative section of the marker from any complex DNA source. This marker becomes a sequence tagged site (STS) and through the use of PCR its presence can be detected in any source of DNA be it an entire genome or a small section of cloned DNA.

Somatic cell hybrids

A large battery of inter-specific somatic cell hybrids have been developed that contain defined sections of the human genome in a rodent cell background. These lines provide very valuable mapping tools as they serve to isolate specific regions of human chromosomes. DNA from these hybrids can be screened using STSs or probed on Southern blots with probes that recognize unique fragments of human DNA. In this way individual markers are assigned within or outside specific chromosomal regions.

A further innovation in this area is radiation hybrid technology. In this method, somatic cell hybrids containing a whole human chromosome are irradiated in order to fragment the genome into subchromosomal sections. These fragments are recovered by fusing the irradiated dead cells with a second rodent cell line. The resultant hybrids contain unselected portions of the primary human chromosome that vary in length and content. DNA probes or STSs that are closer together are less likely to be separated by the fragmentation process and will be contained within the same hybrid line. Those that are far apart will often be separated and be contained within different radiation hybrids. The frequency of occurrence of individual DNA sequences in the same hybrid lines is therefore a measure of the physical distance between them. The mapping resolution of this method depends on the radiation dose, the number of hybrid lines examined and the number of DNA probes used; it can generate maps with as little as a few hundred kilobases between neighbouring sequences. A recent extension of radiation hybrid methodology involves fusion of irradiated human cells, i.e. containing the entire diploid genome, to a rodent cell line. In this case hybrid lines are produced that contain many small sections of the human genome integrated into rodent chromosomes. DNA from large panels (about 100 lines) of hybrids can be examined for the coexistence of human sequences and maps produced in a manner analogous to linkage analysis. Now that a sufficient density of chromosomally mapped human sequences has been generated by more conventional means and many of these loci assigned to radiation hybrids, this is probably the most rapid method for sublocalizing a novel sequence within the human genome.

Pulsed field gel electrophoresis

A critical development for the building of physical maps was the invention of electrophoretic techniques that could resolve fragments of DNA larger than 50 kb.

Many variations on the theme of pulsed field gel electrophoresis (PFGE) have been put into practice and most of them can resolve fragments from a few kilobases to several megabases.

The simultaneous emergence of a wide range of restriction endonucleases that cleave genomic DNA infrequently (the so called 'rare-cutters') paved the way for scaling up restriction mapping. Total genomic DNA is digested with a rare-cutter enzyme and separated on a pulsed field gel. The array of large DNA fragments in the gel is subject to chemical shearing and then transferred to a filter by Southern blotting. Individual small genomic probes are hybridized sequentially to the digested DNA to build up a picture demonstrating which sequences are physically linked within large restriction fragments.

This technique allows a map to be developed across a region of interest before the region has been isolated in overlapping clones. Its success depends in part on the distribution of recognition sites for the rare-cutter enzymes and PFGE maps may contain gaps where sites are unevenly distributed. Figure 6.3 shows an example of a pulsed field gel in which human genomic DNA has been electrophoretically separated alongside whole yeast chromosomes as molecular weight markers.

Fluorescence in situ hybridization

Another way of positioning DNA sequences and ordering them across a subchromosomal region is by hybridization of labelled DNA to intact chromosomes. Traditionally radiolabelled probes were used, but the sensitivity of this technique has been greatly improved by the use of multicoloured fluorescent dyes (Plate 8, facing p. 214). The application of this technique ranges from ordering of small sections of DNA relative to each other on interphase chromatin with a resolution of less than 100 kb to checking the chromosomal location and integrity of large clones of up to 1 Mb in size. A recent innovation is the application of probes to extended DNA, a technique that can order sequences as little as 10 kb apart. Fluorescence *in situ* hybridization (FISH) is also invaluable for detecting and characterizing chromosomal rearrangements that are difficult to interpret by conventional cytogenetic methods.

Cloning genomic DNA across a disease locus

Table 6.3 illustrates the levels of DNA cloning that can now be achieved using a variety of vectors for propagation of recombinant DNA in bacteria or yeast cells. The advent of yeast artificial chromosome (YAC) vectors for cloning large sections of human DNA has revolutionized the characterization of large genomic regions since it represents more than one order of magnitude improvement on the length of DNA that could be obtained from a single recombinant clone.

Yeast artificial chromosomes

The possibility of generating libraries of complex genomes that are represented in DNA inserts exceeding 1 Mb in yeast artificial chromosome (YAC) vectors is a conspicuous development (see Chapter 3). Until recently, the successful isolation of unknown genes implicated in inherited disorders, e.g. cystic fibrosis, has demanded the remorseless application of linkage and physical mapping and cloning methods that are, for practical purposes, limited to approximately 250 kb. Genomic inserts cloned in YACs provide a stable resource that extends the conjunction between subchromosomal mapping and molecular analysis of disease genes.

YAC libraries have been generated from plants, bacteria and several complex genomes including the human. Large fragments of chromosomal DNA, generated by partial digestion with restriction enzymes, are ligated into the vector. The vector arms possess telomeric segments at their flanks as well as centromeric sequences and autonomously replicating sequences that ensure accurate segregation during mitosis and meiosis within a yeast cell host. With average insert sizes approaching 1 Mb, the YAC vector system has the potential for long-range mapping studies of high resolution that bridge the divide between linkage analysis and gene sequencing.

Table 6.3 Scales of genomic cloning.

Vector	Host	Vector structure	Insert size range (kb)
Cosmids	Bacteria (*E. coli*)	Circular plasmid	35–45
P1 clones	Bacteria (*E. coli*)	Circular plasmid	70–100
BACs	Bacteria (*E. coli*)	Circular plasmid	Up to 300
PACs	Bacteria (*E. coli*)	Circular plasmid	100–300
YACs	Yeast (*S. cerevisiae*)	Linear chromosomes	100–2000

(a)

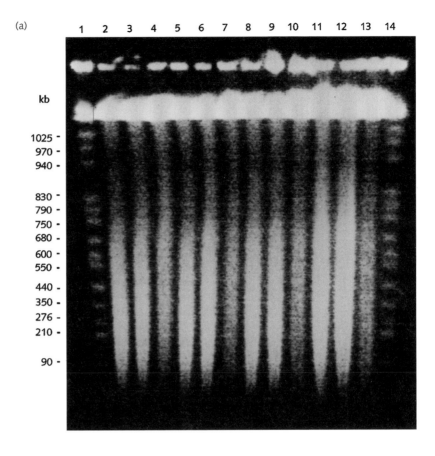

(b)

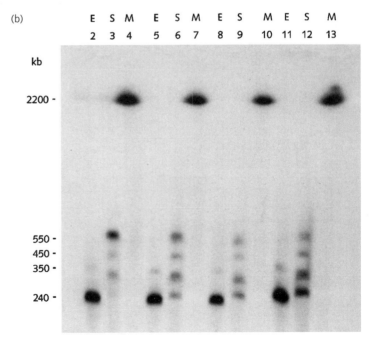

Fig. 6.3 Pulsed field gel electrophoresis. (a) Ethidium bromide staining of restriction enzyme-digested human DNA (lanes 2–13) that has been resolved through a pulsed field gel alongside whole yeast chromsomes (lanes 1 and 14). Yeast chromosome sizes are indicated in kilobases (kb). The restriction enzymes *Eag*I (E), *Sac*II (S) and *Mlu*I (M) were used to cut human DNA samples from four different individuals. (b) An autoradiograph of the same DNA samples after they have been transferred to filters by Southern blotting and hybridized to a unique human sequence from chromosome 3. The sizes of hybridizing fragments was estimated by comparison with the those of individual yeast chromosomes visualized by ethidium staining. Photographs courtesy of Frances Richards, Cambridge University Department of Pathology, Cambridge, UK. These data are part of a set used to generate a restriction map around the locus for Von Hippel–Lindau disease.

Because of this, **large insert size libraries** containing only a few thousand clones may adequately represent the entire human genome. This enables libraries to be stored and screened as an array of individual clones each representing a separate section of DNA.

Libraries of YAC clones containing total genomic DNA are screened either by hybridization with small unique anchor probes from the region or using the PCR to detect STSs on sequentially smaller pools of YAC clone DNA. Individual clones are then characterized with respect to the anchor sequences that they contain and the presence of sites for rare-cutter enzymes (using PFGE). Additional 'fingerprinting' methods are usually required to develop an accurate **map of overlapping YAC clones** and the most common of these relies on an analysis of the repeat sequences present in each clone.

At first inspection it would appear that YAC cloning is all that is required in order to obtain all of the DNA from a region of interest. However, there are several reasons why more conventional cloning vectors with bacterial hosts are used alongside YAC technology. The first is that YAC clones are not always a true representation of a single genomic region. That is, they frequently contain deletions or DNA from more than one chromosomal region (**'chimerism'**). The second is that they are too cumbersome to use in many mapping or gene isolation approaches because of their sheer size, complexity and content of repeated sequences. The genomic inserts from large YAC clones are usually broken down into more manageable pieces by using them to screen cosmid libraries; alternatively, they may be subcloned into these vectors for propagation in bacteria. Recently, several alternative cloning systems have been developed that allow propagation of large genomic fragments in bacterial hosts (P1, PACs and BACs). These systems overcome many of the problems encountered using YACs but provide smaller insert sizes and therefore genomic advantage. Because of the evolving HGP contigs across a region of interest are increasingly available for further characterization.

Refining the position of the disease gene

How does establishing a physical map across a region of a chromosome further the cloning of a disease gene? In the best case the map provides a means of isolating and ordering polymorphic loci that can be used to narrow down the critical region of DNA containing the disease gene to within a few hundred kilobases. This is done by analysing rare meiotic recombination events between the disease gene and flanking polymorphic DNA sequences. On occasion, individual markers will be in linkage disequilibrium with the disease locus, testifying to their proximity. In the worst case, where there is little meiotic recombination, the map provides the material for a large-scale search for candidate genes responsible for the disease.

Isolating coding sequences

Research on the positional cloning of genes responsible for human diseases has had many spectacular successes but the functional gene map remains sparse. When a gene is localized successfully to a few hundred kilobases of a physically mapped region of genomic DNA, a bewildering array of strategies can be used to isolate it. These all rely on the **isolation of expressed sequences** from the region (candidate disease genes) and their subsequent characterization by DNA sequencing. It must be remembered that **less than 5%** of the human genome codes for expressed genes and that this is dispersed amongst a great excess of non-protein-coding DNA. Two main types of procedures are used: those based on structural methods to select for functional elements involved in the expression of genes, such as exons, CpG islands, polyadenylation signals and promoter sequences; and those based on the identification of cDNAs that correspond to mRNA molecules derived from the genomic region of interest, e.g. by direct library selection. As we show later in this chapter, the application of neither type of procedure is mutually exclusive and in most successful positional cloning projects, an opportunistic, combinatorial approach has been used. The structurally based procedures are essentially inferential or suggestive but have the potential to identify all the genes expressed from a given genomic DNA segment. Complementary DNA selection methods are direct but have the intrinsic difficulty that it is often impossible to guarantee a population of cDNA molecules of the gene of interest.

CpG islands

In 1986 Bird made the observation that regions of DNA that are rich in the dinucleotide CpG are often found near the 5′ end of expressed sequences. These clusters or **'CpG islands'** are unmethylated, despite the fact that most of the methylation in the mammalian genome occurs on the cytosine of CpG sequences. An alternative name, 'HTF islands', refers to *Hpa*II *tiny fragments*: these are 1–2 kb islands of genomic DNA, spaced

approximately 100 kb apart, that are released by digestion with the endonuclease *Hpa*II that cleaves unmethylated CCGG sequences. Indeed the reason that the
restriction endonucleases that are used for PFGE analysis cut genomic DNA so rarely is because they contain
CpG dinucleotides in their recognition sequences and do
not cut methylated DNA. These enzymes however will
cut DNA efficiently at CpG islands, where the DNA
remains unmethylated.

The development of a PFGE restriction map across a
region of genomic DNA will therefore highlight the positions of clusters of unmethylated CpG and hence the
likely site of a transcribed gene. These islands can be
selectively cloned from a contig of DNA and used to
screen cDNA libraries of expressed sequences from an
appropriate tissue. Several disease loci have been cloned
by virtue of their association with a CpG, island including the *CFTR* gene which is mutated in cystic fibrosis.
Recently, a biochemical method for direct isolation of
CpG islands from very complex DNA sources has been
devised and provides yet another method for providing
libraries of expressed human sequences.

cDNA selection

This method selects out coding sequences from a region
of genomic DNA by virtue of their complementarity to
sequences within a given cDNA library (Fig. 6.4). DNA
from the genomic region of interest is hybridized to
inserts from an entire cDNA library from a relevant
tissue. Complementary sequences within the two sources
of DNA are selectively amplified by PCR and cloned to
generate a small library enriched for genes from the
genomic region of interest. A limitation of this strategy is
that it depends on identifying a tissue in which the
disease gene is likely to be expressed. For example a
cDNA library made from brain mRNA would be appropriate in the search for a gene responsible for a neurodegenerative disorder; however for many disorders the
appropriate tissue may not be obvious.

Exon trapping

Exon amplification or 'trapping' is a novel procedure
that does not rely on identification of the primary site of
expression of a disease gene. Instead, this strategy
depends on the functional conservation of consensus
sequences surrounding the exons of individual genes, the
so-called donor and acceptor sites recognized by the
hnRNA splicing machinery of the cell nucleus. Small sections of DNA from the genomic region under study are

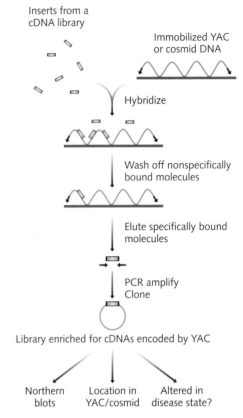

Fig. 6.4 Diagrammatic representation of the cDNA selection
method of cloning gene-coding sequences contained within
genomic DNA clones. cDNA inserts from a tissue-specific
library are generated by PCR amplification using vector-
specific oligonucleotide primers. These are hybridized to
immobilized genomic DNA and only those inserts with
sequence counterparts within the genomic contig are recovered
for cloning (adapted with permission from Hochgeshwender
(1992)).

expressed in a cellular system that promotes recognition
of these sequences and selective recovery of exons (Fig.
6.5). Potential limitations of this technique are the length
of DNA that can be effectively screened for exons and
the possibility of 'cryptic' consensus sequences that
result in recovery on non-exonic sections of DNA.

Conservation between species

Sequences that are conserved between species are more
likely to represent expressed genes than non-coding
DNA and this has been used as a basis for identifying
new genes. Traditionally, these sequences have been

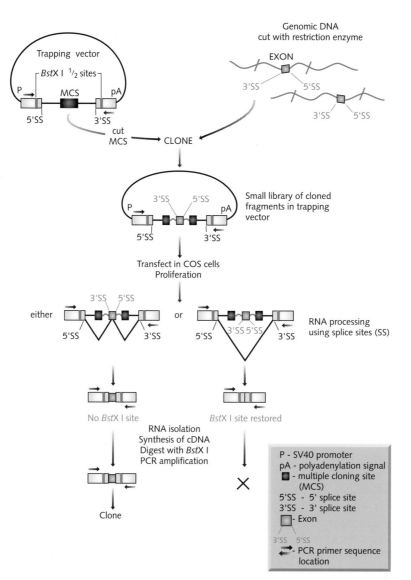

Fig. 6.5 Diagrammatic representation of exon amplification or 'trapping' from cloned DNA. Genomic DNA is subcloned into the trapping vector using one of several enzymes available in the multiple cloning site (MCS). Pools of clones are transfected into mammalian cells (COS) where they replicate and are transcribed under the control of SV40 viral sequences. Transcripts emanating from the SV40 promoter contain the inserted genomic sequence. Splice donor and acceptor sites (SS) in the vector and inserted DNA are used during the production of mature mRNA within the cells. PCR amplification of cDNA generated using total cellular RNA yields fragments that may contain exons from the genomic DNA or vector-only sequences. The latter however will not amplify if the cDNA is predigested with the enzyme *Bst*X 1. Recovered exons are examined by gel electrophoresis and cloned using sites available in the remaining flanking vector DNA.

identified through hybridizing many individual clones to DNA from many species on **'zoo blots'**. A modification of the procedure described above for cDNA selection, where the cDNA is replaced by genomic DNA from a different species, now allows for direct enrichment of sequences conserved between species.

Sequencing of genomic DNA

Recent improvements in sequencing technology have brought the possibility of completing sequencing regions of DNA likely to contain a disease locus, and several laboratories have now reported sequences up to several hundred kilobases. Computer programs have been developed in order to screen for potential **coding sequences** within these large stretches of DNA. A notable success for this strategy was the identification of the Kallmann syndrome gene from 60 kb of completely sequenced genomic DNA.

Identifying the disease gene

Once one or more candidate genes for a disease have been cloned, how can one decide which, if any, corresponds to the true disease gene? Clues to the suitability of a candidate include its profile of expression across a range of human tissues and its nucleotide sequence. It was clear, for example, that a gene with sequence similarity to a known peroxisomal membrane protein represented a good candidate for the gene responsible for adrenoleukodystrophy, a peroxisomal disorder (in real life, the main character of the film *Lorenzo's Oil* suffers from this crippling disease). However, definitive proof of the identity of a disease locus always relies on the detection of causal mutations within the gene in affected patients that are not found in the healthy population. The method of choice for screening for mutations will depend on the size of the gene, its genomic organization and whether it is expressed in an easily available source (such as lymphocytes).

Positional cloning at work

Table 6.4 depicts genes responsible for inherited disorders that have been identified through positional cloning and the remainder of this chapter will discuss some of these examples. Initially, we will describe the identification of novel genes responsible for three major debilitating disorders: DMD, cystic fibrosis and Huntington's disease. Each has a different mode of inheritance and as a group they illustrate different aspects of medical genetics.

Duchenne muscular dystrophy

DMD is an X-linked recessive disorder that affects one in 3500 boys (see Box 6.2 for clinical description). The first clues to the location of the DMD gene were cytogenetic. X: autosome translocations in rare cases of female DMD were found to involve breakage at Xp21, thus implicating this region of the chromosome. This was followed closely by genetic linkage to polymorphic DNA markers in Xp21 and the identification of large cytogenetically detectable deletions in boys with contiguous gene syndromes that included muscular dystrophy. One of these large deletions was used in a unique experiment designed to recover small DNA sequences that normally lay in the

---

Duchenne and Becker muscular dystrophy

Frequency

Approximately one in 3500 males.

Characteristics

Duchenne dystrophy shows progressive severe muscle weakness with associated hypertrophy before the age of 6 years with mild to severe mental impairment and cardiac disease. The patient is usually chair-bound by age 12 and succumbs to respiratory disease (inhalation/pneumonia) or cardiomyopathy disease by the age of 20 years. Becker dystrophy is associated with milder disease. Obligate heterozygous female carriers for either disorder may show segmental muscular hypertrophy and/or weakness together with mild mental retardation.

Transmission

X-linked (Xp21); one-third of affected males arise by *de novo* mutation. The defect represents marked deficiency of a large protein, dystrophin, found in skeletal and cardiac muscle as well as brain. The gene is one of the largest so far described — 2.4 Mb. Large deletions and mutations causing frameshifts are usually responsible for DMD. The milder Becker dystrophy is associated with a truncated or variant polypeptide product in which the mutations may include in-frame deletions.

Treatment

Supportive therapy only is currently available; trials of gene therapy to obtain expression of small sections of the dystrophin gene in myoblasts are proposed.

Box 6.2

---

deleted region. One of these sequences was found to be deleted in several unrelated DMD patients indicating that it lay within or very close to the DMD gene. This was used as a starting point from which to isolate neighbouring sequences that were highly conserved between species and expressed in skeletal muscle. Subsequently cDNA clones corresponding to an mRNA of 14 kb in size were isolated and found to correspond to the DMD gene.

Concurrently, another laboratory utilized the fact that one of the DMD translocations brought a region of chromosome 21 known to house ribosomal genes in juxtaposition with Xp21. Using ribosomal sequences as probes they were able to walk across the translocation breakpoint into the interrupted DMD gene. The sequences isolated by the two laboratories turned out to be several hundreds of kilobases apart, a curiosity that was not resolved until the genomic organization of the DMD gene was determined and it was found to be an extremely

Table 6.4 Disease genes identified by positional cloning.

Disease	Incidence*	Inheritance†	Gene	Primary map tools	Location	Function
X-linked chronic granulomatous disease (CGD)	Very rare	XLR	b-245β	Contiguous gene syndrome, deletions	Xp21	β subunit of cytochrome b-245
Duchenne muscular dystrophy (DMD)	Approx. 1/3500 males	XLR	DYS (Dystrophin)	Translocations, deletions, linkage	Xp21	Cytoskeletal membrane protein
Congenital adrenal hypoplasia (CAH)	Very rare	XLR	DAX-1	Contiguous gene syndrome, deletions	Xp21	Putative nuclear hormone receptor
Cystic fibrosis (CF)	Approx. 1/2500	AR	CFTR	Linkage	7q31	Ion channel
Fragile X syndrome (FRAXA)	Approx. 1/2000–1/4000 males	XL	FMR-1	Linkage, fragile site	Xq27.3	RNA binding protein
Possible mental retardation (FRAXE)	?	XL	?	Fragile site	Xq27	Unknown
Huntington's disease (HD)	Approx. 1/20000	AD	IT15 (Huntingtin)	Linkage	4p16.3	Unknown
Myotonic dystrophy (DM)	Approx. 1/8000	AD	DM	Linkage	19q13.3	Putative protein kinase
Spinocerebellar ataxia (SCAI)	Rare	AD	?	Linkage	6p22–23	Unknown
Dentatorubropallidoluysian atrophy (DRPLA)	Very rare	AD	B37	Linkage	12p	Unknown
Polycystic kidney disease	Approx. 1/1000	AD	PKD1	Linkage	16p13	Unknown
Glycerol kinase deficiency	Very rare	XLR	GK (glycerol kinase)	Contiguous gene syndrome, deletions	Xp22	Kinase
X-linked adrenoleukodystrophy (ALD)	Approx. 1/20000 males	XLR	ALD	Linkage, deletion	Xq28	Peroxisomal membrane protein
X-linked Kallmann syndrome	Approx. 1/10000	XLR	KAL	Contiguous gene syndrome, deletions	Xp	Putative neuronal guidance molecule
Tuberous sclerosis	Approx. 1/10000	AD	TSC2 (tuberin)	Linkage	16p13	Tumour supressor
Menkes disease and X-linked cutis laxa	Approx. 1/40000	AR	Mc1	Translocation	Xq13	Putative cation transporting ATPase
Wilson's disease	Approx. 1/30000	AR	pWD	Linkage	13q14.3	Putative cation transporting ATPase
Neurofibromatosis type 1 (NF1)	Approx. 1/3000	AD	NF1-GRP	Translocation, deletion	17q11.2	GTPase activator protein (GAP)-related protein
Neurofibromatosis type 2 (NF2)	Approx. 1/10000	AD	Merlin	Deletion, linkage	22q11–13	Tumour supressor, putative cytoskeletal linking protein

Table 6.4 *Continued.*

Disease	Incidence*	Inheritance†	Gene	Primary map tools	Location	Function
X-linked agammaglobulinaemia (XLA)	Approx. 1/100 000	XLR	CD19 (atk)	Linkage	Xq21–22	Putative protein kinase
Choroideraemia (TCD)	Very rare	XLR	TCD	Linkage, deletions, translocations	Xq21	Component A of RAB geranylgeranyl transferase
X-linked McLeod's syndrome	Rare	XLR	XK	Contiguous gene syndrome, deletions	Xp21	Putative membrane transporter
Norrie's syndrome	Very rare	XLR	NDP	Linkage, translocations, small deletions	Xp11.4–p11.3	Putative growth factor
Familial Alzheimer's disease (AD3)	Approx. 70% of familial early onset	AD	presenilin1	Linkage	14q24	Unknown, seven transmembrane domain protein
Emery–Dreifuss muscular dystrophy	Rare	XLR	EDMD (emerin)	Linkage	Xq28	Unknown
X-linked hypophosphataemic rickets (HYP)	Approx. 1/20 000	XLD	PEX	Linkage	Xp22	Putative endopeptidase regulating phosphate homeostasis
Oculocerebrorenal (OCRL-1, Lowes syndrome)	Very rare	XLR	OCRL-1	Translocations, linkage	Xq25–q26	Putative inositol polyphosphate-5-phosphatase
Familial breast cancer	1/200 women	AD	BRCA1	Linkage	17q21	Putative DNA binding protein
			BRCA2	Linkage, deletions	13q12–13	Unknown
von Hippel–Lindau disease	Approx. 1/30 000	AD	CHL	Linkage, deletions	3q25–26	Tumour suppressor
Hereditary non-polyposis colon cancer (HNPCC)	Approx. 1/50 000	AD	hMSH2	Linkage	2p16	DNA mismatch repair
Familial adenomatous polyposis	Approx. 1/8000	AD	APC	Linkage, cytogenetics	5q21	Tumour suppressor, cytoskeletal interactions? adhesion?
Retinoblastoma	Approx. 1/30 000	AD	RB1	Deletions, linkage	13q14.2	Tumour suppressor
Wilms' tumour	Approx. 1/10 000	Sporadic	WT1	Deletion	11p13	Tumour suppressor
Ataxia telangiectasia	Approx. 1/40 000	AR	ATM	Linkage	11q22–23	Putative phosphatidylinositol-3′ kinase
Treacher–Collins syndrome	Approx. 1/50 000	AD	Treacle	Linkage	5q32-33	Unknown

* Incidences are taken from individual papers or *McKusick's Mendelian Inheritance in Man*.
† XLR, X-linked recessive; AR, autosomal recessive; XL, X-linked; AD, autosomal dominant; XLD, X-linked dominant.

large gene containing over 100 exons and covering over 2300 kb of genomic DNA. At the time of its discovery the DMD gene was the largest gene identified although it has now been superseded by the neurofibromatosis (NF1) gene.

The complete nucleotide sequence of the DMD gene has been determined and inferences can be made about the structure of its protein product, dystrophin (Fig. 6.6). The 3685 amino acid protein is considered to be rod-like in shape and organized into four domains:

1 a 24 amino acid amino-terminal domain with homology to the actin binding domain of α-actinin;

2 a central domain consisting of 24 repeats showing some similarity to the cytoskeletal protein spectrin;

3 a cysteine-rich domain with homology to a region of α-actinin;

4 a carboxy-terminal domain unrelated to other proteins (with the exception of the related dystrophin-like gene product).

DMD gene expression occurs principally in skeletal, cardiac and smooth muscle as well as, somewhat unexpectedly, in brain. Expression in brain is characterized by the use of promoters and exons that are different from those used in muscle, indicating a role for different isoforms in each tissue. Dystrophin is a cytoskeletal membrane protein located on the cytoplasmic face of the cell membrane. Its function is unknown although it appears to be important for maintaining muscle cell integrity through its interaction with membrane proteins, such as the recently identified dystrophin-associated glycoproteins. Most mutations in the DMD gene are deletions (65%), which may reflect the size of the gene as a target for rearrangement. This high frequency of deletions facilitates **prenatal diagnosis** and **carrier detection** in those families where a deletion is present (Fig. 6.7). Tests have been developed that allow rapid simultaneous detection of multiple exons of the DMD gene in affected cases. However, in the 35% of cases where deletions are not found, the potential for intragenic recombination between the mutation and polymorphic markers within such a large gene makes accurate genetic counselling dif-

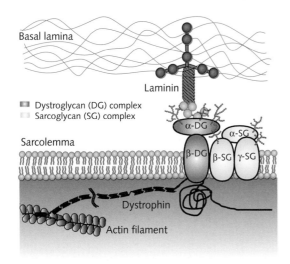

Fig. 6.6 The dystrophin–glycoprotein complex (DGC). Dystrophin has been shown to interact with a variety of molecules beneath the muscle sarcolemma. It is proposed to aggregate as a homotetramer and associate with F-actin at its amino-terminus. A region near the carboxy-terminus interacts with a group of proteins that form the DGC. These comprise dystroglycans and sarcoglycans that form a bridge between dystrophin and the extracellular matrix component laminin. The whole complex is clearly required for the maintenance of normal muscle and mutations in several components have been associated with muscular dystrophies (adapted from Worton (1995)).

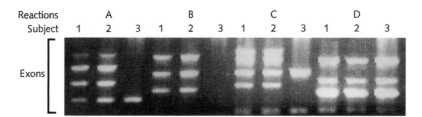

Fig. 6.7 Detection of deletions in the DMD gene. The PCR is used to amplify individual exons of the DMD gene in sets of three or four (multiplexing). In other words, three or four sets of primers are used in a single PCR reaction. The DMD gene consists of a total of 79 exons and therefore combining amplifications is the most efficient way of examining the whole gene. In this example 14 exons of the DMD gene have been analysed in four reactions (A, B, C and D) in three individuals (1, 2 and 3), where 1 is a healthy subject and 2 and 3 are patients with muscular dystrophy. Each band represents the presence of a single exon. Clearly all 14 exons are present in 2 whereas individual 3 has a deletion encompassing at least 6 exons of the DMD gene (data courtesy of Rosalind Clark, Molecular Genetics Laboratory, Addenbrooke's NHS Trust, Cambridge UK).

ficult—a fact that has prompted a search for more subtle mutations.

It is now well established that the less severe Becker muscular dystrophy (BMD) is also due to mutations in the dystrophin gene and is also often associated with large deletions. The difference in phenotype appears to be attributable to the effect of the respective deletions on the translational reading frame. In general BMD deletions, whilst eliminating large internal sections of dystrophin, preserve the reading frame and hence the downstream regions of the protein, whereas DMD deletions destroy the downstream protein coding potential. The observation that large sections of the DMD gene can be eliminated with little phenotypic effect has some interesting consequences for potential gene therapy as the cumbersome full length gene can be replaced by a more tractable, functional **minigene**.

Cystic fibrosis

Cystic fibrosis (CF) is the most common lethal autosomal recessive disease in Caucasian populations, afflicting one in 2000 newborns (see Box 6.3 for clinical description). An imbalance in water and ion transport in secretory epithelia leads to accumulation of a viscid mucus, which obstructs the intestine and the ducts of the biliary system and pancreas *in utero* and accumulates in the distal airways postnatally. The frequency of the disease implies that about one in 25 people of northern European extraction are heterozygotic carriers of a disease allele although they themselves will be completely asymptomatic and therefore unaware of their potential for having a CF child (one in 100).

Direct biochemical analysis did not reveal a malfunctioning protein in CF subjects but provided some clues as to the function of the gene product. As early as 1953 it was noted that CF children have excessive salt loss in their sweat and this observation led to the measurement of sodium and chloride in sweat as a diagnostic standard for the disease. In 1984 it was finally demonstrated that the normal efflux of chloride ions across epithelial cell membranes in response to elevated levels of the intracellular signalling molecule cyclic AMP (adenosine 3′, 5′-monophosphate) is deficient in CF patients. Furthermore, the activation of a cyclic AMP-dependent protein kinase (PKA) was unaffected in CF cells but PKA failed to elicit chloride conductance. This information, however, did not provide a route to identification of the underlying defect and a positional cloning strategy was adopted.

In contrast to DMD, no cytogenetic clues were available for locating the CF gene and its subchromosomal

Cystic fibrosis

Frequency

One in 2000 live births in Caucasian populations. Most common single defect causing premature death in children.

Pathology

Primary defect in chloride secretion by epithelial glands leading to abnormally viscid mucus.

Characteristics

Presents in infancy (meconium ileus) and childhood with failure to thrive, pancreatic exocrine failure, cough due to recurrent bronchopulmonary infection followed by lung destruction and bronchiectasis. Sterility occurs in males due to absence of vasa deferentia. Hepatic cirrhosis due to obstructive biliary disease occurs in both sexes. Diagnosis based on raised sweat sodium and chloride concentrations. Premature death usually occurs in the second to third decade although some patients may now survive to the fifth decade. Death is usually caused by progressive lung destruction and the consequences of pulmonary sepsis.

CF may be diagnosed before or at birth by the finding of reduced tryptic activity in blood and by molecular analysis of *CFTR* genes for the presence of widespread mutations that inactivate the gene product, e.g. ΔF508. The utility of mass screening for CF has not yet been established.

Inheritance

Autosomal recessive disorder representing mutations in the *CFTR* gene on chromosome 7.

Treatment

Supplements of pancreatic enzymes and fat-soluble vitamins, vigorous regular chest physiotherapy and drainage with prophylactic antibiotics. Surgical relief may be needed for small intestinal obstruction due to inspissated mucus. Hepatic transplantation has been used for end-stage biliary cirrhosis and heart–lung transplantation has been successfully applied in patients with terminal respiratory disease and cor pulmonale. Several therapeutic trials of somatic gene therapy in CF are currently in progress.

Box 6.3

position was derived solely through linkage analysis. Although CF is inherited as an autosomal recessive trait the frequency of the disease made this approach feasible and after a period of 5 years the gene was assigned to a region on chromosome 7 (7q31). The genetic location of the gene was ultimately whittled down to a region of less than 1 cM. A combination of chromosome walking and jumping techniques were used to provide DNA clones

(a)

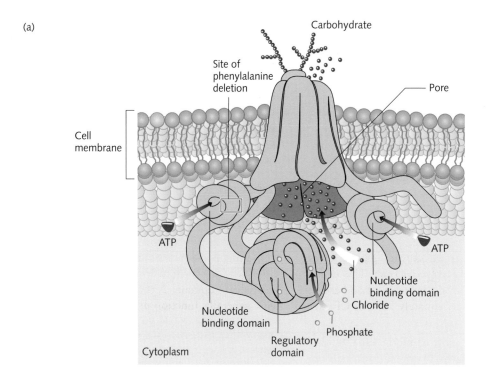

(b)

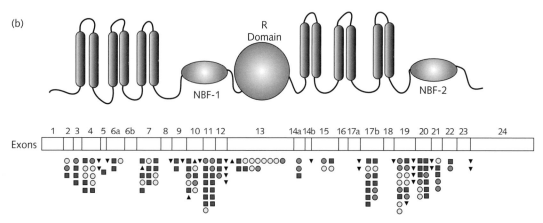

Spectrum of mutations responsible for CF. The location and nature of CF mutations identified by the
Cystic Fibrosis Genetic Analysis Consortium are indicated below a schematic of the CFTR protein

(■) Missense mutation   (▲) In-frame deletion   (●) Nonsense mutation   (○) Frame-shift   (▼) Splicing mutation

Fig. 6.8 The CFTR protein and its spectrum of mutations. (a) A model for the structure of the intact CFTR protein inserted in the cell membrane. Passage of chloride ions through the channel is regulated by the nucleotide binding folds (NBF1 and NBF2) that hydrolyse ATP and the phosphorylatable regulatory (R) domain. The position of the ΔF508 mutation within NBF1 is shown (adapted from Welsh and Smith (1995)). (b) The spectrum of mutations responsible for CF with respect to domains of the unfolded protein (adapted from Collins (1992)).

that could be used for further genetic and physical mapping of the critical region. During this process DNA polymorphisms were identified that were in linkage disequilibrium with the CF locus, that is, over 84% of CF chromosomes were associated with a particular set of alleles (haplotype) at these sites. This indicated that not only were these polymorphic markers likely to be close to the CF gene but also that a single mutation was likely to account for most of the CF alleles.

A candidate for the CF gene was finally identified by its association with a CpG island and expression in sweat glands, lungs and pancreas. This gene was transcribed from a 250 kb region of genomic DNA and its mRNA was about 6.5 kb. Consistent with a role in CF it is expressed almost exclusively in epithelial cells with the highest levels in pancreas, salivary glands, sweat glands, intestine and the reproductive tract. The identity of the gene was confirmed by the presence of a 3 basepair deletion in exon 10 of approximately 70% of CF chromosomes, supporting the suspected homogeneity of most mutant alleles. The 3 basepairs deletion results in deletion of a phenylalanine at position 508 in the mature protein (ΔF508) (Figs 6.8 and 6.9). Furthermore, transfer of full length wild-type gene into CF cells was shown to be suffcient for correction of the chloride channel defect.

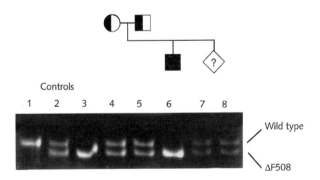

Controls

1   2   3   4   5   6   7   8

Wild type

ΔF508

Fig. 6.9 Prenatal diagnosis for cystic fibrosis. Detection of the common mutation ΔF508 in a family with one affected child. The PCR is used to amplify a section of the CFTR gene surrounding the common 3 basepair deletion ΔF508. Products are resolved on a gel that allows discrimination between deleted (lower) and non-deleted, wild-type alleles. Lanes 1–3 contain controls for homozygous normal (1), homozygous deleted (3) and heterozygous patterns (2). Lanes 4 and 5 indicate that both parents are heterozygous carriers of the deletion and lane 6 shows that the affected child has inherited both defective copies of the gene. Two chorionic villi from an unborn fetus were also analysed (lanes 7 and 8) and a heterozygous pattern indicates that he/she will be an unaffected carrier of the mutation (data courtesy of Rob MacMahon, Molecular Genetics Laboratory, Addenbrooke's NHS Trust, Cambridge, UK).

To reflect what was known about the CF defect at that time, the CF protein was designated CFTR for 'cystic fibrosis transmembrane conductance regulator'. However, subsequent experiments indicate that CFTR itself can function as an ion channel. The predicted amino acid sequence of CFTR reveals homology to a large family of proteins involved in active transport across cell membranes. Member of this highly conserved superfamily, frequently referred to as the ABC (ATP-binding cassette) family, have in common two hydrophobic transmembrane (TM) domains and one or two nucleotide binding folds (NBFs) that bind and cleave ATP providing energy for transport across the membrane. The predicted structure of CFTR is illustrated in Fig. 6.8. In addition to two TM and NBF domains it contains a highly charged central region predicted to be the target for PKA-mediated serine phosphorylation, the R (regulatory) domain. Although the ABC family of proteins generally function as active transporters there is now convincing evidence that CFTR functions as a PKA-activated ion channel. Experiments that examine CFTR in cell-free membrane systems have resulted in a model for CFTR function that involves phosphorylation of the R domain followed by binding of ATP as separable events that lead to opening of the chloride channel.

Many of the mutations found in CF patients, including ΔF508, result in defective intracellular trafficking, i.e. may prevent the translated CFTR protein from being dispatched to its correct location in the cell membrane. Still others prevent the protein from being made at all or specifically disrupt the activity of its functional domains.

While ΔF508 accounts for 70% of mutant CFTR alleles, diverse mutations have been identified amongst the remaining 30%. About 20 of these are common in northern European populations whereas the rest are extremely rare. Mutations have been observed in all functional domains and phenotype : genotype correlations have been attempted. The least disruptive mutations occur in infertile males who have little if any pulmonary or gastrointestinal involvement. The common ΔF508 mutation is associated with severe CF accompanied by pancreatic insufficiency and often meconium ileus. By screening for the most common mutations about 85–90% of CF carriers and 70% of carrier couples can be identified and this has raised the possibility of population screening for couples at risk of bearing CF children. Pilot studies to assess the appropriateness of such screening in view of the inability to detect all mutations and the consequent load on the counselling services are currently under way in several countries. An example of diagnosis based on detection of ΔF508 is shown in Fig. 6.9.

Approaches to CF therapy are focused on the pulmonary consequences of CF since these usually determine the course of the disease. Although improvements in management of CF lung disease in the last few years have led to improved survival, premature death and physical disability are frequent. Cloning of the disease gene offers a route to a better understanding of the disease process and also the possibility of somatic gene therapy. The epithelium of the respiratory tract may prove to be an accessible target for gene delivery, although there is debate as to whether the epithelium itself or the submucosal layer represents the best physiological target for corrective therapy. The efficacy and safety of several delivery systems are being explored ranging from recombinant adenoviruses to liposomes. The recent development of mouse models for CF by transgenic technology provides a system for examining potential therapies. *In vitro* experiments indicate that as few as 6% of cells need be successfully corrected with wild-type CF protein for a physiologically competent cell monolayer to be produced. Important questions still need to be answered, however, before CF gene therapy can become available. As with any inherited disorder for which corrective treatment is considered we need to know if overexpression of CFTR is toxic; how long expression will persist; whether the immune system will intervene; and how safety can be ensured (see Chapter 16).

Huntington's disease

Huntington's disease (HD) is a progressive degenerative disorder of the central nervous system with onset in middle age and death some 15–20 years later (see Box 6.4). Affected subjects exhibit chorea, impaired motor coordination, dementia and a variety of psychiatric disorders. The condition is inherited as an autosomal dominant trait and affects about one in 2500 adults. As for CF, the frequency of the disease and lack of cytogenetic or biochemical indicators prompted the use of linkage analysis for pursuing the gene for this disease. The Huntington locus was the first gene to be localized to a subchromosomal region (4p16.3) by this method, in 1983. Despite its early location the HD gene proved to be particularly elusive, some 10 years elapsing before it was finally isolated in 1993. This was due not only to a lack of cytogenetically detectable changes but also to a scarcity of informative meiotic recombination events.

Isolation of the Huntington's gene thus required the development of a large well-characterized genomic

---

Huntington's disease

Frequency

Three to seven in 100 000 adults.

Pathology

Neurone loss with gliosis in striatum and cortex.

Characteristics

Degenerative disorder of the basal ganglia and cerebral cortex leading to dementia, choreic movements, emotional and cognitive impairment, hallucinations, paranoia, personality changes, agitation. Progression of dementia leads to death within 20 years from the onset. The peak age of onset is 40 years, but onset is occasionally variable and occurs before the age of 20.

Inheritance

The disorder is inherited as an autosomal dominant trait. Sporadic cases arise. The gene maps to chromosome 4p16.3. With successive generations, the age of onset usually decreases — a phenomenon known as 'anticipation' that characterizes autosomal dominant 'triplet-repeat' disorders. Juvenile disease appears to be more frequent in the offspring of males with Huntington's, indicating a sex bias in the stability of the repeat sequence in the gametes.

Molecular defects involve expansion of a trinucelotide repeat sequence, CAG, in affected individuals, The sequence encodes a glutamine residue and there is evidence that the polyglutamine tracts occur in-frame within the Huntington gene translation product. Several homozygous individuals showing a pattern of disease identical to that manifest in affected heterozygotes suggest that the presence of a polyglutamine tract represents a gain of function mutation.

Treatment

Symptomatic for movement disorder and agitation and depression; presynaptic dopamine-depleting agents (e.g. reserpine) may reduce agitation. Huntington's disease raises important ethical questions in relation to carrier testing in affected pedigrees and for counselling first-degree relatives of affected individuals.

Box 6.4

---

contig across the candidate region (over 2 Mb), identification of a region of strong linkage disequilibrium (about 500 kb) and, finally, an exhaustive search for expressed sequences. The HD gene, originally called *IT15*, was finally isolated through exon trapping. The identity of *IT15* came from the observation that a section of the gene encoding multiple copies of the amino acid glutamine (gln) was expanded in all cases of the disorder compared with healthy controls. This was only the third example of a novel mechanism for mutation now called dynamic mutation whereby highly unstable regions of DNA expand and contract in association with disease (see p. 120). The HD gene comprises 67 exons with a coding region of 10 366 basepairs and the unstable CAG, encoding glutamine, resides at the 5′ end.

Unlike CF, the predicted protein sequence of the *IT15* product, huntingtin, has no clear homology to other proteins and little is known of its structure and function. The gene is widely expressed in neural and non-neural tissues and whilst it is highly expressed in brain, its distribution does not correlate with HD neuropatholgy (most prominent in the basal ganglia). Since HD is an autosomal dominant disorder and affected individuals have not yet been found to over- or under-express *IT15*, the pathological effects of the mutation are assumed to be due to a deleterious gain of function by the expanded gene. This is supported by studies in several individuals known to be homozygous for the dynamic mutations: they show no increase in the severity of their condition.

Trinucleotide repeat expansions are the only form of mutation so far found associated with HD. The repeat is naturally polymorphic with a repeat range of 11–36 in healthy individuals compared with 30–100 in affected cases and, in general, the size of the repeated region is inversely correlated with age of onset. The homogeneous nature of mutation type in HD is an obvious advantage for the diagnostic laboratory (Fig. 6.10). Furthermore, spontaneous HD has been shown to arise from expansion of already large alleles in the healthy population meaning that sibs of sporadic cases may be at risk. As with all triplet repeat disorders the mechanism of expansion in HD is unclear although there is a documented sex bias in transmission. Juvenile onset, associated with larger repeat lengths, is paternally determined because the repeat is particularly unstable in developing male gametes.

Finally, although identification of the HD gene will undoubtedly lead to improvements in presymptomatic detection, this must be accompanied by careful counselling and support protocols. Clearly, many complex ethical and social issues will be encountered in the management of this devastating disorder as our methods to diagnose it improve.

Candidate genes

Occasionally, gene searchers find themselves in the fortunate position that a well-characterized, ideal candidate gene has already been placed on the genomic map in the approximate region to which they have localized their disease gene, and they are saved the laborious task of

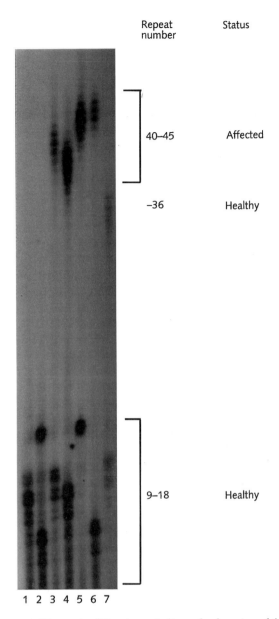

Fig. 6.10 Diagnosis of Huntington's disease by detection of the expanded repeat. The PCR is used to amplify a section of DNA containing the CAG repeat within the *Huntingtin* gene and the products are resolved by gel electrophoresis. Due to the nature of the repeat and its instability, variation in size is seen for any one DNA sample. Lanes 1, 2 and 3 show fragment sizes within the normal range. Lanes 4, 5 and 6 show sizes obtained for individuals with one expanded (disease) allele and one normal allele and lane 7 shows a size that lies at the upper limit of the normal range (36 basepair) (data courtesy of David Rubinstein, Molecular Genetics Laboratory, Addenbrooke's NHS Trust, Cambridge, UK).

Table 6.5 Examples of genes identified through candidate recognition.

Disease	Location	Gene	Gene function
Marfan's syndrome	15q12–21	*FBN*	Extracellular matrix component fibrillin
X-linked hydrocephalus and MASA syndrome	Xq28	*L1*	Neural cell adhesion molecule
Familial hyperekplexia	5q33–35	*GLRA1*	α subunit of receptor for glycine, an inhibitory neurotransmitter
Familial motor neurone disease (amyelotrophic lateral sclerosis, Lou Gehrig's disease)	21q22.1	*SOD1*	Cytosolic Cu/Zn superoxide dismutase
X-linked familial exudative vitreoretinopathy (XLFEVR)	Xp11.4–11.3	*NDP* (Norries disease gene)	Putative extracellular growth factor/ guidance molecule
Retinitis pigmentosa (autosomal dominant)	3q21–qter	*RHO* (rhodopsin)	Photoreceptor eye pigment
X-linked hyper-IgM deficiency (HIGMX-1)	Xq26	*gp39*	CD40 ligand
Charcot–Marie–Tooth neuropathies			
Type 1A	17p11.2–p12	*PMP22*	Myelin component
Type 1B	1q22–23	*Po*	Myelin component
Miller–Dieker lissencephaly	17p13.3	*LIS-1*	45 kb subunit of platelet activating factor acetylhydrolase
Craniosynostoses			
Pfeiffer syndrome	8p11.2	*FGFR1 +2*	Fibroblast growth factor receptors
Crouzon syndrome	10q25–26	*FGFR2*	
Jackson–Weiss		*FGFR2*	
Apert		*FGFR2*	
Craniosynostosis Boston type	5q34–35	*MSX2*	Homeotic gene
Achondroplasia	4p	*FGFR3*	Fibroblast growth factor receptor 3
Waardenberg's syndrome	2q35	*PAX3*	Homeotic gene
Supravalvular aortic stenosis	7q11.2	*elastin (ELN)*	Extracellular matrix component
Gitelman's hypokalaemic alkalosis	16q13	*TSC*	Thiazide-sensitive Na–Cl co-transporter
Usher syndrome 1B	11q13	*Myosin VIIA*	Unconventional myosin
Familial hypertrophic cardiomyopathy (FHC)	14q12	*Myosin H7*	Cardiac myosin heavy chain
Familial aggressive behaviour	Xp	*MOA*	Monoamine oxidase
Familial melanoma	9p21	*p16*	Cyclin-dependent kinase inhibitor

Table 6.5 *Continued.*

Disease	Location	Gene	Gene function
Multiple endocrine neoplasia type 2 (MEN2)	10q11.2	*RET*	Proto-oncogene
Familial Hirschprung's disease	10q11.2	*RET* (*MEN2A* gene)	Proto-oncogene
Muscular dystrophies			
Limb girdle MD2A (LGMD2A)	15q15–22	*CAPN3* (calpain 3)	Cysteine protease
Severe congenital MD (CMD)	6q22–23	Merosin	Laminin subunit
LGMD2D and autosomal recessive MD (ARMD)	17q12–q21	α-sarcoglycan (adhalin or ADL)	Components of dystrophin glycoprotein complex
LGMD2E and ARMD	4q12	β-sarcoglycan	
Severe childhood ARMD (SCARMD)	13q12	γ-sarcoglycan	

mapping and gene isolation across megabases of DNA. Table 6.5 lists some recent examples where positional cloning has been accelerated by this occurrence. For example, the gene for Marfan's syndrome, an autosomal dominant disorder characterized by vascular and skeletal deformities (see Box 6.5), was found by linkage analysis to reside in chromosomal region 15q15–15q21. Histological examination in these patients had revealed a disturbance of connective tissue structure and when the gene for fibrillin (*FBN1*), a connective tissue component, was mapped to the same region it became an obvious candidate for the Marfan's locus. Furthermore, prompted by this association a second related disorder, dominant ectopia lentis, was also found to be due to mutations in the *FBN1* gene.

A similar unexpected revelation was the co-localization of hereditary motor neurone disease (amyotrophic lateral sclerosis (ALS) or Lou Gehrig's disease) with the gene for cytosolic superoxide dismutase (SOD) on chromosome 21. The discovery of mutations in SOD in this familial form of ALS has implications for the progression of sporadic non-hereditary forms and may lead to a greater understanding of the mechanisms that underlie the progression of other forms of motor neurone disease.

Candidate loci will present themselves more frequently as the density of genes on the human map increases. Particularly relevant to this approach is the generation of large databases of partially sequenced cDNA clones during the development of the HGP. Over 30 000 novel cDNAs have now been identified and par-

tially sequenced to produce these 'expressed sequence tags' (ESTs). As these genes become assigned to specific chromosomes they will represent candidates for a wide variety of hereditary disorders, even though the function of many of the cDNAs marked by these annotated partial sequences is quite unknown. The mapping of disease loci will ultimately lead to the discovery of the function of many genes that have been catalogued as cloned cDNAs but despite partial sequence characterization, remain operationally unidentified.

Unusual characteristics of some human genetic disorders

Dynamic mutations

The discovery of the gene responsible for the development of the neurological symptoms associated with fragile X uncovered a new mechanism for disease-causing mutation, the expansion of a region of **unstable DNA sequences**. Since the demonstration that the fragile X syndrome is caused by enormous increases in the numbers of an exonic CGG **trinucleotide repeat**, several other human diseases have been found to be due to a similar mechanism of mutation (Table 6.6).

In most cases these dynamic mutations occur in diseases that display an unusual inheritance pattern such as incomplete penetrance, or increased severity or earlier onset with each new generation (anticipation) in a single pedigree. These unusual features are beginning to be

Marfan's syndrome

Prevalance

The syndrome affects approximately one in 10 000 individuals.

Characteristics

Dominantly inherited, connective tissue disorder with skeletal abnormalities: tall stature, spinal deformity, lax ligaments, spider-like digits; cardiovascular abnormalities: mitral valve prolapse, regurgitation, aortic dilatation with aortic aneurysm and dissection; dislocation of the lens and myopia. Prognosis is related to cardiac manifestations: aortic dissection and regurgitation resulting from dilatation reduces life expectancy by one-third in untreated patients.

Inheritance

Autosomal dominant. Paternal age effect demonstrable with suspected *de novo* mutations responsible for the condition in a proportion of affected subjects. Diverse molecular defects in the fibrillin gene *FBN1*, localized on chromosome 15q21.1. Fibrillin is a 350 kDa protein component of extracellular microfibrils. Most mutations appear to be restricted to single pedigrees and are uniformly distributed throughout the cDNA sequence causing differential effects on fibrillin synthesis and deposition that may show correlation with phenotypic groups. Interestingly, although fibrillin metabolism is abnormal in cultured fibroblasts from patients with Marfan's syndrome, fibrillin synthetic defects were found in fibroblasts cultured from patients showing some Marfanoid features but who do not meet all the established criteria for the diagnosis of the syndrome.

Treatment

Medical: β-adrenergic blockade is effective in slowing the rate of aortic dilatation and significantly reduces the development of aortic complications. Surgical: aortic root replacement with a composite graft is used to treat acute dissection of the ascending aorta but surgical prophylaxis has limited application.

Box 6.5

understood in the context of unstable mutations that can change the length of a stretch of repeat sequences (increase or decrease) within a gene. The number of diseases known to be associated with unstable repeats is rapidly increasing and although the general mechanism for mutation appears similar there are many differences emerging between the characteristics of each repeat (summarized in Table 6.6). For example, the level of expansion of each repeat appears to reflect whether it is contained within a translated (spinal and bulbar muscular atrophy (SBMA), HD, spinocerebellar atrophy type 1 (SCA1)) or untranslated (fragile X syndrome, myotonic

dystrophy (DM)) region of the disease gene. Marked **effects of parental origin** are observed in these disorders so that transmission of congenital or early-onset forms may be either maternally or paternally determined. Differences have also been determined for the timing of expansion. For example, the HD repeat is particularly unstable in male gametes but stable in somatic tissues, unlike the FRAXA repeat which can undergo striking expansion postzygotically. Additional influences on the potential effects of a dynamic mutation include imprinting and increased methylation of the expanded allele; these influences have been demonstrated in the fragile X syndrome.

Finally, although the initial associations between dynamic mutations and disease have been made for a few monogenic disorders and triplet repeats, recent studies on somatic mutations in several forms of cancer demonstrate that variation in repeat copy number may have more general and fundamental importance as a mechanism for mutation. In particular, deficient repair of expanded repeat lesions may predispose to the development of neoplastic change in hereditary cancer syndromes.

Genetic heterogeneity

Analysis of single gene disorders is sometimes complicated by genetic heterogeneity, that is, where mutations in different genes give rise to the same or a similar phenotype. Within individual pedigrees, these disorders are still inherited as simple Mendelian traits but pooling of families for genetic linkage analysis can have misleading consequences. Experiments carried out by Bateson and Punnett with two white-flowered varieties of sweet pea first explored the interactions between different genes that affect the same trait. Crossing the two white varieties of sweet pea gave rise to first-generation flowers that were unexpectedly purple. Self-fertilization of the purple offspring led to purple and white flowers in a ratio of 9 : 7. This was explained by postulating that homozygosity for alleles of two distinct genes inhibited the production of purple pigment; the presence of a product (in this case an enzyme involved in the biosynthesis of anthocyanins) from each gene is necessary for the development of the flower colour. Since the white phenotype results from recessive genes, inheritance of one or more dominant alleles at each locus in nine of the 16 possible genotypes in the second-generation progeny leads to the observed proportion of purple flowers. Bateson termed the interactions of alleles at different loci on observable traits **epistasis**. Epistatic interactions have proved valuable in the analysis of metabolic pathways

Table 6.6 Dynamic mutations.

	Fragile X syndrome (FRAXA)	Spinobulbar muscular atrophy (SBMA)	Myotonic dystrophy (DM)	Huntington's disease (HD)	Spinocerebellar ataxia type 1 (SCA1)	Mild mental retardation (FRAXE)	Dentatorubropallidoluysian atrophy (DRPLA)
Inheritance	X-linked dominant with incomplete penetrance	X-linked recessive, variable severity	Autosomal dominant	Autosomal dominant	Autosomal dominant	X-linked	Autosomal dominant
Anticipation	Possibly	?	Yes	Yes	Yes	?	Yes
Sex bias for transmission of severe form	Maternal	?	Maternal	Paternal	Paternal	?	Paternal
Gene	FMR1	Androgen receptor (AR)	DM	IT15	?	?	B37
Chromsomal location	Xq27.3	Xq11–12	19q13.3	4p16.3	6p22–23	Xq27	12p
Gene expression	Widely expressed	Primarily genital tissue	?	Widely expressed	Widely expressed	?	Widely expressed
Repeat (codon) and location	CCG 5' UTR	CAG (gln) protein coding	CAG 3' UTR	CAG (gln) protein coding	CAG (gln) protein coding	CCG ?UTR	CAG (gln) protein coding
Normal range repeat no.	10–50	11–31	5–35	9–34	25–36	6–25	7–23
Disease range repeat no.	52–200 = pre-mutation 200–2000 = full mutation	40–62	50–80 = proto-mutation 80–2000 = affected	30–100	43–81	?> 25 < 200 = pre-mutation >200 = full mutation	49–75
Protein	Putative RNA binding protein	Androgen receptor	Putative protein kinase	?	?	?	?
Disease-causing mechanism	Transcriptional silencing with abnormal methylation	Abnormal protein—gain of function?	Altered level of mRNA/protein?	Abnormal protein—gain of function?	Abnormal protein—gain of function?	?	Abnormal protein—gain of function?

UTR, untranslated region.

and have allowed the complementary action of genes involved in several biosynthetic processes to be determined.

Epistatic effects provide the explanation for many apparently anomalous observations, e.g. the inheritance of coat colour in animals and the transmission of many human traits. A well-known medical example is provided by the inheritance of recessive deaf mutism: the progeny of parents with deaf mutism that later proves to be due to distinct genetic forms of deafness have often unexpectedly been noted to have normal hearing. This is because of **mutual complementation** of the respective genetic defects in the doubly heterozygous offspring. Table 6.7 lists diseases for which genetic heterogeneity has been recognized in humans and where in some cases

relevant genes have been isolated. A notable example of this phenomenon is familial autosomal dominant Alzheimer's disease where a fraction of families with early-onset disease (~10%) carry mutations in the gene for the β-amyloid gene and others harbour mutations in a gene on chromosome 14 or other as yet unknown loci. Similarly, at least three genetically distinct loci have been found to give rise to the syndrome of peripheral neuropathy associated with Charcot–Marie–Tooth disease and further loci responsible for this disease remain to be defined (Box 6.6).

One locus, several disorders

A phenomenon that represents the counterpart of

Table 6.7 Genetic heterogeneity.

Disease	Inheritance	Phenotype	Gene	Chromosomal location
Familial Alzheimer's disease (FAD)	AD (AD1)	Progressive neurodegeneration	*βAPP* (β amyloid precursor)	21q11.2–q21
	AD (AD2)	Progressive neurodegeneration	*APOE*4* (apolipoprotein)	19q12–q13
	AD (AD3)	Progressive neurodegeneration	*PS1* (presenilin 1)	14q24
	AD (AD4)	Progressive neurodegeneration	*PS2* (presenilin 2)	1q31–42
Charcot–Marie–Tooth (CMT)	AD (CMT1A)	Peripheral neuropathy	*PMP22* (peripheral myelin protein 22)	17p11.2–p12
	AD (CMT1B)	Peripheral neuropathy	*Po* (myelin protein 0)	1q22–q23
	XL	Peripheral neuropathy	*Cx32* Connexin 32 gap junction protein subunit	Xq13
	AR	Peripheral neuropathy	?	8q
Tuberous sclerosis	AD	Tuberous lesions in brain; facial angiomas, other tumours		9q22–q34
			Tumour suppressor	16p13
Polycystic kidney disease (PKD)	AD (PKD1)	Renal cysts		16p13
	AD (PKD2)			4q21–23
Retinitis pigmentosa (RP)	AR	Constriction of visual fields, night blindness, fundus changes	*PDEA* *PDEB* (cGMP phosphodiesterase subunits)	5q31.2
	AD (RP1)		?	8p11–q21
	AD (RP4)		*RHO* (rhodopsin)	3q21–qter
	AD (RP)		*RDS* (peripherin)	6p
	XLR			Xp
Oculocutaneous albinism (OCA)	AR (OCA1)	Hypopigmentation of skin, hair and eyes	Tyrosinase	11q14–q21
	AR (OCA2)		P gene	15q11–q13
Epidermolysis bullosa simplex (EBS)	AD	Epidermal fragility, blistering	Keratin 1	12q11–q13
			Keratin 14	17q12–q21
			Keratin 5	12q11–q13

AD, autosomal dominant; AR, autosomal recessive; XLD, X-linked dominant; XLR, X-linked recessive.

genetic heterogeneity occurs when different mutations at a single locus can give rise to clinically distinct disorders. The most prominent example of this is provided by the androgen receptor gene on the X-chromosome. Diverse mutations that affect the ability of the receptor to respond to androgens have been identified in androgen insensitivity syndromes associated with an astonishingly wide variation of under-virilization in 46XY (genotypically male) individuals. This syndrome includes patients with testicular feminization who are phenotypically indistinguishable from normal females, but who are sterile. However, expansion of a glutamine repeat in the first exon of the gene results in late-onset SBMA with only mild insensitivity to androgens (Table 6.6). The neuropathology in SBMA patients must result from a novel gain of function of the androgen receptor since even complete deletion of the androgen receptor gene in

humans is not accompanied by the development of SBMA.

After cloning: fruits of gene isolation

Single genes and developmental disorders

Intensive investigations of the development of invertebrates such as *Drosophila* and the nematode worm *Caenorhabditis* have provided much information about the molecular code that determines the **formation of the body plan** of an animal from the earliest stages of embryonic development. Studies on the origin of cell lineages have helped to define what determines the fate of each cell in relation to its ancestry and its neighbours. This has allowed for the prediction of the position of each cell in *Caenorhabditis* and its ancestors from a developmental

Charcot–Marie–Tooth disease (hereditary peroneal muscular atrophy syndromes)

Frequency estimates

Autosomal dominant: one in 3000; autosomal recessive: one in 70 000; X-linked dominant: one in 28 000.

Characteristics

Degeneration of spinal nerve roots especially motor roots distally with mixed sensory loss and delayed motor conduction. Pathology shows evidence of distal axonal disease with signs of recurrent segmental demyelination and remyelination associated with concentric (onion-skin) nerve thickening. Clinical features include marked wasting of peroneal (lateral leg) compartment muscles with or without hypertrophy associated with extreme lower limb distal atrophy; deformed feet. In some syndromes, sensory loss (especially of pain and temperature fibres) leads to perforating ulcers especially of feet often associated with unsuspected joint injury and bone fractures. Motor conduction is slowed.

Inheritance

Autosomal dominant, autosomal recessive and X-linked dominant forms have been recognized.

Treatment

Supportive care, pain relief and physiotherapy; specialist foot care is essential.

Box 6.6

tree that follows cell division from the earliest stages of embryonic development.

Developmental genetics in *Drosophila* have by mutational and molecular examination defined determinants for the body plan formation and indicate how mutations change the fate of given cells that determine somatic form. In *Drosophila*, recombinant DNA techniques have allowed many genes that regulate development to be isolated and analysed in terms of expression *in situ* during embryogenesis and by *in vitro* mutagenesis and transduction. Of particular interest in relation to mammalian studies has been the identification of **genes that control segmentation** in the early embryo. These **homeotic** genes control not only the number and organization of segments but also, through expression at different positions along the anteroposterior axis of the developing embryo, determine spatial and temporal patterns of development. Mutations in these genes are associated with monstrous deformations in the appearance of the adult animal and this phenomenon, **homeosis**, was first so designated by

Bateson. In its extreme form, one part of the body becomes converted into another.

Analysis of cloned homeotic genes has shown that they share a conserved 180 basepair segment, the homeobox, encoding a 60 amino acid segment, or **homeo domain**. The homeo domain is capable of binding to DNA in a sequence-specific manner that activates or represses the transcription of specific target genes and appears to confer a specific function on each of the homeotic gene products. Temporal and spatial regulation of these homeotic gene clusters is associated with developmental regulation of segmentation. Once the homeotic genes are activated in their particular cells of expression, they continue to be expressed during the lifetime of the animal.

The discovery of the homeoboxes led to questions about the universality of the developmental programmes that they represent. Southern blotting experiments of genomic DNA from many organisms digested with restriction enzymes and probed with *Drosophila* homeobox cDNA, allowed the recognition of homologous homeobox sequences throughout the animal kingdom, including mice and humans. In mice and humans similar arrays of genes known as *Hox* clusters are located on each of four chromosomes. At the 3′ end of each gene cluster the genes are similar to each other and to one of the insect homeotic genes and similar relationships pertain to other elements of the clusters. It appears that during development of the embryo *Hox* genes are expressed in a continuous block starting at the anterior limit and running posteriorly to the end of the developing vertical column corresponding to the somites. This is also reflected in timing of expression and the order of genes within each *Hox* cluster.

Selective disruption of specific homeobox genes has been carried out experimentally in mice, leading to the birth of animals homozygously disrupted for specific *Hox* sequences (Chapter 3). The phenotype of these mice harbouring targeted knockouts has provided insights into the genetic determination of **segmental identity** during embryogenesis. Clearly the homologues of the *Hox* genes in humans may be implicated in developmental disorders even though these often represent complex syndromes at birth. Of particular interest was the recent identification of mutations in human *pax-3* genes that were found to be causal in Waardenberg's syndrome. Waardenberg's syndrome is associated with pigmentary abnormalities in the iris, face and hair, as well as middle ear defects that could probably be ascribed to disordered branchial arch development in the early human embryo (see Box 6.7). The subsequent identification of another example of a homeotic gene defect (*MX2*) in a rare form of craniosynostosis (Box 6.8) is an indication of the link between single loci and **complex developmental abnormalities.**

Since *Hox* genes confer identity on the segments of the brain and skeleton as well as other tissues and represent a mutually interacting regulatory network, they represent an attractive area for the study of complex developmental abnormalities in humans which may ultimately derive from mutations in single genes. Transgenic inactivation by gene targeting of the *Hox-1.5* gene in mouse embryonic stem cells produces an experimental model of the human developmental syndrome, Di George's syndrome (Box 6.9), further evidence of the potential

---

Waardenberg's syndrome

Characteristics

A diverse syndrome of cranial pigmentary abnormalities, deafness and widening of the nasal bridge due to lateral displacement of the inner canthus of the eyes. Deafness occurs due to cochlear maldevelopment in up to 20% and may be associated with hair lip or cleft palate. White forelock and heterochromia of the irides are the most characteristic pigmentary changes but fundal pigmentation, eyelash colour and facial skin colour may also be abnormal. Waardenberg's syndrome is associated with aganglidosis of the colon (Hirschsprung's disease) in some patients.

Inheritance

Autosomal dominant.

Box 6.7

Craniosynostosis

Characteristics

Craniosynostosis (premature fusion of skull bone sutures) occurs as part of many syndromes: three autosomal dominant forms are well characterized. In the Boston variant, following localization to chromosome 5q a point of mutation in the homeotic gene *MSX2* was identified in all affected individuals in a single pedigree. Crouzon syndrome is characterized by protruding eyes and abnormal skull type. It maps to chromosome 10q25-q26 and is associated with mutations in the fibroblast growth factor receptor 2 gene *FGFR2*. Mutations in *FGFR3*, a related gene, are responsible for the common cause of dwarfism, achondroplasia.

Inheritance

Autosomal dominant forms.

Box 6.8

Di George's syndrome

Characteristics

A defect of branchial arch development principally affecting organs derived from the third and fourth branchial arches of the embryo. Agenesis of thymus and parathyroid glands causes hypocalcaemic tetany and repeated infections due to deficiency of T-lymphocytes. Fetal thymic transplants and vitamin D therapy are beneficial. Associated abnormalities of the first and fifth branchial arches include hyperteleorism, macrognathia, asymmetrical ears, right-sided aortic arch and Fallot's cardiac tetralogy.

Inheritance

Autosomal dominant forms.

Box 6.9

---

importance of homeobox genes. Other well-defined single gene disorders may represent abnormalities of important components of the developmental machinery of specific organs. For example the tuberous sclerosis gene, the von Hippel Lindau gene and the polycystic kidney disease gene, all of which have been recently isolated by positional cloning techniques, promise to shed more light on the control of kidney development and differentiation than might at first have been imagined.

Single genes and behavioural defects

In the 1980s several reports appeared to show that certain psychiatric syndromes in humans, notably manic depressive psychosis (bipolar disorder), could be mapped to individual chromosomes by linkage studies in large kindreds. Later scrutiny of these results failed to confirm the linkage analysis but, nonetheless, there was abundant experimental evidence of a genetic influence in the behaviour of many subhuman species including rodents and *Drosophila*. Despite these early disappointments which probably result mainly from erroneous disease ascertainment in affected pedigrees, **behavioural genetics** remains a tantalizing and important area of human interest.

Genetic determination of behavioural traits is often problematic and even studies of pure bred fruitflies have demonstrated polygenic influences on such traits as 'mobility' or 'roaming'. Nonetheless, a gene *period* has been identified in *Drosophila* that controls the 24 hour circadian rhythm. This gene has been isolated and sequenced, though the means by which it exerts its effect is not understood. Selective disruption of the gene does not affect development in the flies but they show subtle changes in courtship behaviour and in cyclical periods of activity.

Genetic studies have also been carried out in human families showing propensities to abnormal patterns of behaviour. In 1990, it was reported that one particular allele of the dopamine receptor (D2) was present at an increased frequency in individuals with alcoholic proclivities compared with controls. Several other reports appeared in the following few years in relation to alcoholism as well as dependency on other drugs such as cocaine. These have created considerable controversy but no unified view as to the reproducibility of the studies, which at present should perhaps best be interpreted with caution. They certainly require re-evaluation.

Perhaps the most promising finding to date has been the association of an inactivating (nonsense) mutation present in an X-linked gene encoding a specific isoform of the enzyme monoamine oxidase. The defect segregated with aggressive behaviour and psychiatric instability or personality disorder in several apparently psychopathic males within a large Dutch pedigree. The defect correlated with enzymatic changes as shown by abnormalities of urinary catecholamine excretion, previously thought to be associated with psychiatric disorder. At present this single defect of an X-linked gene appears to be the most concrete example of simple hereditary psychiatric disorder in humans and only time will tell whether complex disorders such as schizophrenia, bipolar disorder and Gilles de la Tourette's syndrome will prove to be as simply explained.

The behavioural genetics of alcoholism, drug dependence and even such apparently intractable areas as personality traits, previously thought to belong to the realm of psychology, will be subject to an intensive analysis using the methods of quantitative genetics. The difficulties here still remain those of diagnosis, classification and, of course, the effects of environmental circumstances. The ultimate hope is to understand how gene expression in neural cells is regulated by external experiences and how gene expression may be modified by pharmacological agents. In the behavioural sciences, however, the role of a quantitative approach is beginning to yield fruit in terms of the understanding of behaviour. It may be, however, that an approach involving the search for many genes which contribute to a personality or behavioural trait would be more fruitful than a rigid 'one gene–one behavioural disorder pattern' hypothesis, which may be too simple for an understanding of the complexities of human personality and behaviour.

Molecular genetics becomes human biology and therapeutics

It is clear from the examples given that large-scale gene localization projects require a supreme co-ordination of research effort: the build up of cytogenetic linkage and physical mapping with the ultimate assembly of contiguous cloned segments of DNA related to the disease region is a formidable task. At the same time as the databases containing details about mapped human genes are being assembled, a true picture of the functional integration and organization of the human genome is emerging. This will increasingly permit candidate genes to be tested for causality when they map by linkage to a putative disease locus. This is the refinement of our new molecular anatomy of the human genome.

Nonetheless, the identification of a disease locus, though triumphant, represents merely the beginning of the application of new molecular information to gene function. There is immediately the need to identify causal mutations responsible for disease in pedigrees. Often the availability of genomic DNA or selective expression of genes creates difficulties and here the power of the PCR is invaluable. Later the use of single-strand polymorphisms, denaturing gel electrophoresis, restriction enzme digestion (where the mutations create or abrogate recognition sites for restriction endonucleases) or the amplification refractory mutation system (ARMS) and related techniques help to pinpoint mutations in human genes that are implicated in clinical disease (Box 6.10). Some of these techniques are discussed in Chapter 3.

The identification of the novel gene also raises questions about its function: especially its pattern of developmental and tissue expression as well as biochemical activities. The ability to express proteins in eukaryotic and prokaryotic systems is a powerful method for access to these aspects; it allows also the development of region-specific antibodies for immunocytochemistry. The use of **site-directed mutagenesis** specifically to recreate mutations in a given gene is critical for the definition of mutation causality. Such an approach is particularly valuable where a large gene shows a polymorphic structure in the population and where an individual sequence variation may or may not contribute to the disturbed chemical function and disease phenotype. The ability to synthesize large quantities of recombinant human gene product also has the power to enable detailed structural characterization of the molecular effects of specific

Case study: use of archival analysis to identify the cause of a postoperative death (from Ali *et al.* (1993))

Case history

The occurrence of fatal hepatic and renal failure in a 16-year-old girl, who had received infusions of fructose and sorbitol during minor surgery, led to the suspicion that she had suffered from hereditary fructose intolerance (HFI).

Jaundice, anuria and abdominal pain developed on the first day after routine appendectomy. By the third postoperative day coma with raised blood ammonia concentrations and signs of brain swelling developed: despite assisted ventilation and other intensive life-support measures, liver and kidney function deteriorated and consciousness was not regained. The patient died 5 days after the surgery.

Background

HFI is a recessively transmitted disease caused by the deficiency of a specialized enzyme of fructose metabolism, aldolase B. Aldolase B is expressed selectively in the liver, kidney and small intestine which suffer the main effects of this condition characterized by metabolic disturbances including hypoglycaemia with abdominal pain and vomiting that follow consumption of fructose and related sugars. Symptoms occur at weaning on exposure to sugar: survival beyond this period depends on the exclusion of sugar from the diet and is associated with the development of a marked distaste for sugar-containing foods and drinks. HFI responds favourably to dietary exclusion therapy although food intolerance persists. This, sometimes combined with a family history of the condition, suggests the diagnosis.

Molecular analysis of aldolase B genes in patients with HFI has shown that diverse mutations cause the condition, although several mutations are sufficiently widespread to be of diagnostic significance. Their detection by direct analysis of DNA forms the basis of diagnosis of this condition, using non-invasive methods to obtain genomic samples for amplification of aldolase B sequences in the PCR.

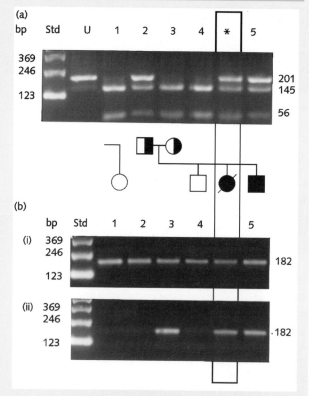

Fig. B Segregation of the mutations in the family. Open symbols represent asymptomatic individuals. (a) *Nco*I-digests of amplified exon 2 using genomic DNA obtained from a healthy individual (Lane 1) and the family members (Lanes 2–5). Lane U represents a 201-basepair undigested PCR product from the control. (b) ARMS analysis of DNA from a healthy control subject (Lane 1) and the family members (Lanes 2–5). (i) The Y203+ oligonucleotide primer. All individuals tested have a wild-type allele (ii) The Y203X oligonucleotide primer. Only the mother and her two affected children have the mutant allele.

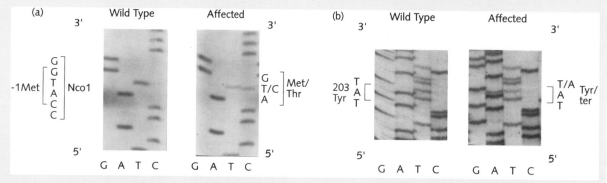

Fig. A Sequence comparison of aldolase B genes from a healthy control subject and the 14-year-old affected boy. (a) Sequence derived from PCR product containing exon 2. There is a T → C transition in the affected individual which changes the methionine start codon to a threonine. Also shown is the position of the *Nco*I restriction sequence destroyed by the point mutation.

(b) Sequence derived from PCR amplified exon 6. The affected individual has a T → A transversion which changes the tyrosine codon at position 203 to a termination codon. This information was used to investigate archival DNA from the deceased sister for compound heterozygosity for the Met^{-1} → Thr and Tyr^{203} → ter mutations (Fig. B).

Box 6.10

Case study: use of archival analysis to identify the cause of a postoperative death

Investigations in the family

After the patient's death, enquiries of the family revealed that she had disliked and avoided fruit and sugary foods since infancy because they induced abdominal pain. There were two surviving brothers, aged 14 and 18. The younger brother shared the proposita's distaste for sweet foods and had also refused these in infancy; both he and his sister had had a striking absence of dental caries. No other family members had symptoms and the parents were not consanguineous.

Although permission for autopsy was not granted, the family consented to the sampling of the patient's liver by needle aspiration *post-mortem*. Histological examination showed absence of surviving liver cells with necrotic collapse of the tissue containing bile ducts and Kupffer cells only (Plate 9a and b, facing p. 214). Five sections were cut from the paraffin block, dewaxed in xylene and the DNA extracted after proteinase K treatment. The PCR was first used to amplify individual coding regions of aldolase B genes using genomic DNA obtained from a blood sample taken from the affected brother. Sequencing revealed two inactivating mutations: at the initiator methionine, a T → C mutation changed the transla-

tion start signal from methionine to threonine; in exon 6, a T → A transversion replaced tyrosine at position 203 by a termination codon, T(U)AA (Fig. A).

To screen for these null mutations in genomic DNA, aldolase B exons 2 and 6 were amplified in the PCR and analysed for Met[1] → Thr and Tyr[203] → ter by restriction endonuclease digestion (Met[-1] → Thr abolishes a unique NcoI site) and by the amplification refractory mutation system (ARMS). In the ARMS, the use of mutant Y203ter primer permitted selective amplification only in the presence of the nonsense mutation (Fig. B). Sufficient DNA was extracted from the archival liver sample embedded in paraffin from the proposita for PCR-based analysis of exons 2 and 6 of the aldolase B gene by the NcoI and ARMS procedure.

The patient and her symptomatic brother were found to share the MIT/Y203ter genotype and hence would have had deficiency of aldolase B associated with hereditary fructose intolerance. Molecular analysis of aldolase B genes obtained from the tiny fragment of fixed liver tissue confirmed the suspected diagnosis and the cause of death. Other cases of inadvertent death in HFI have been recorded as a result of the indiscriminate use of fructose-based solutions and DNA analysis has proved decisive in court.

Box 6.10 *Continued.*

---

mutations to be explored. In the case of the dystrophin gene, detailed investigation of expressed isoforms of the wild-type and mutant protein has not only demonstrated individual polypeptides coded within the dystrophin gene but related genes that interact with them, possibly to form cytoskeletal links between the muscle cell and extracellular matrix. Conventional biochemical analysis had failed to identify any consistent primary protein abnormality in DMD and so no functional integration between the gene locus and the disease phenotype would otherwise have been possible. Furthermore, individual components of the DGC have also been found to be mutated in hereditary forms of muscular dystrophy (see Table 6.5). Thus biochemical investigation of expressed gene products promises to reveal much about the role of newly discovered genes in tissue development and in the molecular physiology of cells.

The ultimate application of gene localization in medicine will be in many cases somatic gene therapy. Clearly a full understanding of the regulation of tissue expression and gene activity will be required so that the effects of mutations in the gene responsible for a given hereditary condition can be decisively alleviated at the physiological site of action. These aspects are further discussed in Chapter 16 and will depend upon safe methods for gene transduction using vector systems. At present, our high expectations for progress towards therapeutic correction of monogenic disorders appear to justify the

heavy costs incurred by positional cloning and molecular analysis of disease loci in terms of protein function and gene regulation.

Further reading

Ahn A.H. and Kunkel L.M. (1993) The structural and functional diversity of dystrophin. *Nature Genetics*, **3**, 283–291.

Ali M., Rosien U. and Cox T.M. (1993) DNA diagnosis of fatal fructose intolerance from archival tissue. *Quarterly Journal of Medicine*, **86**, 25–30.

Buckle V.J. and Kearney L. (1994) New methods in cytogenetics. *Current Opinion in Genetics and Development*, **4**, 374–382.

Collins F.S. (1992) Cystic fibrosis: molecular biology and therapeutic implications. *Science*, **256**, 774–779.

Collins F.S. (1995a) Ahead of schedule and under budget: the genome project passes its fifth birthday. *Proceedings of the National Academy of Sciences of the USA*, **92**, 10821–10823.

Collins F.S. (1995b) Positional cloning moves from perditional to traditional. *Nature Genetics*, **9**, 347–350.

Grompe M. (1993) The rapid detection of unknown mutations in nucleic acids. *Nature Genetics*, **5**, 111–117.

Gusella J.F. and MacDonald M.E. (1995) Huntington's disease: CAG genetics expands neurobiology. *Current Opinion in Neurobiology*, **5**, 656–662.

Guyer M.S. and Collins F.S. (1995) How is the Human Genome Project doing, and what have we learnt so far?

Proceedings of the National Academy of Sciences of the USA, **92**, 10841–10848.

Hochgeschwender U. (1992) Toward a transcriptional map of the human genome. *Trends in Genetics*, **8**, 41–44.

McKusick V.A. (1994) *Mendelian Inheritance in Man: Catalogs of Human Genes and Genetic Disorders*, 11th edn. John Hopkins University Press, Baltimore.

Monaco A.P. (1994) Isolation of genes from cloned DNA. *Current Opinion in Genetics and Development*, **4**, 360–365.

Monaco A.P. and Larin Z. (1994) YACs, BACs, PACs and MACs: artificial chromosomes as research tools. *Trends in Biotechnology*, **12**, 280–286.

On-line Mendelian Inheritance in Man (1996) OMIM(TM) Centre for Medical Genetics. John Hopkins University (Baltimore, MD) and National Centre for Biotechnology Information, National Library of Medicine (Bethesda, MD). World-Wide-Web URI: http://www3.ncbi.nlm.nih.gov/omim/

Prosser J. (1993) Detecting single-base mutations. *Trends in Biotechnology*, **11**, 238–246.

Sutherland G.R. and Richards I.R. (1995) Simple tandem repeats and human genetic disease. *Proceedings of the National Academy of Sciences of the USA*, **92**, 3636–3641.

The Nature Genome Directory (1995) *Nature*, **377**, supplement.

Welsh M.J. and Smith A.E. (1995) Cystic fibrosis. *Scientific American*, December, 36–43.

Welsh M.J., Tsui L.C., Boat T.F. and Beaudet A.L. (1994) Cystic fibrosis. In: *Metabolic and Molecular Basis of Inherited Disease* (eds C.R. Scriver, A.L. Beaudet, W.S. Sley and D. Valle). McGraw Hill, New York.

Worton R. (1995) Muscular dystrophies: diseases of the dystrophin–glycoprotein complex. *Science*, **270**, 755–756.

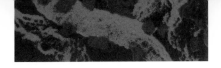

Chapter 7 Polygenic disorders

Introduction

This chapter describes:
• the interaction of genes and environmental factors in common diseases;
• how the contribution of genes to the development of complex disorders can be ascertained;
• genetic influences in the pathogenesis of vascular disease, diabetes mellitus, Alzheimer's disease and other familiar complex disorders.

Humans are enormously diverse in their form, colour, behaviour and ability. This diversity is influenced by environmental factors, but is largely determined by inheritance. Thus while the size and density of the skeleton is undoubtedly influenced by nutrition and the presence or absence of small intestinal disease as well as access to sunlight, these influences do not affect the overall form of the bones or the shape of the face or the likeness of features within a family. Rather, the shape of the face is determined by a specific group of genes (most of them unknown) that must operate through the developmental period *in utero* and during postnatal maturation. While it is certain that the same complement of genes determines the shape of the face of different individuals, it is subtle genetic variation at each of the loci necessary for facial development that decides individual facial appearance and family likeness.

Like facial appearance, disease susceptibility runs in families. Thus common diseases like coronary heart disease, essential hypertension, diabetes mellitus, psychotic illness, senile dementia, cancer and susceptibility to infectious disease tend to cluster in families. Rarely, this familial aggregation is caused by a single gene defect; more usually, it results from the cumulative interaction of a number of genes with environmental factors. These disorders are therefore said to show **multifactorial** or **polygenic** inheritance. The risk of polygenic disease in first-degree relatives is generally less than the one in four risk for Mendelian recessive disorders, being of the order of 5–15% (Table 7.1). The risk of multifactorial disease, however, varies from one disease to another and from one family to another. Within a family, the risk will depend on the severity of the disorder in the proband, the number of affected family members, and the contribution from environmental factors.

Genetic epidemiology and genetic modelling

For any disease it is necessary to establish whether it has a genetic component in its aetiology. Family, twin and adoption studies help to establish the presence and the size of the genetic component, and the risk of disease in the relatives of a **proband** or **index case**. Knowledge of the recurrence risk of a disease in relatives, and curve-fitting of disease parameters such as blood pressure or plasma cholesterol levels between diseased and normal families (**commingling analysis**) may suggest a mode of inheritance. For example, a normally distributed curve is usually indicative of polygenic inheritance, whereas skewness or bimodality may suggest the involvement of major genes or of major environmental factors. Analysis of the segregation of a disease within families (**complex segregation analysis**) using computer programs like PAP (Pedigree Analysis Package) also helps to establish the mode of inheritance of a trait: that is, whether it is likely to be caused by a major gene showing either dominant or recessive inheritance, or is caused by a number of genes, i.e. oligogenic or polygenic inheritance, or whether environmental factors are largely responsible.

Table 7.1 Risks for common polygenic diseases of adults (after Goldstein and Brown (1991)).

Disorder in proband	Risk for first-degree relatives (%)
Coronary heart disease	8 for male relatives
	3 for female relatives
Hypertension	10
Diabetes mellitus	5–10
Epilepsy	5–10
Manic depressive psychosis	10–15
Schizophrenia	15
Psoriasis	10–15
Thyroid disease	10

The number of genes involved in disease

It is necessary to ascertain the genes that participate in a disease. For a complex disorder such as coronary heart disease, in which plasma lipoproteins, the coagulation system and the cellular elements of the blood and the cellular arterial wall play a part, the number of genes may be large. One component of this problem illustrates its complexity. Genes that affect plasma lipids have been the subject of much research, so that a great deal is known about some of these, including those coding for apolipoproteins that carry **cholesterol** and **triglyceride** in the circulation, lipid transfer proteins, receptors for apolipoproteins and key enzymes involved in lipid metabolism (Table 7.2). This list is by no means comprehensive. At least 200 genes have been estimated to be involved in the control of cholesterol uptake by the gut, metabolism in the plasma, liver and peripheral cells, and excretion from the body. The issues here are firstly to establish which of the known genes affect plasma cholesterol concentrations. The extent to which many known genes contribute, if at all, has still to be established. Secondly, it is necessary to identify new loci that contribute to lipid metabolism. Thirdly, genes that con-

Table 7.2 Key proteins associated with lipid metabolism.

Class	Protein	Function
Plasma apolipoproteins	ApoAI	HDL structural protein, LCAT activation
	ApoAII	HDL structural protein
	ApoAIV	Unknown
	ApoB100	VLDL assembly and secretion; ligand for LDL receptor
	ApoB48	Chylomicron assembly and secretion.
	ApoCI	Unknown
	ApoCII	Lipoprotein lipase activation
	ApoCIII	Lipoprotein lipase inactivation
	ApoE	Ligand for chylomicron remnant and LDL receptors
Enzymes	AMP-dependent protein kinase	Inhibits HMG CoA reductase, acetyl CoA carboxylase and hormone sensitive lipase
	Cholesterol 7-α hydrolase	Cholesterol conversion to bile acids
	Cholesteryl-ester hydrolase	Intracellular cholesteryl-ester hydrolysis
	Endothelial lipoprotein lipase	Lipolysis of triglyceride-rich chylomicrons and VLDL
	Fatty acid synthetase	Fatty acid synthesis
	Fatty acyl-CoA cholesterol acyl transferase (ACAT)	Cellular cholesterol esterification
	Hepatic triglyceride lipase	Lipolysis of remnants and HDL
	Hormone sensitive lipase	Hydrolysis of intracellular triglyceride in fat and muscle cells
	HMG CoA reductase	Rate-limiting enzyme of cholesterol synthesis
	Lecithin cholesterol acyl transferase (LCAT)	Plasma cholesterol esterification
	Phosphatidic acid phosphohydrolase	Phospholipid synthesis
	5-, 12- and 15-lipoxygenase	Arachidonic acid oxygenation and oxidization of LDL
Lipid transfer proteins	Acetyl CoA carboxylase	Fatty acid synthesis
	Cholesteryl-ester transfer protein (CETP)	Cholesterol transfer from HDL to VLDL and LDL
	Hepatic fatty acid binding protein	Intracellular fatty acid transport
	Intestinal fatty acid binding protein	Intracellular fatty acid transport
Receptors	ApoE	Remnant clearance
	Low density lipoprotein	LDL and remnant clearance
	Scavenger receptor	Oxidized LDL clearance by macrophages

tribute to other aspects of the problems of atherogenesis must be found.

Genetic variation and susceptibility to disease

DNA sequence variation occurs about every 200–500 basepairs (bp). Thus most genes can be expected to show variation in every human population. Sequence variants (mutations) which have a frequency of >1% in the population are generally called polymorphisms, and those with a frequency of <1% are termed rare alleles (variation at a single gene locus). For the bulk of individuals the risk of developing a disease will depend upon a complex interaction between common alleles, each with small effects which combine additively. Superimposed on the population distribution contributed by polymorphic alleles will be the influence of rare alleles.

Polymorphisms

Common alleles or **polymorphisms** form the basis of human diversity, including our ability to handle environmental challenges, such as exposure to infectious agents or chemical carcinogens or excessive consumption of saturated fat and cholesterol. Such alleles are likely to have increased in frequency in the time since the original mutation occurred, owing to a positive selection acting on variants that confer selective advantage in the heterozygous state. For example, the genetic polymorphisms that contribute to diseases like coronary heart disease, essential hypertension and diabetes mellitus almost certainly have a high prevalence in the population. Perhaps these variants, which once conferred advantage by maintaining blood pressure, and blood glucose and cholesterol concentrations at times when food was scarce for our hunter-gatherer ancestors (the thrifty gene hypothesis of J.V. Neel), now respond to over-nutrition by predisposing to the common diseases that affect modern humans. Is it surprising, in evolutionary terms, that modern humans so crave sugar, salt and fat?

Population association studies and linkage disequilibrium

How are we to establish whether a particular gene contributes to the genetic variation in a trait such as blood pressure or plasma cholesterol concentration? Genetic epidemiology has provided statistical methods for measuring the effect of genetic variation on a phenotypic trait in a population (the so-called measured genotype approach). For example, functional polymorphism of the apolipoprotein (apo) E protein (see below) can be assessed by isoelectric focusing or by the polymerase chain reaction (PCR) and use of allele-specific oligonucleotides. In the normal population these three polymorphisms have a substantial effect on the normal variation in plasma lipid levels (Table 7.3); they account for 16% of genetic variation in cholesterol levels in the population. Yet the effect of these polymorphisms on individual lipid levels and risk of coronary heart disease is small.

In the absence of functional protein polymorphisms, population association studies have been performed using biallelic restriction fragment length polymorphisms (RFLPs) or RFLP haplotypes (closely linked markers on the same chromosome). Highly polymorphic repeats are not useful because their stability in time is uncertain and they are hard to read on gels. Most usually, RFLPs do not mark functional changes in the DNA, but may be closely linked to genetic variation causing a change in phenotype. Association studies with RFLPs usually depend on **linkage disequilibrium**. Linkage disequilibrium is said to exist when two markers, or a marker and a trait, are found in association in a population at a frequency greater than that which would be expected by chance alone (chance being the linkage equilibrium situation). Most usually, this implies that the two mutations are closely linked on the same chromosome and co-segregate in family studies. The finding of disease association with an RFLP implies that natural selection has acted in the heterozygous state to increase the frequency of an allele carrying the marker RFLP and the causal mutation. For this to have occurred, significant inbreeding must have taken place in the founder

Table 7.3 Effect of (apo) E alleles on cholesterol levels [data from Davignon and Mahley (see Scott (1989))].

Allele	Position	Mutation	Receptor binding (%)	Frequency (%)	Cholesterol (mg/dl)	(mmol/l)
E4	112	Arg	100	15	+13	+0.32
E3	112	Arg → Cys	100	72	0	0
E2	158	Arg → Cys	2	13	−8	−0.21

population, where the causal mutation occurred, during a period of population stability after the mutant allele and marker polymorphism first appeared together. Amino acid charge variants are more likely to be direct in their effect, but may also of course mark the mutation causing the trait through linkage disequilibrium.

Association studies have been performed with polymorphic markers for many of the genes believed to be important in determining blood lipoprotein metabolism, blood glucose levels and blood pressure. Not surprisingly, those genes that code for proteins known through metabolic and biochemical studies to be rate limiting in their biochemical pathways, have been found to be subject to genetic variation that substantially contributes to the distribution of the trait they control in the population.

Rare alleles

Rare alleles also contribute to genetic diversity and susceptibility to disease. Indeed, they are the substrate of Mendelian genetic disease. While the effect of such changes may be devastating to the individual and cause genetic disease, in population terms a single rare mutation is insignificant. However, the cumulative effect of each of the rare mutations occurring at each of the loci that confer the risk of a disease may be substantial.

Linkage studies with candidate genes

How can we establish whether a rare allele of a specific gene causes a particular disorder in a family or group of families? The term 'candidate' is used when, for functional reasons, a particular gene has a strong possibility, if defective, of causing a disease. As an example, let us again consider high levels of blood cholesterol. This could be due to either a defect of the low density lipoprotein (LDL) receptor or of its ligand apoB (see below). If genetic modelling suggests that high blood cholesterol with tendon xanthomas and high risk of myocardial infarction (familial hypercholesterolaemia) is likely to be caused by the dominant effect of a major gene, then it would be reasonable to test whether a mutation of the LDL receptor gene (chromosome 19p13) causes this disorder. This can be tested using probes for the LDL receptor gene or nearby flanking markers, and a computer program for linkage analysis. If a mutation of this gene causes familial hypercholesterolaemia, then co-segregation of a specific allele of the gene (marked by an RFLP or other polymorphic repeat) with the disease will occur within a large affected family. If co-segregation does not exist with the allele, the LDL receptor gene can by and large be eliminated as a cause of the disorder in

this family. On the other hand, if consistent co-segregation does exist, a causal role for the gene in the disease is strongly supported.

In fact, the LDL receptor was identified by classical biochemical methods, because the uptake of LDL by cultured fibroblasts was shown to be abnormal in families with severe hypercholesterolaemia. More recently, defects of the apoB gene (chromosome 2p24–p23) have been associated with a similar co-dominantly inherited form of hypercholesterolaemia. If a single very large family was taken in whom the familial form of hypercholesterolaemia was due to a defect of either the LDL receptor gene or of the apoB gene, then linkage would be established. However, if several families with severe hypercholesterolaemia were pooled and some of these had defects of the LDL receptor gene, some of the apoB gene, and some of as yet unknown genes causing severe hypercholesterolaemia, then linkage would not be established. The same phenotypic abnormality being caused by defects at a number of distinct genes is described as **locus heterogeneity**, and is a serious problem in linkage studies.

Positional cloning

How can the new loci that contribute to disease be identified, when the phenotype provides no information about the locus or the biochemical abnormality responsible for the disease? If such a disorder cannot be linked to a candidate gene, then it may be necessary to screen the entire genome for linkage. This strategy has been much simplified by the identification of variable nucleotide tandem repeats (VNTR) and simple di- and tetranucleotide repeats. With such highly polymorphic markers chosen to be spaced at a genetic distance of 10–20 cM, it should be possible to ascertain linkage to a locus which harbours the gene responsible for a disorder. This strategy may be simplified by clues from classical genetic studies, in which chromosome deletions or translocations may provide clues that identify the occult loci responsible for genetic disease. Thus genetic abnormalities of chromosomes such as in trisomy 21 point to possible genes involved in many aspects of the Down's syndrome phenotype. This includes genes causing disorders as diverse as Alzheimer's disease and cardiac septal defects.

Oligo- or polygenic disorders

If computer modelling suggests that the mode of inheritance of a particular disorder is not clear or is due to the interaction of a number of genes, then it is inappropriate to perform classical linkage studies in large families or in pooled small families. In this situation, the affected sib pair or relative pair method have the advantage that linkage can be detected if a disease shows non-Mendelian inheritance due to a number of interacting genes, providing that the origin of each of the four parental chromosomes can be identified in the affected relative pairs — so-called **identity by descent**. This approach is not useful in dominant disorders or when there is genotypic heterogeneity, and has only so far been applied successfully to candidate genes as its power decreases rapidly with increased genetic distance from the affected locus.

Animal models

The study of inbred strains of mice and of other animal models of genetic disease has provided an invaluable tool for analysing the complex patterns of inheritance found in polygenic disease and for identifying occult loci. Most recently, the genetics of insulin-dependent diabetes and of essential hypertension have been the subject of inten-sive study using mouse and rat models, respectively (see below).

Atherosclerosis

Atherosclerosis, the cause of heart attacks, strokes and peripheral vascular disease, affects the walls of large and medium-sized arteries. It is the main cause of death in Europe and North America. Atherosclerosis develops slowly over many years as a consequence of chronic injury to the endothelial cells that line the blood vessels. Abnormal processes involving oxidative damage to LDL, uptake by macrophages, platelet and macrophage adhesion, damage to vascular endothelial cells, re-cruitment of lymphocytes, and proliferation of intimal smooth muscle cells, lead to infiltration of the vessel wall with lipids and formation of fibrocellular atheromatous plaques (Fig. 7.1). The disease does not usually manifest itself until rupture of plaque leads to **thrombosis**, or stable plaque occludes enough of the coronary lumen to cause angina or death of cardiac muscle (**infarction**).

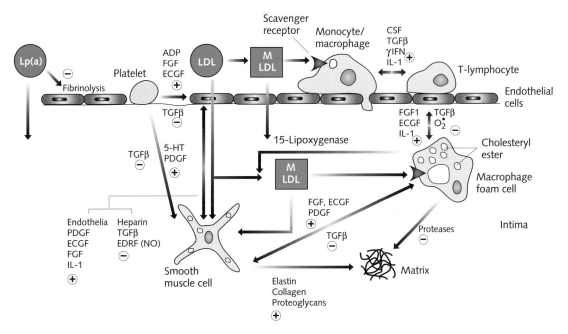

Fig. 7.1 Cellular interactions in atherosclerosis. This figure shows some of the complex cellular 'cross-talk' that occurs between the cellular elements of the blood and the arterial wall during atheroma formation. The diagram has been simplified by not including coagulation factors or arachidonic acid derivatives. Molecules that are stimulatory in their function are accompanied by ⊕, and molecules that are mainly inhibitory by ⊖. The diagram identifies the central role of modified LDL (MLDL) and its uptake by the macrophage, and of the paracrine relationships between macrophages, vascular endothelial cells and vascular smooth muscle cells. The roles of platelets and T-lymphocytes are also shown. ADP, adenosine diphosphate; CSF, colony-stimulating factor; ECGF, endothelial cell growth factor; EDRF, endothelium-derived relaxing factor; 5-HT, 5-hydroxytryptamine; γ-IFN, γ-interferon; IL-1, interleukin-1; NO, nitric oxide; $O_2^{\cdot}$, reactive oxygen; PDGF, platelet-derived growth factor; TGF-β, transforming growth factor-β.

Typically, these events do not occur until the fifth and sixth decades. Coronary heart disease is multifactorial in origin, having many genetic and environmental components. It clusters in families, but does not segregate in a Mendelian fashion. This is not surprising, since any single risk factor is separated from the disease process by the complex chain of events necessary for the disease to manifest itself.

Blood lipids have been prominent in research into atherosclerosis. This has been because of early research which showed the accumulation of cholesteryl-esters in atherosclerotic plaques, and because of epidemiological studies showing the importance of lipids as predictors of risk. More recently, epidemiological studies have shown that blood pressure and blood coagulation factors are important predictors of the risk. Beyond circulating and haemodynamic risk factors, the events that damage the vessel wall are complicated and are only now being understood. For this reason and because of expense and difficulty of measurement, studies which would identify genetic variation in key molecules closer to the disease process have not yet been done.

Genetic variation and lipoproteins

Lipoprotein abnormalities are found in 50–80% of myocardial infarction survivors. Five types of lipoprotein abnormality are common in such persons: increased LDL cholesterol levels; decreased high density lipoprotein (HDL) cholesterol levels, often associated with increased triglycerides; decreased HDL cholesterol levels often associated with increased very low density lipoprotein (VLDL) levels; increased levels of chylomicron remnants and intermediate density lipoproteins (IDL); and increased concentrations of the lipoprotein (a) [Lp(a)].

To comprehend the genetics of dyslipoproteinaemia, normal lipoprotein metabolism must be understood. Three pathways of normal lipoprotein metabolism are described (Figs 7.2–7.4). The exogenous pathway is responsible for the transport of dietary lipid, and uses apoB48. The endogenous pathway is necessary for the transport of triglyceride and cholesterol synthesized in the liver, and involves apoB100. The reverse cholesterol transport pathway carries cholesterol to the liver from the periphery and uses apoAI.

Dietary lipid absorption and exogenous pathway

Within the intestinal absorptive cell, dietary lipid and fat-soluble vitamins are packaged into large (100–500 nm) triglyceride-rich lipoproteins called chylomicrons. The major apolipoprotein of chylomicrons is

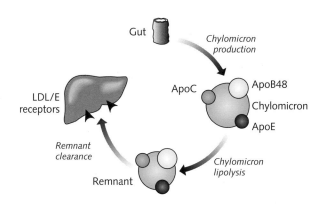

Fig. 7.2 Dietary lipid absorption. The cycle shows the role of apoB48 and apoE chylomicrons in the absorption of dietary lipid, its transport in blood to peripheral capillaries and the clearance of chylomicron remnants by hepatic lipoprotein receptors.

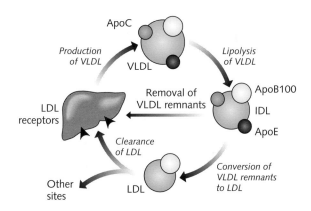

Fig. 7.3 Endogenous lipid transport. The role of apoB100 in the assembly and secretion of VLDL and the metabolism of VLDL to IDL and to LDL is shown. LDL delivers cholesterol to all tissues of the body, and excess is cleared by the interaction of apoB100 with hepatic LDL receptors.

apoB48 (designated on the centile system, because it is 48% of the size of hepatic apoB100 after resolution in SDS-polyacrylamide gels), with small amounts of the apoC peptides (apoCI, apoCII and apoCIII) and of apoAIV. Chylomicrons are secreted into intestinal lymph and pass into the blood through the thoracic duct for transport to peripheral capillaries, where core triglycerides are hydrolysed by endothelial cell lipoprotein lipase and released fatty acids taken up by fat and skeletal muscle cells — apoCII is an essential cofactor for lipoprotein lipase (Fig. 7.3). Loss of triglycerides released from the chylomicron produces a remnant particle, relatively enriched in cholesteryl-esters and con-

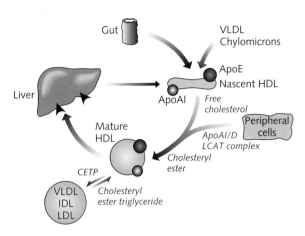

Fig. 7.4 The reverse cholesterol transport pathway. Nascent HDL is secreted as a discoid particle in association with apoAI and apoE. The particle receives material from VLDL and chylomicron metabolism and cholesteryl-ester derived by esterification of the free cholesterol of peripheral cells. Mature HDL transfers cholesteryl-ester to VLDL, IDL and LDL; the triglyceride and phospholipid of HDL is hydrolysed by hepatic lipase. The precise mechanism of clearance of HDL by the liver has yet to be clarified.

taining apoB48 and apoE. This remnant is transported to the liver, where it is taken up both by the LDL receptor and by a chylomicron remnant receptor, that also doubles as a receptor for α_2-macroglobulin.

Endogenous lipid transport

The liver synthesizes triglyceride and cholesterol, which, together with residual dietary lipid and fat-soluble vitamins, are incorporated into VLDL and secreted into the circulation (Fig. 7.3). VLDL contains a single molecule of apoB100 as its major lipoprotein, together with many apoC and apoE molecules. VLDL is transported to the periphery, where the triglyceride is hydrolysed by the same lipoprotein lipase that catabolises chylomicrons. After removal of core triglyceride, VLDL remnants called IDL undergo two distinct fates. Some of the IDL is cleared directly from the liver through the interaction between apoE and the LDL receptor. The remainder is acted on by hepatic triglyceride lipase in hepatic sinusoids. The residual triglyceride is hydrolysed and replaced with cholesteryl-ester. In the course of this conversion, all the apolipoproteins except apoB100 are lost to other lipoprotein particles. The result is a transformation of VLDL remnant particles into cholesteryl-ester-rich LDL, in which apoB100 is the sole apolipoprotein. LDL carries 60–70% of plasma choles-

terol and functions in the delivery of cholesterol to peripheral tissues, where it is required for membrane and steroid hormone biosynthesis, and to the liver for further metabolism or excretion in bile. ApoB100 is the ligand that mediates the cellular uptake of LDL by the LDL receptor pathway.

The reverse cholesterol transport pathway

Newly synthesized HDL is secreted from the liver as disc-shaped particles of apoAI and phospholipid (Fig. 7.4). These particles attract excess free cholesterol from extrahepatic cells and from other lipoproteins. The cholesterol is esterified in the circulation by the enzyme lecithin cholesterol acyl transferase (LCAT) which uses apoAI as a necessary cofactor. This cholesteryl-ester is transferred to the core of HDL, which enlarges in size. Enlargement is facilitated by the transfer of excess surface constituents from triglyceride-rich chylomicrons and VLDL, made available by the peripheral hydrolysis of these particles by lipoprotein lipase. HDL particle enlargement gives rise to an heterogeneous population of particles of different sizes and densities. HDL size can also be reduced by a plasma protein called cholesteryl-ester transfer protein (CETP) which exchanges the cholesteryl-ester of HDL with triglyceride in VLDL and IDL. The triglyceride in HDL is hydrolysed by hepatic lipase, which can also hydrolyse HDL phospholipids. Thus, HDL acts to remove both cholesterol and triglyceride from the blood by the LDL receptor pathway and by hepatic triglyceride lipase, respectively.

Genetic defects in the exogenous pathway

HYPOBETA- AND ABETALIPOPROTEINAEMIA, AND CHYLOMICRON RETENTION DISEASE
Abetalipoproteinaemia and homozygous hypobetalipoproteinaemia are characterized by failure to produce apoB-containing chylomicrons, VLDL and LDL. This causes fat malabsorption and fat-soluble vitamin deficiency, leading to retinal and spinocerebellar degeneration and haemolysis. Abetalipoproteinaemia is a rare autosomal recessive disorder due to a defect in apoB secretion. The genetic abnormality has been found to reside in the gene encoding a microsomal triglyceride transfer protein. Heterozygotes have normal lipoprotein levels. Hypobetalipoproteinaemia is caused by abnormalities of the apoB gene. It is a relatively rare autosomal co-dominant disorder, which leads to low circulating levels of LDL and predisposes to long life in heterozygotes. Heterozygotes have a frequency of around one in 1000.

Chylomicron retention (Anderson's) disease is characterized by intestinal malabsorption, absence of apoB48 from the circulation, and low levels of circulating LDL. It is a rare autosomal recessive disorder and is not caused by a defect of the apoB gene.

LIPOPROTEIN LIPASE AND APOCII DEFICIENCY
Defective processing of triglyceride-rich chylomicrons and VLDL occurs in lipoprotein lipase deficiency and apoCII deficiency. Both disorders are characterized by very high levels of chylomicrons and VLDL. Other features may include acute pancreatitis and eruptive xanthomas. Atherosclerosis risk is not apparently increased. Both are rare autosomal recessive disorders. A number of defects in the lipoprotein lipase (chromosome 8p22) and apoCII (chromosome 19q13) genes have been described. Genetic variation at both of these loci contributes significantly to normal plasma lipid variation.

REMNANT CLEARANCE
Chylomicron remnants and IDL are markedly elevated in dysbetalipoproteinaemia or type III hyperlipoproteinaemia. This disorder is invariably associated with defects of the apoE gene (chromosome 19q13) with the apoCI and CII genes; most usually, this is homozygosity for a common protein polymorphism designated E2, which is defective in binding to the LDL and chylomicron remnant receptors (Table 7.3).

Common alleles of the apoE gene produce three polymorphic proteins, designated E2, E3 and E4 (Table 7.3). These variants have occurred due to mutation of the unstable CpG dinucleotide in arginine codons 112 and 158 to form cysteine. The three apoE alleles have similar frequencies in most populations throughout the world. The average effects of each of the alleles on circulating cholesterol levels are shown in Table 7.3. The high frequency of the apoE alleles was probably determined by selective pressure acting on cholesterol levels, or possibly on the neural regeneration or immunological processes in which apoE is also involved. Selection may have been balanced by the high mutation rate occurring at the unstable arginine codons.

In dysbetalipoproteinaemia there is failure to clear chylomicron and VLDL remnants producing profound hypertriglyceridaemia, moderate hypercholesterolaemia and premature coronary heart disease. Failure to clear remnant particles is due to complete absence of an effective apoE on the surface of these particles. Homozygosity for the E2 allele is found in one in 100 individuals. This condition is necessary, but not the sole cause of dysbetalipoproteinaemia. The frequency of dys-betalipoproteinaemia is 50–100-fold less than that of homozygosity for E2. The presence of diabetes mellitus, hypothyroidism, or of another, possibly dominant, gene defect is necessary to manifest this disorder. ApoE deficiency may also cause this disorder. Alleles of apoE have been described that produce a co-dominant form of remnant clearance disease.

Genetic defects in endogenous fat transport

FAMILIAL COMBINED HYPERLIPIDAEMIA
Familial combined hyperlipidaemia (FCHL) is characterized by the presence in individuals of a single kindred of hypercholesterolaemia, hypertriglyceridaemia, or both abnormalities, and this phenotype can vary in an individual. It has a prevalence of around 1%. Individuals characteristically overproduce apoB100 from the liver and have LDL which is small and dense. Small dense LDL is unduly susceptible to oxidative damage and is highly atherogenic. Certain individuals with a *forme fruste* of this disorder called hyperapobetalipoproteinaemia do not show elevated lipid levels, but have increased circulating levels of apoB100 and small dense LDL. The mode of inheritance of FCHL is not completely clear. It was originally described as an autosomal co-dominant disorder with reduced penetrance. Other work suggests an oligogenic mode of inheritance. The apoB gene is not defective. Reduced levels of lipoprotein lipase have been described, and a linkage study has suggested that defects of the apoCIII (an inhibitor of lipoprotein lipase) gene cause combined hyperlipidaemia in some families.

FAMILIAL HYPERCHOLESTEROLAEMIA AND
FAMILIAL DEFECTIVE APOB100
Familial hypercholesterolaemia (FH) is characterized by tendon xanthomas and elevation of LDL and IDL cholesterol. It is an autosomal co-dominant disorder caused by defects of the LDL receptor gene (Fig. 7.5). Numerous mutations of this gene have been described. These mutations variously perturb the itinerary of the LDL receptor in the cell, including transport, ligand (apoB100 and apoE) binding, clustering in clathrin-coated pits and recycling through endosomes. The overall frequency of heterozygosity for these mutations is one in 500 in the general population, where they account for one in 50 individuals with cholesterol above the 90th percentile. Increased frequency of FH is seen in South African, French Canadian, Lebanese and Finnish populations, due to founder effects. It is a serious cause of premature coronary heart disease. Expression of the disease is wors-

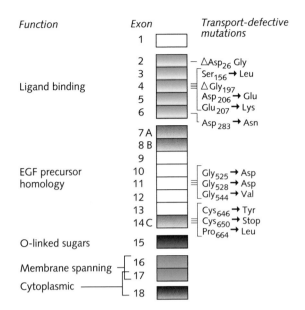

Function	Exon	Transport-defective mutations
	1	
Ligand binding	2	— $\triangle Asp_{26}$ Gly
	3	$\lceil Ser_{156} \rightarrow Leu$
	4	$\equiv \triangle Gly_{197}$
	5	$Asp_{206} \rightarrow Glu$
	6	$\lfloor Glu_{207} \rightarrow Lys$
		$\lfloor Asp_{283} \rightarrow Asn$
	7 A	
	8 B	
	9	
EGF precursor homology	10	$\lceil Gly_{525} \rightarrow Asp$
	11	$\equiv Gly_{528} \rightarrow Asp$
	12	$\lfloor Gly_{544} \rightarrow Val$
	13	$\lceil Cys_{646} \rightarrow Tyr$
	14 C	$\equiv Cys_{650} \rightarrow Stop$
		$\lfloor Pro_{664} \rightarrow Leu$
O-linked sugars	15	
Membrane spanning	16	
	17	
Cytoplasmic	18	

Fig. 7.5 The intron/exon organization of the LDL receptor gene, together with the domain organization of the protein. Mutations are shown which cause defective transport of nascent LDL receptor through the endoplasmic reticulum and Golgi apparatus to the cell surface.

ened by certain alleles of apo(a), and ameliorated by another, as yet poorly defined, dominant LDL-lowering locus, that is not the LDL receptor or apoB genes. Homozygosity for LDL receptor defects causes heart attacks with certainty in the first and second decades and death before the age of 20 without treatment by plasma exchange or plasma apheresis. It is the only genetic condition causing heart attacks with complete penetrance.

LDL hypercholesterolaemia is also produced by defects in apoB100 (Fig. 7.6). Mutation of a CpG dinucleotide in amino acid codon 3500 changes an arginine to glutamine. This causes complete failure of the binding of the variant LDL to its receptor. The defect has a heterozygous frequency of one in 500 to one in 1000 in the general population. It affects one in 50 individuals with LDL cholesterol levels above the 90th percentile. Homozygosity for the apoB defect has not yet been described. The extent to which coronary heart disease and tendon xanthomas are prevalent in familial defective apoB100 depends on the height of the blood cholesterol. The cholesterol level in blood tends to be higher in FH, because IDL clearance is defective as well as LDL.

Although defects of the apoB gene and of the LDL receptor gene have profound effects on individual LDL cholesterol levels, they are not sufficiently frequent in the population to affect the general risk of coronary heart disease. However, polymorphic alleles of the LDL receptor locus also contribute to the variation in cholesterol levels and are linked to the presence of small dense LDL in the general population. Polymorphic mutations of the apoB gene have a more marked effect on the variation of cholesterol levels and confer increased risk of coronary heart disease and obesity in the general population.

An additional insight into the biology of weight control and obesity has been gained with the cloning of the murine 'fat gene' — a gene encoding the leptin protein that controls body weight in mice. The subsequent cloning of the murine receptor for this protein has allowed isolation of the human homologue and the race is on to determine if obese people have defects in their leptin receptors or in the signalling pathway that the receptor turns on, and for drugs that may increase receptor activity in the hope of controlling body weight.

LIPOPROTEIN (A)

Numerous studies have found that plasma Lp(a) concentrations above 0.3 g/l (total Lp(a) mass) which are found in one in five people are associated with increased coronary heart disease and stroke. Lp(a) consists of LDL with an additional protein, apo(a), linked to apoB100 by a disulphide bridge (Fig. 7.7). Apo(a) is related to plasminogen, the precursor of the enzyme plasmin that hydrolyses fibrin blood clots (Fig. 7.8). It is released by the enzyme tissue plasminogen activator from its precursor. The apo(a) molecule is composed of an amino-terminal variable repeat of plasminogen kringle (a disulphide bonded domain shaped like a Danish cake) IV, a single kringle V, and the plasminogen protease domain. The protease domain in apo(a) is probably not active,

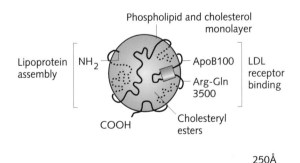

Fig. 7.6 Plasma LDL. A schematic view of the organization of apoB100 in the context of LDL is shown, together with the lipid composition of LDL. The position of $Arg_{3500} \rightarrow Gln$ is shown.

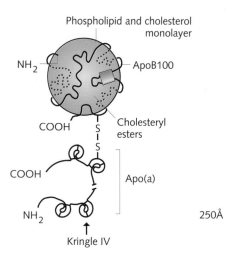

Fig. 7.7 Plasma Lp(a). A schematic view of the organization of plasma Lp(a) is shown.

because the activation site found in plasminogen is absent. The apo(a) and plasminogen genes are close together on chromosome 6q26–q27.

In the apo(a) gene the kringle IV region is repeated a variable number of times. This gives rise to allelic size variation of the protein (280 to 830 kDa) which is inversely correlated with Lp(a) levels in the circulation. Individuals with a small protein have much higher levels and are at greater risk of coronary heart disease. The size polymorphism accounts for more than 40% of the variability in plasma Lp(a) concentrations. Other sequence differences in the apo(a) gene, which presumably change mRNA or protein processing, also substantially alter Lp(a) plasma concentrations.

In LDL receptor-defective familial hypercholesterolaemia, but surprisingly not in familial defective apoB100, the concentration of Lp(a) is much increased, and this greatly compounds the risk of coronary heart disease.

Lp(a) appears to have a number of atherogenic prop-

erties: it blocks the access of plasminogen to its receptor on vascular endothelial cells and inhibits local fibrinolysis, thereby producing a prothrombotic state; it enhances the secretion of plasminogen activator inhibitor-1 (PAI-1) from the vascular endothelial cells; and kringle IV binds to fibrin at sites of vascular injury and may serve to deliver cholesterol to these sites. The shared structures of these functional domains in Lp(a) with components of the coagulation system provide the operational link between the lipid transport pathway and thrombotic disease.

Genetic defects in reverse cholesterol transport

A number of rare defects of the apoAI gene have been described. Some of these may interfere with LCAT activation and/or HDL production and metabolism. Those individuals with low HDL develop premature coronary heart disease and corneal clouding, and heterozygotes have half normal HDL levels. Individuals with disruption of the apoAI, CIII, AIV gene cluster (chromosome 11q23–q24) are susceptible to premature atherosclerosis.

Defects in lipoprotein processing caused by abnormalities of the lipoprotein lipase and apoCII genes may cause low levels of HDL. This is probably due to failure to transfer the products of triglyceride lipolysis to HDL. Abnormalities of the enzymes LCAT (chromosome 16q22), hepatic triglyceride lipase (chromosome 13q21–q23) and CETP (chromosome 16q13) affect HDL levels and composition because of defective cholesteryl-ester formation, hydrolysis and transfer, respectively. Tangier disease is a rare disorder with abnormally rapid clearance of HDL and low HDL levels. This may be due to failure in the normal regulation of HDL uptake and retroendocytosis. The precise genetic defect in this disorder is not known. Collectively these disorders of HDL do not explain the common genetic variation in the HDL levels of the population. Their combined frequency is only of the order of one in 10 000. Variation at these

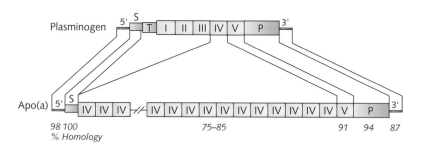

Fig. 7.8 Comparison of the structure of plasminogen and apo(a) is shown. The domains are: signal peptide (S), amino-terminal tail region (T), kringles I–IV, protease domain (P) (after McLean *et al.* (1987)).

various loci does however substantially affect plasma lipid levels in the normal population.

Other genetic variation

Coagulation factors

Although work on coagulation factors has lagged behind work on lipoproteins because of lack of appropriate methods of measurement, it is now clear that elevated levels of fibrinogen (chromosome 4q28) and of coagulation factors VII and VIII are important risk factors for atherosclerosis and its complications. Preliminary studies suggest that genetic variation at these loci (chromosomes 4q28, 13q34 and Xq28, respectively) may affect the level of their gene products. Defects of the factor V gene (chromosome 1q21–25) with a high frequency in the population markedly increase the risk of deep vein thrombosis (Factor V Leiden, R506Q). This variant was first described in Leiden, Holland, and involves a missense mutation that changes arginine at position 506 in the protein by replacing it with a glutamine residue.

Homocystinuria is an autosomal recessive condition, usually due to a defect of the gene encoding the pyridoxine-dependent enzyme cystathionine-β-synthase (chromosome 21q22), which is required for the conversion of homocystine, derived from dietary methionine, to cystathionine. Persons homozygous for homocystinuria have ocular, skeletal and neurological disease. They are at high risk for premature atherosclerosis and venous thromboembolism but may respond to pharmacological doses of pyridoxine (vitamin B_6). This appears to be explained by the reduced affinity of the mutant cystathionine-β-synthase for its essential cofactor. Heterozygosity for this disorder, which has a prevalence of 1–2% of the population, causes risk of premature atherosclerosis. High levels of homocystine in the blood are toxic to vascular endothelium, may potentiate oxidative damage to LDL, and promote thrombosis.

New targets for genetic research

Investigation of the molecular and cellular mechanisms that lead from a risk factor such as hypercholesterolaemia or hypertension or smoking to atheromatous plaque formation and its complications, narrowing of the arterial lumen and stable angina or rupture, and either healing or thrombosis and unstable angina or myocardial infarction, are only now being understood. Yet each step in the pathogenetic process and each molecule involved will have been subject to genetic variation which alters the risk for developing atherosclerosis. New targets for investigation are shown in Fig. 7.1.

Hypertension

Hypertension affects some 20–30% of individuals in the modern world. It is a major risk factor for atherosclerosis and its complications, and for haemorrhagic stroke. Genetic epidemiology suggests that the inheritance of hypertension is, with rare exceptions, polygenic. Abnormalities of the renin–angiotensin–aldosterone system are common in hypertension, but the extent to which these are primary or secondary is not clear. The importance of this system in the control of blood pressure is shown by the production of fulminant hypertension in transgenic rats harbouring the mouse renin gene. While plasma renin levels in these animals were low, overexpression of the renin transgene in the adrenals suggests steroid hormone overproduction.

Adult polycystic kidney disease

Adult polycystic kidney disease is characterized by numerous bilateral renal cysts. It gives rise to renal failure in middle life and in 50–75% of cases is associated with serious hypertension. The mutant gene that causes more than 95% of adult polycystic kidney disease has been localized to chromosome 16p13 and the gene cloned, but in 4% of families the disorder is caused by unknown mutations elsewhere in the genome. The disorder is inherited as an autosomal dominant, and affects one in 1000 individuals. It is responsible for 5–10% of end-stage renal failure in Europe and North America. The renin–angiotensin–aldosterone system is stimulated substantially more in hypertensive patients with polycystic kidney disease than in comparable patients with essential hypertension. The increased renin release, possibly due to renal arteriolar attenuation and ischaemia caused by cyst expansion, probably contributes to the early development of hypertension in this disease. Angiotensin converting enzyme (ACE) inhibitors are therefore likely to be of great value in preventing the onset of hypertension in adult polycystic kidney disease; they are dangerous agents to use in conditions where hypertension results from the adaptive response of the kidney to narrowing of the renal arteries.

Glucocorticoid-remediable hyperaldosteronism

Glucocorticoid-remediable hyperaldosteronism is an autosomal dominant form of hypertension characterized by a variable degree of hyperaldosteronism and elevated levels of the abnormal adrenal corticosteroid, 18-oxycortisol and 18-hydroxycortisol. Each of these hormones is under the regulation of adrenocorticotropic hormone and can be suppressed by glucocorticoid. This disorder has been linked to chromosome 8q21–22, where the genes encoding aldosterone synthase and steroid 11-β-hydroxylase reside. In one case these genes, which are 95% identical, have been shown to undergo duplication due to unequal crossover involving fusion of the 5′ regulatory region of 11-β-hydroxylase to the coding sequences of aldosterone synthase. This mutation accounts for all the physiological abnormalities of glucocorticoid-remediable hyperaldosteronism, and can cause hypertension in otherwise normotensive individuals.

Animal models

Chromosome mapping of genes involved in hypertension has focused on the spontaneously hypertensive rat as a stroke-prone model of human disease. In this animal a major locus has been identified on rat chromosome 10, a region closely linked to the rat gene encoding ACE. This enzyme plays a major role in blood pressure homeostasis and is an important target for anti-hypertensive drugs. In humans this gene resides on chromosome 17q23. Other loci involved in hyperten-sion have been found on rat chromosome 18 and the X-chromosome. Other rat strains with raised blood pressure should prove valuable in mapping additional disease loci.

New candidates for genetic susceptibility to hypertension

Recent understanding about the biochemical control of vascular smooth muscle tone and of blood volume provides new candidates for involvement in the genetics of hypertension. These include the pathways involved in the generation and metabolism of endothelium-derived relaxing factor (nitric oxide), endothelin, its processing enzymes and receptors, and atrial natriuretic peptide, its metabolic regulators and receptors. Recent studies in genetically manipulated mice homozygous for null alleles of one isoenzyme of nitric oxide synthase provide further evidence for the role of endothelium-derived relaxing factor in blood pressure control. Homozygous 'knockout' mice have sustained arterial hypertension and the existence of a human counterpart of this is actively being sought. Abnormalities of ion transport are also implicated by genetic studies that have indicated the involvement of a major susceptibility gene that is identified by abnormal sodium and lithium countertransport out of lithium-loaded red cells. This locus has still to be found; it is not Na+, K+-ATPase.

Diabetes mellitus

Diabetes mellitus is characterized by an elevation of blood glucose. Uncontrolled diabetes causes polyuria, polydipsia, weight loss, prostration, coma and even death from shock and ketoacidosis. It is a cause of premature atherosclerosis and of small vessel disease leading to blindness, neuropathy and renal failure. There are two main forms of diabetes. Insulin-dependent diabetes (IDDM or type 1) is caused by an absolute deficiency of insulin due to immunological destruction of insulin-secreting β-cells in the pancreatic islets of Langerhans. These patients require insulin treatment to survive. In this sense, non-insulin-dependent diabetes (NIDDM or type 2) is a milder disorder but the overall complication rate in the long term is similar. The islets of Langerhans are intact and secrete insulin. Patients with NIDDM may have relatively reduced production of insulin, or be unable to use insulin appropriately and so have paradoxically high levels. The overall prevalence of diabetes in the Western world is around 5%. Both forms of diabetes result from polygenic and environmental factors.

Insulin-dependent diabetes

The HLA locus

As with other **autoimmune diseases** in humans (see Chapter 11), population association and affected sib pair studies have identified causal genes in the major histocompatibility complex (MHC) in IDDM. The relative risk of IDDM in human leukocyte antigen (HLA)-identical siblings is 15% compared with 1% in non-HLA-identical siblings. Particular alleles of at least three MHC class II genes, HLA-DQA1, -DQB1 and -DRB1 on chromosome 6p21, predispose to IDDM. The presence of a non-charged residue at position 57 of the DQβ chain correlates most consistently with susceptibility, whereas non-diabetogenic alleles have asparagine at position 57. Amino acid residue 57 of the DQβ chain is necessary for its structure and function. Three-dimensional modelling of MHC class II molecules puts residue 57 at the end of an α helix in the β chain, which is accessible to the peptide binding grove and to the T-cell antigen receptor, and near enough to arginine residue 79 of the α chain to form a salt bridge if there is a negatively charged asparagine residue at position 57.

The insulin gene and other loci

The insulin gene has been implicated in IDDM in population association studies, but family studies have failed to demonstrate linkage. This paradox is explained by work showing that HLA-DR4-positive diabetics have an increased risk of IDDM with certain alleles at the insulin *IGFII* locus (chromosome 11p15). This effect is transmitted preferentially to HLA-DR4-positive diabetic offspring from heterozygous parents. The effect is most strong from paternal meioses, suggesting a role for maternal imprinting (i.e. markedly reduced expression of one parental allele that is stably transmitted to the offspring—as a consequence of hypermethylation of the C in the dinucleotide CpG). Maternal imprinting in this region has also been implicated in the origin of the Beckwith–Weiderman syndrome of neonatal macrosomia and increased risk of Wilms' tumour. Several other minor loci have also been identified.

Animal models

The non-obese diabetic (NOD) mouse that spontaneously develops IDDM has remarkable similarities to the human disorder. In both species there is autoimmune islet cell destruction, autoantibodies raised against β-cell components, and defects in T-cell activity, as well as susceptibility genes in the MHC. The NOD mouse shares the same HLA association, with serine at position 57 in the β chain. In addition to the mouse MHC locus on mouse chromosome 17, linkage studies in the NOD mouse have identified loci designated *idd-3*, *idd-4* and *idd-5*, on chromosomes 3, 11 and 5. These probably correspond to loci on human chromosome 1 or 4 for *idd-3* and 17 for *idd-4*. *Idd-5* maps close to the interleukin-1 receptor, which mediates resistance to bacterial and parasitic infection, and affects the function of macrophages. As with other autoimmune disorders susceptibility to infection is considered to be a component in the aetiology of IDDM.

Non-insulin-dependent diabetes

Studies in HLA-identical twins and other evidence from genetic epidemiology has shown that inheritance plays a more important role in NIDDM than in IDDM. However, the mode of inheritance of NIDDM has still to be elucidated, and the genes involved have yet to be characterized.

Association studies with candidate genes

Association studies have been performed in NIDDM in a variety of populations using candidate genes. HLA associations have not been identified in most populations, but positive association has been found with some HLA alleles in American Indians, certain tribes of southern Africa and in Finns. Rhesus factor (chromosome 1p36–p34), haptoglobin (chromosome 16q22) and insulin receptor (chromosome 19p13) have population associations in some studies of Mexican Americans, but not in others. Rhesus factor has also been associated with gestational diabetes in Italians. The apoAI and the apoB genes have been associated with diabetes in Chinese. Genetic variation in or near one of the facultative glucose transporter gene (chromosome 1p33) has been associated with NIDDM in Europeans and Japanese. In one study in North Americans of the same extraction, this association has not been found. All of these associations must be regarded as tentative. At best, population association studies have identified genetic components that modify the expression of the diabetic phenotype or are linked at some distance from the primary susceptibility genes.

Linkage studies

Maturity-onset diabetes of the young (MODY) is an autosomal dominant form of diabetes for which multi-generation pedigrees have been described. Prevalence varies between 0.2% in the general population and 18% in certain inbred populations. The hormonal and metabolic characteristics of MODY suggest that it is heterogeneous and that different genes may be responsible in different families. A recent linkage study in one large pedigree has demonstrated tight linkage to the glucokinase gene. A large number of glucokinase mutations have now been found.

Insulin and insulin receptor gene abnormalities

Mutations that affect the insulin gene have been identified (Fig. 7.9). Most have been in heterozygotes who appear to have increased risk of developing NIDDM. The frequency of these mutations is low, and other factors are also necessary to produce diabetes.

Several syndromes of extreme insulin resistance, including leprechaunism, Rabson–Mendenhall syndrome, type A severe insulin resistance with acanthosis nigricans and congenital lipodystrophy, are associated with mutated insulin receptors. The phenotype varies with the mutation involved. In general, mutations which affect the extracellular portion of the insulin receptor have a recessive mode of inheritance (Fig. 7.10). Mutations that affect the intracellular tyrosine kinase domain have a dominant mode of inheritance, as the defective allele impairs the function of the normal allele.

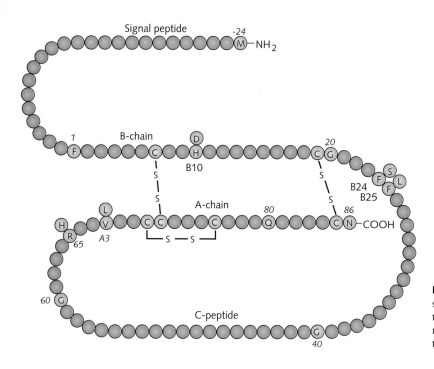

Fig. 7.9 The insulin molecule. A schematic view of the organization of the insulin precursor, together with mutations that cause defects in activity of the hormone (after Bell *et al.* (1991)).

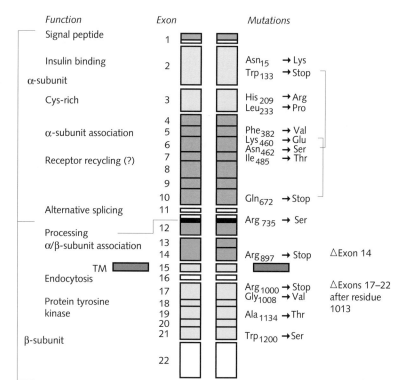

Fig. 7.10 The insulin receptor. The intron/exon organization is shown, together with functional domains and mutations which affect function (after Bell *et al.* (1991)).

Animal models

On mouse chromosome 4 an autosomal recessive muta-tion is associated with profound obesity and hyperpha-gia, increased metabolic efficiency and insulin resistance — interbreeding with different mouse strains markedly modulates this phenotype.

Respiratory disease

Asthma and atopy

Asthma is a disorder of the airways that is characterized by increased responsiveness of the tracheobronchial tree to many stimuli, particularly those that enhance airway permeability. Clinically it is manifested by widespread narrowing of the air passages. It is associated with paroxysms of dyspnoea, cough and wheezing. It has a prevalence of around 3% in the West, and is the cause of some 2000 deaths per year in Britain.

Atopy is the state of allergic hyperresponsiveness of the skin (eczema) and mucous membranes (asthma and hay fever) to protein antigens that underlies the allergic form of asthma. This form of asthma is frequently asso-ciated with a family history and produces lifelong mor-bidity. It is likely to result from a complex reaction between genetic and environmental factors. An essential component of the atopic state which distinguishes it from non-atopic asthma is the presence of immunoglob-ulin E (IgE) directed against allergens. Atopic individuals differ from normal individuals because they produce IgE in response to minute doses of allergens. Despite the familial aggregation of asthma, studies that have focused on disease expression or the total amount of serum IgE for phenotype analysis have not elucidated a genetic model for the inheritance. By assay of IgE responsiveness to skin prick tests and the assay of serum IgE in response to a variety of allergens, a dominant mode of inheritance for atopic allergy responsiveness has been suggested. Linkage studies map this abnormality to chromosome 11q13. This linkage has been confirmed by some workers, but not all.

The origin of those forms of asthma which do not show IgE hyperresponsiveness is probably heteroge-neous and they are not obviously associated with an allergic or genetic component.

α_1-Antitrypsin deficiency

Emphysema is the most common clinical complication of α_1-antitrypsin (α_1AT) deficiency. Disease generally only manifests in the homozygous state, though het-erozygotes may be at increased risk if other risk factors are present. It is one of the commonest lethal hereditary disorders of Caucasians of European descent, with a prevalence of around one in 2000. Symptomatically, dys-pnoea, particularly with exercise, becomes evident by the third and fourth decade. There is characteristic panacinar cystic disruption of lung parenchyma, particu-larly at the bases, which progresses to respiratory failure and death. The condition is markedly exacerbated by cigarette smoking. Certain mutations of the α_1AT gene (chromosome 14q31–q32) aggregate irreversibly and can also give rise to hepatic disease and cirrhosis (Fig. 7.11). One mutant has been described in which the aber-rant form of α_1AT formed an antithrombin, leading to uncontrollable haemorrhage and death after trauma. α_1AT is the major inhibitor of neutrophil elastase, a pro-tease capable of destroying most extracellular matrix components. Mutations that cause α_1AT deficiency reduce its secretion and hence serum levels. The most common disease mutations, designated S and Z, were originally identified as charge variants by isoelectric focusing (Fig. 7.11). There is some evidence that emphy-sema but not the liver disease can be prevented by inter-mittent infusion of α_1AT. More importantly, gene therapy could be effective in preventing this disorder by supplying the necessary α_1AT. This might provide a supply of the inflammatory modulator in the lung but it would not readily prevent the heat-induced aggregation of mutant α_1AT molecules in the hepatic cytosol.

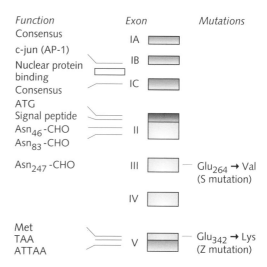

Fig. 7.11 The α_1-antitrypsin gene. The intron/exon organization of the α_1-antitrypsin gene, together with the functional regions of the protein and the common mutations S and Z are shown.

Psychiatric disorders

Affective illness

This group of illnesses is characterized by disturbance of mood, varying from extremes of despair to euphoria. There is associated disturbance of awareness, judgement, sleep, appetite, psychomotor function and sexuality. Typically they affect young adults, but also occur in very young children and the elderly. They are separated into the manic-depressive disorders (bipolar) and depressive disorders (unipolar). Five per cent of the population are estimated to be affected at any one time. Family, twin and adoption studies strongly support a genetic contribution to affective disorders. Segregation analysis has not elucidated a mode of genetic transmission, and there is little evidence for a single major gene.

Linkage studies

Affective illness was reported to be linked to the Harvey *Ras* oncogene and insulin loci on chromosome 11p15 in an Older Order Amish pedigree. These genes are close to the tyrosine hydroxylase gene—an important candidate gene because of its involvement in dopamine metabolism. This linkage has now been firmly refuted. Linkage to red–green (proton–deutan) colour blindness, to the Xg blood group and to glucose 6-phosphate dehydrogenase deficiency on chromosome Xq28 has been reported in some families. Linkage has also been reported to the HLA system.

Schizophrenia

Schizophrenia is a disturbance of thinking, characterized by disordered content and process, and by looseness of association. There may also be auditory hallucinations and persecutory delusions. It is usually divided into a number of subtypes, depending on the manifestations. The prevalence is around 1%. Genetic studies of this disorder have been fraught, because of lack of uniformity of definition, a heterogeneous cluster of symptoms, and lack of measurable medical or biological markers. Nevertheless, there is general agreement that the disorder is strongly inherited. The mode of heritance is unclear, but it is unlikely to be due to a single major gene. Chromosomal microdeletions of 22q11 have recently provided clues to one gene in families with velocaudiofacial syndrome and paranoid schizophrenia. There is, in addition, a substantial non-genetic component.

Linkage studies

Classical genetic studies demonstrating a translocation chromosome provided a candidate locus on chromosome 5 for a gene that may contribute to schizophrenia. This locus appeared to be confirmed in linkage studies, identifying the region of chromosome 5q11–q13 in Icelandic families. This linkage has not been confirmed in British, American or Scandinavian families.

The linkage assignments in the major psychiatric disorders are controversial and tentative. Although major genetic components exist to affective disorders and schizophrenia, the mode of inheritance is unclear and environmental factors contribute.

Dementia

Alzheimer's disease (previously divided into senile and presenile dementia) is the most common primary dementing illness. In persons over the age of 65 it is responsible for 60–80% of dementias. Multi-infarct dementia and stroke are also common, but have their root in hypertension and atherosclerosis. Other less common causes of dementia with a major genetic component include depression ('pseudodementia'), prion disease and Huntington's disease.

Alzheimer's disease

Dementia characterized by the presence in the brain of senile plaques and neurofibrillary tangles is the most prevalent (5–10% of the population over 65, and 50% of the population over 85) cause of failure in cognitive ability in late life in most developed countries. Typically, recent memory and attention are impaired early, before loss of other cognitive abilities. Ultimately the process affects language, abstract reasoning, judgement and spatial/visual orientation. Frequently there is lack of insight, often with paranoid or delusional content. Later, global confusion with motor and extrapyramidal signs, and occasionally epilepsy, occur. The disorder progresses relentlessly over 4–12 years to death in a debilitated, vegetative state. Atypical presentation with progressive aphasia, isolated sensorimotor or visual deficits has been reported. *Most* late-onset Alzheimer's disease occurs sporadically, and no pattern of inheritance has been elucidated. This may be because in late-onset disease it is difficult to establish a genetic component. Certain forms of early-onset disease show dominant inheritance—so-called familial Alzheimer's disease (FAD). In addition, people with Down's syndrome, who are born with three copies of chromosome 21 instead of the normal two, almost invariably develop brain lesions typical of Alzheimer's disease in their fifth and sixth decades.

Neurofibrillary tangles and senile (amyloid) plaques

Electron microscopy has demonstrated that fibrillary tangles are composed of 10 nm filaments wound in a helix — 'paired helical filaments' of the microtubule-associated protein tau. Antibody studies have suggested that it is an abnormally phosphorylated form of tau that forms neurofibrillary tangles.

The main constituent of senile plaques is β-amyloid peptide (β-AP; Fig. 7.12), the gene for which resides on chromosome 21q21. This is generated by proteolytic cleavage of a larger transmembrane glycoprotein, the amyloid precursor protein (APP). Differential splicing of heterogeneous nuclear RNA pre-mRNA for this precursor generates forms of 695, 751 and 770 amino acid residues. The 751 and 770 residue forms contain conserved sequences characteristic of the Kunitz protease inhibitors. A secreted form of APP is identical to the protease inhibitor, protease nexin-II. These observations have led to the suggestion that APP is involved in the regulation of protease activity.

β-AP of plaques is generated by an abnormal internal clip of the precursor (residue 16 of β-amyloid and residue 612 of the 695 amino acid residue precursor). Proteases that potentially produce this abnormal clip

have been identified from human brain and some of these appear to be lysosomal in origin. The β-amyloid protein precursor is expressed in other tissues, including the skin, intestine and adrenal medulla, and in some of these sites in patients with Alzheimer's disease and Down's syndrome, β-amyloid immunoreactivity has been detected. This has led to the suggestion that Alzheimer's disease is a component of a more generalized amyloidosis.

A direct pathogenetic role for β-amyloid in Alzheimer's disease is suggested by the observation that the protein is toxic to neuronal cells *in vivo* and in culture. The toxic region of the protein has been identified to a discrete region which is homologous to an 11 amino acid segment of the tachykinin family of neuropeptides (Fig. 7.12). This family of neuropeptides has one receptor to which the β-AP does not bind, and a second receptor of the serpin class of protease inhibitors to which tachykinins and β-AP bind (Fig. 7.12). Abnormal sequestration of this protease inhibitor could impair cellular capacity for the clearance of extracellular proteases and lead to neuronal degeneration.

Animal models of Alzheimer's disease include a rhesus monkey model that develops the disease spontaneously in old age, and transgenic mice models in which overexpression of the entire amyloid protein, as opposed to the β-AP sequence alone, causes the histopathological features of the disease to develop.

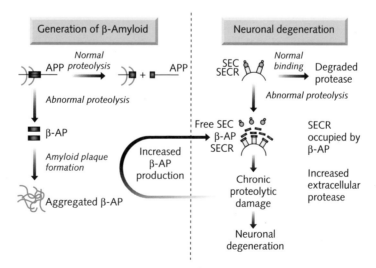

Fig. 7.12 A model for the pathogenesis of Alzheimer's disease. A change in the protease cleavage pattern of the amyloid precursor protein generates the β-amyloid protein (β-AP). β-AP is able to bind to the receptor for the serpine–enzyme complex (SECR) and compete for the normal serpine–enzyme complex (SEC) ligand. This leads to an increase in extracellular protease activity and may predispose to chronic damage to neuronal membranes and degeneration. In addition, abnormal cleavage may exacerbate the production of β-AP from its precursor, providing a positive feedback loop (after Yankner and Mesulam (1991)).

Molecular genetics

The finding that the gene for APP resides on chromosome 21 led to investigation of the possible role of this gene in the disease. Certain families were shown not to co-segregate with the disorder, whereas some early-onset FAD was linked to the β-AP gene. Several FAD families have now been identified with the same mutation in the β-AP sequence. This is a conservative substitution of isoleucine for valine, 4 residues from the β-AP sequence. This substitution results in a subtle alteration in the metabolism of APP. Additional mutations have now been associated with FAD.

Another disorder associated with amyloid deposition and mutation of the β-amyloid precursor protein gene is hereditary cerebral haemorrhage with amyloidosis of the Dutch and Icelandic type. In this disorder the mutation falls in the extracellular domain. Other diseases of the nervous system that give rise to amyloid deposition are the Gerstmann–Straussler–Scheinker (GSS) syndrome which results from mutation of the prion protein gene (see below) and familial amyloidotic polyneuropathy, which is caused by defects of the plasma prealbumin (transthyretin) and apoAI genes.

Thus, a genetic basis for Alzheimer's disease is established, as is a role for abnormal proteolysis in the generation of the neuropathology. In the sporadic form of the disease it is likely that both genetic and environmental factors may also be detected. Aluminium poisoning and a history of major head trauma have both been implicated, but neither has been proved. The role of proteases in the causation of Alzheimer's disease, and the possible role of protease inhibitors in its prevention, may lead to new modalities of treatment.

A remarkable recent disovery was the association between the apoE4 allele and hereditary Alzheimer's disease. Linkage established the involvement of this polymorphism with the disease, and aopE has been found in physical association with Alzheimer's plaques. Further recent discoveries have been the identification of genes for FAD on chromosome 14 and chromosome 1. Both genes encode novel proteins with 7 transmembrane domains. Their functions have still to be ascertained.

Prion disease

Creutzfeldt–Jacob disease (CJD) is a rapidly progressive degenerative disease of the cortex, basal ganglia and spinal cord that affects middle aged and elderly people. It is characterized by mental deterioration and movement disorders, which include startle myoclonus. Until recently it was believed to be caused by a spongiform virus that could be transmitted through improper sterilization of neurosurgical instruments, or in pituitary extract, once used as the source of human growth hormone. It is closely related to the disorder kuru, which was transmitted by cannibalism between the tribes in the Fore highlands of New Guinea, and to scrapie in sheep and its cattle counterpart, bovine spongiform encephalopathy. Autosomal dominant inheritance of CJD and of the related disorder GSS is also described.

Molecular genetic studies

Despite their evident transmissibility by ingestion and by inoculation, no nucleic acid component has been identified in material capable of transmitting any of these diseases. This has led to the proposition by Prusiner that they are transmitted by a protein only, or prion (small *pro*teinaceous *in*fectious particles) component. Prion protein turns out to be a normal cell surface glycoprotein found in neuronal cells, lymphocytes and other tissues. In subjects with CJD and GSS and dementias clinically like Alzheimer's disease, and other neurodegenerative diseases like fatal familial insomnia, several dominant missense mutations of the prion gene (chromosome 20pter–p12) have been identified (Fig. 7.13). There is now much evidence that when the prion protein carries one of these mutations it undergoes conformational change that can be transmitted to other prion proteins carrying the same mutation and even to normal prion protein, and that this progresses relentlessly to cause prion disease. This conjecture is strongly supported by transmission studies between transgenic mice.

The sporadic form of CJD occurs in individuals who are homozygous for a common polymorphism of the prion gene, which substitutes valine for methionine at position 129. This observation and the finding of prion mutations in persons previously classified as having

Pathogenic mutations in familial prion disease

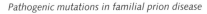

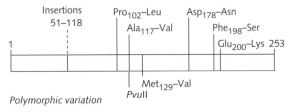

Fig. 7.13 The prion protein. Rare alleles and common polymorphisms of the prion protein that are associated with spongiform encephalopathy are shown (after Palmer *et al.* (1991)).

Alzheimer's disease suggest that the disease may be much more common than previously considered.

Conclusions

Many, if not all, common diseases show genetic differences in their susceptibility. Most usually this is due to a complex interaction between environmental risk factors and the multiple genetic components that come together to cause the disease. The methods of epidemiology and genetics have focussed in on the loci responsible for common diseases, and molecular biology has elucidated the structure and genetic variation of the specific molecules involved—as has been demonstrated for the plasma lipoproteins. This approach has led to a burgeoning of information about the pathogenetic processes and the molecular defects that cause disease. For the main part, genetic susceptibility is conferred by common polymorphic alleles present at each of the gene loci responsible for the disease. More rarely and more significantly, in those persons affected, rare alleles at certain key loci have a heritable effect and lead more directly to disease. Knowledge about the rarer, more heritable forms of common disease leads to new knowledge about the more common forms of the same disease and this in turn may lead to improved diagnosis and new treatment.

Further reading

Bahary N., Leibel R.L., Joseph L. and Friedman J.M. (1990) Molecular mapping of the mouse *db* mutation. *Proceedings of the National Academy of Sciences of the USA*, **87**, 8642–8646.

Becker A.B. and Roth R.A. (1990) Insulin receptor structure and function in normal and pathological conditions. *Annual Review of Medicine*, **41**, 99–115.

Bell G.I., Wu S.-H., Newman M., Fajans S.S., Seino M., Seino S. and Cox N.J. (1991) Diabetes mellitus: identification of susceptibility genes. In: *Etiology of Human Disease at the DNA Level* (eds J. Lindsten and U. Pettersson), pp. 93–113. Raven Press, New York.

Breslow J.L. (1989) Genetic basis of the lipoprotein disorders. *Journal of Clinical Investigation*, **84**, 373–380.

Breslow J.L. (1991) Lipoprotein transport gene abnormalities underlying coronary heart disease susceptibility. *Annual Review of Medicine*, **42**, 357–371.

Ciaranello R.D. and Ciaranello A.L. (1991) Genetics of major psychiatric disorders. *Annual Review of Medicine*, **42**, 151–158.

Clarke R., Daly L., Robinson K., Naughten E., Cahalane S., Fowler B. and Graham I. (1991) Hyperhomocysteinemia: an independent risk factor for vascular disease. *New England Journal of Medicine*, **324**, 1149–1155.

Cornall R.J., Prins J.-B., Todd J.A., Pressey A., DeLarato N.H.,

Wicker L.S. and Peterson L.B. (1991) Type 1 diabetes in mice is linked to the interleukin-1 receptor and *Lsh/Ity/Bcg* genes on chromosome 1. *Nature*, **353**, 262–265.

Davies J.L., Kawaguchi Y., Bennett S.T., Copeman J.B., Cordell H.J., Pritchard L.E., Reed P.W., Gough S.C.L., Jenkins S.C., Palmer S.M., Balfour K.M., Rowe B.R., Farrall M., Barnett A.H., Bain S.C. and Todd J.A. (1994) A genome-wide search for human type 1 diabetes susceptibility genes. *Nature*, **371**, 130–136.

European Polycystic Kidney Disease Consortium (1994) The polycystic kidney disease 1 gene encodes a 14 kb transcript and lies within a duplicated region on chromosome 16. *Cell*, **77**, 881–894.

Fuster V., Badimon L., Badimon J.J. and Chesebro J.H. (1992) Mechanisms of disease: the pathogenesis of coronary artery disease and the acute coronary syndromes. *New England Journal of Medicine*, **326**, 242–251, 310–319.

Goldstein J.L. and Brown M.S. (1991) Genetic aspects of disease. In: *Principles of Internal Medicine*, 12th edn (eds J.D. Wilson *et al.*). McGraw-Hill, New York.

Hilbert P., Lindpaintner K., Beckmann J.S., Serikawa T., Soubrier F., Dubay C., Cartwright P., De Gouyon B., Julier C., Takahasi S., Vincent M., Ganten D., Georges M. and Lathrop G.M. (1991) Chromosomal mapping of two genetic loci associated with blood-pressure regulation in hereditary hypertensive rats. *Nature*, **353**, 521–529.

Hyman B.T. and Tani R. (1995) Molecular epidemiology of Alzheimer's. *New England Journal of Medicine*, **333**, 1283–1284.

Jacob H.J., Lindpaintner K., Lincoln S.E., Kusumi K., Bunker R.K., Mao Y.-P., Ganten D., Dzau V.J. and Lander E.S. (1991) Genetic mapping of a gene causing hypertension in the stroke-prone spontaneously hypertensive rat. *Cell*, **67**, 213–224.

Julier C., Hyer R.N., Davies J., Merlin F., Soularue P., Briant L., Cathelineau G., Deschamps I., Rotter J.I., Froguel P., Boitard C., Bell J.I. and Lathrop G.M. (1991) Insulin-IGF2 region on chromosome 11p encodes a gene implicated in HLA-DR4-dependent diabetes susceptibility. *Nature*, **354**, 155–159.

McLean J.W., Tomlinson J.E., Kuang W.J. *et al.* (1987) cDNA sequence of human apolipoprotein(a) is homologous to plasminogen. *Nature*, **330**, 132–137.

Palmer M.S., Dryden A.J., Hughes J.T. and Collinge J. (1991) Homozygous prion protein genotype predisposes to sporadic Creutzfeldt-Jakob disease. *Nature*, **352**, 340–342.

Propping P. and Nothen M.M. (1995) Schizophrenia: genetic tools for unraveling the nature of a complex disorder. *Proceedings of the National Academy of Sciences of the USA*, **92**, 7607–7608.

Scott J. (1987) Molecular genetics of common diseases. *British Medical Journal*, **295**, 769–771.

Scott J. (1989) The molecular and cell biology of apolipoprotein-B. *Molecular Biology and Medicine*, **6**, 65–80.

Scott J. (1991) Lipoprotein(a): thrombotic and atherogenic. *British Medical Journal*, **303**, 663–664.

Shoulders C.C., Brett D.J., Bayliss J.D., Narcisi T.M.E., Jarmuz A., Grantham T.T., Leoni P.R.D., Bhattacharya S., Pease R.J., Cullen P.M., Levi S., Byfield P.G.H., Purkiss P. and Scott J. (1993) Abetalipoproteinaemia is caused by defects of the gene encoding the 97 kDa subunit of a microsomal triglyceride transfer protein. *Human Molecular Genetics*, **2**, 2109–2116.

Todd J.A. (1990) Genetic control of autoimmunity in type 1 diabetes. *Immunology Today*, **11**, 122–129.

Todd J.A., Aitman T.J., Cornall R.J., Ghosh S., Hall J.R.S., Hearne C.M., Knight A.M., Love J.M., McAleer M.A., Prins J.-B., Rodrigues N., Lathrop M., Pressey A., DeLarato N.H., Peterson L.B. and Wicker L.S. (1991) Genetic analysis of autoimmune type 1 diabetes mellitus in mice. *Nature*, **351**, 542–547.

Tuddenham E.G. (1994) Thrombophilia: the new factor is old *factor V* (comment). *Lancet*, **343**, 1515–1516.

Yankner B.A. and Mesulam M.-M. (1991) β-amyloid and the pathogenesis of Alzheimer's disease. *New England Journal of Medicine*, **325**, 1849–1857.

Chapter

8 Molecular biology of cancer

Introduction

The evidence that cancer has a genetic basis originates from three observations: first, carcinogens cause DNA mutations; second, tumours frequently display specific chromosomal abnormalities; third, in rare cancer syndromes, a predisposition to the development of cancer is inherited. The study of molecular genetics has demonstrated the links between mutation and cancer by identifying the target genes for mutations that are implicated in malignant transformation. These genes can be divided into two operational classes, **oncogenes** and **tumour suppressor genes**. Oncogenes are predominantly components of pathways that activate cell division in response to growth factor stimulation. Malignant transformation can be a consequence of mutations that increase their activity or expression (gain-of-function mutations). The functions of these positive effectors are in contrast to the second operational class, the tumour suppressor genes. Mutations that inactivate tumour suppressor genes (loss-of-function mutations) are commonly found in human tumour samples. The role of these genes is to encode proteins that **constrain** proliferation, in some cases by direct interactions with members of the oncogene family.

In this chapter we begin by discussing the link between somatic mutation and cancer, and show how oncogenes and tumour suppressor genes were discovered and how they are affected by carcinogenic mutations. We emphasize the observations that demonstrate that cancer cells must bear multiple genetic lesions in order to become fully malignant.

Definitions of cancer and transformation

Unicellular organisms must respond to changes in the environment that favour growth, compete effectively with surrounding cells for resources and continue cell division until the nutrient supply is exhausted. The evolutionary step that created multicellular organisms (metazoa) required the imposition of a different set of cellular priorities. Rather than compete, neighbouring cells must grow in a way that favours the survival of the whole organism. To do this, complex signalling mechanisms have evolved, so that cell growth and differentiation is coordinated and an internal environment maintained. A failure in cellular coordination is catastrophic, as the unrestrained growth of just one cell, by competing with its neighbours for space and nutrients, will disrupt and eventually destroy the organism (Fig. 8.1). Cancer is the term used to describe this event and examples have been documented in many metazoan species. It is perhaps surprising, given the complexities of multicellular organisms, that cancer is not more frequent. It seems likely that evolution has furnished metazoa with regulatory mechanisms that prevent aberrant cell growth.

The 'transformed' cell is the *in vitro* counterpart of the cancer cell. Normal cells in tissue culture require exoge-

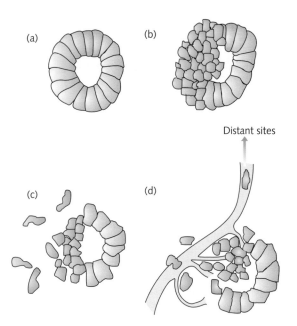

Fig. 8.1 Cancer is a disorder of cellular organization. Building even the simplest structures from single cells requires a complex biological programme so that each constituent cell maintains its orientation with respect to neighbouring cells and grows in a regular manner. The duct structure, depicted in (a), illustrates this principle. In (b), a single clone of cells have lost their ability to co-ordinate growth with neighbouring cells and have begun to compete for space, growing into the duct. In (c), further expansion of the clone has led to growth beyond the confines of the duct, breaching the basement membrane (invasion). Further expansion requires the induction of a new blood supply (angiogenesis) (d). Ultimately, cells are carried away by the lymphatics and the bloodstream to lodge in other organs and disrupt structure and function at distant sites (metastasis).

reflects the more complex environment *in vivo* which selects for other characteristics beneficial to a cancer cell's survival, such as the ability to acquire a blood supply, or escape from immune recognition.

Somatic cells and germ cells

As well as the need for co-operative rather than competitive growth, a key difference between metazoa and protozoa (nucleated single cell organisms) is the division between **germ cells** and **somatic cells**. All members of a protozoan species can, in the right circumstances, undergo genetic recombination. In metazoa, genetic recombination (sexual reproduction) is the function of a subpopulation of specialized cells—germ cells. The cells that constitute the rest of the organism, the somatic cells, do not contribute genetic material to reproduction. This cellular division is important in terms of the consequences of a mutation that disrupts growth regulation. A mutation in a germ cell that disturbs cellular growth may not be compatible with normal formation of the embryo and because the developing organism is not viable such mutations will be deleted from the germ line. However, mutations that are lethal when they are present in all cells during organogenesis may not be so when they arise by somatic mutation in the occasional cell in mature organs. Indeed, populations of somatic cells bearing mutations that increase growth or modify cell survival persist and accumulate in adult life.

Carcinogenesis and the rate of somatic mutation

In humans and laboratory animals, epidemiological evidence suggests that cancer arises through a number of steps. In humans, measurements of the age-related incidence of common cancers demonstrates kinetics dependent on the fourth or fifth power of elapsed time. This suggests four or five independent events must take place before a cell is fully malignant. If each of these steps represents a somatic mutation, there is a strong theoretical argument, based on the rate of somatic mutation, that these mutations must arise sequentially rather than simultaneously.

Experimental estimates of the frequency of somatic mutation are of the order of one in 10^6 per gene per cell cycle. If we assume that mutations in two genes in any given cell are required for oncogenesis, the rate for this combined event occurring in the same cell cycle is one in 10^{12} cell divisions. Estimates of the number of mitoses that occur during the lifetime of a human being are of the order of 10^{16}. Thus, the estimated frequency of muta-

nous growth factors to proliferate and have a limited life span before they senesce and die. They also demonstrate contact inhibition, so that once the tissue culture dish is covered in a monolayer of cells, proliferation ceases. In contrast, cancer cells in culture have some or all of the following characteristics:

1 reduced requirement for **growth factors**;
2 **loss of contact inhibition**, so that cells have the tendency to pile up and form foci;
3 The capacity to **divide indefinitely**, i.e. the cells are immortal;
4 **anchorage-independent growth** — usually demonstrated by the capacity to grow in soft agar.

The acquisition of these characteristics in tissue culture does not, however, always guarantee that an experimentally transformed cell will grow as a tumour when transplanted into an appropriate host. This presumably

tions affecting any two given genes in a single cell cycle is 10^4 times per lifetime. For three mutations in a single cell cycle, the chance falls to one in every 100 human beings, and for four or more, the chance of a single cell receiving the number of mutations necessary for malignant transformation is totally incompatible with observed cancer rates.

These calculations suggest that somatic mutation can only be the basis of cancer if cells bearing carcinogenic mutations undergo positive selection. In this model (Fig. 8.2), a primary mutation takes place that causes a cell to either grow more quickly than its neighbours, or to survive longer than is physiologically appropriate. As a result, a population (or **clone**) of cells arises, each replicating the mutation. Once the clone approaches 10^6 cells in size, the chance of a cell receiving a second mutation that confers a further growth or survival advantage becomes significant. The cell bearing such a 'double hit' will then go on to outgrow the first clone. In this way, a tumour could continuously evolve with time, accumulating increasing numbers of growth-stimulating mutations by somatic mutation and clonal outgrowth.

We know from clinical experience that tumours continue to evolve after detection. Major determinants of patient survival such as seeding of tumour cells around the body (metastasis) and drug resistance also arise through mutation and clonal selection. A factor that may affect tumour evolution is the possibility that the somatic mutation rate in tumours is greater than 10^{-6} per gene for each cell cycle. This would be the case if either (i) the target genes are very large, (ii) the tissue is exposed to repeated doses of a mutagen, (iii) there is an increased rate of misrepair or replication error (i.e. mutations in genes controlling these processes) or (iv) there is a defect in the ability of the cell to detect or respond to genetic damage, allowing cells with unrepaired DNA damage to enter the cell cycle, with consequent loss, translocation or duplication of chromosomal material.

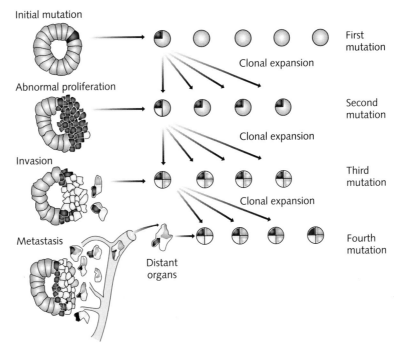

Fig. 8.2 Tumour development by sequential somatic mutation and clonal outgrowth. The somatic mutation and clonal outgrowth theory predicts that all cancers arise from a single progenitor cell that undergoes a somatic mutation in a gene that results in enhanced growth or survival. By successfully competing with normal cells, a population (or clone) of cells arises, replicating the mutation. Eventually a second mutation takes place in a single cell within this clone that further enhances growth or survival, generating a second population of double mutant cells that outgrow the original single mutant clone. In this way, cells can accumulate mutations over time. It is estimated that at least four or five mutations have to take place before full transformation takes place. Studies of premalignant conditions such as Barrett's oesophagitis (a forerunner of adenocarcinoma of the oesophagus) have demonstrated that a number of clones with varying numbers of somatic mutations and malignant potential can co-exist in the same tissue.

Tumours are monoclonal

A prediction of the somatic mutation and clonal selection model is that tumours are monoclonal in composition. The analysis of X-linked genes in females provided the first evidence of tumour clonality. Although all cells in a female contain two X-chromosomes, one is inactivated by a random process that takes place early in embryogenesis. Thus every female is a mosaic in the sense that her cellular composition is a mixture of cells that have one or other X-chromosome inactivated. These two sets of cells can be distinguished if the genes on one X-chromosome are different from the other. This was first done by taking advantage of the observation that certain (principally African) populations carry a high incidence of mutations in the X-linked gene for the enzyme glucose-6-phosphate dehydrogenase (G6PD; Fig. 8.3). In individuals that are heterozygotes, with a wild-type gene on one X-chromosome and an inactive mutant on the other X-chromosome, X-inactivation can be identified by a cell staining method that relies on the activity of G6PD. In this situation, tissues have a mixture or mosaic of cells containing either active or inactive G6PD. Cancers arising in these individuals express only one G6PD allele, and are therefore monoclonal. Studies on B- and T-cells demonstrate that clonal rearrangements in immunoglobulin or T-cell receptor genes take place early in lymphoid differentiation, providing another unique marker to demonstrate tumour monoclonality (see Chapter 10). On this basis, B- and T-cell tumours must arise from a single progenitor cell, since all the cells in any particular T-cell lymphoma bear the same T-cell receptor rearrangement, and in the case of B-cell tumours (myeloma), an antibody of a single type. More

recently, the clonal nature of tumours has also been confirmed by the direct analysis of mutated oncogenes and tumour suppressor genes in cancerous rather than noncancerous tissue, in material obtained by biopsy or surgical resection, using such techniques as fluorescent *in situ* hybridization (FISH) in which fluorescent probes specific for certain DNA sequences can be hybridized to specific chromosomes.

The germ line contribution to carcinogenesis

The somatic mutation and clonal selection hypothesis needs to accommodate the observation that an individual's inherited gene complement appears to influence susceptibility to cancer. There are many examples of familial cancer syndromes where a predisposition to the development of cancer is inherited (see Chapter 9). Studies of these syndromes have demonstrated two mechanisms by which inheritance can influence the development of cancer.

1 The germ line can contribute directly to malignant transformation through mutations that are compensated for during embryogenesis by the presence of a normal allele. The mutation is unmasked by a second, somatic mutation that disrupts the remaining healthy allele later in an individual's (postnatal) life. A well-defined example of this is familial retinoblastoma, which is transmitted in Mendelian dominant fashion.

2 Inherited conditions exist that increase the chance of cancer by increasing the rate of somatic mutation. Here the inheritance pattern is usually recessive. Defects in DNA repair such as ataxia telangectasia, Bloom's syndrome and xeroderma pigmentosum fall into this category. Other classes of inherited conditions that increase cancer risk include certain immune deficiencies that are associated with an increased incidence of cancers such as lymphoma and skin tumours, and polymorphisms in genes encoding for enzymes that affect the metabolic activation of xenobiotic carcinogens, such as the cytochrome P450 superfamily.

Carcinogens and mutagenesis

The discovery that a chemical or physical agent is a **carcinogen** (causes cancer) nearly always preceded the observation that it was a **mutagen** (mutates DNA). X-rays were discovered in 1895. Seven years later a skin cancer was observed on the hand of a man whose occupation was to make and test X-ray tubes. Another 25 years elapsed before X-irradiation was shown to cause mutagenesis in fruit flies. Similarly, the high incidence of

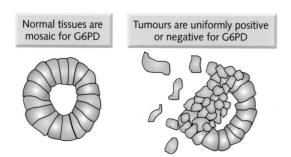

Fig. 8.3 Experimental support for tumour monoclonality by examining the expression of G6PD in tumours arising in females heterozygous for G6PD deficiency. Cancers arising in these patients are uniformly either positive or negative for G6PD, whereas normal tissues are a mixture or mosaic of positive or negative cells (see text for further explanation).

cancer amongst workers in the chemical industry had been noted as long ago as 1902, but the link between chemical carcinogenesis and mutagenesis was not made until 1941, when mustard gas was shown to be a mutagen.

The first demonstration in 1915 that cancer could be induced in the skin of mice by the repeated application of coal tar initiated 50 years of intensive research into experimental animal carcinogenesis. An important finding resulted from the purification and testing of each of the components of coal tar. Whilst some of the substances purified are capable of initiating skin cancers if repeatedly painted onto mouse skin, others appear to be more irritant than carcinogenic, causing a transient increase in the proliferation of skin cells after application but few cancers. Applied together, the two classes of chemical induce many more tumours than when applied separately. In fact, a single dose of a chemical capable of initiating cancers will induce tumours if mouse skin is subsequently subjected to repeated applications of the non-carcinogenic irritant. Experimentalists labelled this two-step process **initiation** and **promotion**, and the substances involved initiators and promoters. A similar pattern can be demonstrated in organs other than skin, for example liver tumours can be induced in rodents fed a single dose of an initiator, if this is followed by a 'tumour-promoting' stimulus to hepatocyte proliferation such as partial hepatectomy or a dose of a hepatotoxin.

Further studies have shown that the initiators are mutagens, and that there is a direct relationship between their activity in initiating tumours in mouse skin and their ability to interact with DNA and cause mutation. The biological basis of tumour promotion remained controversial for many years, but it is now acknowledged that tumour promoters affect the physiological state of the tissue from which the tumour arises. They do this by interacting with cellular components involved in the regulation of cellular proliferation. The distinction between promoters and initiators is somewhat blurred by the fact that tumour promoters themselves are weakly carcinogenic in experimental animals. This is assumed to be because the action of the tumour promoter reveals the presence of 'background' mutations that occur at low frequency in the absence of exogenous mutagens.

Tumour viruses

Whilst experiments on animal carcinogenesis pointed towards a close link between somatic mutation and cancer, the key to progress lay in the identity of the genetic targets for transforming mutations. The existence of these target genes, **oncogenes**, had long been postulated, but the technology that allowed a systematic search of the human genome has been available only recently. A major obstacle to their identification is the complexity of the human genome — up to 50 000 functional genes buried within 3×10^9 basepairs of sequence.

A direct route to the identity of at least some oncogenes has been furnished by the so-called **tumour viruses**. These viruses can be divided into two groups based on the rapidity at which they induce tumours: the first group induces tumours after chronic infection of the host, with a long interval between infection and the appearance of the first tumour; the second group causes tumours very rapidly — within weeks of infection. Two biologically distinct types of tumour viruses have been identified that cause tumours after chronic infection of the host, RNA tumour viruses and DNA tumour viruses, a division based on whether the genome of the infecting particle is composed of RNA or DNA (see Chapter 13). Viruses that induce tumours after a very short interval have exclusively an RNA-based genome. The transforming capacity of these 'acutely transforming' RNA tumour viruses is all the more remarkable for the fact that the genome of these viruses consists of only a few kilobases, and encodes only three known viral genes.

Acutely transforming RNA tumour viruses

The first acutely transforming RNA tumour virus was described by Peyton Rous, in 1911, as a filterable agent that induces sarcomas in chickens (Rous sarcoma virus, or RSV). Subsequently over 40 have been identified, capable of inducing several tumour types in a variety of species, including rats, mice, chickens and cats. Although RNA tumour viruses are known that induce tumours in primates, a direct link between these viruses and human cancer has only been established in the case of the HTLV-1 virus, which causes a form of adult T-cell lymphoma/leukaemia that occurs endemically in parts of Japan, the Caribbean and sporadically throughout the world. The observation that RNA tumour viruses apparently induce tumours in a single step following infection at first seems incompatible with the hypothesis that cancer arises in a series of steps, and we will return to this issue later. This fact, taken with the observation that RNA tumour viruses are not a major cause of human malignancy, led to transient questions about the relevance of tumour virus research. These objections were soon overcome by the demonstration that RNA tumour viruses provide a remarkably effective route to the direct cloning of genes involved in viral as well as non-viral carcinogenesis.

The structure of the RNA tumour viruses is outlined in

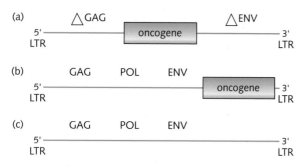

Fig. 8.4 The structure of transforming RNA tumour viruses. Three classes of RNA tumour viruses have been implicated in experimental tumorigenesis. (a) The most frequently observed arrangement of an oncogene inserted into the retrovirus genome disrupting viral replication genes. Such viruses need a 'helper virus' that provides the required replication proteins. (b) The exceptional arrangement of the avian sarcoma virus v-*src* oncogene in the 3′ LTR, generating a replication-competent transforming virus. (c) A retrovirus that does not carry an oncogene, e.g. mouse mammary tumour virus and avian leukosis virus. In these cases, insertion of viral regulatory sequences (promoters) in the cellular genome disrupts the normal regulation of adjacent cellular oncogenes leading to overexpression and transformation.

Fig. 8.4. Upon infection a viral enzyme, reverse transcriptase, transcribes double-stranded DNA from the RNA virus genome (the general name for such viruses that replicate through this 'reverse' movement of genetic information from RNA to DNA is **retrovirus**). The DNA copy of the virus then integrates into the host cell chromosome. Transcription ensues from a promoter at the end of the viral genome, within a sequence termed the long terminal repeat (LTR) present at either end of the integrated virus genome. LTRs also provide regulatory signals ensuring that viral mRNAs are correctly polyadenylated and translated. Transcription is driven by cellular transcription factors that recognize sequence elements in the LTR that are homologous to sequences that control cellular genes (see Chapter 4). Some RNA viruses encode genes that enhance LTR function, for example the HTLV-1 *tax* gene. The principal structural genes *gag* and *env* are concerned with packaging nascent viral RNA into infectious particles that bud from the cell surface to infect other cells.

Investigation of these acutely transforming retroviruses reveals a genome structure that includes novel sequences unrelated to genes previously associated with the viral genome. Studies on non-tumorigeneic revertants demonstrated mutations in these novel sequences, supporting the hypothesis that they conferred transforming capability on the virus. In RSV, the transforming

sequence is found in the 3′ end of the virus, leaving the virus replication genes intact. In most other acute retroviruses, the transforming sequences disrupt viral genes, and the virus can only replicate in the presence of a 'helper' virus that provides the essential virus gene products that are otherwise missing. The transforming gene is called the **retroviral oncogene**.

The identification of the origin of retrovirus oncogenes was the first breakthrough in the identification of the target genes in malignant transformation. Hybridization of retrovirus oncogenes to cellular RNA and DNA demonstrated that these sequences originated from cellular genes, expressed in normal healthy and uninfected cells. During passage in and out of the host cell's chromosomes, the occasional non-transforming virus, through chance recombination with surrounding host cell DNA, acquires host sequences — a process known as **viral transduction**. On occasion, these sequences are from genes that, when inappropriately expressed in the context of viral regulatory sequences, or mutated by fusion with viral genes, cause a loss of growth control in the infected cell. A general theme has emerged in which acutely transforming retroviruses are found to carry sequences that are related to highly evolutionarily conserved cellular genes. This evolutionary conservation suggests that the cellular counterparts of the retroviral oncogenes are involved in critical functions common to all eukaryotes.

The name of each oncogene generally refers to the species in which it was identified and the type of tumour it induces. When referring to the viral gene the suffix v is used, and for the cellular homologue, c. For example, the v-*sis* gene is an oncogene from the *si*mian *sar*coma virus. The cellular homologue is the c-*sis* gene (Table 8.1). A

Table 8.1 Nomenclature of some retroviral oncogenes.

Oncogene	Retrovirus
abl	Abelson murine leukaemia
erb	Avian erythroblastosis
fes	Feline sarcoma
fms	McDonough feline sarcoma
fos	FBJ murine osteosarcoma
mos	Moloney murine sarcoma
myb	Avian myeloblastosis
myc	MC29 avian myelocytom atosis
ras	Rat sarcoma
ros	Rochester VRII avian sarcoma
sis	Simian sarcoma
src	Rous sarcoma
yes	Yamaguchi avian sarcoma

detailed comparison of viral oncogenes and their cellular counterparts indicates that in the course of the transfer of these genes into the retrovirus, many mutations have taken place. In addition to point mutations, the viral genes are often truncated and fused to retrovirus genes generating chimeric virus–host fusion genes. The result of these mutations is to change the expression or activity of the viral protein with respect to the cellular counterpart (homologue). Indeed viruses engineered to express the wild-type cellular gene are frequently unable to induce tumours, emphasizing the importance of 'activating' mutations in viral transforming genes.

DNA tumour viruses

For a decade the study of tumour viruses has been dominated by RNA tumour viruses. Epidemiology, however, strongly indicates that some DNA tumour viruses are more important in terms of the causes of human cancer. For example, the human papilloma viruses are linked to cervical cancer, Epstein–Barr virus is linked to B-cell lymphoma and nasopharyngeal cancer, and hepatitis B virus is a significant factor in the aetiology of liver cancer. As with the RNA tumour viruses, critical discoveries have not come from studies on viruses directly implicated in human cancer, but from viruses that are carcinogenic in experimental animals. These investigations have turned out not only to impact on how DNA viruses might cause human cancer, but also on the mechanisms of carcinogenesis through somatic mutation, just as in the study of RNA tumour viruses.

Five DNA tumour viruses have been subject to intensive investigation: (i) simian virus 40 (SV40), discovered as a contaminant of polio vaccine preparation; (ii) polyoma virus, which has a similar structure, but whose natural host is the mouse rather than the monkey; (iii) adenovirus, which also can induce tumours in mice if they are infected when newborn; (iv) human papilloma virus (HPV); and (v) Epstein–Barr virus (EBV). Adenovirus, EBV and HPV have considerably more complex genomes than either polyoma or SV40. This made the simpler viruses more attractive in initial studies. Experiments with these viruses in tissue culture cells show that they all stimulate host cell DNA synthesis during the course of lytic infection. Presumably they do this to facilitate their own replication as they require many components of the host cell's replicative machinery in order to reproduce their own genomes. To achieve activation of the host cell and to trigger their own replication, tumour viruses encode 'early genes', expressed in the early phases of infection. The proteins encoded by these genes are multifunctional, and serve to stimulate expression of both host cell and viral genes as well as DNA replication. They also turn out to be the key genes that confer the capacity of these viruses to transform cells. The transforming genes of SV40 and polyoma are referred to as viral 'tumour antigens' or **T antigens** as their expression can elicit a strong immune response. The adenovirus transforming genes *E1a* and *E1b* have the suffix E to emphasize that they are expressed early after infection.

Exactly how the transforming genes of DNA tumour viruses transform cells is a question addressed by many laboratories around the world. The driving concept in these studies is that DNA virus oncogenes must directly interact with critical cellular components involved in replication and transcription. In keeping with this idea, investigators demonstrated that antibodies raised against tumour antigens co-precipitate cellular proteins. Co-precipitation experiments with antibodies against SV40 large T antigen led to the identification of a cellular protein, p53 (so named on the basis of its apparent size). Once cloned, the gene for p53 turned out to be a dominant acting oncogene. For a while the story rested on the assumption that the interaction with SV40 large T antigen somehow activated the transforming capacity of the *p53* proto-oncogene. Subsequent analysis of somatic mutations in *p53* in human tumours demonstrates this model as incorrect. First, the *p53* clone initially isolated turned out to be a mutated form. The wild-type gene has no transforming capacity, and has the paradoxical property of *inhibiting* transformation in some assays. Second, human tumours not only show clusters of point mutations in the *p53* gene, but also deletions in *p53* that completely eliminate expression of the affected allele. In fact, a deletion is frequently accompanied by a point mutation in the other allele so that the transformed cell does not express any wild-type *p53*. In extensive studies of large numbers of breast, lung and colon tumours, *p53* is the most frequently mutated gene described so far. Recently, in a rare autosomal dominant condition characterized by the occurrence of diverse mesenchymal and epithelial neoplasms at multiple sites, the Li–Fraumeni syndrome, a *p53* point mutation has been shown to be inherited in affected individuals in the family.

Taking into account all these lines of evidence, the current view is that *p53* is a member of a family of tumour suppressor genes whose functions are inactivated when a cell is transformed. The data from families with point mutations indicate that a *p53* mutation can be the initiating event in carcinogenesis, but since cancer develops after a lag period of several decades, other genetic changes are required before a cancer develops. One of the most frequent secondary changes is a deletion of the wild-type *p53* allele. An understanding of how *p53* might be involved in transformation comes from the observation that p53 operates in a complex, both with itself and other cellular proteins. In a cell that expresses one mutated and one wild-type allele, complexes form between mutated and wild-type proteins. These wild-type–mutant complexes are thought to be inactive, thus mutants of *p53* sequester wild-type protein into non-functional complexes, reducing the availability to the cell of functional wild-type p53 complexes. This type of mechanism is termed a 'dominant negative effect', as the wild-type protein is inactivated by the presence of a mutated protein.

It has recently become clear that in the absence of p53, in cells that have both alleles deleted, the introduction of at least some of the mutant *p53* alleles can increase the rate of proliferation. This suggests that not all the activity of mutant *p53* alleles can be explained in terms of a dominant negative effect, as this experiment clearly indicates that mutant *p53* is active in the absence of wild-type *p53*. This idea is further supported by the observation discussed earlier, that tumours frequently contain one deleted *p53* allele and one mutated allele, again suggesting there is some growth advantage to the cancer cell in expressing mutant *p53* in the absence of the wild-type gene. In addition to SV40 large T, oncogenes expressed by both adenovirus (*E1b*) and human papilloma virus (*HPV E6*) complex with *p53*. The common action of these tumour antigens is to inactivate *p53* in a complex, reducing the effective free p53 concentration in the cell. In the case of *HPV E6*, complex formation accelerates the proteolytic degradation of p53.

The normal function of p53 is discussed further in subsequent sections on the cell cycle and programmed cell death (p. 167). The role of p53 in cell cycle control, an involvement in inherited cancer syndromes, and activity as a tumour suppressor gene have parallels with another cellular gene targeted by tumour antigens, *Rb*.

Proteins encoded by oncogenes are components of signalling pathways that regulate cell proliferation and differentiation

As the number of identified oncogenes increases, a common theme has emerged concerning the mechanisms by which these genes transform cells. The cellular homologues—termed **proto-oncogenes** to underline their capacity to act as oncogenes in particular circumstances—encode components of the cellular machinery that regulates cell growth and differentiation. Whilst the first proto-oncogenes were discovered through homology to retroviral oncogenes, a number of other proto-oncogenes have since been defined during other investigations into cellular signalling and gene regulation. Most retroviral oncogenes have been ascribed functions in signal transduction pathways (Table 8.2), and fall into four broad categories:

1 intercellular signalling molecules (e.g. polypeptide growth factors);

2 cell surface receptors for these growth factors;

3 cytoplasmic signalling components that transmit (transduce) the signal from the ligand-activated receptor to the nucleus;

4 nuclear proteins that receive signals from the cytoplasm, and convert them into changes in the expression

Table 8.2 Functional classes of oncogenes (retroviral oncogenes in italics).

Growth factor	
sis	PDGF β- chain growth factor
int-2	
hst	FGF-related growth factor family
FGF-5	
Receptor protein tyrosine kinases	
erb-B	Truncated EGF receptor
kit	Truncated haemopoietic stem cell growth factor receptor
fms	Mutant CSF-1 receptor
Receptor protein tyrosine kinases ligand unknown	
ros, neu, trk, met	
Non-receptor protein typosine kinases	
Membrane associated	
src, yes, fgr, lck	
Not membrane associated	
fps, abl/bcr-abl	
Serine-threonine protein kinases	
raf, mos, pim 1	
Membrane associated G proteins	
H-ras, K ras, N ras, gsp and gip α subunits.	
Transcription factors	
Regulators of proliferation	
myc, N-myc, L-myc, fos, jun,	
Regulators of differentiation	
erb A, Gli, ski, retinoic acid receptor	
Cell cycle regulators	
PRAD 1 (cyclin related)	

of genes involved in regulating cellular proliferation and/or differentiation.

To understand how growth control and differentiation is subverted by mutations in oncoproteins, we must first understand their normal biochemistry. For this reason, we outline below the major mechanisms through which oncoproteins transfer information from the external environment to the cell's nucleus to elicit a cellular response (Fig. 8.5).

Protein phosphorylation

One biochemical function of some oncogene products is the phosphorylation of proteins. Oncogenes that do this

can be divided into two broad categories according to the amino acids that they phosphorylate:
1 the tyrosine kinase family;
2 the serine–theonine kinase family.

Members of the protein tyrosine kinase family fall into three further types according to their cellular location: (i) spanning the cell membrane, with a large ligand binding extracellular domain (e.g. c-*erbB* oncogene); (ii) located within the cytoplasm, attached to membranes (e.g. the c-*src* gene product); and (iii) in the nucleus (e.g. the c-*abl* gene product).

The ability of growth factor receptors such as epidermal growth factor receptor (EGFr) (Plate 10, facing p. 214) to phosphorylate tyrosine is activated upon binding

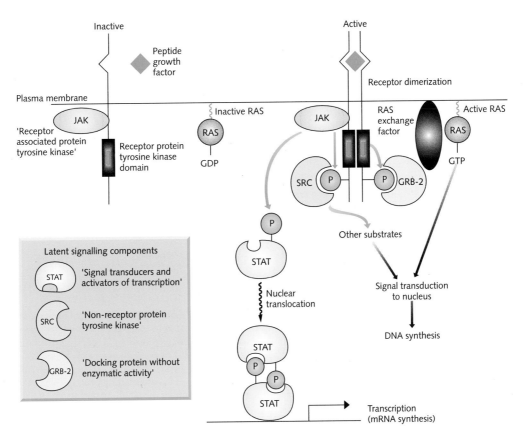

Fig. 8.5 Examples of signalling mechanisms via ligand-activated receptor protein tyrosine kinases. Binding of a growth factor to its cognate receptor leads to receptor dimerization and activation of the protein tyrosine kinase (PTK) domain in the intracellular portion of the receptor. This results in the receptor tyrosine kinase domain phosphorylating both the receptor itself (autophosphorylation) and associated signalling proteins. Phosphotyrosine residues stimulate receptor binding to a variety of signalling molecules, of which two examples are given in this figure: (1) 'docking proteins' that assist in the formation of multiprotein signalling complexes with RAS, but do not themselves have enzymatic activity—an example of this class is the 'GRB-2' protein (see Fig. 8.6); (2) cytoplasmic enzymes directly involved in signal transduction, for example the SRC gene product (another protein tyrosine kinase). Another class of receptor-associated signalling molecules are the 'Janus' protein kinases (JAKs). In the presence of ligand, JAKs phosphorylate latent cytoplasmic transcription factors (STATs) leading to dimerization and nuclear translocation. Phosphotyrosine reactions are indicated by blue arrows.

the growth factor ligand e.g. EGF. High energy phosphate is transferred to tyrosine residues in a number of substrates including the receptors themselves (autophosphorylation) and cytoplasmic signal transduction components. Once phosphorylated these proteins stimulate a cascade of biochemical events that eventually leads to the activation of cell division (see below). Oncogenic mutations affecting growth factor receptors give rise to deregulated tyrosine kinase activity. This may, for example, be due to mutations in the receptor kinase domain that affect autophosphorylation, or overexpression of intact receptors due to gene amplification. Substrates for protein tyrosine kinases, other than signal transduction components, include the integrin family, where phosphorylation may decrease cellular adhesiveness, and connexin, a component of gap junctions, whose functions in cell–cell communication may be inhibited by tyrosine phosphorylation.

The second class of protein kinases involved in transformation comprises the threonine–serine kinases. The normal forms of these genes encode proteins that have functions such as the regulation of the stability of protein complexes that control the meiotic and mitotic cell cycle (c-*mos*), or cytoplasmic signal transduction. An example of a threonine–serine kinase that acts as a signal transduction component is the protein encoded by the c-*raf* oncogene. The phosphorylation of the RAF (by convention oncogenes are referred to in italics and the proteins encoded by these genes in capital letters) protein increases rapidly on stimulation of resting cells with mitogens, leading to an increase in serine–threonine kinase activity. It has recently been determined that RAF is a critical signalling intermediary between RAS (see below) and the MAP kinases (mitogen-activated protein kinases) that directly phosphorylate nuclear proteins that modulate gene expression.

G proteins

Mutation and overexpression of another class of cytoplasmic signalling molecules, the GTPases, constitute a second mechanism by which RNA tumour viruses can transform cells (Fig. 8.6).

The role of RAS GTPases was first appreciated through the study of the *ras* oncogenes. These genes encode several members of a family of GTPases, generally known as **G proteins**, which bind GTP and thereby activate components further down the signalling cascade. The persistence of the 'onward' signal is determined by the ability of RAS to hydrolyse the bound GTP, and thereby switch itself into an inactive GDP-bound form. *ras* genes capable of transforming cells have mutations that inactivate their GTPase activity. The effect of

this is to leave the G protein permanently bound to GTP so generating a constitutive signal. Other oncogenes in the G protein family, *gsp* and *gip* (for G stimulatory protein and G inhibitory protein), have been identified as a result of studies on signal transduction. Mutations in *gsp* and *gip* α subunits have been found in a number of

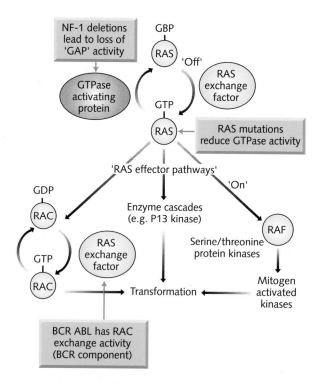

Fig. 8.6 Activation of RAS signalling. RAS and RAS-related proteins can either be in the active GTP-bound form or the inactive GDP-bound form. The rate of exchange of GDP for GTP is stimulated by 'exchange factors' that are themselves activated by non-receptor and receptor tyrosine kinases via a bridge provided by proteins such as GRB-2. RAS reverts to the inactive form by hydrolysing GTP to GDP, and this process is activated by GTPase-activating proteins, or GAPS. RAS in turn activates a number of signalling pathways, including the serine–threonine kinase cascade (RAF and MAP kinase), phosphatidyl inosinol 3-kinase, and other G proteins such as RAC and RHO. Activation of these 'downstream' pathways leads to phosphorylation of a series of nuclear targets that activate the cell cycle. In addition, phosphorylation of cytoplasmic targets leads to other aspects of the transformed phenotype, for example loss of contact inhibition of growth and morphological changes. Oncogenic mutations have been shown to occur in a number of genes encoding components of the RAS pathway, including in the RAS proteins themselves (leading to an inability to hydrolyse GTP), loss of GAP activity (loss-of-function mutations in NF1) and unregulated GTP exchange factor activity (the BCR component of the BCR–ABL fusion gene has exchange activity for RAS-activated G protein RAC, but has lost associated GAP activity).

human tumours. An important recent contribution to the understanding of G protein signalling is the identification of a group of proteins that activate the GTPase activity of RAS proteins — GTPase activating proteins (GAPs). These enzymes mediate the return of the G protein switch to the 'off' GDP-bound form. Mutations which inactivate GAP proteins can be themselves oncogenic (e.g. the neurofibromatosis gene *NF1*; see Chapter 9). In another recent development, cellular components have been identified that directly link tyrosine kinase receptors to RAS signalling. The presence of phosphotyrosine on tyrosine kinase receptors triggers a series of protein–protein interactions that leads to an increase in the rate of RAS GTP exchange.

Transcription factors

A third major theme in the cellular function of oncoproteins is their influence on gene expression by **transcriptional control**. Oncoproteins have been shown to bind directly to regulatory sequences that flank the coding sequences of target genes (enhancer and promoter sequences) and thereby modulate the activities of RNA polymerases. Broadly speaking, these oncogenes can be divided into two operational classes:

1 transcription factors involved in the activation of cellular proliferation in response to growth factors;
2 transcription factors involved in the regulation of differentiation.

Transcription factor proto-oncogenes involved in cellular proliferation are members of the 'immediate early' gene family whose expression is rapidly activated when growth-arrested cells are exposed to mitogens. Immediate early genes encode proteins that are required to initiate the cascade of events that lead the cell through G1 into S phase of the cell cycle (p. 167). Cellular activation by growth factors does not always involve the stimulation of transcription factor synthesis. Some oncoproteins, e.g. the REL family — members of the NFκB family of proteins — are expressed in resting cells but prevented from activating transcription by cytoplasmic inhibitors. Stimulation with growth factors leads to the release of REL proteins from cytoplasmic inhibitors with subsequent nuclear translocation and transcriptional activation.

Differentiation and cancer

The main focus of discussion has thus far been the concept of malignancy as a disorder of cellular growth, but an equally important aspect of the malignant phenotype is loss of the capacity to differentiate. This is particularly well illustrated in the **leukaemias**. Each type of

leukaemia causes arresting at a different stage in blood cell differentiation, which provides a clinico-pathological basis for a classification of these diseases. A small group of oncogenic transcription factors have been demonstrated to be inhibitors of blood cell differentiation, rather than activators of stem cell proliferation. Two leukaemias, one experimental and one clinical, are good examples of this.

The oncogene v-*erbA* was discovered in an acutely transforming retrovirus that causes a leukaemia (erythroblastosis) in chickens. v-*erbA* is a fusion protein between thyroid hormone receptor and the viral *gag* gene, and transforms cells in conjunction with the v-*erbB* oncogene, co-expressed by the same virus (v-*erbB* is related to epidermal growth factor receptor, see Plates 11 and 12, facing p. 214). Normal thyroid hormone receptors are nuclear located transcription factors. In the absence of thyroid hormone (T3), they act to suppress expression from genes that have thyroid hormone response elements in their promoters. In the presence of T3, expression from these genes is strongly activated. v-*erbA* has lost the ability to respond to T3 and acts as a constitutive repressor. The effect of an infection of chicken bone marrow stem cells with the retrovirus is to cause differentiation arrest in the erythrocyte lineage, presumably by blocking the expression of erythrocyte-specific genes that normally respond to T3. In clinical studies, retinoic acid (vitamin A) is an effective treatment of the human malignancy acute promyelocytic leukaemia (PML) by forcing terminal myeloid differentiation. Like the T3 receptor, the receptor for retinoic acid is a nuclear located transcription factor that regulates differentiation. Intriguingly, all cases of PML have a chromosomal translocation involving the α retinoic acid receptor (RARα). As a result, PML cells express a fusion gene comprised of truncated RARα sequences and a gene on the reciprocal chromosome (see p. 160 for a discussion of chromosomal translocations). The effect of this abnormal protein is to arrest myeloid differentiation in cells exposed to physiological levels of retinoic acid. Higher, therapeutic levels of retinoic acid overcome this block, which may reflect the fact that leukaemia cells are heterozygous for the translocation. Normal receptors, encoded by the non-translocated αRAR allele, are probably functionally repressed by the fusion gene so that higher levels of retinoic acid are required for activation.

Human tumours frequently carry mutations and chromosome rearrangements

If proto-oncogenes are implicated in human carcinogenesis, the somatic mutation hypothesis predicts that tumours must carry mutations that occur in these genes. Furthermore, the mutations have to be the result of non-retroviral mutagenesis, i.e. compatible with the epidemiological evidence that does not implicate such infectious agents in most human cancers. Somatic, non-viral mutations have indeed been demonstrated in many, but not all the proto-oncogenes identified in studies on acutely transforming retroviruses. Mutations in c-*src*, for example, have never been documented in human tumours (although the normal allele has been found to be overexpressed in some colon cancers). Extensive studies reveal that a restricted number of oncogenes are regularly mutated during human carcinogenesis (see Table 8.3). Mutations in cancers take the form of one of six types (Fig. 8.7):

1 point mutation, leading to either amino acid substitution (missense), or premature termination of translation (nonsense);

2 chromosome translocation or other rearrangement, for example inversion;

3 amplification of a specific area within a chromosome to produce multiple gene copies;

4 loss of chromosomal material;

5 insertion of external DNA through the action of viruses;

6 expansion of nucleotide repeat sequences due to defective DNA repair.

Point mutation

Point mutation appears to be a common form of activating mutation. Many examples are seen in the *ras* family of oncogenes. A large number and variety of human tumours have been found to bear point mutations in one or other *ras* genes. The mutations are restricted in their localization to a number of specific amino acids and recent analysis of the crystal structure of RAS indicates that all would inhibit the coordination of a GTP molecule in the catalytic site and therefore compromise GTP hydrolysis. A link between experimental carcinogenesis and human disease is afforded by study of these genes, as mutation of *ras* has been demonstrated in tumours induced by the application of carcinogen to mouse skin. In general the types of mutation accord with the chemical action of the carcinogen, in keeping with the view that tumorigenesis involves direct mutation of *ras* genes.

Chromosome translocation

Although an increasing number of cytogenetic abnormalities have been documented in human cancer, chromosome translocations are particularly associated with leukaemias and lymphomas. An example is Burkitt's lymphoma (see Chapter 10). This tumour occurs in two forms, an endemic form in equatorial Africa and a sporadic form. In both types, the distal end of the long arm of chromosome 8 is translocated to chromosome 14, 22 or 2. Armed with the knowledge that the chromosomal site of c-*myc* had recently been mapped to chromosome 8, several groups considered the possibility the c-*myc* might be the key cellular gene involved in the Burkitt's translocations. Careful analysis of the translocations demonstrated this to be the case. c-*myc* is involved in reciprocal translocations with the immunoglobulin loci in 100% of cases. The effect of this translocation appears to be an alteration in c-*myc* regulation. Under the influence of the transcriptional activity of the immunoglobulin locus, MYC becomes constitutively expressed and does not respond to the signals that normally regulate MYC expression. These translocations are of course only seen in the genesis of B-cell tumours as the immunoglobulin loci are transcriptionally inactive in non-B-cells.

Table 8.3 Examples of oncogenes consistently altered in human cancers.

Oncogene	Neoplasm	Alteration
abl	Chronic myeloid leukaemia	Translocation
erb-B1	Squamous cell carcinoma Astrocytoma	Amplification
neu/erb-B2	Adenocarcinoma of breast stomach and ovary	Amplification
gip	Ovarian and adrenal carcinoma	Point mutation
gsp	Pituitary adenoma, thyroid carcinoma	Point mutation
myc	Burkitt's lymphoma Lung, breast and cervical carcinoma	Translocation Amplification
L-*myc*	Lung carcinoma	Amplification
N-*myc*	Neuroblastoma and small cell lung cancer	Amplification
H-*ras*	Colon, lung and pancreatic carcinoma, melanoma	Point mutation
K-*ras*	Acute myeloid and lymphoblastic leukaemia Thyroid carcinoma	Point mutation
N-*ras*	Bladder, thyroid carcinoma, melanoma	Point mutation

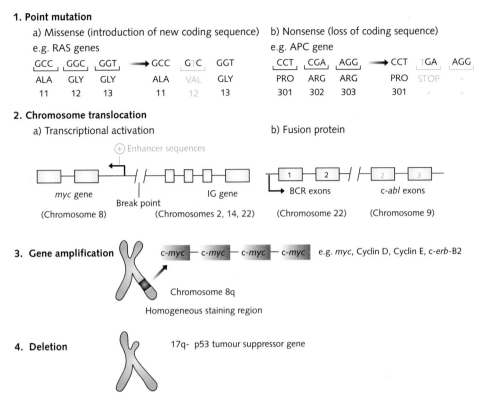

1. Point mutation

a) Missense (introduction of new coding sequence)

e.g. RAS genes

GCC   GGC   GGT   →   GCC   GTC   GGT
ALA   GLY   GLY   ALA   VAL   GLY
11   12   13   11   12   13

b) Nonsense (loss of coding sequence)

e.g. APC gene

CCT   CGA   AGG   →   CCT   TGA   AGG
PRO   ARG   ARG   PRO   STOP   -
301   302   303   301   -   -

2. Chromosome translocation

a) Transcriptional activation

(+) Enhancer sequences

myc gene   IG gene
(Chromosome 8)   Break point   (Chromosomes 2, 14, 22)

b) Fusion protein

BCR exons   *c-abl* exons
(Chromosome 22)   (Chromosome 9)

3. Gene amplification

c-*myc* — c-*myc* — c-*myc* — c-*myc*   e.g. *myc*, Cyclin D, Cyclin E, *c-erb*-B2

Chromosome 8q

Homogeneous staining region

4. Deletion

17q- p53 tumour suppressor gene

Fig. 8.7 Mutations in human cancers. (1) Point mutations. The consequences of point mutation can be either to cause an amino acid substitution (missense mutation) that alters the function of the encoded protein, or to cause premature termination of transcription by disrupting the reading frame (nonsense mutations) with subsequent loss of coding sequence. (2) Chromosome translocation. There are two principal consequences of translocation. The abnormal juxtaposition of chromosomal material either (i) brings new regulatory sequences (promoter and enhancer elements) near to the location of proto-oncogenes leading to inappropriate gene expression, or (ii) results in the formation of a fusion gene that encodes a novel protein that contains amino acids from two different genes. (3) Gene amplification. Gene amplification is a frequent event in the later phases of malignant transformation and leads to protooncogene overexpression. The presence of gene amplification may be indicated by characteristic cytogenetic abnormalities including homogeneously staining regions and double minute chromosomes. (4) Deletions. Loss of DNA in cancer cells varies from single nucleotide deletions to losses of large sections of chromosomes that are visible by cytogenetics. Deletions are typical of mutations associated with tumour suppressor genes.

The combination of cytogenetic analysis and molecular genetics has provided insight into the pathogenesis of leukaemia, notably chronic myeloid leukaemia (CML). In CML the characteristic cytogenetic abnormality is a translocation between the distal end of chromosome 9 and chromosome 22. This leaves a smaller than normal chromosome 22, the 'Philadelphia' chromosome. The oncogene c-*abl* is involved in this translocation in 95% of cases. The result is a fusion protein between ABL and the product of a gene, *bcr* (*b*reak point *c*luster *r*egion), located in the reciprocal chromosome. The functional result of fusing these proteins is to produce a constitutive tyrosine kinase, although how exactly this is responsible for the CML phenotype is unclear.

Why should translocations be such an apparently common mechanism of transformation in haemopoietic malignancies? B- and T-cells undergo a programme of controlled somatic mutation to create diversity in immune recognition (see Chapter 10). Sequence analysis of the break points in both sporadic and Burkitt's B-cell lymphomas suggests that the characteristic translocation takes place in pre-B-cells, when the process of V-D-J joining is taking place. The enzyme VDJ recombinase, critical to this process, seems to be involved in joining the ends of the translocated chromosomes. This mechanism is suggested by several lines of evidence: first, the translocations involve the J segment region; second the characteristic recombinase signal sequence is present on both sides of the break point; and finally extra nucleotides are found around the join, just as in normal VDJ recombination. Translocations might not be expected to be common in malignancies arising from cells lineages that do not express VDJ recombinase. Whilst it is true that in other cancers translocation is perhaps a less common form of karyotypic abnormality, there are still examples, such as Ewing's sarcoma and neuroepithelioma. The mechanism involved in these cases is not clear, but investigation may well reveal novel recombination mechanisms at work.

How do translocations involving c-*myc* and the immunoglobulin loci fit into our understanding of the pathogenesis of endemic Burkitt's lymphoma in equatorial Africa? The heavy epidemiological association with malaria and Epstein–Barr virus (EBV) has led to the following pathogenic model. EBV infection of young African children leads to an expansion of the pool of B-cells rearranging their immunoglobulin genes. These EBV-infected B-cells persist as T-cell immunity is suppressed by malaria infection. The chance of a mistake during VDJ recombination increases as the infected B-cell pool expands, and aberrant ligation events causing chromosome translocation are selected for by the increased growth potential of cells with Burkitt's translocations.

Characteristic translocations are not restricted to Burkitt's lymphoma and CML. The well-differentiated follicular lymphoma, a less aggressive 'indolent' type of lymphoma, is characterized by a 14:18 translocation. One of the genes disrupted by this translocation, *Bcl-2* (for B-cell lymphoma gene 2), has been shown to enhance the survival rather than the proliferation rate of lymphoma cells in comparison with normal B-cells. Thus cells accumulate, not because of increased growth, but because the cells do not die when physiologically appropriate. The concept that there are cellular pathways that control cell death as well as cell growth is an important one that will be returned to later.

Gene amplification and polyploidy

Amplification in a segment of a chromosome is a relatively common event in tumour cells in the later stages of their development. Amplification occurs under the selective pressure of tumour evolution, as a mechanism that increases the expression of genes that give the cell a growth advantage. At a karyotypic level, the presence of gene amplification is indicated by homogeneous staining regions and double minute chromosomes. Interestingly, not all amplified loci in cancer samples contain previously identified oncogenes with increased or altered

expression patterns and this may indicate the presence of unidentified oncogenes. For example, in a number of breast cancers, a locus that includes members of the fibroblast growth factor family is amplified, however none of the known genes in the amplicon is expressed. A recently identified gene involved in a chromosome 11 inversion in parathyroid adenomas, *PRAD1* (*parathy-roid ade*noma), has been mapped to this region. The inverson involves chromosome 12q21 and results in the parathyroid hormone promoter being relocated next to the *PRAD1* gene, leading to activated expression in parathyroid cells. The same gene is in the breast cancer chromosome 11 amplicon and is expressed at high levels. *PRAD1* is therefore a new candidate oncogene in breast cancer, and is of particular interest as it is a member of the cyclin family (cyclin D1), involved in cell cycle regulation (p. 167).

The exact mechanism of amplification is unknown. Amplification does not take place in normal cells, but becomes more common as cells progress towards malignancy. It is possible that activated oncogenes induce amplification by disrupting the S phase of the cell cycle, so that S phase either starts in the presence of DNA damage, or signals from the genome fail to indicate that DNA replication is complete (see below). In general, transformed cells *in vitro* go through a 'crisis' involving a transition from a normal diploid complement of chromosomes to a polyploid state where the number of chromosomes per cell can greatly exceed the normal number. This event is associated with a marked increase in the malignant potential of the cancer, and for patients bearing polyploid tumours, a poorer prognosis.

Deletion of chromosomal material

The genes for retinoblastoma, neurofibromatosis and familial adenomatosis coli are prominent successes in the identification of genes responsible for inherited cancer predisposition. These genes were relatively easy to track down due to large, cytogenetically observable deletions in a few patients that served to pinpoint chromosomal locations for gene mapping approaches (see Chapter 3). Recent efforts to map the human genome (Chapter 6) have led to the availability of increasing numbers of **sequence tagged sites** or genetic markers with known chromosomal locations. These markers are now being used to map deletions and rearrangements in cancers that are not big enough to be detected by standard cytogenetic techniques. Many of the most useful markers contain **simple tandem repeats** (STRs), sometimes referred to as **minisatellites** (Fig. 8.8a). These are sequences containing repeating motifs of between two

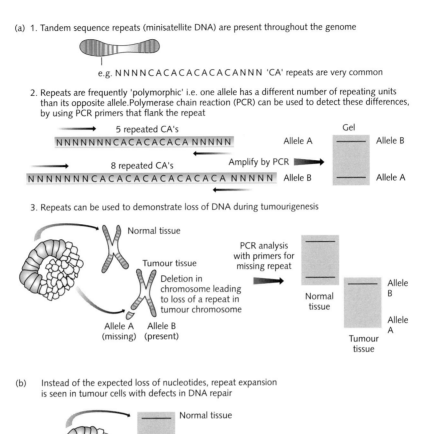

(a) 1. Tandem sequence repeats (minisatellite DNA) are present throughout the genome

e.g. N N N N C A C A C A C A C A C A N N N   'CA' repeats are very common

2. Repeats are frequently 'polymorphic' i.e. one allele has a different number of repeating units than its opposite allele. Polymerase chain reaction (PCR) can be used to detect these differences, by using PCR primers that flank the repeat

5 repeated CA's
N N N N N N C A C A C A C A N N N N N   Allele A

8 repeated CA's
N N N N N N C A C A C A C A C A C A N N N N N   Allele B

Amplify by PCR

Gel
Allele B
Allele A

3. Repeats can be used to demonstrate loss of DNA during tumourigenesis

Normal tissue

Tumour tissue

Deletion in chromosome leading to loss of a repeat in tumour chromosome

PCR analysis with primers for missing repeat

Allele A (missing)   Allele B (present)

Normal tissue

Allele B

Allele A

Tumour tissue

(b)   Instead of the expected loss of nucleotides, repeat expansion is seen in tumour cells with defects in DNA repair

Normal tissue

Increase in number of nucleotides in repeat in tumour cells

Tumour tissue

Fig. 8.8 (a) Demonstration of loss of chromosomal material using minisatellite DNA. Examination of repeat sequences (minisatellite DNA) is a powerful way of identifying submicroscopic deletions in DNA, and for mapping the exact boundaries of deletions to identify the precise genes lost. The utility of repeat sequences lies in the fact that (i) the actual number of nucleotides in each repeat is frequently heterozygous, i.e. the number of nucleotides in any particular repeat is not the same on both chromosomes; and (ii) there are large numbers of these repeats throughout the human genome. By comparing normal tissue with cancer tissue from the same individual, the loss of one repeat (loss of heterozygosity) indicates the presence of a deletion at that particular minisatellite locus. (b) Examination of repeat sequences in cancer samples occasionally demonstrated an increase in the number of nucleotides or repeat expansion, rather than the expected deletions (a). These tumours have been shown to have mutations in genes that encode proteins that repair mistakes in replication. Replication errors are particularly prevalent in repeat sequences, expansion resulting from inaccurate repair of mismatched nucleotides. Inherited mutations in these repair genes (e.g. *MSH2*) have been associated with an increased risk of colon cancer.

and five nucleotides. A common example is the dinucleotide repeat AC, for which over 2000 polymorphic markers are known. The value of these markers is that the size of the STR repeat is frequently heterozygous, allowing one allele to be readily distinguished from another. Loss of one allele — referred to as **loss of heterozygosity (LOH)**—is taken to indicate the presence of a tumour suppressor gene, i.e. one in which a loss-of-

function mutation will provide an advantage for the evolving cancer (see below). STR analysis and cytogenetics, as well as more sophisticated approaches using fluorescent hybridization techniques, have demonstrated that deletion of DNA is a very common event in the evolution of the common solid tumours (lung, breast, prostate, colon, cervix and ovary cancers). For example, more than 20 sites have been defined in breast cancer as regularly showing LOH. Numerous laboratories are working to identify the genes disrupted at these locations. The *DCC* gene (*d*eleted in *c*olorectal *c*arcinoma) on chromosome 18 is an example of a gene that was identified by LOH studies.

Insertional mutagenesis

A further mechanism of transformation exhibited by viruses is 'insertional mutagenesis'. Latent or chronically transforming RNA viruses and DNA tumour viruses integrate into host cells' chromosomes and can disturb the expression of cellular genes in the vicinity. A good example in experimental animal systems is the mouse mammary tumour virus (MMTV) where proviral insertion activates members of the fibroblast growth factor family to cause mammary tumours. Hepatitis B virus is a DNA virus that integrates into chromosomes, although unlike the MMTV retrovirus, it is far from clear whether this is how hepatitis B virus induces liver cancer. Examples of genes found near to or within integrated hepatitis B genomes in hepatoma samples includes c-*myc*, retinoic acid receptors and cyclin A.

Genomic instability and expansion of nucleotide repeats

A search for sites of LOH using markers containing STRs revealed a surprising finding. In a number of cases of colorectal cancer, rather than the expected loss of chromosomal material, expansion of the number of repeats was observed (with respect to adjacent normal material; Fig. 8.8b). The explanation for this observation relates to the action of the DNA polymerases. During replication of the billions of nucleotides that constitute the human genome, occasional errors are made. STRs are particularly prone to error, due to the tendency of the polymerase to slip, missing the occasional nucleotide in repeated sequences. Normally this does not matter as there is a system of repair enzymes that recognize the mismatch created in the newly synthesized strand and replaces the whole segment, matching it to the template strand. It turns out that in cancer cells that have a tendency for STR instability, there are loss-of-function mutations in genes that either recognize the mismatch or are involved in repairing it (*MSH1* and *MSH2* for Mut S Homologue after homologous genes in yeast). When these genes were mapped, their positions were very close to polymorphic markers that pinpointed the chromosomal sites of several cancer predisposition syndromes, Lynch syndrome 1 (non-polypopsis inherited colon cancer) and Lynch syndrome

2 (inherited colon, breast and uterine cancer). It has recently been confirmed that mutations in the *MSH1* and *MSH2* genes are present both in affected individuals in Lynch syndrome cancer families, as well as in cancers arising in individuals without a family history (sporadic cancer).

The *Rb* gene and its function

The *Rb* protein is located in the nucleus and has the properties of a cell cycle control element. Its function is regulated, at least in part, by changes in phosphorylation during the cell cycle, and is affected by interaction with other specific cellular and viral proteins.

Several lines of evidence have contributed to a picture of *Rb* function.

1 The *Rb* protein (pRB) is relatively underphosphorylated in cells in the G1 phase of the cell cycle, and overphosphorylated in S, G2 and M cells. The phosphorylation occurs on serines or threonines, and may be effected by cyclin-regulated kinases such as cdc2. The underphosphorylated form of pRB appears to be strongly bound within the cell nucleus; the phosphorylated form is not.

2 The DNA tumour virus transforming proteins E1a, SV40 large T and papillomavirus E7 each bind directly to pRB. Mutants of these proteins that are defective in binding pRB are also defective for transformation.

3 Mutant pRB from tumours have lost their ability to bind to the viral transforming proteins; site-directed mutagenesis of pRB cDNA clones shows that two polypeptide domains which together form a binding 'pocket' on the pRB molecule are critical for binding.

4 Mutations which interfere with the pRB binding 'pocket' also cause loss of the nuclear binding of underphosphorylated pRB.

5 The viral transforming proteins bind exclusively to underphosphorylated pRB.

Of course, the viral transforming proteins are not normally present in cells, and we must presume that they are usurping a set of normal cellular proteins, the binding of which is critical for the tumour suppressor functions of pRB. Thus, the scheme that emerges is as follows (Weinberg, 1995): on emergence from mitosis, the cell dephosphorylates pRB, which is then available to suppress further growth. The suppression is achieved by interaction, through the binding 'pocket', with a complex of cellular proteins. If conditions are suitable for continued growth, cyclin-regulated kinases will phosphorylate pRB, which prevents binding to cellular proteins required for G1 progression, and the cell cycle can proceed. pRB mutations, or the presence of the viral transforming proteins, also prevent binding and abolish growth-suppressing activity.

How pRB signals its control of the cell cycle is not yet clear. A link with components of the cell circuitry involved with proliferation comes from the observation that pRB can suppress expression of FOS and MYC, transcription factors involved in cell proliferation which respond to growth factor stimulation. This suggests a possible role for pRB as a negative regulator of factors that trigger cell proliferation. In this model, the pRB is hypophosphorlyated in quiescent cells and prevents progression through the cell cycle. In normal cells growth factor stimulation allows a controlled phosphorylation of pRB, permitting the cell cycle to proceed in an orderly manner. After a cycle is completed, the pRB is again dephosphorylated and prevents another round of DNA synthesis, unless there is a continuing growth factor signal. Presumably, in cells that lack pRB, there is a lack of this restraining influence on the cell cycle. A link between pRB and transcriptional regulation has also been demonstrated by the observation that the cellular proteins that complex with pRB are transcription factors such as the transcription factor E2F. This transcription factor is involved in regulating the expression of genes such as c-*myc* and EGF receptor. When complexed with pRB, E2F is non-functional, but when pRB becomes

phosphorylated, functional E2F is released resulting in a general 'switch on' of genes regulated by this transcription factor—many of which are genes involved in the cell cycle (see below).

Clearly the observation that T antigens—adenovirus E1a, polyoma large T, SV40 large T and HPV E7—interact with both p53 and pRB emphasizes a common mode of action of DNA tumour viruses in targeting both these cell cycle regulatory proteins (Fig. 8.9).

DNA virus oncogenes interact with the products of cellular proto-oncogenes as well as with p53 and pRB. Polyoma middle T has been shown to complex with a number of cytoplasmic enzymes involved in signalling, including (at least) three members of the tyrosine kinase family, phosphatidylinositol 3-kinase, and a protein phosphatase. Intriguingly, many of the proteins that form complexes with viral T antigens have yet to be isolated and their respective genes cloned. Currently great emphasis is being placed on this problem as identification of other proteins in the T antigen–cellular protein complex will provide further important insights into the mechanisms of both viral and non-viral carcinogenesis. A recent example of this is the recognition that the p60, adenovirus E1a binding protein is the cell cycle regulator, cyclin A. Cyclin A is expressed in S phase in association with the mitosis triggering gene, cdc2

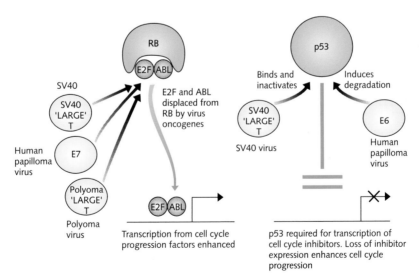

Fig. 8.9 DNA tumour viruses encode oncogenes (tumour antigens) that alter the function of a number of cellular proteins. Two frequently targeted cellular proteins are the retinoblastoma gene product (RB) and p53. When tumour antigens interact with RB, they displace cellular proteins such as the transcription factors C-ABL and E2F. Once liberated from the restraining action of RB, C-ABL and E2F stimulate the transcription of genes that initiate the cell cycle. p53 is a transcription factor that stimulates the expression of genes that suppress cell cycle progression. Tumour antigens bind and inactivate p53, preventing the expression of cell cycle inhibitors.

kinase. The function of the E1a/cyclin A/cdc2 complex is speculative, but it may drive premature S phase and mitotic starts (see Fig. 8.10 for an outline of the cell cycle and examples of oncogenes that interact with cell cycle regulators).

Tumour suppressor genes

The discussion of p53 and pRB has already introduced the idea that the genesis of cancer can involve the inactivation of tumour suppressor genes. This hypothesis has been propounded for many years on the basis of three lines of evidence: (i) somatic cell hybrids; (ii) familial cancer; and (iii) the loss of heterozygosity in tumours. Cloning of tumour suppressor genes based on these observations involves technology that allows the manipulation of relatively large pieces of chromosome to search for genes that are affected by cytogenetically observable deletions.

Hybrid cells formed by fusion between tumorigenic and non-tumorigenic cells do not give rise to tumours when injected into suitable hosts, unless chromosomes have been lost from the hybrids to generate tumorigenic revertants. The conclusion of these experiments is that tumorigenicity is suppressed in the hybrid by genes provided by chromosomes from the non-transformed partner in the cell fusion. Thus 'normal' cell behaviour is usually dominant over transformed cell behaviour, establishing the idea that transformation must involve loss of a function, which can then replaced by the normal gene in the hybrid. At first sight, this model seems to conflict with the concept of dominant acting oncogenes, which implies that the chromosomes from a malignant cell should be dominant over those from a normal cell. The resolution of this paradox pivots on studies that unravel the intricate relationship between positive-acting oncogenes and tumour suppressor genes in the regulation of common pathways.

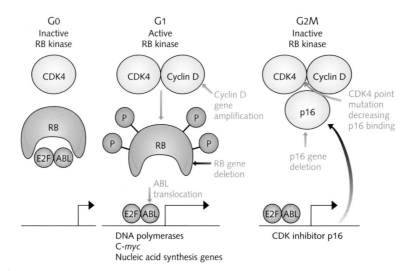

Fig. 8.10 Oncogenes, tumour suppressor genes and the cell cycle. The cell cycle is regulated by the activity of protein complexes that have at their core a member of the cyclin family and a cyclin-dependent protein kinase (CDK). Each phase of the cell cycle is characterized by a unique combination of family members. In addition, other proteins are present in the cyclin–CDK complex that act to modulate CDK activity. The link between the cell cycle and somatic mutations in oncogene and tumour suppressor genes is most striking in G1, the phase of the cell cycle concerned with the timing of the onset of the S or DNA synthetic phase. During G1, cyclin D complexes with CDK4 to form a complex that phosphorylates RB ('RB kinase'). RB phosphorylation leads to the release of transcription factors E2F and C-ABL. These proteins stimulate the transcription of a number of genes that include (i) c-*myc* (which also acts as a transcription factor); (ii) genes involved in DNA synthesis; and (iii) a feedback inhibitor of CDK4 kinase activity called p16. In this scheme it can be appreciated that RB and p16 oppose G1 progression and cyclin D, CDK4, E2F and C-ABL promote G1 progression. This defines RB and p16 as tumour suppressors, supported by the observation that somatic mutations in cancer lead to 'loss-of-function'. In contrast cyclin D, CDK4 and C-ABL are oncogenes and somatic mutations lead to 'gain-of-function'. In the case of cyclin D somatic mutation leads to gene amplification; for CDK4, a point mutation has been described that reduces p16 inhibitor binding; and the C-ABL oncogene is characterized by a translocation that constitutively activates the nuclear protein tyrosine kinase activity. The net result of these mutations is to lose cell cycle control, a cardinal feature of malignancy.

Despite the attraction of cell fusion experiments, no tumour suppressor genes have been cloned by this route. However, the development of microcell fusion has allowed single chromosomes or parts of chromosomes to be transferred into malignant cells and, in a large number of experiments, different chromosomes have been assigned the capacity to suppress tumours of different types. By defining the segment of the chromosome that can suppress the malignant phenotype in a microcell hybrid it may be possible to identify the suppressive genes. The slow progress in the somatic cell hybrid field, hampered by technical difficulties, is in contrast to the rapid progress in the identification of a number of tumour suppressor genes by studying the chromosomal deletions present in familial cancer syndromes and in samples of human tumours. This is because the presence of a deletion makes it immediately possible to investigate an area of a chromosome to search for genes that are modified in tumours.

The cell cycle and tumour suppressor gene function

The ability of oncogenes to stimulate cell proliferation and tumour suppressor genes to inhibit cell proliferation demonstrates that these genes have key roles in the regulation of the cell cycle. An outline of the cell cycle is given in Fig. 8.10. The cell cycle is divided into a series of phases. The S, or synthetic, phase refers to the time when the cell replicates its DNA, and the M or mitotic phase is when the cell divides. Between these phases of the cell cycle are two G or growth phases: G1 precedes S, and G2 precedes M. The boundaries between G1 and S and G2 and M are 'check points' that cannot be transversed until the conditions are appropriate. During G1 the cell is setting up for DNA replication, a process that requires a large repertoire of gene products, from enzymes involved in nucleotide biosynthesis to the DNA polymerases themselves. The M phase programme is set in motion during G2. Proteins such as tubulin (required for the formation of the mitotic spindle) are synthesized so that physical division of the cell can take place.

Progress of cells though the cell cycle is governed by a set of protein kinase complexes involving regulatory subunits called **cyclins**, and catalytic subunits called **cyclin-dependent kinases** (CDK). The level of each member of the cyclin family peaks at a different phase of the cell cycle: cyclin D in early G1, cyclin E at the G1/M boundary, cyclin A during S phase and cyclin B at the G2/M boundary. Each cyclin interacts with several characteristic CDKs so that each phase is distinguished by a particular pattern of cyclin expression and a restricted set of CDKs.

In order to transverse the G1/S checkpoint and enter S phase, the cell has to integrate multiple signals from the external environment, and growth factor receptors play a large part in this. However, the internal environment of the cell, particularly the integrity of the genome, is also a key determining factor for S phase entry. Exposure to radiation or cytotoxic drugs leads to cell cycle arrest—as DNA repair is the priority for the cell exposed to these agents, not replication. This has a clear survival advantage for the organism, as an attempt to replicate the genome in the presence of DNA damage would have disastrous consequences for the cell. Initial studies of p53 and pRB emphasized a potential role in growth factor-mediated cell cycle arrest by peptide growth factors such as TGF-β. The discovery that cells that expressed mutated *p53* did not show cell cycle arrest after irradiation indicates an important function of p53 in the cellular response to DNA damage. Radiation stabilizes the p53 protein (how this takes place is unclear), and stimulates p53-dependent transcription. One of the genes transcriptionally activated by p53 encodes a protein called p21. p21 interacts with the cyclin–CDK complexes that form during G1 to inhibit CDK activity and thus prevents cell cycle progression so that DNA repair can take place. Several other inhibitors functionally similar to p21, such as p16, have recently been identified. Mutations in the *p16* gene have been identified in a number of cancers, suggesting that loss of expression of CDK inhibitors can also lead to unregulated cell proliferation.

Apoptosis

If DNA is irrevocably damaged by radiation or chemical insults, the cell undergoes a process called **programmed cell death** or **apoptosis**. Apoptosis is an energy-requiring process, characterized by morphological changes, nuclear condensation, plasma membrane blebbing and the action of an endonuclease that digests DNA into small fragments (Fig. 8.11). The presence of a 'cell death' pathway was mentioned earlier in the context of the *Bcl-2* gene and has only been appreciated recently. Clearly the integrity of a multicellular organism benefits from the selective suicide of cells with damaged genomes. Apoptosis must, therefore, represent a major protective mechanism against cancer. Given this, it is not surprising that several oncogenes and anti-oncogenes impact on the rate of apoptosis. DNA tumour virus T antigens that target RB, such as adenovirus E1a, sensitize normal diploid cells to apoptotic stimuli such as radiation. This

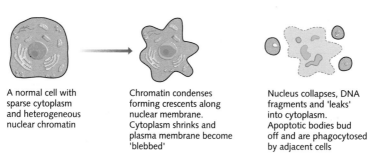

A normal cell with sparse cytoplasm and heterogeneous nuclear chromatin

Chromatin condenses forming crescents along nuclear membrane. Cytoplasm shrinks and plasma membrane become 'blebbed'

Nucleus collapses, DNA fragments and 'leaks' into cytoplasm. Apoptotic bodies bud off and are phagocytosed by adjacent cells

Fig. 8.11 Apoptosis or programmed cell death. Apoptosis is a mechanism for maintaining normal cell numbers in tissues and also deletes cells with severe DNA damage, thus protecting the organism from the persistence of cells with potentially transforming mutations. Furthermore the sensitivity of a cell to cancer chemotherapy is determined in part by how readily the tumour cells undergo apoptosis. Apoptosis is characterized by specific morphological features and by the action of an apoptosis-specific nuclease that cleaves DNA at internucleosomal sites, giving rise to a characteristic 180 basepair ladder.

may be due to an effect on c-*myc* expression, as c-*myc* overexpression also increases the rate of apoptosis. In contrast, T antigens that target p53 such as E1b inhibit apoptosis. Similarly, it is becoming clear that a number of cellular factors such as BCL-2 also act to inhibit apoptotic cell death like E1b, and that cells also contain apoptotic inducers such as the Bax protein which physically and functionally interact with BCL-2. Thus p53 has a dual role in the response to DNA damage, both inhibiting cell cycle progression and being critical for the onset of apoptosis if DNA damage is overwhelming. From this it can readily be seen that cells that contain mutations in *p53* will replicate despite the presence of DNA damage, and although many cells will not survive this, a subpopulation of cells with greatly deranged genomes results with a consequential exacerbation of the malignant phenotype. This may be the basis for the crisis referred to earlier when the chromosomal complement of a normal diploid cell becomes polyploid during malignant transformation. Furthermore, the state of the *p53* gene may determine the responsiveness of a tumour to cytotoxic drugs and radiation.

DNA damage and inappropriate oncogene expression are not the only stimuli that activate apoptosis. Programmed cell death is critically important to normal embryogenesis, occurring, for example, in the web spaces between digits during the formation of the hands and feet, and when T-cell clones are being deleted from the immune repertoire due to recognition of self-antigens (see Chapter 10). The recent observation that some growth factors, such as the insulin-like growth factors, act as cell survival factors, as distinct from growth factors, is beginning to suggest that apoptosis may be a process that could be accelerated or inhibited by hormones in a therapeutically meaningful way.

Oncogene co-operation

The evidence for the multistep nature of carcinogenesis (so-called multiple hit theory) has been described and a number of genes involved in transforming cells have been discussed. To be consistent with the idea of a multistep process, evidence is required for multiple mutations in oncogenes and tumour suppressor genes accumulating over time and acting in concert to produce an increasing 'malignancy'. The first direct evidence for oncogene co-operation came from studies on the polyoma DNA tumour virus. It was demonstrated that neither polyoma large T nor polyoma middle T is able to transform cells on its own, yet the two together can. The observation that large T has a nuclear location and middle T has a cytoplasmic location led workers to try other pairs of oncogenes, one cytoplasmic, one nuclear, in co-operation assays. The first such successful pair tested was *ras* and *myc*, with many later examples confirming the general concept. Each partner in the collaboration provides distinct aspects of the transformed phenotype. *ras* oncogenes induce morphological changes, anchorage independence and increased growth factor secretion. *myc* provides the capacity for unlimited growth in tissue culture—'immortalization'.

Thus, as expected, primary cells in culture do require more than one activated oncogene to demonstrate malignant behaviour in tissue culture and *in vivo*. The experiments outlined above generally consider the result of combinations of activated oncogenes, but examples of naturally occurring tumours containing two activated oncogenes are uncommon, so that this may not be a general mechanism for transformation. The search for evidence of multiple genetic lesions in cancer cells is now beginning to suggest that a more frequent combination of lesions is the inactivation of a tumour suppressor gene combined with activation of an oncogene. Once again the DNA tumour viruses provide a model. As described above, E1a acts to stimulate DNA synthesis through its ability to stimulate transcription of G1 phase genes, but also sensitizes the cell to apoptosis, a potential limitation to tumour formation. However the adenovirus E1b oncogene inhibits the action of p53, preventing both apoptosis and the expression of proteins that limit the action of cyclin–CDK complexes.

Clinical applications

Although there have been dramatic advances in the management of patients with several types of cancer, we are still limited by a lack of selectivity of many of our drugs when used against common solid tumours. Whilst surgery and radiotherapy can be effective in treating localized disease, the frequent occurrence of metastases means that some form of systemic therapy is vital to increase the chances of cure. Most anticancer drugs have been identified by screening large numbers of chemicals for their antiproliferative effects on cells followed by trials on animal tumours. Our rapidly increasing knowledge of the molecular genetics of cancer has led to a new phase in the design of drugs which are designed to selectively counter the abnormal growth processes involved. Furthermore, by understanding the details of the molecular pathogenesis of malignancy it is likely that diagnosis and screening can be made more effective. This will increase the rate of early cancer detection.

Prognosis

Already there are hints that new technology is having an impact on the diagnosis and separation of patients into different prognostic categories (see Table 8.4). In chronic myeloid leukaemia, for example, reagents that can identify the fusion product of the c-*abl* gene with the *bcr* gene are proving valuable in monitoring the effectiveness of intensive chemotherapy and bone marrow transplantation, aimed at eradication of the last remaining clones of malignant cells in the bone marrow. In breast cancer, antibodies which detect the overexpression of the c-*erb*-B2 gene product are proving useful as an indicator of prognosis in breast cancer (Plate 11, facing p. 214). The chances of a woman surviving 5 years after surgery are considerably reduced if the presence of high levels of this surface receptor is detected immunohistologically on tumour biopsies. This group of patients may benefit from the use of intensive chemotherapy given soon after the diagnosis has been made. As importantly, it may

Table 8.4(a) Oncogenes and prognosis.

Tumour	Gene	Prognostic lesion
Adenocarcinoma of lung	k-ras	Point mutation
Carcinoma of breast	erb-B1	Overexpression
	erb-B2	Overexpression
	PRAD1	Amplification
	myc	Amplification
Myelodysplasia	n-ras/k-ras	Point mutation
Neuroblastoma	n-myc	Amplification

Table 8.4(b) Anti-oncogenes and detection of predisposition.

Tumour	Gene	Prognostic lesion
Retinoblastoma	RB	Deletions
Tumours at multiple sites	p53	Point mutations
Colorectal carcinoma	APC	Point mutations
Breast cancer	BRAC1	Point mutations

help to define groups of patients that have a very good prognosis, in whom chemotherapy of this type is *not* beneficial. Monoclonal antibodies that recognize tumour-specific antigens may also allow the delivery of radiopharmaceuticals selectively to cancerous cells (Plate 13, facing p. 214). Recently, evidence is accumulating that certain types of *ras* mutation are associated with prognosis in lung cancer. These examples suggest that reagents that detect oncogene mutations and expression may soon become routine tools to gauge prognosis and guide cancer treatment. As yet the prognostic significance of deletions in tumour suppressor genes is unclear, but as with oncogenes, studies are under way.

Screening

Population screening to detect mutations that predispose to cancer may be possible in the longer term. Particular emphasis will be on individuals with several relatives affected by cancer. Carriers of defined cancer-predisposing mutations could be specifically targeted for early detection, e.g. colonoscopy and mammography, prevention (smoking behaviour and diet) and administration of cancer-preventing agents. Examples of cancer-preventing drugs include retinoids, tamoxifen in the case of women at risk from breast cancer, and prostaglandin synthesis inhibitors in patients with familial adenomatous polyposis (sulindac has recently been shown to

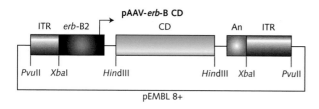

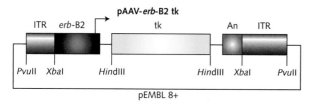

Fig. 8.12 Drug activating vectors for gene therapy. Many different viral and non-viral vectors are being developed for gene therapy. This picture shows two engineered adeno-associated viruses. The top diagram shows the c-*erb*-B2 promoter region upstream of the bacterial enzyme cytosine deaminase whilst the lower diagram illustrates the same promoter upstream of herpes simplex thymidine kinase. c-*erb*-B2 negative cells will not express the enzyme but positive cells will, so giving a highly selective method of destroying cancer cells.

retard the development of colonic polyps). Definitive identification of carriers would be a significant advance over the current approach of regular screening of all members of an affected family, only a proportion of whom are at increased risk.

Therapy

The molecules outlined in this chapter are promising targets for logical drug design. On the cell surface, growth factor antagonists which mimic the ligand's binding action but lack its stimulatory activity have been constructed. Other potential receptor inhibitors include blocking antibodies and tyrosine kinase inhibitors. Within the cytoplasm, molecular modelling of *ras* has led to the development of compounds that stabilize *ras* in the inactive GDP binding state. In the nuclear compartment, the artificial regulation of gene expression is a major goal. It may be possible to switch genes off or on using 'informational drugs' that incorporate DNA or RNA sequences to allow recognition of defined genes, directing a specific block or activation in transcription or translation. Finally, technology that corrects genes deleted during tumour evolution is an attractive prospect, and virus vector systems designed specifically to render tumours susceptible to cytotoxic drugs are currently under intense investigation (Figs 8.12 and 8.13) (see Chapter 16). In certain cases tumour nodules can be the target for direct administration of gene therapy vectors (Plate 10, facing p. 214). Without doubt, our increasing understanding of genetic lesions in the cellular circuitry that disrupt cell growth and differentiation in cancer cells holds great promise, both for the development of novel therapies in the future, and for better, more 'individually tailored' use of the ones currently available.

ACKNOWLEDGEMENTS
We are grateful to Dr Gerard Evan for critical reading of the manuscript, and thank the Imperial Cancer Research Fund, and the Vincent T. Lombardi Cancer Research Center for their support.

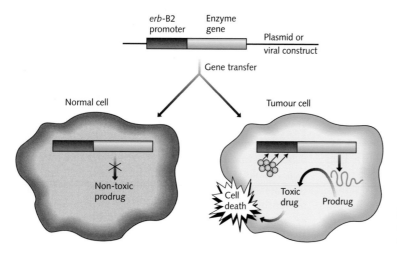

Fig. 8.13 Drug activation gene therapy for cancer. Discriminating between normal and cancer cells by selective drug activation.

Further reading

Bishop J.M. (1985) Viral oncogenes. *Cell*, **42**, 23–38.

Bishop J.M. (1991) Molecular themes in oncogenesis. *Cell*, **64**, 235–248.

Cell Cycle Review Issue (1994) *Cell*, **79**, 547–582.

Fearon E.R. and Volgelstein B. (1990) A genetic model for colorectal tumorigenesis. *Cell*, **61**, 759–767.

Hartwell L. (1992) Defects in a cell cycle checkpoint may be responsible for the genomic instability of cancer cells. *Cell*, **71**, 543–546.

Knudson A.G. (1986) Genetics of human cancer. *Annual Reviews of Genetics*, **20**, 231–251.

Marshall C.J. (1991) Tumour suppressor genes. *Cell*, **64**, 313–326.

Radman M. and Wagner R. (1993) Missing mismatch repair. *Nature*, **366**, 722.

Signal Transduction Review Issue (1995) *Cell*, **80**, 179–276.

Sutherland G.R. and Richards R.I. (1994) DNA repeats—a treasury of human variation. *New England Journal of Medicine*, **331**, 191–193.

Weinberg (1995) The retinoblastoma protein and cell cycle control. *Cell*, **81**, 323–330.

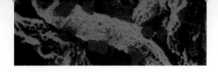

Chapter 9 Inherited cancers

Introduction

There are three main reasons to study the molecular biology of inherited predisposition to cancer:

1 cancer families provide a way in to identify the predisposing genes and so to improve our knowledge of the events in carcinogenesis;

2 individuals in cancer families are a high risk group who may benefit from early diagnosis and prevention, approaches to which will ideally be based on knowledge of the predisposing genes;

3 understanding cancer at the molecular level will give insight into processes controlling normal growth and development.

Inheritance and carcinogenesis

When cancer is thought of as a genetic disease, it is usually in terms of genetic events at the level of the somatic cell—activation of **oncogenes** or loss of **suppressor genes** as a result of mutation (Chapter 8). How do ideas about inherited risk fit into this scheme?

The conversion of a normal cell to a cancer cell requires the accumulation of several changes (so-called multiple hits), most, if not all of which involve mutation. **Predisposition** implies that this series of events is more likely to be completed, leading to cancer. This could come about either (i) because one of the mutational steps inherited is already complete and present in the germ line, so that each cell in the target tissue has a 'head start' towards completing the full set of mutations; or (ii) because of a genetic trait (such as defective repair of DNA damage) which makes the mutations more likely, or enhances their effects (Fig. 9.1). The basic set of mutations is probably the same in cancers of the same type, whether inherited or not. Among the few inherited cancers in which the mechanism of predisposition has so far been elucidated, it seems that inheritance of one of the mutational steps itself is the more usual reason for predisposition. Such mutations are rare, but have strong effects. In the future, however, it is likely that more cases will be found in which common genetic variants influence the likelihood or the consequences of the mutations which lie on the direct pathway to cancer (Fig. 9.1). This is the same distinction as was made between rare single genes and polygenic effects in susceptibility to coronary heart disease (Chapter 7). Although currently attention is focused on the rare inherited cancer syndromes (see below) where single predisposing genes of strong effect can easily be identified, in the future the polygenic component of predisposition may well prove more important in terms of preventing deaths from cancer.

The contribution of inheritance to cancer incidence and the search for predisposing genes

The recognition of inherited predisposition is often difficult. From a practical point of view, one can think of three categories of predisposition, from the easiest to recognize to the most difficult (Table 9.1).

The inherited cancer syndromes (Table 9.2)

This is the most easily recognized group. Strong genetic predisposition gives rise to extensive family histories in a pattern consistent with the effects of a single gene (Fig. 9.2). There are often characteristic associated phenotypes as well, which signal the cancer to be of the inherited type (Fig. 9.3). Because the families are easily recognized, and the presence of the cancer or the associated phenotype is a reliable indication of inheritance of the predisposing gene, these syndromes are easily accessible to genetic linkage analysis to locate and identify the genes involved. Most of the 'inherited cancer genes' so far identified therefore belong in this group, and they will occupy most of this chapter. In aggregate these rare

Different mechanisms for inherited susceptibility to cancer

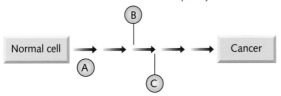

The sequence of 5 arrows represents the accumulation of successive events within a single cell, resulting in its transformation into a cancer cell. In principle this sequence could be accelerated in any of three ways.

(A) By inheritance of one of the steps already completed.
(B) By inheritance of a trait which made the occurrence of one or more of the steps more likely.
(C) By inheritance of a trait which increases the effect of one of the steps and thereby the likelihood that the next step will occur.

Fig. 9.1 To illustrate idea of multiple steps, inheritance of one of the steps (A) or a factor which increases likelihood (B)/effect (C) of step.

syndromes probably account for well under 1% of all cancer incidence — perhaps 200 cases a year in the UK. Their main interest lies in the opportunity they provide to identify genes which are important in the normal control of cell growth and development and to determine how disruption of this function leads to cancer. While the identification of these genes has made possible genetic diagnosis for the families involved, these families are uncommon. The analysis of this type of inherited

predisposition to cancer therefore does not directly address in any major way the public health problem of reducing deaths from cancer.

Familial cancers

Up to 5–10% of cancers at commonly affected sites such as breast and colon occur in individuals who have a family history of similar cancers. Because these cancers are common, one could argue that the family clusters are

Table 9.1 Categories of inherited predisposition.

Inherited cancer syndromes
Easily recognized by multiple case families and/or characteristic phenotype
Examples: familial polyposis of the colon, multiple endocrine neoplasia syndromes

Familial clusters of cancer
Common cancers, no characteristic phenotype; may be difficult to decide whether a given family history is significant or not
Examples: breast cancer, colorectal cancer outside polyposis syndromes

Predisposition without evident familial clustering
Predisposition by common weakly predisposing genes; not much familial clustering so difficult to recognize by family history
Examples: metabolic polymorphisms determining response to exogenous or endogenous carcinogens

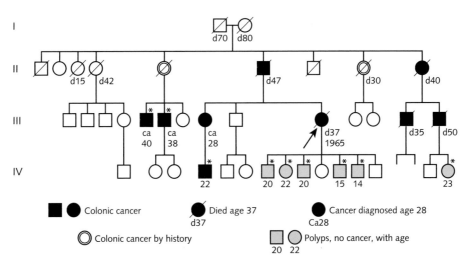

Fig. 9.2 Pedigree of a dominantly inherited cancer, e.g. familial polyposis of the colon (FAP). The family was recognized when the individual in generation III (arrowed) presented with colonic cancer and was found to have multiple colonic polyps. Subsequently, other members of the family (indicated by asterisk) have been screened by sigmoidoscopy. Three were found to already have cancer; five siblings and a cousin in generation IV had polyps and were treated by prophylactic colectomy.

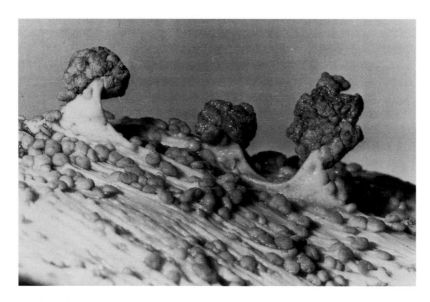

Fig. 9.3 Polyps in the colonic mucosa of an individual with FAP. Polyps measure a few millimetres to a few centimetres in size and may number from a hundred to several thousand in the colon.

Two large polyps and a smaller one are shown arising from the surface of the colonic epithelium. (Photograph provided by the ICRF Colorectal Cancer Unit, St Mark's Hospital, London.)

Table 9.2 Some features of inherited cancer.

- The pattern of inheritance in the families is in most cases autosomal dominant
- Predisposition is to one or more specific types of cancer, not to cancer in general
- Characteristic phenotypic abnormalities may be present in a variety of specific tissues, often with no clear relationship to the target tissue for the cancer
- The pattern of cancers and of phenotypic abnormalities may vary markedly both between and within families
- The age at onset of the cancers may vary between and within families
- In a few cases, the expression of the inherited predisposition may be influenced by the sex of the transmitting parent—'genomic imprinting'

simply chance. However, studies in the population show that the risk of cancer at most sites is increased in the close relatives of a patient with that cancer, generally by a factor of 1.5–3 (Table 9.3). This indicates that at least some family clustering is real, though not necessarily due to inheritance. Evidence for the role of inheritance comes from analyses, in larger series of families, of the patterns in which the cancers occur. Different patterns would be expected for inherited, environmental or chance effects. The results indicate a major contribution of inherited predisposition, for the most part in the pattern expected for a dominant gene. Epidemiological studies of this type lead to the conclusion that 5–10%, and possibly more, of the incidence of the common cancers may result from strong inherited predisposition. Epidemiology, however, although suggestive, is not proof. Proof of inherited pre-

disposition can come only from the demonstration of the association of the cancer with a genetic marker in the family.

Such an association is generally sought by the methods of genetic linkage, described in Chapter 6. Linkage is based on proving a significant association between the inheritance of a phenotype (in this case, the cancer) and a genotype (nowadays, usually a DNA polymorphism). The cancer phenotype is being used as an indicator of the supposed susceptibility gene. The linkage is being sought between this gene and the polymorphic DNA marker, to demonstrate their proximity (or otherwise) on the chromosome (Fig. 9.4). The whole process therefore relies on the assumption that the cancer phenotype does accurately reflect the presence of the susceptibility gene in that individual. In the inherited cancer syndromes, in general it does. Because the genetic predisposition is

Table 9.3 Estimates of relative risks of the same cancer in first-degree relatives of individuals affected with various common cancers.

Site	Relative risk
Breast	2.2
Ovary	3
Endometrium	2.7
Melanoma	2.5
Lung	2.7
Colon	3.4
Stomach	2.6

Adapted from Easton and Peto (1991).

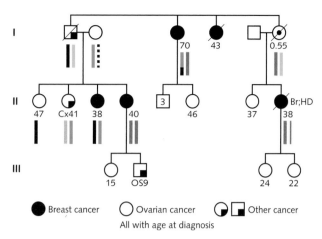

Fig. 9.4 A family with breast and ovarian cancer showing linkage to the BRCA1 locus on chromosome 17, but with one affected individual who is a phenocopy—that is, she does not share the BRCA1 chromosome with the other affected family members, and she has developed breast cancer by chance. Vertical lines represent copies of chromosome 17 in each individual, defined by DNA polymorphisms lying either side of the locus for BRCA1. The copy of chromosome 17 shown in black is consistently present in affected family members, with the exception of the individual I-3 who developed breast cancer at age 70. The association of the black chromosome with the disease in this family is sufficient to provide moderately strong evidence that the disease is linked to the BRCA1 locus. On this basis, the affected 70-year-old is a phenocopy; and the unaffected 47-year-old, II-1, who turns out to have inherited the predisposing chromosome is an example of a gene carrier in whom the gene is not yet penetrant —that is, she has not manifested the disease.

strong, most individuals who have the predisposing gene will develop the cancer, or at least the associated phenotype (polyps, for example). Moreover, in many of the syndromes the cancers are of a type which is rare outside predisposed families, so that the reverse error will also be rare: there will be few if any 'phenocopies' — cases of cancer which do not reflect inherited predisposition.

In the familial cancers, linkage analysis is more difficult. The occurrence of cancer is likely to be a much less reliable indicator of the inheritance of the susceptibility gene, for several reasons.

1 Because the susceptibility is in general less strong, a significant proportion of family members who carry the predisposing gene do not develop cancer.

2 Conversely, because the cancers are common, there may be several family members with cancer who do not have the predisposing gene. Examples are shown in Fig. 9.4. Although allowances can be made for this in the mathematical linkage analysis, the analysis is usually considerably weakened.

3 Possibly more important, there is also the problem of genetic heterogeneity. Evidence for genetic linkage requires that a certain level of significance be reached for the association between phenotype and genetic markers; and unless large families are available (which in the familial cancers they generally are not) this can be achieved only by combining the results from several families. If different genes are predisposing in different families, the combining of results from dissimilar families is likely to obscure linkage associations even when they are present.

The molecular genetic analysis of inherited predisposition in familial clusters of the common cancers therefore has lagged somewhat behind similar analysis of the well-defined inherited cancer syndromes. However, over the next decade, further epidemiological and clinical studies which result in the description of large family sets, improvements in the human gene map, and possibly the recognition of associated phenotypes (like colonic polyps) which will distinguish inherited from sporadic forms of the common cancers, will lead to further progress.

Inherited predisposition without evident familial clustering

Although most attention is naturally given to families with multiple cases of cancer, the most significant inherited contribution to cancer incidence may in fact never be apparent in the form of obvious familial clustering. Take, for example, a common recessive allele (frequency 0.7) which is associated with a 50-fold increase in cancer risk, from one in 1000 in individuals with one or zero copies of the allele to one in 20 in homozygotes. This allele would result in the occurrence of 99% of the incidence of that cancer in the 49% of the population who

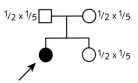

Fig. 9.5 Low penetrance alleles will seldom cause an obvious family history. If the affected woman shown by the filled-in circle has developed her cancer because of a dominantly inherited predisposing allele which confers a lifetime risk of 1 in 5, each of her close relatives has a 50:50 chance of having inherited the same allele, and therefore a risk of that specific cancer of 1 in 10. Families with more than two affected close relatives will therefore be uncommon.

were homozygotes; and yet the increased risk to close relatives of a case (1.49-fold) would only be detectable by careful epidemiological studies. Similar conclusions can be reached for recessive or dominant predisposing alleles over a range of allele frequencies. The essential point is that if the predisposing allele is incompletely penetrant—that is, most people who inherit it still do not get cancer—it is unlikely often to give rise to multiple-case families (Fig. 9.5). If the cancer in question is common, a low degree of family clustering will be even harder to detect.

If cancer is the same as other diseases, such as coronary artery disease, the risk to an individual is likely to be the result of the combined effects of several such genes, and the interaction of these genes with factors in the environment. In this respect, the principles of investigation of inherited risk of cancer are the same as for the investigation of any polygenic disease, described fully in Chapter 7. The practical distinction between the investigation of inherited predisposition of this type, and the familial clusters of inherited cancers described above, is that in the familial cases the existence of multiple-case families allows the use of linkage methods to search for the predisposing genes empirically, without prior knowledge of what they may be. Without family clustering, genetic linkage becomes impossible and it is necessary to adopt different strategies. These are based on a search for differences in the frequency of mutations (or at least genetic variation) in 'candidate genes' between cancer cases and controls. A candidate gene is any gene that is thought for some reason to have a possible role in carcinogenesis. Shortage of ideas for good candidates to test have so far limited progress in this area. However, this type of predisposition is likely to be numerically by far the most significant, and the genes involved are likely to include many whose effects are modulated by interaction with extrinsic factors and which could therefore conceiv-

Table 9.4 Some features of the inherited cancer syndromes which require explanation at a molecular and cellular level.

- *Recessive mutations give rise to dominant pedigrees*. This paradox is explained in the section on retinoblastoma.
- *Tissue specificity*. Even though the predisposing gene may be expressed in many different tissues, cancers are often restricted to specific tissues with no obvious developmental or physiological link between them.
- *Variable expression*. Mutations in the same predisposing gene may result in a different spectrum of abnormalities in different individuals, in different families and even in the same family. Some individuals may also be severely affected, whereas others have no manifestations at all.
- *Differences between the effects of mutations in the germ line and in somatic cells*. In a number of cases, somatic mutations of a particular gene are commonly seen in non-familial tumours, yet inherited (germ line) mutations in the same gene appear to predispose weakly or not at all to the same tumour. Conversely, for example in the case of *BRCA1*, germ line mutations confer a strong predisposition to breast cancer, but sporadic breast cancers seem rarely if ever to arise from somatic *BRCA1* mutation.

ably be open to manipulation. It may be that, in terms of overall prospects for cancer control, this is where the future lies.

The molecular biology of inherited cancers

In this section, examples of several inherited cancers will be described under the headings:
- clinical description;
- mapping and identification of the predisposing gene;
- description of the gene and its function;
- mechanisms of development of cancers and preneoplastic lesions;
- special features or problems;
- prospects for clinical application.

A number of features which are shared to some degree by all the inherited cancers are summarized in Table 9.4 and described in more detail under each cancer. Each of these features must eventually be explained in molecular terms. For the most part, such an explanation is still beyond reach, but some speculation and possible lines of investigation will be discussed.

Retinoblastoma

Clinical description

Retinoblastoma is a cancer of the developing retina which presents in early childhood. It can occur in unilateral or bilateral form, with or without a family history. Analysis of the proportion of cases in each category led Knudson to important conclusions about mechanisms, described below. In about 30% of cases the tumours are multiple and affect both eyes; in 70% the tumours are single, affecting only one eye, and these develop at a later average age than the multiple tumours. Some patients with retinoblastoma have a family history of the disease, consistent with autosomal dominant inheritance. In about 68% of familial cases the tumours are bilateral, and in 32% unilateral. Families sometimes show skipped generations, in which an individual who must have inherited the gene does not develop any tumour. Of cases with no family history, all of those with bilateral tumours and about 10% with single tumours can transmit susceptibility to their offspring. These heritable sporadic cases are presumably the result of new germ line mutation.

Individuals with the inherited form of retinoblastoma have a substantially increased risk of developing osteosarcoma, especially in the field of radiation treatment for a retinal tumour; they are also at increased risk for the later development of a variety of other cancers including melanoma, bladder, lung and possibly breast cancer.

Knudson's two-hit hypothesis

Analysis of the numbers and age at diagnosis of tumours in sporadic and familial retinoblastoma led Knudson to formulate the **two-hit model**, which has become the paradigm for the mechanism of tumour development in the inherited cancer syndromes. The key observations were:

1 the numbers of tumours in hereditary cases fitted a Poisson distribution, suggesting that each arose from an independent stochastic event;

2 the distribution of age at first diagnosis of the tumours in these cases fitted a mathematical model of the occurrence of a single stochastic event;

3 the average age at diagnosis in unilateral cases was later and fitted a model requiring two events;

4 unilateral sporadic cases are rare (one in 30 000 of the population).

Together, these suggested a model in which two events must occur in a single retinal cell for a tumour to

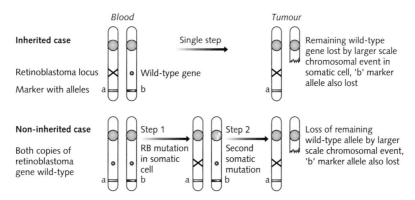

Fig. 9.6 Knudson's hypothesis and its experimental verification. Two copies of chromosome 13 are shown, bearing the retinoblastoma gene locus. In individuals with inherited predisposition to retinoblastoma, Knudson postulated that one *Rb* allele would already be inactivated by mutation in the germline. Thus every cell in the retina would carry an inactive *Rb* allele. A single somatic mutational event in one retinal cell would be sufficient to result in loss of all *Rb* activity, and tumour formation (top line). In individuals without inherited predisposition, by contrast, both *Rb* alleles would have to be lost in the same retinal cell as a result of somatic mutation events. This coincidence of two somatic mutations in a single cell would be expected to be much less common (bottom line), and so sporadic tumours would on average develop at older ages.

The experimental verification of this came from studies of the loss in tumours, compared with blood, of alleles at polymorphic loci distal to *Rb* on chromosome 13 (a, b). The second somatic mutation event in the development of both hereditary and sporadic tumours is expected often to involve loss of a large region of the chromosome (by a variety of mechanisms which are not relevant here). Thus, Knudson's hypothesis would predict that (i) in sporadic retinoblastoma, one allele at a locus distal to *Rb* on chromosome 13 would commonly be lost in tumours, and (ii) in hereditary retinoblastoma, the same would be true, and moreover the allele lost would be that which was carried on the wild-type chromosome (i.e. the chromosome not inherited through the family with the *Rb* mutation). These predictions were confirmed by analysis of DNA from blood and tumour of retinoblastoma patients.

develop: in unilateral sporadic cases both events must occur by somatic mutation, whereas in bilateral or hereditary cases, one event is already present in the germ line and so in every retinal cell; and only one further event, in any cell, is required. These predictions have subsequently been confirmed at the molecular level.

Mapping and identification of the Rb-1 gene

The *Rb-1* gene is at chromosome 13q14. The first clue to location came from cytogenetic deletions involving this region in retinoblastoma tumours, and in the normal somatic cells of a few familial cases. Proof of the involvement of a gene at 13q14 came from the demonstration of linkage of retinoblastoma in families to the inheritance of polymorphisms at the locus for esterase D, which maps to this region. The chromosomal deletions at 13q14 suggested that the inherited mutation resulted in loss of activity of one copy of the *Rb-1* gene; a reasonable guess as to the section step postulated by Knudson was that it should involve loss of the second copy of the gene. Using RFLP (see Chapter 5) markers for several loci on chromosome 13q (Cavenee *et al.*, 1983), it was shown that indeed, in many familial retinoblastoma tumours, the copy of chromosome 13q which was inherited from the unaffected parent (and should therefore still carry an active copy of the gene) had been lost (Fig. 9.6). Knudson's two-hit hypothesis could now be refined: *Rb-1* was postulated to be a *suppressor* of tumorigenesis, and both copies of the gene must be inactivated for suppressor activity to be lost and tumour development to occur.

The chromosomal deletions indicated the region of chromosome 13q14 where the gene must lie. A systematic search for genes in this region led to the isolation of several cDNAs, which were used as hybridization probes on restriction digests of DNA from tumours and blood from familial cases, and on Northern blots of RNA from tumour and other tissues. One cDNA clone, *Rb-1*, represented a gene that was expressed in normal tissue and unrelated tumours, but which was absent (or expressed in altered form) in all retinoblastomas examined.

Subsequently, the *Rb-1* gene (whose function is detailed in Chapter 8) has been shown to consist of 27 exons spread over some 200 kb of genomic DNA, encoding a 928 amino acid protein of 106 kDa. Inactivating mutations range from gross deletions (a minority) to point mutations resulting in missense or nonsense, or splice donor or acceptor mutations: in every case, the result is failure to express a normal *Rb* gene product. Final proof of identity is given by experiments in which restoring the wild-type *Rb* gene to tumour cells results in suppression of tumorigenicity.

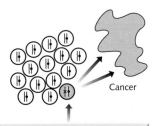

| All the cells in the tissue carry a recessive mutation in (for example) the RB gene. The tissue is apparently normal because the effect of the recessive mutation is masked by the remaining wild-type copy | A single, somatic, mutation occurs in a **single cell**. Normally this would probably be unnoticed, but in this case it develops into a cancer, and so the phenotype is clearly manifest. Since the probability that this will happen in at least one cell in any individual bearing the recessive mutation is high, the inheritance of the single recessive mutation is associated with the phenotype – and the inheritance of one copy of a mutant gene has the characteristics of dominant inheritance in the pedigree: |

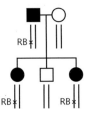

Fig. 9.7 The recessive mutation/dominant pedigree paradox.

The development of retinoblastomas, and preneoplastic lesions

There is no clear-cut preneoplastic lesion in the development of retinoblastoma, analogous to the polyps of familial adenomatous polyposis (FAP; see below); nor are there associated phenotypes characteristic of the hereditary form.

Although the development of retinoblastoma is described in terms of the two-hit model, it should be noted that all tumours examined have shown some cytogenetic abnormality other than on chromosome 13, which suggests that further genetic events are needed for tumour progression.

Special features

Hereditary retinoblastoma exemplifies some of the questions posed in Table 9.4.

1 If the *Rb* mutation is recessive at the cellular level (both copies have to be lost for a tumour to develop), why is the disease dominant in its inheritance? This paradox is easily resolved. It arises from the property of cancer, that a single mutant cell (which would not ordinarily be detected) can grow and give rise to a detectable phenotype, the cancer (Fig. 9.7).

2 The pRB protein is ubiquitously expressed, so why is predisposition mainly to retinoblastoma and osteosarcoma?

3 Since somatic *Rb-1* mutation is a feature of sporadic tumours of many types, why does germ line mutation not have a stronger effect in predisposing to these cancers also?

The answers to these questions are still not known.

Mouse model of retinoblastoma

Transgenic mice have been constructed with inactivation of the mouse *Rb-1* homologue. Heterozygotes develop not retinoblastomas but pituitary tumours; homozygotes die at day 12 of embryonic development with impaired differentiation in lineage of the central nervous system and erythrocytes. These results suggest that the critical function of *Rb-1* may not be in the control of cell division in general (the embryo has undergone many cell divisions by day 12), but in the arrest of proliferation associated with terminal differentiation.

Clinical application

Genetic diagnosis of the inheritance of the *Rb-1* gene is now possible using either linked genetic markers or direct identification of mutations in the *Rb-1* gene.

Wilms' tumour

Clinical description

Wilms' tumour accounts for 90% of childhood kidney tumours, and about 8% of childhood cancers overall. Although fewer than 1% of cases are familial, about 10% of cases present with bilateral tumours, and these occur on average about 2 years earlier than sporadic unilateral cases. These data suggest a similar model to retinoblastoma, in which bilateral cases are the result of a heritable germ line mutation: however, since very few of the bilateral cases have a family history of the disease, one must assume that almost all are new mutations, and that their ability either to reproduce or to transmit the gene is very low.

Wilms' tumours consist of undifferentiated 'blastemal' cells, and stromal and epithelial elements. The tumours are thought to arise from malignant transformation of a persistent renal stem cell which has failed to undergo correct differentiation. About 5% of cases are associated with genitourinary abnormality, most often cryptorchidism, hypospadias or structural abnormalities of the urinary tract. Four syndromes of congenital abnormalities have been associated with Wilms' tumours (Table 9.5).

Table 9.5 Wilms' tumour and associated syndromes of congenital abnormalities.

	Wilms' tumour–aniridia	Denys–Drash syndrome	Beckwith–Wiedemann syndrome	Perlman syndrome
Proportion of Wilms' tumour cases	Approx. 1%	<1%	0.5%	Very rare
Risk of Wilms' tumour	30–50%	High (also other tumours: rhabdomyosarcoma, adrenal cortical cancer, hepatoblastoma)	3–5%	High
Mode of inheritance	*De novo* mutation in germ line (rare autosomal dominant)	*De novo* germ line mutation	Autosomal dominant	Autosomal recessive
Chromosomal locus	11p13	11p13	11p15.5	Not known
Disease gene	*WT-1* and adjacent aniridia gene ('contiguous gene syndrome')	*WT-1*	Not known	Not known
Associated abnormalities	Aniridia	Nephropathy, male pseudohermaphroditism	Hemi-hypertrophy, genitourinary and cardiac malformations, macroglossia	Gigantism, cryptorchidism

Mapping and identification of the Wilms' tumour genes

At least three genes are thought to be involved in predisposition to Wilms' tumour.

The location of the 11p13 gene was first suggested by constitutional deletions of this chromosomal region in a few patients who also had aniridia, in some cases with the other defects of the Wilms' tumour-aniridia-genitourinary abnormalities-mental retardation (WAGR) syndrome (Table 9.5). Positional cloning using deletions in both constitutional and tumour DNA as a guide led to the identification of a gene which was expressed in fetal kidney, and the sequence of which showed it to encode a transcription factor of the zinc finger family (see Chapter 4). Mutations in the zinc finger regions of this gene in patients with Wilms' tumours provide strong evidence that it is indeed the 11p13 Wilms' (WT-1) gene.

The existence of another gene at 11p15 is indicated by (i) the finding that in about one-third of Wilms' tumours, chromosomal losses are restricted to the region of 11p15 and do not include 11p13, and (ii) the increased risk of Wilms' tumour in Beckwith–Wiedemann syndrome (Table 9.5), the locus for which maps to 11p15. This putative Wilms' tumour gene has not yet been identified.

A third Wilms' tumour gene must also be postulated because the rare multiple-case families show clear evidence against linkage to markers on chromosome 11p13–15. The chromosomal location of this gene is also unknown.

Description of the WT-1 gene and its function

The WT-1 gene contains 10 exons spanning 50 kb of DNA, and encodes a 3 kb transcript. The predicted protein is 46–49 kDa (there are four alternative splice patterns). The carboxy-terminus contains four zinc finger motifs, typical of the DNA binding domains of transcription factor, and the N-terminus contains a proline- and glutamine-rich region also seen in other transcription factors, which may be involved in transducing the signal received by WT-1. The role of the different spliced forms is unclear but good evidence exists to suggest that some spliced forms of WT-1 are involved in post-transcriptional processing of RNA by interacting with splicing factors.

The expression of the WT-1 gene is restricted in time and space. This, and the association of developmental anomalies of the genito-urinary tract with Wilms' tumour, suggests a developmental role for the gene. In the kidney, in situ hybridization studies show WT-1 expression in the cells of the metanephric blastema for a brief period as they condense around the ureteric bud and develop into the podocytes of the renal glomerulus. In the developing gonad, WT-1 is expressed initially in coelomic epithelium, then in the sex cord stromal cells which become the Sertoli cells in the testis, and the cells surrounding the follicle in the ovary. Unlike Rb, WT-1 is not widely expressed.

Mechanisms of development of cancers

The finding of deletions in WT-1 in both germ line and tumour DNA suggests that inactivation of the gene is required for tumour development. The demonstration of deletions involving both WT-1 alleles in some tumours suggests a two-hit mechanism, similar to retinoblastoma. However, some pieces of evidence suggest that this may be an oversimplification.

1 The ages at diagnosis and proportions of bilateral and unilateral tumours do not fit very well with expectations of the classical two-hit model, as seen in retinoblastoma.
2 Multicentre disease appears to be more often unilateral than bilateral.
3 The proportion of survivors of Wilms' tumour who have children who themselves developed Wilms' tumour is much smaller than would be expected.
4 Some tumours in WAGR syndrome individuals (therefore with a germ line mutation of the 11p13 gene) appear to have allele loss restricted to the 11p15 region in the tumour, suggesting that the effects of loss of activity of the 11p13 and 11p15 genes may interact in some way.

These problems are still unresolved.

Wilms' tumour is thought to arise from metanephric stem cells at different stages in commitment along the normal pathway of nephrogenesis. A plausible model for tumorigenesis is that WT-1 normally acts as a transcriptional regulator in the inductive events occurring in metanephric stem cells during kidney formation — either to suppress genes which would maintain cell proliferation, or to activate genes involved in differentiation. Consistent with this is the observation that WT-1 is known to negatively regulate cell proliferation in the developing kidney by repressing expression of insulin-like growth factor genes.

Special features

Many Wilms' tumours show losses of alleles for loci on chromosome 11p, reflecting the loss of a large segment of chromosome presumably as the result of somatic mutation, the 'second hit' in tumour development. Remarkably, in about 90% of cases, the chromosome which is lost is the one which was originally derived from the mother. Events which are non-random with respect to the parent of origin of a chromosome suggest the involvement of genomic imprinting (see Chapter 5). Imprinted genes are modified by some as yet unknown mechanism in the germ line, so as to reduce or abolish their subsequent expression during embryogenesis. If the paternally derived copy of WT-1 was inactivated by imprinting, this would be functionally equivalent to a mutation, and only one further event—a somatic mutation of the maternally derived allele—would be required for tumorigenesis. Support for this scheme comes not only from (i) the preferential involvement of the maternal chromosome in allele losses in tumours, but also (ii) from evidence that genes which map to this chromosomal region (or its homologue in the mouse) are indeed subject to imprinting, and (iii) from the finding that duplications of the chromosome 11p15 region in Beckwith–Wiedemann syndrome patients (Table 9.5) are exclusively of paternal origin.

A fault in the imprinting mechanism might account for familial Wilms' tumour. Imprinting of the 11p13–15 region might be regulated by another gene, not on chromosome 11p. Mutation of the regulating gene might result in inappropriately strong or prolonged inactivation of the Wilms' tumour genes on chromosome 11p, equivalent to an inherited loss-of-function mutation at these loci. This explanation, for which there is as yet no proof, could account for both the failure to find linkage to chromosome 11p13–15 in familial cases, and the otherwise possibly surprising observation that these tumours nevertheless show allele losses in the 11p13–15 region.

Clinical application

Genetic prediction of risk is an issue only in the very rare familial cases, where it is at present impossible because the gene has not been located.

Neurofibromatosis type 1

Clinical description

Neurofibromatosis type 1 (NF-1) is one of the commonest autosomal dominant disorders. The manifestations are very varied (Table 9.6; Fig. 9.8; Plate 14, facing p. 214), but mostly involve tissues of neural crest origin.

Table 9.6 Some features of NF-1.*

	Approximate % of gene carriers affected	Probable cell of origin	Comments
Diagnostic features			
Café au lait spots (more than 5)	>95	Melanocyte	1 cm or larger pigmented skin patches
Skin neurofibromas (up to 500 or more)	>90	? Schwann cell (multiple cell types)	Develop at puberty. Nonmalignant. Contain Schwann cells, axons, fibroblasts, mast cells, perineural cells and blood vessels
Lisch nodules	>90	?	Nodular developmental abnormalities of iris
Less common problems			
Learning difficulties	25	?	
Short stature	15	?	
Large head	25	?	
Skeletal abnormalities			
Scoliosis	30	?	
Pseudoarthrosis	2	?	Failure of development of one segment of a long bone (usually tibia)
Epileptic fits	<5	?	
Tumours			
Plexiform neurofibromas	20	? Schwann cell (multicellular like skin neurofibromas)	Can cause severe deformity; may become malignant; may be associated with local hypertrophy
Neurofibromas of spinal and peripheral nerves†	5	? Schwann cell (multicellular like skin neurofibromas)	

(Continued on p. 182)

Table 9.6 *Continued.*

	Approximate % of gene carriers affected	Probable cell of origin	Comments
Schwannomas of peripheral nerves	<5	Schwann cell	Occasionally become malignant
CNS tumours (glioma, ependymoma, occasional meningioma)	3	Glia, ependyma, arachnoid	Optic nerve gliomas relatively frequent, often non-progressive
Phaeochromocytoma	1	Chromaffin cell of adrenal medulla	Usually benign
Neurofibrosarcomas (malignant, schwannoma)	2	? Schwann cell	Malignant: usually develop from plexiform NF or Schwannoma

* Neurofibromatosis type 2 (NF-2) is genetically distinct (the gene maps to chromosome 22) and consists of schwannomas of the VIII cranial nerve, meningiomas, spinal nerve root tumours, few cutaneous neurofibromas, and lens opacities.
† These tumours are prominent in some families with a variant form of NF-1 which maps to the *NF-1* locus.

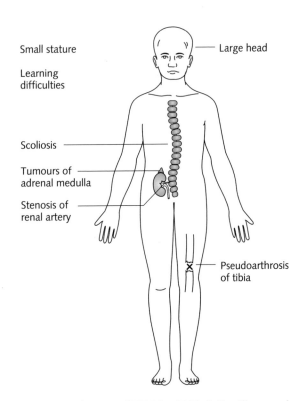

Fig. 9.8 Some features of NF-1 (see Table 9.6) to illustrate the diffuse nature of the abnormalities, many of which cannot plausibly be ascribed to second somatic mutations in a single cell, on the retinoblastoma model.

Benign and malignant tumours (Table 9.6) are a relatively minor feature.

Variation in the spectrum and severity of expression is a prominent feature of *NF-1*, just as in the extracolonic features of FAP. About two-thirds of patients are mildly affected, but 10–15% are severely incapacitated. Apart from its biological interest, this variability has clinical importance. DNA-based antenatal prediction of inheritance of the *NF-1* gene is now possible, but prediction of the severity of the disease is not. Under these circumstances, most parents in the UK have so far decided against genetic testing because they would not wish to terminate an affected pregnancy.

Mapping and identification of the NF-1 gene

The *NF-1* gene was mapped to chromosome 17q12 by linkage. The location of the gene was subsequently revealed by two independent constitutional chromosome translocations in *NF-1* patients, the breakpoints of which turned out to interrupt the gene.

The gene and its function

The *NF-1* gene is unusual for its large size (11 kb of coding sequence extending over 300 kb of genomic DNA), and for having three genes, transcribed in the opposite direction, embedded within a large intron. The *NF-1* gene contains a so-called GAP domain (GTPase-activating protein) which has strong homology with similar domains in GAP proteins in yeast (IRA1, IRA2) and mammals. This suggests that it may be part of the signal transduction pathway involving the *ras* and related families of oncogenes, whose activity is regulated by switching between the GTP (active) and GDP (inactive) forms (see below). This cannot, however, be the whole story as large regions of the rest of the gene are highly conserved between species, suggesting that they are important for function, and moreover very few mutations of the gene in *NF-1* patients have been shown to lie in the GAP homology region.

The NF-1 protein, neurofibromin, has been shown by immunoelectron microscopy and *in vitro* binding studies to be associated with the tropomyosin fibres of the cytoskeleton. Although the *NF-1* message can be detected by PCR methods in all tissues examined, the relative abundance and distribution of neurofibromin in different tissues is controversial. The observation of association with tropomyosin is, however, consistent with a recently postulated role for proteins of the *ras*-related families as transducers of signals through the cell membrane to the cytoskeleton.

Development of cancers and preneoplastic lesions

The tumours in NF-1 fall into two groups.
1 The phaeochromocytomas, neurofibrosarcomas and probably the gliomas, which are clonal and which consist of a neoplastic population of cells which are derived from a single cell which has undergone a somatic mutation leading to loss of activity of the remaining allele at the *NF-1* locus. The development of these tumours appears to follow the two-hit model of retinoblastoma.
2 The cutaneous and plexiform neurofibromas. These are benign tumours which are composed of a mixture of Schwann cells, fibroblasts, vascular endothelium and other cells. It is still not entirely clear whether these tumours contain a clonal neoplastic cell population (with the implication that they arose from a somatic mutation in a single cell) or whether they are truly poly-clonal in origin, the result of disorganized paracrine and autocrine interactions. If there is a single neoplastic cell

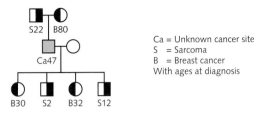

Fig. 9.9 Pedigree of a Li–Fraumeni family to illustrate astonishing diversity of young individuals suffering from cancers.

type in these tumours—the others being bystanders—the Schwann cell is the likeliest culprit: but even this is not known.

Special features and problems

NF-1 illustrates strikingly the gulf that still exists between the cloning and description of a disease gene, and an explanation of all the manifestations of the disease. The tumours—gliomas, phaeochromocytomas, sarcomas — are relatively straightforward: the cells involved are known and *NF-1* seems to be acting as a classical suppressor gene. But in the case of short stature, learning difficulties or pseudoarthrosis, for example, even the critical cells in which the defect is primarily expressed are not known, and the mechanism for the local expression of these defects is completely obscure. Since these abnormalities presumably result directly from the loss of activity of only one copy of the gene, a mechanism involving sensitivity to gene 'dosage', similar to that described for FAP (see below), must be involved.

One aspect of the NF-1 phenotype, the variability, is especially amenable to analysis because the cutaneous neurofibromas and café au lait patches can be counted, and so provide a convenient quantitative measure of *NF-1* gene effect. Variations in expression of *NF-1* within a family might in principle be due to chance, environmental factors or modifying genetic factors. In each of these cases, the degree of similarity in expression between affected relatives would be different: for example, monozygotic twins should be identical in expression of the disease if 'genetic background' factors are paramount, whereas they should be no more similar than siblings or dizygotic twins if chance or environmental factors predominate. Limited analysis indicates that most of the phenotypic variation is indeed probably the result of 'genetic background' (Table 9.7).

Prospects for clinical application

Genetic prediction of the inheritance of the *NF-1* gene,

Table 9.7 Correlations between pairs of relatives with NF-1 for numbers of café au lait patches.

Relative pair	Number	Correlation coefficient
Monozygotic twins	6	0.85*
Siblings	76	0.34**
Parent–offspring	60	0.37**
2nd degree	54	0.17
3rd degree	43	−0.32

The closest correlation is seen between monozygotic twins, and the degree of correlation diminishes with increasing distance of relationship. This is the pattern expected of a 'genetic background' effect.
From Easton *et al*. (1993).
* $p < 0.05$, ** $p < 0.01$.

but not of the severity of disease expression, is possible using linked markers or in principle by direct testing for the mutation. In practice, it has proved very difficult to identify most *NF-1* mutations: 2 years after the cloning of the gene, in only about 10–15% of individuals analysed had the mutation been identified.

Inherited *p53* mutation: Li–Fraumeni syndrome

Clinical description

Li–Fraumeni syndrome (LFS) is an uncommon autosomal dominant cancer syndrome in which the commonest cancers are *s*arcomas, young-onset *b*reast cancer and *b*rain tumours, *l*eukaemia and *a*drenal cortical cancer (hence the alternative name SBLA syndrome; Fig. 9.9). Cancers at several other sites are also probably involved. In a large series of families, the risk of cancer at some site was 50% by age 40 in those who had inherited the gene.

Arbitrary definitions have been made, so that to be an 'LFS family' there must be a certain number of cancers of certain types below the age of 45. Some of the families which meet these criteria are found to have a constitutional mutation of one copy of the *p53* gene. Some have no detectable mutation: possibly they are due to mutations in other genes, such as *MDM2*, which may be in the same regulatory pathway as *p53* or have related functions. Many families have a clustering of cancers typical of LFS but falling outside the strict definition. *p53* mutations have been found in a few of these families, but the basis for the majority remains unclear.

Mapping and identification of the predisposing gene

The *p53* gene was known as a cancer gene some years before it was implicated in LFS. Because of the problems of finding sufficiently large families to search for the LFS gene by genetic linkage, a candidate gene strategy was used. Plausible genes were analysed for germ line mutations in a series of unrelated LFS individuals; *p53* mutations were identified and shown to be present in the affected members of several families. It is interesting that, at the time of writing, this is the only successful guess of a candidate gene in the inherited cancers. This contrasts with, for example, the genetics of coronary artery disease, where knowledge of mechanism, and thus of possible candidate genes, has been better.

The p53 gene and its function

The *p53* gene encodes a 393 amino acid protein which can bind to DNA and probably acts as a transcription factor. Its function is to regulate progression from the resting phase of the cell cycle into DNA synthesis, preventing entry into DNA synthesis unless conditions are suitable—that is, an adequate supply of growth factors is available and there is no unrepaired DNA damage. Failure of this function would lead to DNA synthesis and replication under adverse conditions, leading to genomic instability and cancer.

The role of *p53* mutation in cell cycle control, apoptosis and tumorigenesis has been described in Chapter 8. *p53* acts as a tumour suppressor gene, with the complication that mutant forms of the protein may interfere with the function of the wild-type protein—in this case, the mutation is said to have a 'dominant negative' effect.

Mechanisms of development of cancers

The cellular mechanism of action of mutant *p53* when it acts as an inherited predisposing gene is presumably the same as in sporadic tumours. Different cancers show a different spectrum of *p53* mutations, reflecting either different carcinogens or different selective effects of the p53 mutations in different tissues. The spectrum of germ line mutations in LFS is slightly different again, possibly because certain mutations are filtered out because they are incompatible with normal embryonic development.

Special features or problems

As with other inherited cancer syndromes, the particular spectrum of cancers that is seen in LFS, and the variation that is seen within that spectrum in different individuals and families, is unexplained. It is puzzling that some cancers in which *p53* mutations are common in the non-familial form are hardly increased in frequency in LFS. If *p53* mutation is important in development of the sporadic cancer, why does germ line *p53* mutation not increase the incidence?

Animal models of LFS

Transgenic mice carrying two wild-type and one mutant *p53* allele develop cancers at a greatly increased frequency, although the range of histological types does not correspond closely with that seen in humans. Whether breeding onto different genetic backgrounds will alter the pattern is yet to be seen. Transgenic mice have also been bred which are homozygous for a null *p53* mutation (no *p53* product): surprisingly in view of the central role ascribed to *p53* in cell cycle control, these mice appear to develop normally. It is reported, however, that cells from these mice are more mutable than normal, and that the mice have a high incidence of tumours.

Clinical application

Because *p53* is not a large gene, and most of the mutations occur within a fairly small region, screening for inherited *p53* mutations is feasible on a clinical as well as a research basis. Because of the wide and unpredictable range of cancers, lack of information about the penetrance of the gene outside selected series of large families, and lack of proven methods for screening or prevention, however, it is far from clear in what circumstances such screening will be of benefit to the individual or family. The discovery, for research purposes, that an individual or family carries a germ line *p53* mutation therefore raises difficult questions of responsibility in the disclosure of this information.

Mutant *p53* and its effects are currently attracting much attention as targets for cancer therapy, but no effective schemes have yet been reported.

Colorectal cancer

Clinical description

Several types of familial colon cancer have been described (Table 9.8). For the most part, these seem to be clinically distinct and to 'breed true' in families, indicating that they are the result of predisposition by different genes. There are, however, some grey areas—in particular, families which seem to be intermediate between full-blown FAP and familial site-specific colorectal cancer, and a variety of 'family cancer syndromes' which comprise familial associations of colorectal cancer with ovarian, endometrial, breast and other cancers in differing proportions. Evidence is emerging that the attenuated forms of FAP are indeed due to 'weak' mutations at the FAP locus. The genetic classification of the other familial cancer syndromes will become clearer with the identification of the predisposing genes and information about the involvement of these genes in families of different types.

The main features of FAP are the very large numbers of intestinal polyps, which first appear at 10–15 years (mostly, but not exclusively, in the large intestine), and the development of one or more colorectal cancers in the majority of cases by the age of 50. There may also be abnormalities in a variety of other tissues (Table 9.8). Of these, congenital hypertrophy of the retinal pigment epithelium (CHRPE) is sufficiently frequent to be used in the recognition of gene carriers in early childhood,

Table 9.8 Familial colon cancer syndromes.

Polyposis syndromes
Familial adenomatous polyposis
- FAP: multiple intestinal polyps; CHRPE
- Gardner's syndrome variant: FAP, CHRPE plus soft tissue tumours, sebaceous cysts, thyroid tumours, hepatoblastoma
- Attenuated FAP variant: autosomal dominant inheritance of right-sided flat adenomas and risk of colonic cancer

Turcot syndrome
- Intestinal polyps and adenocarcinoma, CNS tumours, skin lesions including café au lait spots

Hamartomatous polyp syndromes
- Peutz–Jegher's syndrome: autosomal dominant, mucocutaneous pigmentation, hamartomas of small and large bowel, risk of gastrointestinal, genitourinary and other cancers
- Cowden syndrome: autosomal dominant, multiple hamartomas and risk of breast and thyroid cancers
- Juvenile polyposis: non-premalignant small and large bowel polyps

'Non-polyposis' colon cancer syndromes
HNPCC
- Lynch I—site-specific colon cancer
- Lynch II—colon cancer with endometrial, urothelial and other cancers in the family

before intestinal polyps have developed. The fibroblastic 'desmoid' tumours typically involve the abdominal and chest wall. Although not metastatic, they may be progressive and deeply infiltrating, and in several cases are extremely difficult to treat. When these features are present, the clinical picture is sometimes referred to as Gardner's syndrome.

Members of families at substantially increased risk of colorectal cancer are recommended to have regular endoscopic screening of the bowel for polyps. It is probable (though not formally proven) that such screening will prevent deaths from colorectal cancer.

Mapping and identification of the gene

The predisposing gene for colorectal cancer in FAP has been mapped to chromosome 5q21 and identified. The FAP gene was identified by the usual methods of positional cloning, starting from the finding of a 5q21 deletion in a man with FAP and mental retardation. Further localizing information came from the identification of small overlapping regions of deletion in a set of colorectal cancers. The history of the final identification of the gene is instructive because it illustrates the difficulty of proving that alterations in a gene are actually causally related to a disease, and that the gene is therefore the 'disease gene'. The first gene in the 5q21 region to be identified as a candidate was thought to be the FAP gene because it was mutated in some colon cancers (it was called *MCC* for this reason). However, despite a frantic search, no mutations could be found in this gene in constitutional DNA from FAP patients. The puzzle was solved when a neighbouring gene, *apc* (for adenomatous polyposis of the colon), was found to be mutated in DNA from both sources, making it a more credible candidate. The conclusion that *apc* is the gene for FAP has been strengthened since by the consistent finding of mutations in a large number of FAP patients, and in the *apc* homologue in a mouse strain with polyposis.

The apc *gene and its function*

The *apc* gene encodes a 8.4 kb mRNA, corresponding to a protein of 2844 amino acids. The protein has a predicted coiled coil motif similar to that of intermediate filament proteins. Heptad repeats within the protein structure may be capable of mediating protein–protein interactions and recently it has been shown that the APC protein interacts with proteins that bind the E-cadherin cell adhesion protein suggesting a link between tumorigenesis and cell adhesion. The *MCC* gene contains a similar sequence, raising the possibility that the protein products of these genes may interact with each other.

The spectrum of mutations in the *apc* gene reported so far includes (in addition to a few large deletions) base changes leading to stop codons, frameshifts or splicing mutations, but not amino acid substitutions. The mutations are largely clustered in the 5′ half of the gene. There is evidence that the 'attenuated' forms of FAP mentioned above may result from mutations at the 5′ extremity of the gene (perhaps allowing some reinitiation downstream of the mutation and so production of a limited amount of *apc* product); there is also evidence of correlations between specific mutations and the presence or absence of extracolonic abnormalities. These observations indicate a specific functional role of different domains of the *apc* protein in different regions.

Hereditary non-polyposis colon cancer

At least four genes are responsible for hereditary non-polyposis colon cancer (HNPCC) which is characterized by instability at short tandem DNA repeats or microsatellite sequences (see Chapter 3). One of these genes has been mapped to chromosome 2 and cloning and analysis of the gene (*MSH2*) suggests it is involved in

DNA repair due to its sequence homology to the bacterial DNA mismatch repair gene, *mutS*. Three other genes also responsible for HNPCC (*MLH1*, *PMS1* and *PMS2*) are homologues of the bacterial DNA mismatch repair gene *mutL*. Mutations in each of these four genes have been found in the germ line of HNPCC families. Knockout mice (see Chapter 3) deficient in the *MSH2* gene develop lymphoid tumours with microsatellite instabilities.

Mechanisms of development of cancers and preneoplastic lesions

The earliest recognizable phenotypic abnormality in the colonic epithelium is an alteration in the balance between proliferation and maturation in the intestinal crypts. Normally, proliferating cells are confined to the lower one-third of the crypt, but in FAP the proliferating compartment is considerably expanded. This change affects all crypts, not just a few, and must presumably therefore reflect the direct effect of the inherited mutation even though this only affects one copy of the *apc* gene. In other words, the *apc* mutation appears (unlike mutations in *Rb-1*, but like *NF-1*) to have direct phenotypic expression. During late childhood, polyps develop on the surface of the epithelium: since these are discrete lesions, they probably do result from additional somatic mutations in one or more genes which are critical for the progression towards colorectal carcinoma. The accumulation of further mutations results in the evolution of the polyp until eventually an invasive cancer results. Mutation of the second allele at the FAP locus occurs at some stage in this process in many, but possibly not all, colorectal cancers. Similar genetic changes are seen in sporadic colorectal cancers and those from FAP patients.

The additional genetic events, if any, which are involved in the development of the extracolonic manifestations of FAP are still not known.

Special features and problems

FAP provides one of the clearest examples of an inherited cancer where, in distinction to retinoblastoma, it seems that the inherited mutation has a phenotypic effect even when present only in a single copy. Since at least some FAP mutations involve deletion of a whole copy of the gene, and others lead to premature termination of transcription, the most likely explanation is that the reduced 'dose' of the gene leads to a reduced concentration of the protein and this reduction is sufficient to cause an effect. One plausible mechanism of the effect would be that the *apc* product is involved in interaction with another protein, and the reduced concentration destroys the stoichiometry. Alternatively, the mutation might sometimes result in production of an altered protein which could interfere with the building of a multi-protein complex in the same way that a triangular brick will not fit into a regular wall. This so-called 'dominant negative' effect, in which a mutant gene interferes with the action of the normal allele, is also thought to result from some mutations in the *p53* gene (see above).

Another striking feature of FAP, seen also very clearly in *NF-1* (see above), is the variation in expression of the phenotype even within a family. This variation is probably the result of modifying effects of the genetic background in *apc* expression. Evidence for this idea was described briefly under *NF-1*.

Animal models of FAP

A mouse strain, the 'min' mouse, which has a point mutation in the murine homologue of the *apc* gene, has been identified as a result of large-scale experiments in which germ line mutations were systematically induced with the mutagen ethylnitrosourea. Crossing these mice onto different genetic backgrounds has a marked effect on the development of intestinal polyps, consistent with the idea of modifying gene effects described above. The first of the modifying genes has now been mapped to a specific mouse chromosome by genetic linkage.

Prospects for clinical application

Linked genetic markers and mutation testing of the *apc* gene are now in routine use for the prediction of inheritance of the predisposing gene in FAP families.

Breast and ovarian cancer

Clinical description

Breast cancer and ovarian cancer have long been known to cluster in families (Table 9.3), but extensive families with a clear inherited basis proved difficult to identify. There are three possible reasons:
1 males will seldom contribute to the pattern of cancers in the family;
2 there is no recognized phenotype akin to the polyps of FAP which indicates a hereditary case;
3 breast cancer, at least, is common so that only the most striking family clusters will rise clearly above the background.

Nevertheless, several striking families with young-onset breast cancer and ovarian cancer in different combinations have now been identified (Fig. 9.10), and proof that they reflect the action of a single highly penetrant gene has come from linkage analysis and the identification so far of one of the predisposing genes, *BRCA1*.

Mapping of the predisposing gene

After an extensive search using linkage markers systematically covering the chromosomes, linkage was obtained to a locus in 17q12–21. The locus was designated *BRCA1* and it is probably responsible for about 40% of families with multiple cases of breast cancer and over 80% of families with cases of both ovarian and breast cancer. If several different genes account for the remaining 60% of families, and if these genes are less highly penetrant than the 17q gene (80% by age 70),

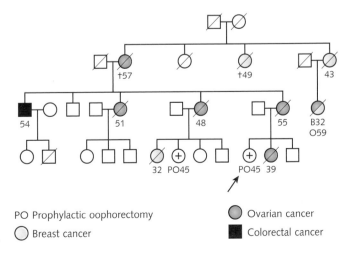

Fig. 9.10 A family with breast/ovarian cancer syndrome due to mutation in the *BRCA1* gene on chromosome 17q.

PO Prophylactic oophorectomy
○ Breast cancer
● Ovarian cancer
■ Colorectal cancer

Model	Proportion of population who are gene carriers	Risk of breast cancer by age 60 (%)	Proportion of all breast cancer <60 years in gene carriers (%)
Rare high risk gene	1:250	50	10
Common lower risk gene	1:4	10	86

Table 9.9 Possible genetic models to explain the epidemiological observation that the risk of breast cancer is 3% by age 60 in the general population, and this risk is two-fold greater in the sibling of a case.

These models are hypothetical. The table is intended to illustrate that, if it is assumed that the observed familial clustering of breast cancer is due to dominantly inherited genetic effects, in principle these could result from either a rare gene of strong effect, or a common gene of less effect. The implications of the two models for individuals and for strategies for breast cancer prevention are clearly different.

mapping them by linkage will prove very difficult. However, a second predisposing gene — BRCA2 — has recently been mapped to chromosome 13q12–13. This gene may be of equal importance to BRCA1 in conferring risk of early-onset breast cancer, although it seems to be less important than BRCA1 in ovarian cancer for, so far, undetermined reasons.

Description of the BRCA1 gene and its function

Extensive work from a number of laboratories has recently led to the cloning of BRCA1. BRCA1 comprises some 21 exons and is distributed over more than 100 kb of DNA. Analysis of the predicted amino acid sequence of the gene suggests it contains a zinc finger domain which is present in a number of transcription factor proteins but also in many other proteins as well. Analysis of mutations in BRCA1 and allele loss data from familial cancers also suggests BRCA1 may be a member of the tumour supressor family of proteins, possibly acting on the retinoblastoma model.

Special problems

Breast cancer illustrates the problem of determining how much of inherited predisposition to a given cancer is accounted for by rare highly penetrant genes, and how much by polygenic effects. This is important because it affects the total proportion of breast cancer which is attributable to inherited predisposition, and thus the scope for applying knowledge of inherited predisposition to prevention.

The only measure we have of the magnitude of predisposition is the relative risk to close family members. If, for the sake of argument, the familial risk has an entirely inherited basis, there are two extreme possibilities (Table 9.9). It could be the result of strong effects in a very small proportion of the population, accounting for a small minority of total cancer incidence, or the result of weaker effects in many people, accounting for a substantial fraction of cancer incidence. The public health implications are clearly different. The real situation will lie somewhere between these extremes; but where? We know from linkage analysis that some rare strongly predisposed families exist, but there is no way to tell how much of total inherited predisposition these families account for. The search for polygenic predisposing effects, as described in Chapter 7 and the Introduction to this chapter, is wide open.

Clinical applications

In families where there are sufficient affected individuals available to provide evidence for linkage to 17q or where mutations in the BRCA1 gene itself have been identified, genetic prediction of inheritance of the predisposing gene is possible. Whether, in view of the limited possibilities for prevention, families will want this information remains to be seen.

Inherited defects in DNA repair and chromosomal instability

Since the development of cancer requires the accumulation of mutations in a single cell, disorders which involve defects in the repair of DNA damage or hypersensitivity to the effects of DNA damaging agents through other mechanisms would be expected to be associated with an increased risk of cancer. Several such disorders have been recognized (Table 9.10). Except for HNPCC, which we have discussed above, all are rare.

Heterozygotes for these rare disorders will of course be much less rare. For example, ataxia telangiectasia (AT) heterozygotes may be as many as one in 200 of the population. If they have increased sensitivity to DNA damage, these individuals may be at increased risk of

Table 9.10 Some human syndromes with DNA repair abnormalities and a predisposition to cancer.

Syndrome	Clinical features	Cancers	Cellular characteristics	Genes
Xeroderma pigmentosum	Sun-sensitive skin, neurological abnormalities	Skin cancer	UV hypermutable defective in early stage of nucleotide excision repair	Several complementation groups, some cloned
Ataxia telangiectasia	Progressive ataxia telangiectasias, sensitive to ionizing radiation	Lymphomas	Hypersensitive to ionizing radiation	Cloned
Bloom syndrome	Retarded growth, sun-sensitive	Early-onset cancers of several types	Elevated sister chromatid exchange, hypermutable	Cloned
Hereditary non-polyposis colon cancer	No abnormal clinical phenotype	Familial colon, endometrial, urothelial and other cancers	Defective DNA mismatch repair, instability of simple repeat sequences	Probably several, some cloned
Fanconi's anaemia	Small stature, anaemia due to bone marrow failure	Myeloid leukaemia	Chromosome aberrations, hypersensitive to DNA cross-linking agents	Several, some cloned

cancer. Epidemiological studies of relatives of AT homozygotes suggest that this may indeed be true, and that as much as 5% of breast or ovarian cancer below the age of 50 could occur in this group. Proof, however, awaits a reliable assay for the AT mutation and careful measurement of the frequency of the gene in cases and controls. Maybe polymorphism in DNA repair genes is one source of polygenic variation in cancer susceptibility.

Metabolic polymorphisms

The progression of a cell towards cancer involves interaction with the environment in the form of potential mutagens and the effects of potential regulators of cell growth such as steroid hormones. Genetically determined individual differences in metabolic pathways will clearly influence these processes (Fig. 9.1). It is therefore logical to look for inherited determinants of cancer susceptibility in genetic variation in the enzymes which metabolize exogenous and endogenous carcinogens, and in the genes which might be expected to regulate different aspects of cellular growth. Compared with the search for determinants of atherosclerosis, however (Chapter 7), the knowledge of plausible candidate genes for cancer susceptibility is very limited. Effort has focused on:

1 the genes of the cytochrome P450 mono-oxygenase family, which are involved in the metabolism of foreign compounds, as well as in the synthesis of endogenous steroid hormones;

2 glutathione S transferases, which catalyse the detoxification of mutagenic electrophiles by conjugation to glutathione;

3 acetyltransferases, which among other reactions, catalyse the detoxification of potentially mutagenic aromatic amines present in food.

A number of possible associations have been reported, for example between a polymorphism at the cytochrome P450 *CYP1A1* locus and lung cancer susceptibility, levels of glutathione S transferase and susceptibility to chemical carcinogens in animals, and rapid acetylator phenotype and colon cancer. All require to be confirmed, and none has yet led to practical application in terms of cancer prevention. Nevertheless, as knowledge of candidate genes increases, and the techniques are developed for rapid identification and analysis of DNA polymorphisms in large population-based series of cases and controls, identification of predisposed subgroups of the population is likely to become possible. If the environmental component of the susceptibility can also be identified and reduced, this may provide a rational strategy for cancer prevention.

Conclusion

'Inherited predisposition' is currently top of the list of cancer research priorities in many countries. This enthusiasm probably reflects the spectacular advances in the past 10 years in which study of families has led to the identification of genes such as *Rb-1*, *WT-1* and *NF-1* which in turn have yielded important insights into the processes of normal growth controls. The same is expected of the inherited cancer genes such as *apc*, the function of which is still to be elucidated in detail.

How far this biological insight will translate into better prevention or treatment of cancer is unclear. The inherited cancers which are most open to this type of genetic analysis are also rather rare. In the coming decade, improvements in epidemiology and in genome analysis will open up the analysis of the polygenic contribution to individual susceptibility to the common cancers. This may suggest approaches to prevention on a much larger scale. Whether people will wish to follow this route remains to be seen.

Further reading

Cavenee W.K., Dryja T.P. and Phillips R.A. (1983) Expression of recessive alleles by chromosomal mechanisms in retinoblastoma. *Nature*, 305, 779–789.

Easton D. and Peto J. (1991) The contribution of inherited disposition to cancer incidence. In: *Cancer Surveys, Vol. 9, Genetic Predisposition to Cancer* (eds W. Cavenee, P. Ponder and E. Solomon), pp. 395–415. Oxford University Press, Oxford.

Easton D.F., Ponder M.A., Huson S.M. and Ponder B.A.J. (1993) An analysis of variation in expression of neurofibromatosis (NF) type 1 (NF1): evidence for modifying genes. *American Journal of Human Genetics*, 53, 305–313.

Chapter 10
Molecular biology of the immune response

Introduction

The immune system has evolved to protect the host against infection by micro-organisms. It has the capacity to recognize the different macromolecules (**antigens**) of invading pathogens, and to direct immune responses against these antigens in a way that minimizes damage to the host itself. Some of the macromolecules of micro-organisms are structurally quite different from those of the host, such as the complex polysaccharide components of bacterial cell walls, which can themselves directly trigger the activation of the host complement system. However, many pathogens have macromolecules that closely resemble those of the host. To be able to recognize and respond appropriately to micro-organisms, through evolution the host has acquired an array of sophisticated **antigen receptors** that can distinguish subtle differences in the primary, secondary or tertiary structure of polypeptides. These antigen receptors are highly polymorphic — different receptors recognize different antigens. The interaction of a given antigen receptor with its antigen ligand is very specific, i.e. each receptor can bind with high affinity to one particular antigen but not other closely related molecules. Because this recognition of antigen is so specific, indiscriminate damage to host tissues can be avoided during immune responses directed against foreign antigens.

Antigen receptors are expressed on the surface of **lymphocytes**, enabling these cells to **recognize and respond** to antigen. Unlike most other cells in the body, lymphocytes have a distinctive clonal organization which is based on the antigen receptor. Each lymphocyte has a single antigen receptor; by repeated cell division, each lymphocyte can give rise to a large population of genetically identical daughter cells, all of which express on their surface the same distinctive antigen receptor characteristic of that particular clone of cells. Different lymphocyte clones express a different antigen receptor and therefore are capable of recognizing different antigens. Because it is possible to generate an enormous **diversity** of antigen receptors, the immune system contains a vast number ($>10^7$) of different **lymphocyte clones** (from 10^2 to 10^4 cells per clone), which collectively are capable of recognizing a huge range of different antigens exhibited by invading micro-organisms.

Upon **first exposure** to a given antigen, only a small number of lymphocyte clones whose antigen receptors specifically recognize the antigen are stimulated to proliferate into an enlarged population of effector cells and long-lasting memory cells. Thus an immune response is amplified by increasing the number of cells in selected clones — the cellular composition of the immune system changes in response to exposure to antigen. Upon subsequent exposure to the same antigen, there is a stronger, more rapid **secondary response** directed against the antigen, brought about by the expanded population of antigen-specific **memory cells** (the cellular basis of immunological memory).

There are **two classes of lymphocyte** within the immune system that are capable of specific recognition of antigen, namely **B-cells** and **T-cells**. B-cells produce antibodies (immunoglobulins), which in membrane-bound form act as the **B-cell antigen receptor** and which in secreted form serve important effector functions. T-cells carry out diverse regulatory and effector functions, including helping B-cells to produce antibody. The **T-cell receptor** is found only in membrane-bound form. It recognizes antigen which has been processed and presented on the surface of other cells by major histocompatability complex (MHC) molecules.

Figure 10.1 shows a simplified scheme of the immune system.

How does the immune system generate such enormous diversity of antigen receptors? There is a challenge

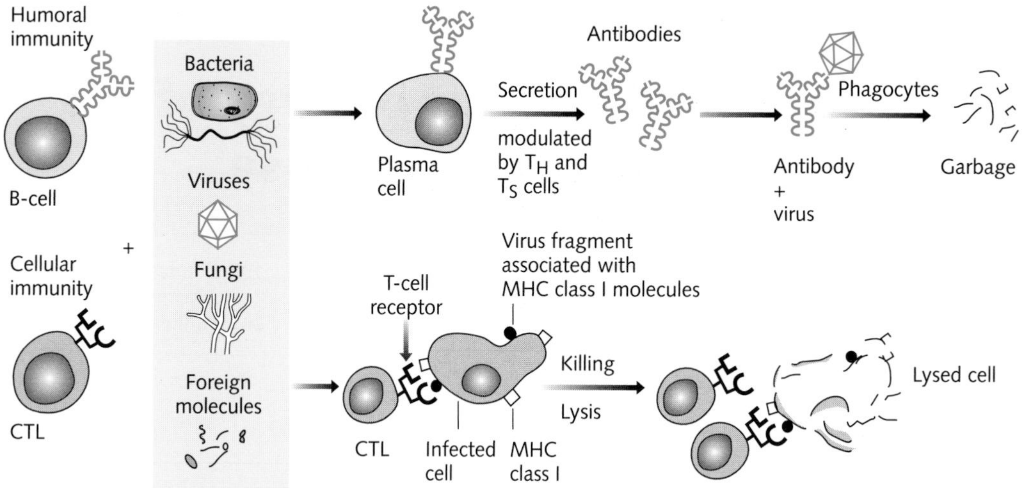

Fig. 10.1 Simplified scheme of the immune system. Antibodies are secreted by B-cells. They arise from stem cells in the bone marrow and have IgM or IgM and IgD on their surface. Eventually, the interaction of the surface antibody with antigen (from e.g. foreign molecules) leads to B-lymphocyte activation and maturation into plasma cells that secrete antibody. In the early phase of B-cell development, diversity is generated by an organized succession of recombination events that modify random multiple genes in the germ line DNA. Cell-mediated immunity is brought abought by cytotoxic T-lymphocytes (CTL) that kill cells bearing foreign antigens (e.g. viral antigens) specifically in the context of self-derived class I major histocompatibility antigens. T-cell recognition is brought about by T-cell receptors on the surface of T-lymphocytes that are genetically distinct two-chain molecules that resemble antibodies and specifically recognize MHC and antigen molecules jointly. Subsets of T-lymphocytes, T-helper (T_H) and T-suppressor (T_S) cells, regulate and modify the immune response and secrete activators of macrophages and other antigen-presenting cells.

in that the resources available are finite, and are restricted by the information encoded in the genomic DNA of each cell. The elegant solution is a genetic mechanism that applies both to antibody molecules and to T-cell receptors. An outline of the molecular pathways of **gene recombination** and **somatic mutation** by which this is achieved forms the first part of this chapter. The mechanisms involved are subject to error, which may lead to the development of **lymphoid tumours**. The processes by which this occurs offer a fascinating insight into the molecular basis of oncogenesis and normal cell growth in lymphoid tissue, and are described in the later section.

Structure and rearrangement of human antigen receptor genes

Antigen receptors are long, folded polypeptide chains with a definite modular tertiary structure, in which distinct parts of the receptor (called domains) carry out different biological functions. The polymorphic receptor region recognizes and binds to antigen, while other non-polymorphic domains can interact with a variety of common effector mechanisms, e.g. they connect cell-surface antigen receptors to intracellular signalling pathways, and enable secreted antibody to interact with receptors on mast cells and phagocytic cells and to activate complement. This modular domain structure is achieved by the presence in germ line DNA of linear arrays of many different variable region genes and also a smaller number of constant region genes on the same chromosome. During lymphocyte development, the variable and constant gene segments on the same chromosome rearrange and join to each other in many different combinations (with loss of the intervening chromosomal DNA) to produce a novel recombined gene encoding the full-length receptor. Such gene rearrangements are stable and inheritable from cell to cell, so that each daughter cell inherits the same single antigen receptor characteristic of that lymphocyte clone. As might be expected, the structure and rearrangement of the genes encoding immunoglobulin and T-cell receptor have much in common. There are also significant differences, such as the presence of somatic mutation in the development of the antibody repertoire which has important consequences for self-tolerance (see Chapter 11).

Immunoglobulin

The structure of an immunoglobulin molecule is depicted in Fig. 10.2. The basic structure consists of paired heavy and light chains, both of which have variable and constant regions. These chains are encoded at three separate immunoglobulin (Ig) gene loci: one heavy (H) chain locus and two light (L) chain loci. The five different classes of immunoglobulin molecules (IgA, IgD, IgE, IgG and IgM) each have a particular heavy chain (α, β, ϵ, γ and μ, respectively). Light chains belong to two classes, κ or λ; a given antibody molecule contains either κ or λ light chains. The light chains may assemble with any heavy chain type to form the complete antibody molecule. Each of the three loci are encoded by separate chromosomes (Table 10.1). A summary of the organization of these loci appears in Figs 10.3 and 10.4.

Variable genes

The heavy chain locus (Fig. 10.3) is the most complex, consisting of a set of variable (V) region, diversity (D) region and joining (J) region segments, which rearrange and join to create the active heavy chain V gene. The

Table 10.1 Chromosome location of antigen receptor genes in humans.

Gene	Chromosome location
Immunoglobulin genes	
H chain	14q32.3
L chain	
κ	2p12
λ	22q11
T-cell receptor genes	
TCR α	14q11
TCR δ	14q11
TCR β	7q35
TCR γ	7p15

downstream end of each V segment is flanked by sequences recognized by the enzyme (recombinase) responsible for carrying out the **gene rearrangement** (see below). The size of the heavy chain V region repertoire is estimated at 100–200 genes, lying in a region of 2500 kb on human chromosome 14.

The two light chain loci only have V and J segments (neither has D segments). Thus, only V-J joining occurs to create the active loci. There are approximately 80 V_κ and 30 V_λ genes.

The assembled heavy chain V region and the assembled light chain V region come together to form the antigen binding site of the complete immunoglobulin molecule, which confers antigen specificity.

Constant genes

The constant region of immunoglobulin heavy chains influences the tissue distribution of Ig molecules (e.g. IgG can cross the placenta; IgA is delivered onto mucosal surfaces) and also their effector function (e.g. IgM can activate complement; IgE can trigger mast cell degranulation).

Of the three immunoglobulin loci the most complex is the heavy chain constant (C_H) locus. In humans, this contains 11 constant region genes contained within about 200 kb, the organization of which is represented in Fig. 10.3. All but one C_H gene has immediately upstream a switch or S sequence responsible for the heavy chain class switch (see below); the C δ segment is the exception. The C_H gene segments, unlike C_L, have domains represented by exons which are separated by introns (Fig. 10.3). Apart from the exons encoding the transmembrane region, the C_μ and C_ϵ genes have four domains, C_δ has three (including a hinge), the γ genes

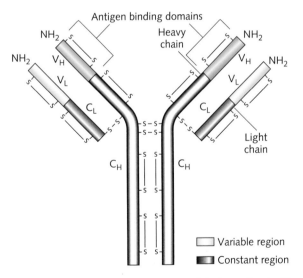

Fig. 10.2 Representation of an immunoglobulin molecule. The molecule is made up of two light (L) and two heavy (H) polypeptide chains, each of which bears variable (V) and constant (C) regions. The variable regions make up the immunoglobulin antigen binding domain. These polypeptide chains are encoded by three genes: κ and λ (for light chain loci) and the heavy chain locus (H), which has several subtypes (see text). Multiple disulphide bonds (S–S) bridge between these protein chains.

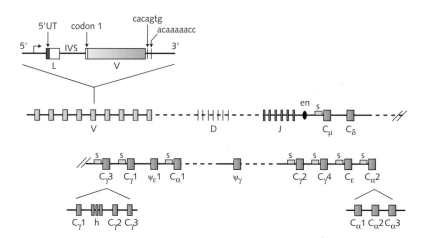

Fig. 10.3 Organization of the human immunoglobulin heavy chain locus. The schematic picture depicts the clusters of V, D, J and C segments. There are of the order of 100–200 segments; the detailed organization of individual V gene is shown above. A cluster of D elements exists upstream of J, but other D elements (not shown) occur within the body of the V cluster. The major H transcription enhancer (En) is located between C_μ and J. Switch (S) region elements are indicated near each C gene which undergoes the class switch. The domain structure of exons (boxes) and introns (lines) of the C genes is illustrated in detail for C_γ (h, hinge exons) and for $C_\alpha 2$. Pseudogenes are indicated by (Ψ).

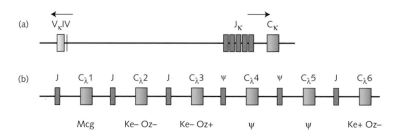

Fig. 10.4 The human light chain constant region genes. (a) The single human C gene has five associated J elements. No D elements exist for the light chains. The V gene nearest to the C_κ is $V_\kappa IV$, and this V gene is organized in the opposite transcription orientation to the C_κ gene (as depicted by the arrows). The five J segments are shown as striped boxes. (b) The C_λ gene cluster. Six C_λ genes, each with associated J segments, are shown (not to scale). Four of the C_λ segments are allelic genes and two are pseudo (Ψ) genes.

have four domains (one of these being a hinge which is quadruplicated in γ) and the α genes have three domains, with the hinge as part of the second domain.

There is a single C_κ gene about 3 kb from the set of J_κ segments (Fig. 10.4a). The λ light chain locus contains at least four expressed C_λ genes (Fig. 10.4b), each of which apparently has one (or more) associated J_λ segments.

Immunoglobulin gene rearrangement programme

The immunoglobulin genes exhibit **allelic exclusion**, i.e. normally only one of the two parental alleles at each locus is expressed. This seems to be the result of impre-cise joining during rearrangment; for example, the protein translation frames of the V and J regions after joining may not coincide. Therefore only one allele is expressed as a polypeptide product.

A sequence of gene rearrangements occurs during the development of B-cells. The heavy chain locus appears to be the first to rearrange: sequences between V and J are deleted, producing a V-D-J join and allowing expression of μ heavy chains. The κ light chains undergo rearrangement next, resulting in the production of κ light chain protein. Alternatively, in B-cells which ultimately produce λ light chains, the κ genes are usually deleted, following which λ gene rearrangement takes place and λ light chains are produced. The production of light chains permits the assembly of mature immunoglobulin as IgM and IgD (the co-expression of the same variable region with either a μ or δ constant segment is achieved by alternative RNA splicing of a common precursor molecule). The functionally rearranged V_H segment can subsequently be expressed with one of the other downstream C_H genes (γ, ε or α giving rise to IgG, IgE and IgA antibodies, respectively) by the heavy chain class switch (see below). It is also possible for a germ line V_H to join to the rearranged J_H, deleting the previously joined V_H; this may be a mechanism for expanding the Ig repertoire and for ensuring full usage of the germ line V_H genes.

Sequence requirements for gene rearrangement

There are two forms of gene rearrangement. The first, V-D-J joining, is common to immunoglobulin and T-cell receptor genes; the second, H class switching, is restricted to the immunoglobulin heavy chain genes.

V-D-J joining is mediated by an enzyme, 'recombinase'. This enzyme system has not yet been fully characterized but its sequence requirements have been deduced and are shown in Fig. 10.5. The spacer sequences must be 23 basepairs (two turns of the DNA helix) and 12 basepairs (one helix turn) on opposite sides of the join.

The Ig heavy chain class switch allows the switching of a variable heavy gene segment from expression with the C_μ constant region to one of the other C_H genes. In this way, the same antigen binding region can be linked to a heavy chain with a different spectrum of biological effector functions. This process results from a recombination event between so-called switch or S sequences, which are found upstream of all C_H genes except C_δ (see Fig. 10.3).

The generation of immunoglobulin diversity

It is now possible to see how the multiple germ line V, D and J region segments, together with the rearrangement programme, contribute to the generation of a very large immunoglobulin repertoire. The extent of theoretical diversity that can result from the rearrangement of antibody gene segments is the product of the number of V, D (if present) and J segments; this calculation could, for example, lead to a minimum of about 6×10^3 different human V_H segments, i.e. $10^2\,V \times 10\,D \times 6\,J$. Similar calculations can be performed for V_L segments, and, as the binding site of an antibody has contributions from both light and heavy chains, the number of possible combinations is the product of V_H and V_L diversity. This enormous combinatorial diversity is further enhanced by the processes of junctional diversity and somatic mutation.

There are two forms of **junctional diversity**: imprecision of V-J, V-D and D-J joining, and the addition of random nucleotides at the junction of sequences (N-region diversity). An example of the consequences of imprecise joining is provided by residue 96 of the κ light chains. This is a highly variable residue, even though it is normally encoded by the first codon of the J. This is because V-J joining can occur in such a way that only the second or third residue to the triplet comes from J, the first or second respectively coming from the incoming V. In addition, codon 96 can be deleted entirely, or out-of-frame joins can be compensated by base deletions upstream of the join.

Somatic mutation is a process which introduces additional diversity not encoded by germ line genes, within the immunoglobulin of B-cell clones that have been stimulated by antigen. It plays an important role in producing the increasing affinity of antibody found during an immune response (affinity maturation). There appears to be a specific enzymatic hypermutation process which acts on rearranged V genes. The resulting alterations have a tendency to cluster within or close to the regions involved in antigen binding rather than in framework regions. This gives rise to a set of B-cell subclones whose antigen receptors have a range of slightly different affinities for the antigen, some of higher affinity than the original B-cell clone and some of lower affinity. During the later stages of an immune response, antigen can select for those mutated B-cell clones which express antibody with higher affinity, leading to expansion of these clones and a higher aggregate affinity of the mixed population of different antibodies.

T-cell receptor

The T-cell receptor, like the immunoglobulin molecule, consists of variable and constant regions; the overall structure, particularly the position of cysteine residues, resembles that of immunoglobulin light chains and thus a very similar domain structure can be predicted (Fig. 10.6). There are two types of T-cell receptor. Bone marrow-derived T-cell precursors enter the thymus and become functional T-lymphocytes carrying either an α-β **heterodimer** (the 'classical' T-cell receptor) or a γ-δ **heterodimer**. T-cells with the α-β receptor predominate on T-cells in peripheral blood, whereas in mice epithelial and epidermal T-cells almost exclusively bear γ-δ complexes. The chromosomal locations of the genes for the four human T-cell receptor proteins are shown in Table

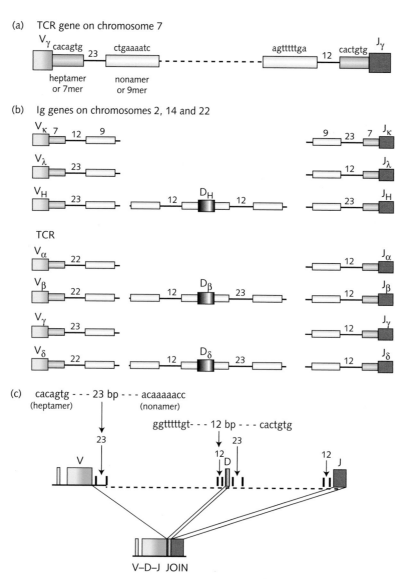

Fig. 10.5 Organization of recombinase signal sequences within the various human antigen receptor loci. (a) The downstream recombinase signals are shown with typical sequences of heptamers and nanomers for the T-cell receptor locus of humans. (b) Each of the rearranging genes within immunoglobulin and T-cell receptor loci are depicted, with D elements where applicable, with appropriate spacing of the signal sequences (12 or 23 basepairs). (c) Mechanism of gene rearrangement (deletional). A hypothetical V gene joins to a D and to a J. Spacing of heptamer and nanomer signals complies with the 12–23 rule. Note that in this case, a direct join from V to J would be possible by this rule.

10.1; the loci encoding the α and δ chains appear to overlap. A summary of the organization of these loci appears in Fig. 10.7.

Variable genes

T-cell receptor α and γ chains use V and J elements to form the variable region gene, whereas β and δ chains use V, D and J elements. The V genes contain two conserved cysteine residues that are probably involved in the formation of intramolecular disulphide bridges and the generation of an immunoglobulin-like fold. An estimated 100 V_α genes can be grouped into 12 families defined operationally as having more than 50% sequence homology at the amino acid level. More than 100 V_β genes are divided among 14 families, with three

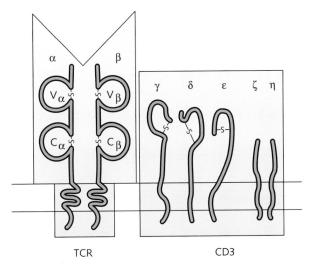

Fig. 10.6 Representation of T-cell receptor. Unlike the immunoglobulin molecule and membrane-bound B-cell receptor, the T-cell receptor is a transmembrane heterodimer of α and β polypeptide chains, which are linked by disulphide bonds (S–S). Each chain possesses a relatively invariant domain (c) (resembling the immunoglobulin Ig fold); and a highly variable domain (V). The T-cell antigen receptor is closely associated with a CD3 complex consisting of the non-covalently linked polypeptides, γ, δ, ε, ζ and η that are involved in transduction of the signal generated by antigen binding. Thus the functional T-cell receptor can be considered as a five-membered complex of the α/β heterodimer and CD3.

families having only one member. The V_δ gene pool in humans is not yet fully defined.

The human D elements of the T-cell receptor β locus are very similar to each other, both in sequence and in length. The D elements in the δ locus are shorter and very dissimilar. A comparison of J elements from the T-cell receptor loci reveals that they are slightly longer than immunoglobulin J elements, but all very homologous to each other.

Constant genes

The constant region genes of the T-cell receptor polypeptides are associated with their corresponding D (for β and δ) and J elements, as shown in Fig. 10.7. The constant regions generally contain three cysteine residues (for exceptions, see below), two of which reside in the first exon and again are believed to be involved in creating an immunoglobulin-like fold. The third cysteine residue, encoded in a separate exon, is thought to be involved in interchain disulphide bonds.

A hydrophobic stretch of about 20 amino acids in the carboxy-terminal part of the T-cell receptor is believed to be the membrane spanning region. The cytoplasmic tail is rather short (approximately 5 residues) in α and γ chains, and longer (approximately 15 residues) in β and δ chains.

Patterns of rearrangement and expression in T-cell receptor loci

The sequence requirements for T-cell receptor gene rearrangements appear similar to those of immunoglobulin genes: the heptamer/nonamer signal sequences are the same, and the 12/23 spacer rule also applies. This strongly suggests that the same recombinase machinery acts on both immunoglobulin and T-cell receptor genes. Mature T-cells sometimes carry abortive immunoglobulin gene rearrangements, suggesting that control over which locus is rearranged is not absolutely tissue specific. This is emphasized by the observation that leukaemias of pre-B- or pre-T-cell phenotype may have antigen receptor gene rearrangements of both lineages.

Allelic exclusion in the β chain locus is probably due to an inhibition of V-D-J rearrangements by the presence of β chain polypeptides. In contrast, productively rearranged γ chain alleles are generally not expressed in cells bearing α/β receptors. This suggests that γ chain gene transcription is tightly controlled, and subject to negative regulation; it seems that γ expression is the biological consequence of δ expression, and that these are intimately linked.

Rearrangements in the δ locus appear to be the earliest events in T-cell ontogeny. Owing to the unique geometry of the T-cell receptor α/δ loci, rearrangement of a V_α element to a J_α element invariably deletes the δ chain D, J and C genes on that allele. Therefore, V_α rearrangements can be considered as a mechanism for the elimination of δ chain expression. The expression of productive V_α rearrangements seems to be controlled in several ways at the levels of transcription and translation; the level at which allelic exclusion appears is unclear.

The generation of T-cell receptor diversity

The structure of T-cell receptor polypeptides is clearly homologous to that of immunoglobulins, and a similar process of **combinatorial rearrangement** contributes to the generation of diversity. Thus diversity of α variable regions is brought about not only by a relatively large number of V_α elements but also by an estimated 100 J_α elements with which they can rearrange. However, the relatively small number of V elements in δ and γ genes

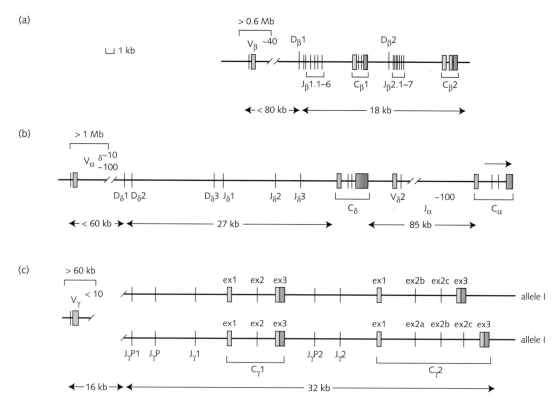

Fig. 10.7 Genomic organization of T-cell receptor D, J and C complexes in humans (drawn to scale). (a) T-cell receptor β chain locus. Each of the highly homologous C_β genes (encoded in four exons) is associated with a single D element and a number of closely linked J elements. An estimated 40 V_β genes are located within 0.6 Mb, with the most 3′ member less than 80 kb away from $D_\beta1$. All V_β genes so far analysed lie upstream of the DJC complexes. The transcriptional orientation of C_β genes is from left to right; that of V_β genes is presumed to be the same. (b) T-cell receptor α and γ chain locus. Two related C complexes are located in tandem with similar transcriptional orientation (arrow above exons). A single V_α element is known to be located 3′ of C_α and shows opposite transcriptional orientation. The J_α region is about 80 kb in length and contains an estimated 100 J_α segments. Three D_δ and three J_δ elements have so far been described. An estimated 100 V_α and 10 V_δ genes are located in a region of about 1 Mb upstream of $D_\delta1$; the distance between the first $V_{\alpha/\delta}$ and $D_\delta1$ is thought to be less than 60 kb. The transcriptional orientation of V elements is presumed to be similar to that of C regions. (c) T-cell receptor γ chain locus. The two haplotypes thus far described in humans are depicted. The $C_\gamma1$ gene has three associated J elements, the $C_\gamma2$ gene is preceeded by two J elements. In allele I, the $C_\gamma2$ gene occurs as a gene with a duplicated exon 2, whereas the $C_\gamma2$ gene in allele II carries a triplicated second exon. The V gene cluster is located less than 20 kb upstream of J_γP1.

limits the combinatorial diversity in heterodimers based on these V elements alone. In this context junctional diversity is of particular importance, and is greatly enhanced as compared with the immunoglobulin genes. The δ chain is the prime example for this phenomenon; only about 10 V, 3 D and 3 J elements suffice to generate about 10^{15} different δ chains, because of N-region diversification, usage of D elements in all three reading frames and flexibility in the 3′ joining position of V elements.

In contrast to immunoglobulin genes, somatic mutation does not occur in the T-cell receptor genes. This is probably because the T-cell receptor must preserve both the ability to recognize foreign antigen in the context of major histocompatibility molecules, and the ability not to react with self (see Chapter 11). Both of these abilities could be destroyed by random somatic mutation, rendering the T-cell either useless or dangerous (autoreactive).

Chromosomal abnormalities in lymphoid tumours

The presence of chromosomal abnormalities in lymphoid tumours has been established for many years. The fact that characteristic chromosomal changes occur **consistently** in specific tumour types suggests that the tumour phenotype is predisposed by the development of the chromosomal abnormality. These abnormalities can occur by mistakes in the normal process of antigen receptor chromosomal DNA rearrangement, resulting in attachment of part of a different chromosome (translocation), rather than the normal V-D-J joining or class switching which occurs within the same chromosome. When a chromosome translocation occurs, genes on the translocated chromosome near the abnormal junction are placed immediately downstream of a strong lymphocyte-specific promoter/enhancer and the active transcription initiation site for the antigen receptor. This alteration is critical for the formation of lymphoid tumours, and the affected genes on the translocated chromosome are therefore operationally defined as oncogenes. These oncogenes include previously known oncogenes (such as c-*myc* in **Burkitt's lymphoma**) and newly discovered ones (such as *Bcl-2* in **follicular lymphoma** and *rhombotin* in **T-cell acute lymphoblastic leukaemia**).

Chromosome abnormalities in B-cell tumours

Burkitt's lymphoma

Burkitt-type lymphoma (Plate 15, facing p. 214) is a B-cell tumour which is found in the malarial belt of Africa (endemic Burkitt's lymphoma, which is associated with infection by **Epstein–Barr virus**) and sporadically elsewhere. This tumour carries a chromosome translocation which involves the c-*myc* proto-oncogene at 8q24 and either the immunoglobulin heavy chain (about 90% of cases), κ light chain or λ chain genes (Fig. 10.8).

Most endemic Burkitt's lymphoma samples have chromosome 8q24 breakpoints far upstream of c-*myc*, whereas sporadic cases show breaks close to the 5′ end of c-*myc* or within the gene itself. There is also a difference in breakpoints at the immunoglobulin heavy chain locus. In endemic Burkitt's lymphoma the predominant site of breakage is within the J region, whereas switch region breakpoints are most frequently observed in sporadic cases. This difference probably reflects the stage at which B-cells are afflicted during their development. Endemic Burkitt's lymphoma is associated with Epstein–Barr virus, and occurs in cells which do not secrete IgM. Presumably, translocation occurs here during the process of V-D-J joining. **Sporadic Burkitt's lymphoma** is found in cells which are capable of IgM secretion. These are more mature cells undergoing the Ig heavy chain class switch (which occurs after V-D-J joining) during which translocation presumably takes place.

B-cell follicular lymphoma with translocation t(14;18)

B-cell follicular lymphoma is a common B-cell neoplasm in humans. A cytogenic hallmark of this disease is the presence of a translocation, t(14;18)(q32;q21). The chromosome 14 junction of this translocation is within the J segment cluster of the immunoglobulin heavy chain locus, and indeed is usually found at positions adjacent to the normal site of DNA rearrangement associated with V-D-J joining.

A gene, *Bcl-2*, has been identified close to be chromosome 18 junction of the translocation. The biological characteristics of the *Bcl-2* gene and the consequences of 'activation' of this gene in follicular lymphoma are particularly interesting. Recent work has shown that expression of *Bcl-2* blocks programmed cell death (apoptosis). Deregulated expression of *Bcl-2* in transgenic mice induces a polyclonal expansion of small resting B-cells which also have the property of prolonged survival. In addition, *Bcl-2* can co-operate with c-*myc* in doubly transgenic mice to produce hyper-proliferation of pre-B- and B-cells, with resulting tumour development.

Chromosome abnormalities in T-cell tumours

Transcription factors as oncogenes in chromosome translocations

The molecular analysis of chromosome translocations in acute T-cell leukaemias has provided consistent evidence that activation of transcription factors is implicated in the development of T-cell tumours. Several identified translocation oncogenes carry a protein motif called the basic helix-loop-helix motif (b-HLH). This motif is common to many transcription factors and mediates binding to DNA as well as protein–protein interaction (dimerization). Thus the *lyl-1* and *tal/SCL/TCL5* genes belong to a family of b-HLH genes and both have been found in translocations involving T-cell receptor genes in some cases of T-cell acute lymphoblastic leukaemia.

Another example is provided by a translocation found in lymphoid leukaemia that fuses the *E2A* gene encoding Ig enhancer binding proteins (which carry the b-HLH motif) with a transcribed gene designated *prl-1*. Sequence analysis of the *prl-1* gene product suggests that it has the capacity to bind DNA. The fusion gene created by this translocation is therefore most likely to a chimeric transcription factor in which the activation domain of *E2A* has been linked to a new DNA binding domain.

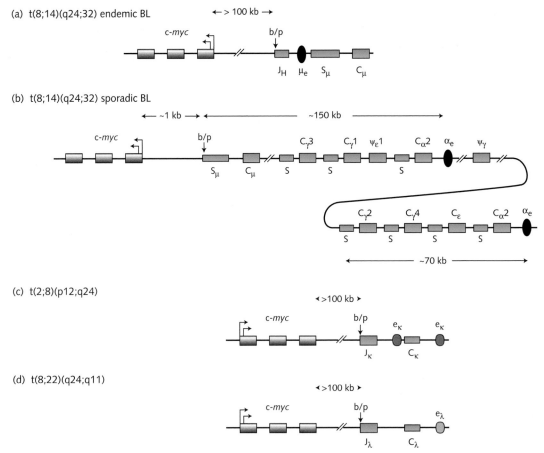

Fig. 10.8 Diagrammatic representation of chromosomal translocations found in Burkitt's lymphoma. The c-*myc* gene on the long arm of chromosome 8q is associated with translocations resulting from chromosome breaks either upstream (centromeric) or downstream (telomeric) to the gene itself. (a,b) Following a chromosome break upstream of c-*myc*, translocation of the distal end of chromosome 8q onto the Ig heavy chain locus at 14q32 leads to the long arm of chromosome 14 bearing c-*myc* and IgH sequence in opposite orientations. The exact position of the breakpoint (b/p) on chromosomes 8 and 14 differs between endemic and sporadic Burkitt's lymphoma. (c,d) Variants of Burkitt's lymphoma can involve either the κ light chain locus (translocation of the short arm of chromosome 2 onto the long arm of chromosome 8 telomeric to the c-*myc* gene (c)) or the λ chain locus (translocation of the long arm of chromosome 22 onto the long arm of chromosome 8 telomeric to the c-*myc* gene (d)). Both of these translocations result in an extended 8q in which the c-*myc* and Ig genes are in the same orientation. In both of these variants, the breakpoint is generally not immediately adjacent to c-*myc*, but rather in a region designated the pvt-like region at least 100 000 basepairs from the c-*myc* gene.

A new and different family of proto-oncogenes has been discovered with the detailed analysis of the *rhombotin* gene. This gene was first found at the site of a rare translocation in T-cell acute lymphoblastic leukaemia (Plate 16, facing p. 214) involving the T-cell receptor δ chain locus. The major normal site of expression of *rhombotin* is the brain, and this has reinforced the idea that genes important for differentiation can be important in tumour development when subverted by translocation. A second related oncogene, *rhom-2*, is also affected by translocations found in T-cell tumours. It has been postulated that proteins of this family may form complexes with each other and subsequently affect transcriptional activity.

The master gene mechanism of leukaemogenesis

Most oncogenes implicated in chromosomal translocations have rather limited potential for acting in the transformation process; they might be termed 'low grade' oncogenes compared with the 'high grade' oncogenes encoded by **retroviruses**. A common feature of these genes is their activity as transcription factors of one type or another, either acting by DNA binding (e.g. *lyl-1*) or protein interaction (e.g. as proposed for *rhombotin*). The genes can thus be regarded as '**master**' genes whose role is to influence the activity of a set of other genes. The effect of the chromosomal abnormality involving such master genes is clearly to increase the rate of subsequent mutations in other loci that contribute to the development of the tumour phenotype.

T-cell leukaemia: a paradigm for tumour development

The study of chromosomal abnormalities in human T-cell leukaemias has illustrated some of the general processes involved in tumour progression. The creation of the abnormal T-cell clone with a chromosomal translocation occurs as an early event before or after the cell has entered the thymus, in many cases due to aberrant activity of the VDJ recombinase. The contribution of this chromosome abnormality to the eventual phenotype of the tumour may only be slight, e.g. translocations involving genes such as the b-HLH genes may only subtly affect transcription equilibria. However, these changes provide a susceptible target cell in which further destabilizing genetic changes may subsequently occur. Since the chromosomal abnormalities are usually acquired early in thymic maturation of T-cells, it is possible for the T-cell receptor gene on the allelic chromosome to rearrange and produce a functional receptor. This allows pre-leukaemic T-cells to undergo the normal selection processes within the thymus. They can then form a pool of lymphocytes in the periphery that is responsive to different antigens but also remains a target in which mutations may subsequently occur. Thus the early acquisition of T-cell chromosomal abnormalities is followed by a long period during which clonal derivatives of the initial cell accumulate. Presumably the longevity of the initial translocation clone increases the opportunity for accumulation of successive mutations, which may eventually result in the emergence of the overtly malignant clone.

Further reading

Berek C. and Milstein C. (1987) Mutation drift and repertoire shift in the maturation of the immune response. *Immunology Reviews*, **96**, 23–41.

Davis M.M. and Bjorkman P.J. (1988) T-cell antigen receptor genes and T-cell recognition. *Nature*, **334**, 395–402.

Mossalagi M.D. and Debré P. (1994) Human early T-cell differentiation; 56th Forum in Immunology. *Research in Immunology*, **145**, 119–158.

Rabbitts T.H. and Boehm T. (1991) Structural and functional chimerism results from chromosomal translocation in lymphoid tumours. *Advances in Immunology*, **50**, 119–146.

Schatz D.G., Oettinger M.A. and Baltimore D. (1992) V(D)J recombination: molecular biology and regulation. *Annual Review of Immunology*, **10**, 359–383.

Strominger J.L. (1989) Developmental biology of T cell receptors. *Science*, **244**, 943.

Tonegawa S. (1983) Somatic generation of antibody diversity. *Nature*, **302**, 575–581.

Chapter 11 Human autoimmunity

Introduction

The fundamental specific recognition molecules of the immune system are the **antibody** molecule and the **T-cell receptor**. Autoimmunity implies the existence of antibodies and T-cells that are capable of recognizing elements of self, either directly in the case of antibody, or in the context of **major histocompatibility complex** (MHC) products in the case of the T-cell receptor. It is important to realize that such recognition need not necessarily lead to disease, and may indeed be physiological. Thus autoantibodies, albeit at low concentration, are found in all individuals and may play a vital role in the normal development of the antibody repertoire by a process of cross-reactive stimulation of other antibodies. It is also possible to isolate autoreactive T-cells from normal individuals, although the putative physiological role of such cells is even more speculative.

However, as usually understood, autoimmunity is equivalent to autoimmune disease, in which autoreactivity (by antibody and/or T-cell) produces tissue damage. This means that there has been a breakdown in the normal mechanisms of **tolerance**, whereby potentially autoreactive antibodies or T-cell receptors are either eliminated or controlled. This chapter will review what is known of the molecular mechanisms by which tolerance is imposed, and illustrate how these might be circumvented to produce autoimmune disease. This will be followed by a brief examination of the effector mechanisms that actually produce damage; these are not, of course, unique to the autoimmune response. Finally, a selection of the main human autoimmune diseases is reviewed from a molecular perspective.

Mechanisms of tolerance and the aetiology of autoimmunity

Because specific immunological recognition is performed by B-cells and T-cells it is these cells that must be rendered tolerant during normal development. Of the two, the T-cell compartment is probably by far the most important. In general, T-cell help is required to make a high-titre, high-affinity antibody response, and therefore without a helping autoreactive T-cell, autoreactive B-cells probably do little harm. In addition, the process of somatic mutation, so important during affinity maturation of the antibody response (see Chapter 10), must be constantly generating autoreactive B-cell clones; without T-cell help, these are not stimulated to further development. Consistent with this view is the lack of somatic mutation during T-cell development (which might generate autoreactive cells capable of causing damage without further help), and the fact that **autoantibodies** (e.g. rheumatoid factors) are readily found in normal individuals. However, there is no doubt that a degree of tolerance does occur within the B-cell compartment, and this is considered first.

B-cell tolerance

It has been known for some time that if the surface receptors (immunoglobulins) of B-cells are cross-linked at a certain critical stage of their development, then the cell is inactivated or deleted; which event occurs probably depends on the extent of cross-linking. This provides an obvious tolerizing mechanism as shown by the production of inactivated B-cells in an elegant experiment employing transgenic mice (Fig. 11.1). One strain is created that is transgenic for hen egg lysozyme (HEL), and which expresses this protein in the peripheral blood. A second strain is produced that is transgenic for the immunoglobulin genes that code for an anti-HEL antibody. As is characteristic of such transgenic animals, a high proportion of their antibody repertoire consists of the anti-HEL antibody. What happens when the two strains are crossed? The resulting hybrids still have a

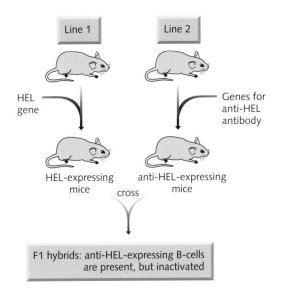

Fig. 11.1 B-cell tolerance. Hen egg lysozyme (HEL) is a useful antigen for study (see text).

large proportion of B-cells that express the transgenic antibody, but the cells have been inactivated.

It is probable that B-cell tolerance only occurs for self proteins above a certain concentration threshold. Below this threshold, a potentially damaging autoreactive response may be produced if the B-cells can be stimulated by a T-cell-independent mechanism. This might consist of polyclonal stimulation, as is found during infection by the Epstein–Barr virus. Alternatively, there might be neoplastic or paraneoplastic transformation within this compartment, resulting in a frankly malignant condition such as chronic lymphocytic leukaemia, or a relatively benign disease such as essential cryoglobulinaemia. All of these conditions may be associated with the production of clinically relevant autoantibodies.

T-cell tolerance

The thymus

For the reasons outlined above, tolerance within the T-cell compartment is of particular importance. Experimental work over the last few years has produced a much clearer picture of the events occuring during T-cell ontogeny within the thymus (Fig. 11.2). Two main processes are involved, both of which involve the interaction between T-cell receptor on the one hand and ill-defined self peptides bound to self major histocompatibility complex (MHC) molecules on the other. One

process involves the **positive selection** of T-cells whose T-cell receptor has an affinity for its ligand greater than a particular threshold. T-cells recognize antigen in the context of self MHC molecules, and therefore a certain affinity for self MHC is required for efficient recognition. On the other hand, too high an affinity for self MHC would lead to autoreactivity, and there is therefore a process of **negative selection** in which T-cells that have an affinity for their ligand greater than a particular threshold are eliminated. The order in which these steps occur, the mechanism(s) by which the programmed death (apoptosis) of non-selected cells is induced, and the nature of the self peptides involved (are these thymus specific?) remain uncertain, but the principal processes are clear.

These events within the thymus may explain much of the most important immunogenetic association of autoimmunity, namely that with the MHC. Many autoimmune diseases (and others of a questionable autoimmune nature such as narcolepsy) demonstrate associations with particular MHC alleles, and some of these are dealt with in greater depth later in the chapter. The usual form of association is between possession of a particular allele and increased predisposition to the development of disease. This can be understood in terms of the positive selective process: those T-cells selected because of a particular affinity for an MHC molecule are those capable of recognizing the relevant autoantigen involved in the pathogenesis of the autoimmune condition associated with that particular MHC gene. This

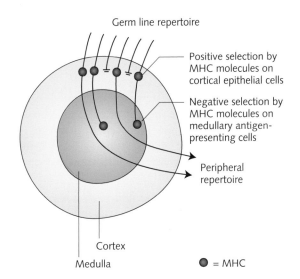

Fig. 11.2 Thymic T-cell tolerance.

explanation is not mutually inconsistent with the mechanism of determinant selection: the MHC molecule associated with the disease is able to bind and present the relevant autoantigen to the autoreactive T-cell, whereas other MHC molecules are less efficient at this.

A rarer form of association is between possession of a particular allele and relative protection from development of disease. The best example of this in humans is insulin-dependent diabetes mellitus, in which certain DQ alleles confer a strong protective influence (see below). The mechanism(s) involved in this type of association are much less clear, but the process of negative selection is one possibility: those T-cells eliminated because of affinity for a particular MHC molecule are those required to mount an autoimmune response.

The periphery

It is now clear that non-thymic or peripheral mechanisms are also important in the production and maintenance of T-cell tolerance. The need for such mechanisms is implied by the considerable potential for self-renewal possessed by the peripheral T-cell pool; individuals who have had a thymectomy, or in whom the thymus has atrophied, do not develop any obvious T-cell deficiencies. Experimentally, **peripheral tolerance** can be demonstrated using mice that express transgenic MHC molecules solely in the periphery; such mice are usually tolerant of the transgenic molecule (see p. 207). Other work has shown that presentation of the T-cell ligand (MHC molecule plus bound peptide) by a 'non-professional' antigen-presenting cell, or even a lipid membrane, will produce long-lasting non-responsiveness (**anergy**) in the relevant T-cell. The molecular mechanisms underlying the production of this anergic state are uncertain, but it presumably involves the failure to deliver a critical second signal, such as a particular lymphokine produced by professional antigen-presenting cells or activation via the CD28–B7 pathway. More generally, it has been suggested that any factors that decrease the strength of interaction between the T-cell and antigen-presenting cell, or that result in a reduction in concentration of responding T-cells below a critical threshold, will generate a tolerogenic as opposed to an immunogenic signal.

The active maintenance of tolerance

The mechanisms of tolerance outlined above are essentially passive in the sense that potentially autoreactive T-cells are eliminated or rendered unresponsive. It is,

however, possible to isolate autoreactive T-cells from apparently normal individuals; the lack of disease would seem to require some more active mechanism (such as **suppression**) for keeping these cells in check. This is a controversial area; the extent to which suppressive mechanisms contribute to the maintenance of self-tolerance, and whether a breakdown in such mechanisms can be a critical factor in the generation of autoimmunity, are unresolved issues. A defect in autoantigen-specific suppression has been found in a few autoimmune diseases, but there is doubt as to the significance of these findings. Nothing is known about the possible molecular mechanisms that might be employed by such putative suppressor cells.

The sequestration of autoantigens

The induction of tolerance, be it by passive or active means, is only necessary if an autoantigen is likely to interact with a T-cell receptor or an antibody molecule. For many self antigens, notably intracellular components, such interaction is most unlikely, and a state of tolerance does not need to exist. The consequences, of course, are that an autoimmune response may be induced if such intracellular components are released by tissue injury. A good example of this is lens-induced uveitis, in which release of lens material into the aqueous humour is followed by inflammation of the iris and ciliary body, probably mediated by a local Arthus reaction. It is easy to see how this mechanism could also be involved in the perpetuation, even if not the initiation, of a variety of autoimmune diseases.

There are two more recent variants on this idea of sequestration of potential autoantigens. As mentioned above, T-cells can only recognize antigens in the context of MHC molecules. Of the two principal classes of MHC molecules, class I molecules interact with CD8+, mainly cytotoxic, T-cells, whereas class II molecules interact with CD4+ helper/inducer T-cells. This latter subset of T-cells is of particular importance, as in general an effective immune (or autoimmune) response requires help from this subset. It may therefore be significant that although class I MHC molecules have a wide tissue distribution, class II molecule expression is normally confined to specialized antigen-presenting cells. As a result the CD4+ helper/inducer T-cell is effectively blind to other cell types. If upregulation of class II molecules is induced on such cells, perhaps by γ-interferon (IFN) produced as a result of a viral infection, then an autoimmune response may result. This concept is discussed further below in the context of insulin-dependent diabetes mellitus and autoimmune thyroid disease. However, it is worth noting here that although such aberrant expression of class II molecules certainly occurs, it is far from clear whether this is the cause of the autoimmune response, is simply an irrelevant effect of cytokines released during the inflammatory process, or even is a protective mechanism to provide a tolerogenic signal.

The other variant arises from a consideration of the normal role of the complement system in the handling of immune complexes. Such complexes are being generated constantly under normal circumstances, both in response to exogenous antigens (e.g. food antigens) and in response to self antigens released during normal cell turnover (remember that low concentrations of autoantibodies are normal). In the presence of a normal complement system, these complexes activate the classical pathway of complement which results in the attachment of C3 molecules. These complexes can then bind to the CR1 receptor on red blood cells and be carried to the liver for disposal (Fig. 11.3); as a result they are effectively sequestered, and do not provide a sustained stimulus to the immune system. If there is an abnormality of the complement system, either due to hereditary deficiency of one of the classical pathway components or perhaps an acquired defect, then this mechanism is disrupted. The complexes may then deposit in tissues where they can set up an inflammatory response; this leads to further release of autoantigens and perpetuation of the process (Fig. 11.3). It has been suggested that this mechanism is an important cause of systemic lupus erythematosus, which is strongly linked to certain complement component deficiencies.

Hyperacute rejection of xenografts is also mediated by the complement pathway and a possible solution to reducing at least hyperacute rejection is being addressed using transgenics. Attempts are in progress to generate transgenic pigs expressing the human complement regulatory proteins 'decay accelerating factor' (DAF) and 'membrane cofactor protein' (MCP) in the hope that transplantation of pig organs expressing these proteins will downregulate complement activation and increase the chances of graft survival.

The aetiology of autoimmunity

Some of the many ways in which a breakdown of tolerance can occur have been mentioned above. We will conclude this section with a brief mention of other mechanisms that may be involved.

The importance of T-cell tolerance has been stressed above. One way in which this might be circumvented is via **molecular mimicry**. In this situation, T-cell help may be supplied, but it is directed to foreign T-cell epitopes on a molecule that shares B-cell epitopes with self components. These T-cells, behaving correctly in responding to non-self antigens, can then provide help via the classical hapten-carrier mechanism to the linked autoreactive B-cell. A similar process could also provide help for autoreactive cytotoxic T-cells. There are now many examples of mimicry by pathogens of self antigens (see, for example, p. 221, ankylosing spondylitis).

There are undoubtedly many other factors involved in the aetiology of autoimmunity. These include variations in the target organ, the influence of sex, and ill-defined polygenic contributions to high and low immune responsiveness. Although there may be examples of autoimmunity that have a relatively 'pure' aetiology, this is likely in most cases to be multifactorial.

Effector mechanisms in the autoimmune response

These effector mechanisms, with the exception of certain autoantibodies that have an activating or stimulatory effect, are not unique to the autoimmune response, and are just the same as those used in the immune response to foreign antigens. This section will aim to provide a general overview; in some cases a more detailed exposi-

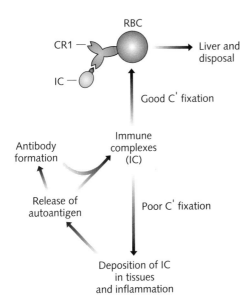

Fig. 11.3 Role of complement in disposal of immune complexes.

tion of particular mechanisms is provided below in the context of certain diseases.

Broadly speaking, effector mechanisms may be classified into specific and non-specific; this is not a rigid distinction, as in many cases the specific mechanisms subsequently engage non-specific processes. The specific effector mechanisms are those involving the specific recognition molecules of the immune system, namely antibody molecules and the T-cell receptor.

Antibody-mediated mechanisms

Antibodies, once bound to their target antigen, may trigger a variety of events. Some of these are (for practical purposes) confined to the response to exogenous antigens; examples would be the activation of mast cells by the cross-linking of surface IgE (for which mast cells have specific receptors), and the Arthus reaction which occurs under conditions of relative antibody excess. Two properties of particular relevance to the pathogenicity of autoantibodies are the activation of the complement system, and the ability to bind to Fc receptors on a variety of effector cells.

The complement system is a series of serum proteins activated by two main pathways (Fig. 11.4). The classical pathway may be initiated by a single bound molecule of IgM or two molecules of IgG bound in close proximity. The subsequent binding of C1q then leads to the formation of the classical pathway C3 convertase and the consequent activation of C3, the pivotal component of the complement system. The alternative pathway may

be activated directly by substances such as bacterial polypeptides, and can also serve as a feedback amplification loop for the classical pathway. Activation of further complement components leads to the assembly of the membrane attack complex, which produces transmembrane channels in the target cell and eventual death, although sublethal complement injury may be equally important, as this can lead to metabolic alterations and release of inflammatory mediators by attacked cells. Other biological activities of the complement system are opsonization and the generation of a variety of chemotactic and anaphylotoxic cleavage products.

Effector cells with receptors for the Fc portion of antibodies include polymorphonuclear leukocytes and macrophages. In addition to their phagocytic activity, these cells are capable of producing a variety of proteolytic enzymes and other potentially injurious compounds such as reactive oxygen species. Macrophages in particular also have significant procoagulant activity (see below).

Lastly, as mentioned above, a unique pathogenetic property of certain autoantibodies (i.e. not shared by antibodies to exogenous antigens) is their ability to stimulate receptors or activate other endogenous processes. The best example of the former is the stimulation of thyroid hormone release by autoantibodies to the thyroid-stimulating hormone (TSH) receptor in Graves' disease (p. 212). The activation of endogenous processes is exemplified by the activation of the alternative pathway of complement (see above) by the autoantibody nephritic factor (NeF). This antibody, found in certain types of renal disease (notably mesangiocapillary glomerulonephritis type II) and in partial lipodystrophy, binds to the alternative pathway C3 convertase (C3bBb) and prevents its inactivation. As a result the alternative pathway is permanently activated and hypocomplementaemia results. Of possible relevance to the connection between NeF and partial lipodystrophy is the recent fascinating observation that a serine protease produced by fat cells, adipsin, is probably identical to the complement component factor D, the key enzyme involved in the activation of the alternative pathway of complement. Despite this clue, it must be admitted that the pathogenetic connection (if any) between NeF and the associated diseases is obscure, but the molecular details of the interaction are well defined.

Cellular mechanisms

Both main classes of T-cells, CD4+ and CD8+, may serve as effector cells in an autoimmune response. CD8+ T-cells function mainly as **cytotoxic** cells. After specific

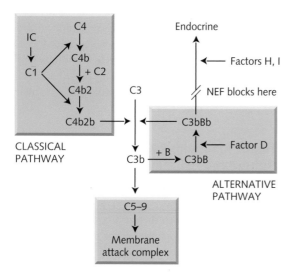

Fig. 11.4 The complement system.

recognition of their target antigen (**epitope**) in the context of an MHC class I molecule, and possibly with help from CD4+ T-cells, the cytotoxic T-cell delivers a lethal hit to the target cell. The precise mechanisms involved in this are uncertain, but the assembly of perforin molecules to form transmembrane channels with very similar appearances to those produced by the membrane attack complex of complement (see above), and with similar effects, may play a major role. CD4+ T-cells, as well as having an indirect role by providing help for cytotoxic T-cells, also produce a variety of cytokines themselves which, particularly via the recruitment of macrophages, participate in the production of tissue damage.

Non-specific mechanisms

Several of these have been mentioned above (e.g. complement, polymorphonuclear leukocytes) as their recruitment is in part responsible for the effects of more specific mechanisms. Involvement of the clotting system may be of particular importance in the mediation of certain forms of autoimmune glomerulonephritis. Certainly in some experimental systems the procoagulant activity of macrophages plays a major role, and in humans the defibrinating agent ancrod appears to improve the glomerulonephritis of systemic lupus erythematosus.

Products of arachidonic acid metabolism such as prostaglandins, thromboxanes and leukotrienes are important vasoactive and inflammatory mediators. These molecules are of particular interest, as the relative balance of pro- and anti-inflammatory species is susceptible to manipulations such as alterations in dietary lipids, as well as a variety of drugs. They thus provide attractive therapeutic targets.

The molecular biology of human autoimmune diseases

This section is not a comprehensive survey of human autoimmunity, but instead concentrates on those diseases that are of particular interest from the molecular viewpoint; it will be seen that work with animal models has contributed enormously to our understanding of the development of these disorders. The impact of recent techniques for the molecular analysis of autoimmunity has varied. For instance, attention has focused predominantly on autoantigen epitope mapping and T-cell receptor usage in models of multiple sclerosis and on immunogenetics in type 1 diabetes mellitus. Where there is sufficient material we have followed a common

pattern, dealing with autoantigens, immunogenetics and pathogenesis in turn.

Type 1 diabetes mellitus

Three main types of diabetes exist in the UK: type 1 (also known as juvenile-onset or insulin-dependent), type 2 (maturity-onset or non-insulin-dependent) and diabetes secondary to some other disorder (pancreatic disease or glucose counter-regulatory hormone excess). Only the type 1 form has an autoimmune aetiology, which is evident from the lymphocytic infiltrate in the islets of Langerhans (**insulitis**) and the occurrence of autoantibodies to β-cell autoantigens. Observations on spontaneously occurring diabetes in animals provide further proof for autoimmunity being the cause of β-cell destruction (Table 11.1).

Type 1 diabetes mellitus is an important disease, with an annual incidence of 15.6 cases per 100 000 of the population under 21 years in the UK. Presentation is usually due to the consequences of insulin deficiency, with hyperglycaemia leading to glycosuria, polyuria and thirst. There is often general tiredness and malaise. Occasionally the initial presentation is with severe ketoacidosis.

The mainstay of treatment is with insulin replacement. There is considerable current interest at present in two other broad strategies. First, the autoimmune nature of the disease suggests that immunosuppressive treatment might be appropriate. It is indeed possible to secure short-term remissions in newly diagnosed diabetics using agents such as cyclosporin A. The problem is that by the time of diagnosis so much of the β-cell mass in the pancreas has been destroyed that the potential for this strategy is limited. Current interest is therefore focused on transplanting functioning islet tissue. Some success has been achieved with whole pancreas allografts, but the

Table 11.1 Features of diabetes in the NOD mouse, BB rat and human.

	NOD mouse	BB rat	Type 1 diabetes
Hyperglycaemia	Yes	Yes	Yes
Weight loss	Yes	Yes	Yes
Polydipsia/polyuria	Yes	Yes	Yes
Ketoacidosis	Occasional	Common	Common
Insulitis	Yes*	Yes*	Yes
Islet cell antibodies	Yes*	Yes*	Yes*

* Known to precede the onset of diabetes.

future probably lies with isolated islet transplantation. Methods are being developed for protecting such islet preparations from rejection and promising initial results have been reported. The hope must be that this form of treatment will help protect from the devastating long-term complications of diabetes involving blood vessels, especially those supplying eyes, kidneys and nerves (Plates 17–19, facing p. 214).

Autoantigens

GLUTAMIC ACID DECARBOXYLASE

Most interest has centred on autoantibodies against a 64 kDa protein which are found in more than 80% of newly diagnosed diabetics. The presence of antibodies against this 64 kDa antigen in relatives of diabetic patients is a powerful predictor of subsequent diabetes, predating overt disease by several years. Similar antibodies are found in the NOD mouse and BB rat. Immunoprecipitation studies have shown that the 64 kDa antigen is present in the β-cells; elsewhere, a similar protein can only be detected in brain tissue. The observation led to identification of the 64 kDa protein as the enzyme glutamic acid decarboxylase (GAD), which synthesizes γ-aminobutyric acid from glutamic acid.

Autoantibodies against GAD had previously been identified in patients with a rare neurological disorder, the stiff-man syndrome, almost all of whom also have islet cell antibodies demonstrable by immunofluorescence. A significant proportion of these patients become diabetic. Complete cross-reactivity was observed between anti-GAD sera from these patients and anti-64 kDa sera from diabetics, GAD activity was precipitated by antibodies in diabetic sera, and similar properties of GAD in brain and β-cells were demonstrated, thus proving the identity of the 64 kDa antigen.

It seems likely that different GAD epitopes are recognized by the immune system in patients with the stiff-man syndrome and type 1 diabetes to account for the incomplete concordance between the two disorders. Other factors may contribute, including the need to breach the blood–brain barrier in autoimmune disorders affecting the central nervous system. GAD appears to be confined to the cytoplasm of β-cells, being localized particularly in synaptic-like microvesicles. As the antigen is not present on the surface of intact β-cells, autoantibodies against GAD probably have only a secondary role in pathogenesis. However, specific T-cells could initiate an autoimmune response by recognition of GAD peptides bound to MHC molecules, and such cells have been identified in the circulation of newly diagnosed diabetic patients, and in their relatives at risk of developing disease.

GAD antibodies have strong predictive value for the development of diabetes and, in combination with analysis of HLA genes (see below), may in the future identify individuals whose risk of diabetes warrants immunological intervention. This is important because the β-cell reserve is already too low at the time of presentation to allow recovery of normal glucose control, even if the autoimmune process could be reversed. Any attempts at successful treatment will need to be instituted early in the process, in individuals at risk.

OTHER ANTIGENS

Islet cytoplasmic and cell surface antibodies are found in about 75% of newly diagnosed diabetics. The antigens to which these bind are unknown but seem to be shared with other islet cell types besides the β-cell, making their pathogenic significance unclear. More recently two components of the insulin secretory granule, a 38 kDa protein and 52 kDa carboxypeptidase H, have been identified as T-cell autoantigens. Antibodies against insulin and, less commonly, the insulin receptor occur in type 1 diabetes, but are also associated with separate, rare autoimmune conditions. Insulin antibodies, which may be monoclonal, can result in a syndrome of spontaneous reactive hypoglycaemia and insulin receptor antibodies can produce the type B insulin resistance syndrome. Other β-cell antigens of uncertain significance exist. It is possible that this diversity of autoantigens is the result of 'spreading' of the immune response. The autoimmune process may be directed against a single autoantigen initially, but with chronic inflammation and β-cell damage within the islet, other autoantigens become targets for the autoimmune process.

Immunogenetics

GENETIC CONTRIBUTION

Monozygotic twins are only 20–30% concordant for diabetes. This contrasts with the still lower 10% concordance seen in dizygotic twins and in HLA-identical siblings. However, the risk of diabetes is at least fourfold greater in completely HLA-mismatched siblings of diabetic patients than in the general population, in which the prevalence is 0.2–0.4%. From these observations it is clear that type 1 diabetes is a polygenic disease, with some susceptibility conferred by genes within the MHC, some conferred by genes lying outside the MHC and some conferred by a separate environmental component. The impact of a non-genetic factor is emphasized by the recent increase in disease incidence in Europe.

Viruses and other infectious agents have long been thought to be involved in the aetiology, as discussed below. Another possible environmental trigger is cow's milk, resulting from cross-reactivity between bovine albumin and a 69 kDa β-cell autoantigen. On the other hand, recent evidence from NOD mice and BB rats suggests that particular viral and other infections may actually prevent diabetes: in germ-free conditions the prevalence of disease in these strains increases from 40–75% to almost 100%. Such effects are probably due to non-specific enhancement of weak immunoregulatory mechanisms, for instance by stimulating release of cytokines with inhibitory activity. Therefore, environmental factors may have both permissive and inhibitory effects, with disease being the result of the interplay between these effects and genetically-determined susceptibility.

MHC CLASS II GENES ASSOCIATED WITH TYPE I DIABETES

About 95% of Caucasian type 1 diabetics are HLA-DR3 and/or -DR4, compared with around 50% of healthy individuals. A weak positive association with HLA-DR1 also exists, whereas HLA-DR2 and -DR5 are under-represented in the diabetic population. There is a considerably greater risk of developing diabetes for DR3/4 heterozygotes than individuals with only one of these two alleles. However, analysis of families with two or more affected siblings demonstrated that the primary disease susceptibility loci are not these particular DR genes. Instead, there appear to be two separate loci in linkage disequilibrium with DR3 and DR4 which confer genetic predisposition (together with a contribution from non-MHC genes discussed below).

Further evidence that DR3 and DR4 are not the key loci came from the observation that only certain haplotypes bearing these alleles were associated with type 1 diabetes. Initial attempts to delineate the crucial genes in linkage disequilibrium with DR4 on these disease-related haplotypes used restriction fragment length polymorphism (RFLP) analysis. A *Bam*H1 restriction fragment of 3.7 kb, hybridizing with a DQB gene probe, was found in over 30% of controls but in less than 2% of diabetics. The difference persisted when only DR4-positive individuals were considered. Cloning this fragment revealed that the *Bam*H1 sites lie in the regions of the DQB1 gene encoding the first and second domains of DQ β chain.

DQB1 GENES INFLUENCE SUSCEPTIBILITY

More complex analysis of DQB1 gene RFLP patterns in DR4-positive individuals revealed two subsets, only one of which was associated with diabetes. Two major DQB1 loci in linkage disequilibrium with DR4 were identified corresponding to these RFLP subsets. These were originally termed DQw3.1 and DQw3.2 and are now known as DQB1*0301 and DQB1*0302. Only the latter is positively associated with diabetes whereas DQB1*0301 is almost never present in such patients.

Sequence analysis of the polymorphic DRB1 and DQA1 genes ruled out the existence of mutant class II alleles in diabetic patients. However, comparison of the DQB1 sequences in those haplotypes positively and negatively associated with diabetes revealed a striking difference in the codons for the amino acid at position 57 of the DQ β chain first domain. All of the alleles negatively associated with diabetes encode a negatively charged aspartate (Asp) residue at this position, whereas those that are positively associated encode the neutral residues alanine, serine or valine, which are relatively conservative substitutions (Table 11.2). Amplification of the DQB1 first domain sequence by the polymerase chain reaction (PCR) and hybridization with allele-specific oligonucleotide probes covering the region around position 57 confirmed these results. The amino acid residue at position 57 is situated in the antigen binding cleft of the assembled DQ molecule and the presence or absence of Asp-57 may be critical to the structure and function of the molecule, especially with regard to antigen presentation. One possible explanation for the protective effect of Asp-57 is that diabetogenic T-cells may be deleted in individuals with alleles encoding this type of DQ β chain. Alternatively, Asp-57-containing DQ molecules may act

Table 11.2 Amino acid substitutions in the DQ β chain correlate with susceptibility or resistance to type 1 diabetes.

HLA-DR type	HLA-DQ type*	Amino acid 57 on DQ β chain	Association†
1	w5	Valine	+
2 (w16)	w5	Serine	+
3	w2	Alanine	+
4	w8	Alanine	+
7	w2	Alanine	±
2 (w15)	w6	Aspartic acid	−
4	w7	Aspartic acid	−
5	w7	Aspartic acid	−
w6	w6	Aspartic acid	−

* HLA-DQ allele in linkage disequilibrium with DR.
† + = positive; − = negative; ± = neutral.

as restriction elements for suppressor T-cells capable of preventing diabetes.

INFLUENCE OF OTHER MHC GENES

Similar effects of substitutions at position 57 have been found in the homologues of the DQ β chain in NOD mice, BB rats and their related strains, but it is clear from these animal models that other MHC genes also influence susceptibility. For instance, failure to express I-E, the homologue of HLA-DR, is an important determinant of diabetes in NOD mice, and rat strains related to BB do not develop diabetes despite having a serine residue at position 57. The contrasting positive and neutral associations of DR3 and DR7 with diabetes in Caucasians, despite their sharing linkage disequilibrium with the same DQB1 allele (DQB1*0201), also indicates that DQB1 genes alone do not account for MHC-encoded susceptibility.

Trans-racial mapping has shown that the DQA1 locus is another important determinant of diabetic susceptibility (Fig. 11.5). In Jamaicans, a unique DR7 haplotype is positively associated with type 1 diabetes, in which the DQ α chain is encoded by the DQA1*A3 specificity (compared with A2 in Caucasians). A3 is also present on the DR8, DQw2 haplotype, again positively associated with diabetes in Jamaicans. This haplotype is very rare in Caucasians, accounting for the apparent lack of any association with diabetes. In the Japanese, the effect of DQA1*A3 is greater than any other MHC allele in predisposing to diabetes.

The DRB1 genes themselves may modify the risk generated by DQA1 and DQB1 alleles. In particular DR3-positive healthy individuals have immunological properties which could enhance autoimmune responses generally (Table 11.3). This non-specific effect would account for the association of HLA-DR3 with many other autoimmune disorders besides type 1 diabetes. It is also possible that DR3 is in linkage disequilibrium with other susceptibility genes telomeric to the D region. One candidate is the gene encoding tumour necrosis factor-α (TNF); as discussed below, TNF is believed to be an important cytokine in the pathogenesis of diabetes.

NON-MHC GENES AND TYPE 1 DIABETES

At least 13 genetic loci contribute to the development of diabetes in NOD mice and lie outside the MHC. One of these genes is essential to the initiation of insulitis, while a second acts with the MHC class II genes to exacerbate β-cell destruction, resulting in diabetes. Furthermore, an important determinant of diabetes in the BB rat is a non-MHC gene which is also responsible for producing lymphopenia. The exact location and function of these

Table 11.3 Immunological features in HLA-DR3-positive healthy subjects.

- Delayed Fc receptor-mediated clearance of immune complexes.
- Altered circulating lymphocyte subsets.
- Reduced degradation of endocytosed antigen by macrophages *in vitro*.
- Altered lymphocyte responses to mitogens *in vitro*.
- Decreased IL-1 production *in vitro*.

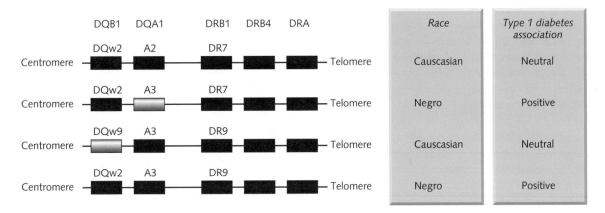

Fig. 11.5 Association of type 1 diabetes with *HLA* haplotypes depends on race. The upper figure shows that replacement of the DQA1 locus A2 allele with the A3 allele changes the association of DR7 with diabetes from neutral to positive. In the lower figure, changing the DQB1 locus DQw9 allele to DQw2 also alters the DR9 association (reproduced with permission from Todd (1990)).

mouse and rat genes are unknown but analogous genes almost certainly modify susceptibility in human diabetes. The genes encoding immunoglobulins, T-cell receptors and insulin have all been suggested as candidates, but no conclusive data have yet emerged although one incompletely characterized gene in the insulin-IGF2 region on chromosome 11p is clearly linked to diabetes susceptibility. The effects of maternal imprinting on this latter gene have been proposed to account for the increased risk of disease in the offspring of diabetic fathers compared with diabetic mothers, although some studies have found no effect of parental sex on the linkage of the insulin-region gene and diabetes. These interactions demonstrate how complex the effects of genetic susceptibility are in diabetes (and other autoimmune diseases).

Pathogenesis

VIRUSES AS AN ENVIRONMENTAL FACTOR

A protective effect of viruses and other mico-organisms has already been mentioned. Viruses could also initiate diabetes: (i) by altering β-cell structure or function; (ii) by molecular mimicry, if there is sequence homology between viral and β-cell epitopes; and (iii) by inducing a breakdown of tolerance as a result of these two processes. There have been many attempts to incriminate viruses as aetiological agents in diabetes but, apart from the strong association of type 1 diabetes with congenital rubella, there is little direct evidence in humans.

Nevertheless the potential for viral infections to induce diabetes has been strikingly demonstrated in transgenic mice expressing the haemagglutinin of influenza virus on their β-cells. Specific targeting was effected by using constructs containing the insulin enhancer and promoter fused to the cDNA encoding haemagglutinin. Diabetes developed in about a quarter of such animals and this was accompanied by the development of insulitis and autoantibodies against β-cell antigens, including GAD. Varying expression of haemagglutinin between and within individual animals may explain the relatively low prevalence of disease and differing ages of onset in such transgenic mice.

EXPRESSION OF MHC MOLECULES BY β-CELLS

The hallmark of type 1 diabetes is selective destruction of β-cells with sparing of the other cell types within the islets of Langerhans. Clearly a virus with exclusive tropism for the β-cell could initiate its singular destruction. A second possible mechanism capable of conferring appropriate specificity was suggested by the demonstration of MHC class II molecules on the surface of remaining β-cells in diabetic patients. Normally β-cells are class II negative but can be induced to express class II *in vitro* by culture with the cytokines TNF and γ-IFN, which are derived from activated macrophages and T-cells, respectively. This aberrant expression of class II could be sufficient to convert the β-cells into antigen-presenting cells, capable of stimulating autoreactive CD4+ T-cells by virtue of their surface class II molecules containing self peptides, including β-cell autoantigens.

However, other islet cells, secreting glucagon and somatostatin, express class II *in vitro* in response to TNF and γ-IFN, yet only insulin-containing islet cells appear to be class II-positive in diabetic islets. In diabetic BB rats such cells have in fact turned out to be macrophages, which constitutively express class II and ingest β-cell fragments to account for their staining with insulin antiserum. It is also doubtful whether the β-cells in diabetic NOD mice express class II. Together, these findings provide circumstantial evidence against class II expression being an initiating event in type 1 diabetes.

A direct approach to address the possible role of β-cell class II expression has been the creation of transgenic mice expressing MHC class II molecules on their β-cells, again targeted by using constructs containing the insulin promoter and enhancer. Such animals certainly developed diabetes but, surprisingly, this was not accompanied by insulitis. Moreover, the T-cells from these transgenic mice were tolerant of the transgenic class II molecule despite its lack of expression in the lymphoid system. Tolerance is not an inevitable consequence of β-cell class II expression in transgenic mice, but may arise in some lines because T-cells do not receive a necessary co-stimulatory signal for activation (Fig. 11.6). However, insulitis never develops, even in those transgenic lines in which there is no peripheral tolerization of T-cells. Class II expression by β-cells is therefore insufficient to induce an autoimmune response, because these cells lack a critical second signal with a co-stimulatory function which is present on 'professional' antigen-presenting cells such as dendritic cells.

Why do these animals develop diabetes? The answer is not yet clear but must accommodate the similar development of diabetes by a non-immune mechanism in transgenic mice hyperexpressing syngeneic class I MHC molecules on their β-cells. One possibility is that qualitatively or quantitatively inappropriate expression of class I or class II MHC molecules could interfere with important intracellular functions, leading to β-cell death. Whether similar, detrimental effects occur in human diabetes is unknown, although hyperexpression of class I

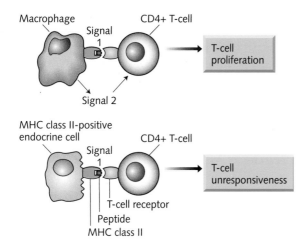

Fig. 11.6 Pathways of T-cell stimulation or tolerance. MHC class II-positive macrophages can present antigenic peptides to CD4+ T-cells because they can also supply an essential co-stimulatory second signal (upper). MHC class II-positive endocrine cells may be unable to deliver this second signal: in its absence, recognition of MHC class II-positive plus peptide by the T-cells induces a state of tolerance.

molecules by β-cells is a feature of this disease. The converse situation, of animals with insulitis but not diabetes, has been found in mice whose β-cells express a TNF transgene. This mirrors the clinical observations of insulitis without diabetes in some individuals and shows that several steps are required to accrue sufficient β-cell damage for diabetes to occur.

EFFECTOR MECHANISMS IN β-CELL DESTRUCTION
There is good evidence that cytotoxic T-cells and macrophages destroy β-cells in NOD mice and BB rats; antibodies against β-cells may only have a pathogenic role in the later phases of disease. Cytokines may also affect β-cell function and viability. Certainly TNF, γ-IFN and interleukin-1 (IL-1) can be shown to reduce β-cell insulin content and release and to induce ultrastructural degenerative changes *in vitro*. These effects are particularly impressive with IL-1, but there is disagreement over the β-cell specificity of its action. Cytokines induce nitric oxide and oxygen radical formation and β cells may be particularly sensitive to the toxic effects of such metabolites. Both diabetes and insulitis develop in transgenic mice whose β-cells produce γ-IFN, although the exact pathogenic mechanisms involved are unknown. It is unclear how this model and the TNF transgenic animals mentioned above relate to human diabetes, in which such cytokines will only be synthesized by infiltrating mononuclear cells.

Summary

Type 1 diabetes mellitus is a paradigm for the impact of molecular biology on the investigation of autoimmunity. Within a very short time, the structure of a major antigen has been determined, a comprehensive immunogenetic analysis has been undertaken and major advances in understanding the pathogenesis have been made. It is now clear that genes in the HLA-DQ subregion have an important role in determining susceptibility or resistance to diabetes, although there is a hierarchy for these effects which depends on the whole MHC haplotype, in turn implicating other loci in modifying disease expression. The additional role of non-MHC genes is currently being analysed. Experiments with transgenic mice have suggested previously unsuspected pathogenic mechanisms, compatible with epidemiological and histological data demonstrating heterogeneity within the syndrome currently termed type 1 diabetes mellitus.

Thyroid autoimmunity

Hashimoto's thyroiditis, primary myxoedema and Graves' disease affect around 2% of women, with men having a 10-fold decrease in frequency of disease (Fig.

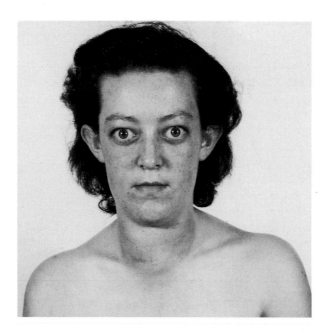

Fig. 11.7 A patient with Graves' disease. This patient has an enlarged thyroid (goitre) despite a previous thyroidectomy as shown by the neck scar. She also has the eye signs (thyroid-associated ophthalmopathy) found in 30–50% of patients with Graves' disease.

11.7). These are the prototypes of organ-specific autoimmune disease in humans. Patients with Hashimoto's thyroiditis present with a goitre or hypothyroidism; goitre is absent in primary myxoedema and these patients are recognized by hypothyroid features. Graves' disease causes hyperthyroidism and usually a goitre and around half the patients will have the eye signs of Graves' ophthalmopathy. It is also associated with skin infiltration: pretibial myxoedema (Plate 20, facing p. 214).

The same thyroid antigens are targets for the response in all three conditions, but with qualitative and quantitative differences. In Graves' disease the key feature is the presence of thyroid-stimulating antibodies (TSAb) which activate thyroid cells and result in hyperthyroidism (Plate 21, facing p. 214). By contrast, Hashimoto's thyroiditis and primary myxoedema produce hypothyroidism as a result of humoral and cell-mediated destruction of thyroid cells (Plate 22, facing p. 214). Antibodies blocking activation of the TSH receptor also contribute.

Autoantigens

THYROGLOBULIN

This is a large homodimeric glycoprotein (molecular weight 660 kDa) whose amino acid sequence is characterized by a pattern of imperfect repeats derived from three cysteine-rich motifs. Thyroglobulin (TG) acts as a prohormone. Tyrosine residues on the molecule are iodinated and coupled by the enzyme thyroid peroxidase, located at the apical surface of the thyroid cell, to form thyroxine and triiodothyronine, as well as mono- and di-iodotyrosines. TG is then stored in the follicular colloid; thyroid hormone secretion depends on endocytosis and lysosomal hydrolysis of TG, as freshly formed thyroid hormones are not released directly from the thyroid cell. This tortuous method of secretion presumably evolved to conserve iodine, which is a scarce element in many parts of the world.

Autoantibodies against TG in humans are usually polyclonal and predominantly recognize only two major and one minor epitope. Because these epitopes are widely spaced on this large molecule, no cross-linking of IgG molecules is possible when autoantibodies bind, and so TG antibodies do not fix complement. This may limit their pathogenic role. There is a significant sequence homology between TG and acetylcholinesterase, including similar hydropathy profiles and conserved disulphide bonds. Because acetylcholinesterase is found in muscle, immunological cross-reactivity between this molecule and TG could explain the association of ophthalmopathy with Graves' thyroid disease.

THYROID PEROXIDASE

This is the haem-containing enzyme central to thyroid hormone synthesis. The gene for thyroid peroxidase (TPO) gives rise to two co-existing proteins by alternate splicing. TPO is located mainly at the apical microvillar border of the thyroid cell. Antibodies present in patients with thyroid autoimmunity react with a microsomal fraction of thyroid cells and also bind to a surface antigen at this microvillar site. The identification of this microsomal antigen as TPO was achieved by immunoprecipitation and immunoblotting studies.

Autoantibodies against TPO are polyclonal and react with at least six epitopes. One is the catalytic site for peroxidation and antibodies against it may inhibit enzyme function, thus contributing to hypothyroidism. Another epitope may be shared with TG, which could explain the frequent concurrence of these two autoantibodies. However, the distinctive feature of TPO antibodies, compared with those against TG, is complement fixation, indicating an important pathogenic role. There is no single immunodominant T-cell epitope in TPO.

TSH RECEPTOR

The structure of the TSH receptor eluded discovery until recently because of the low abundance of this molecule (about 2000 receptors per thyroid cell). The activated TSH receptor stimulates adenylate cyclase via the G protein, G_s, and there is sequence similarity in all known G protein-coupled receptors. Therefore, to obtain the TSH receptor sequence, degenerate oligonucleotide primers corresponding to conserved sequences for transmembrane regions of known receptors were used in a PCR to amplify and clone new G protein-coupled receptors from genomic DNA. One such clone hybridized with a thyroid cDNA clone. This turned out to contain the TSH receptor sequence.

The primary structure reveals all the features of G protein-coupled glycoprotein hormone receptors: a large extracellular amino-terminal domain (398 residues in humans) with five glycosylation sites and a carboxy-terminal domain (346 residues) with seven transmembrane regions. Alternative splicing gives rise to two separate forms of the receptor. Glycosylation is important for high-affinity TSH binding. Different regions of the receptor are binding sites for TSH, TSAb and TSH receptor-blocking antibodies. X-ray crystallography will be required to determine the exact nature of these binding sites.

There is accumulating evidence that TSAb have a pauciclonal or even monoclonal origin, unlike antibodies against TG and TPO. The majority of TSAb are λ light chain restricted, all are of the IgG_1 subclass and isoelectric focusing shows that activity is confined to one or two fractions of separated sera. Sequencing of the appropriate immunoglobulin V region genes will be required to reveal the exact degree of restriction involved and how TSAb differ in their effects on the receptor from TSH receptor antibodies which block TSH. Clonal restriction of TSAb may have therapeutic implications: if sharing of TSAb V region sequences occurs in Graves' disease patients then anti-idiotypic antibodies could be developed to control production of the pathogenic idiotypes. Finally, there is some evidence that the extracellular domain of the TSH receptor is present in the extraocular muscles which are the key site for the autoimmune process causing ophthalmopathy. This is, therefore, another antigen which could cause cross-reactivity and account for the association between the thyroid and eye disease.

Immunogenetics

HLA ASSOCIATIONS

As in diabetes, there is greater concordance for Graves' disease in monozygotic than in dizygotic twins (30–50% versus 10%). Graves' disease is associated with HLA-DR3 in Caucasians but the relative risk is only moderate (around 3.0). Apart from DQw2, which is in linkage disequilibrium with DR3, no other DR, DQ or DP alleles appear to confer any additional susceptibility. It is possible that the association with DR3 simply reflects a non-specific immunological effect, present in all such individuals (Table 11.3). Primary myxoedema is also associated with HLA-DR3, with a similar relative risk to that in Graves' disease. There is no consensus regarding Hashimoto's thyroiditis; DR3, DR4 and DR5 have all been associated with this disorder in Caucasians. Recent studies in the UK suggest that the only association is with DR3. Whether the previously described DR4 and DR5 associations reflect ethnic or temporal differences in susceptibility is unclear.

NON-MHC GENES

The concordance for Graves' disease in HLA-identical siblings is 7%, at least seven-fold higher than the random population prevalence of this disorder and confirming an important effect of HLA loci on susceptibility. However this figure is much less than the concordance seen in monozygotic twins. Thus, non-MHC genes must play a role in Graves' disease and, from similar kinds of studies, in autoimmune hypothyroidism.

At least three loci determine susceptibility in an animal model of spontaneous autoimmune thyroiditis, occur-

ring in the obese strain of chicken. Only one of these lies in the MHC; another has an effect on T-cell regulation and the third results in a variety of thyroid abnormalities which presumably render the gland prone to autoimmune destruction. There is no evidence as yet for a genetically determined thyroid abnormality in patients with autoimmune thyroiditis.

Pathogenesis

ENVIRONMENTAL FACTORS

The incomplete concordance in monozygotic twins suggests that endogenous and environmental factors in part determine susceptibility to thyroid autoimmunity. Female sex hormones cause the increased prevalence of thyroid disease in women and fluctuations in endocrine function during and after pregnancy may be responsible for the exacerbation of thyroiditis postpartum. A role for infection is suggested by the failure of experimental thyroiditis to develop in susceptible strains of rat raised in specific pathogen-free conditions. Transfer of gut microflora from normal animals reverses this protective effect. There is much less evidence for a role of infection in human disease, although Graves' disease has been associated with previous *Yersinia* infections. This organism contains a protein capable of binding TSH-mimicking the TSH receptor, and this could trigger formation of TSH receptor antibodies. Finally, a high iodide intake leads to intrathyroidal synthesis of heavily iodinated TG molecules. These have increased immunogenicity compared with poorly iodinated TG in experimental models of thyroiditis. There are epidemiological data to support an aetiological role for increasing iodide intake in human thyroid autoimmunity.

MHC CLASS II MOLECULE EXPRESSION BY THYROID CELLS

The thyroid is a major site for the autoimmune response in Graves' disease and Hashimoto's thyroiditis and there are several reasons for this. Thyroid cells in both conditions unequivocally express class II molecules, a phenomenon which can be reproduced *in vitro* by culture with γ-IFN. This could convert thyroid cells into autoantigen-presenting cells, as discussed above with regard to β-cells, leading to localization of autoreactive T-cells in the gland. Normal thyroid cells are equally susceptible to the class II-inducing effects of this cytokine. Immunohistochemical analysis of gland sections from patients with thyroid autoimmunity reveals that class II expression is confined to follicles adjacent to areas of lymphocytic infiltration, and sequential studies in

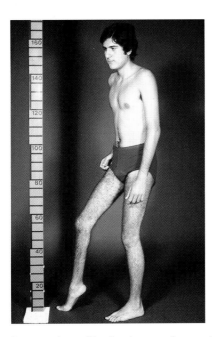

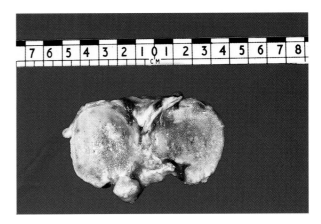

Plate 2 Tibial condyles removed at operation for total knee replacement. Note granular dull surface due to loss of cartilage.

Plate 1 Deformities due to bleeding in severe haemophilia A. The patient who grew up with little treatment for bleeding has fixed flexion due to ankylosis of his right elbow, and right knee. He also has talipes due to ischaemic necrosis of his right calf muscles consequent on bleeding within the muscle compartment.

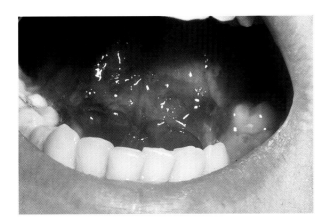

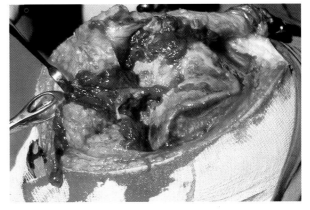

Plate 3 Dangerous sublingual bleeding, which spread to the tissues around the larynx with compression threatening the patient's breathing.

Plate 4 Knee joint opened to remove extensive synovial overgrowth, a consequence of repeated bleeding in the joint.

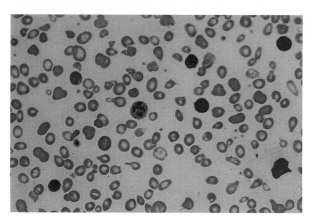

Plate 5 Homozygous β-thalassaemia. Blood film from patient with homozygous β-thalassaemia. This disorder is caused by defective β-globin chain synthesis leading to defective haemoglobinization of red cells and their precursors as well as premature destruction of abnormal young red cells caused by precipitation of excess α-globin chains with oxidation injury caused by increased free haem pigments. The consequent anaemia provides further erythropoietin-stimulated red cell formation with expansion of the marrow cavity and the ejection of immature red-cell forms into the bloodstream. The film shows marked variation in the size and shape of red cells many of which show poor pigmentation associated with defective haemoglobin synthesis. The blue unnucleated cells show polychromasia related to their high content of residual mRNA. Apart from the normal polymorphonuclear leukocyte in the centre of the film, several immature nucleated red-cell precursors (later normoblasts) are present on the film. Note also the bizarre structure of many of the red cells.

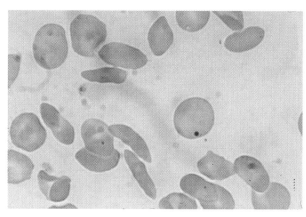

Plate 6 Sickle cell anaemia. Blood film shows characteristic irreversibly deformed red cells due to the formation of haemoglobin aggregates under conditions of deoxygenation. The large cell just to the right of the middle of the blood film is an immature erythrocyte containing residual nucleic acid (Howell–Jolly body) caused by failure of the spleen to remove this material. As a result of recurrent episodes of red cell sludging within the tiny blood spaces of the spleen in sickle cell anaemia, the organ shrinks and patients are at increased risk from bacterial infection as a result. Recurrent infarction episodes due to sludging of red cells causes skeletal pain and deformity due to death of bone tissue and similar episodes of lung infarction—sometimes associated with chest infections.

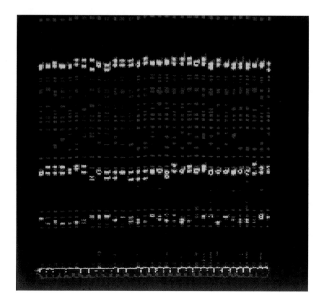

Plate 7 Multiplex fluorescent VNTR analysis of the genome. Figure shows multiple polymerase chain reaction (PCR) amplification products after priming with fluorescent dye-labelled oligonucleotides. The products have been illuminated after electrophoretic separation in an agarose gel. Automated procedures based on detection of these labelled products enable allele sizes of PCR products from genomic DNA templates to be analysed in a single track.

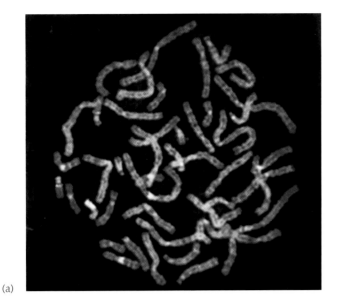

(a)

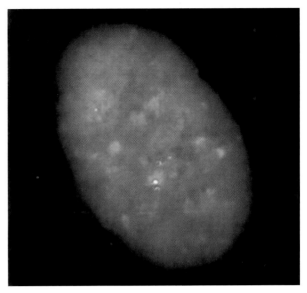

(b)

Plate 8 Fluorescent *in situ* hybridization (FISH) of sequences from human chromosome 22 to either metaphase (a) or interphase (b) chromatin.
(a) Hybridization of two cosmid clones from chromosome 22 to a metaphase spread. Chromsomes are counterstained to produce a banded appearance that allows unambiguous assignment of individual chromosomal subregions. Hybridizing clones are labelled with different fluorochromes, red or green. The relative position of red and green signals is determined for a series of similar spreads and order can be resolved for clones separated by

more than 1000–2000 kb on the chromosome. Clearly, these two sequences are very close together.
(b) Hybridization of three clones derived from chromosome 22 to an interphase nucleus. Clones are labelled either red, green or a mixture of red and green (orange) and span a distance of 2000 kb. The chromosomes in a non-dividing nucleus are less compact than they are in metaphase and so clones separated by as little as 50 kb can be resolved. (Photographs courtesy of Margaret Leversha, The Sanger Centre, Hinxton Hall, Cambridge.)

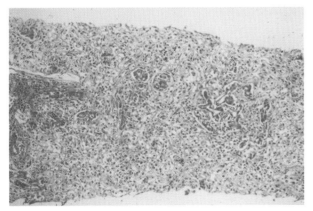

(a)

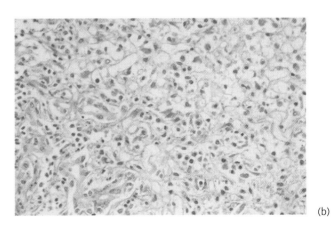

(b)

Plate 9 Pathohistological examination of liver cells in a patient with hereditary fructose intolerance (HFI). Note the absence of surviving liver cells with necrotic collapse of the tissue containing bile ducts and Kupffer cells. (a) ×50; (b) ×200.

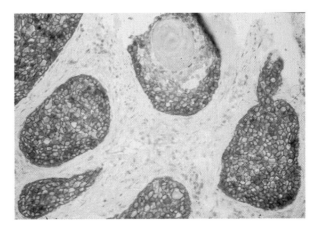

Plate 10 Epidermal growth factor receptor overexpression in head and neck cancer. Epidermal growth factor receptor genes are often amplified in tumours of the head and neck region. This example is from a 64-year-old man with oropharyngeal tumour with lymph node involvement. (Courtesy of William Gullick.)

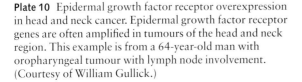

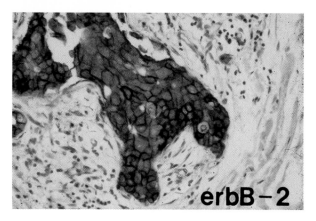

Plate 11 c-*erb*-B2 in breast cancer. The expression of an oncogene product of c-*erb*-B2 in breast cancer. An immunoperoxidase stain showing abundant expression of this tyrosine kinase cell surface receptor. Overexpression carries an adverse prognosis. (Courtesy of William Gullick.)

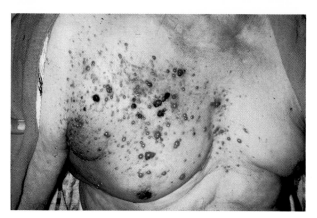

Plate 12 Nodular recurrent c-*erb*-B2 positive breast cancer. Direct injection of virus or plasmid into such nodules can result in localized drug activation.

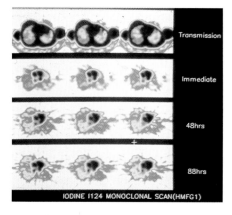

Plate 13 Monoclonal antibody targeting. A monoclonal antibody which reacts with a surface antigen on breast cancer cells has been labelled with iodine-124 and injected intravenously. Eighty eight hours after injection, the antibody, detected by scanning the patient, can be seen accumulating in the primary breast tumour—to the upper left of the transverse sections. (Courtesy of Agamemnon Epenetos.)

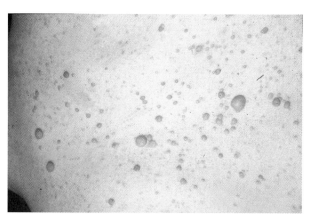

Plate 14 Neurofibromas of the skin on the back of a patient with NF1.

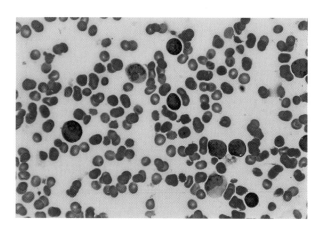

Plate 15 Burkitt's lymphoma. The bone marrow aspirate obtained from a young white man indigenous to Europe. He had presented with anaemia, nosebleeds and general malaise over the last few months and was noted to have splenic enlargement and small haemorrhages (purpura) in the skin. The marrow smear shows many abnormal B lymphocytes with a high nuclear to cytoplasmic ratio and strikingly basophilic (purple–blue staining) cytoplasm showing vacuolation. Cytogenetic studies confirm the typical presence of the chromosome 8 : 22 translocation characteristic of Burkitt's lymphoma. The patient made a good response to cytotoxic chemotherapy and returned to work as a hospital porter. (Courtesy of Drs A. Green and S. John, Department of Haematology, Addenbrooke's Hospital, Cambridge.)

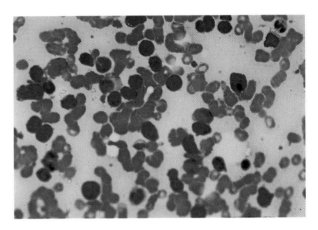

Plate 16 T-cell acute lymphoblastic leukaemia. Bone marrow aspirate obtained from 45-year-old woman presenting with a short history of recurrent infection, nosebleeds, conjunctival haemorrhage and skin bruising with pallor. Blood count determination showed marked pancytopenia (reduction in the counts of all formed elements of the blood). The aspirate shows multiple lymphoblasts showing characteristically clefted nuclei. Although the patient improved on treatment with combination chemotherapy, the prognosis for adult T-cell acute lymphoblastic leukaemia is not as favourable as for the childhood forms, where a cure rate in excess of 80% is now to be expected.

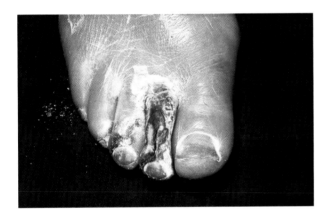

Plate 17 Diabetic gangrene.

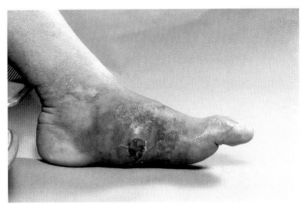

Plate 18 Charcot deformity with ulceration in diabetes.

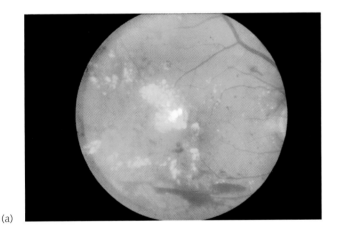

(a)

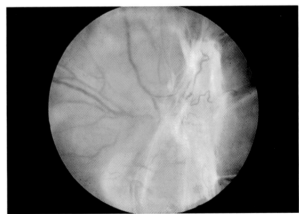

(b)

Plate 19 (a,b) Diabetic retinopathy showing consequences of microvascular disease in the eye. Note the exudates, vessel proliferation and haemorrhages.

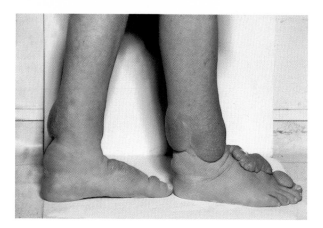

Plate 20 Pretibial myxoedema.

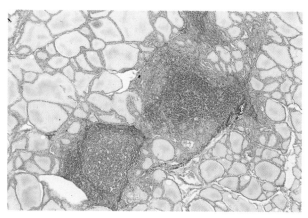

Plate 21 Graves' disease showing lymphoid follicles in the centre of the picture surrounded by stimulated thyroid follicles full of colloid. This patient had been treated with antithyroid drugs prior to thyroidectomy (original magnification ×100).

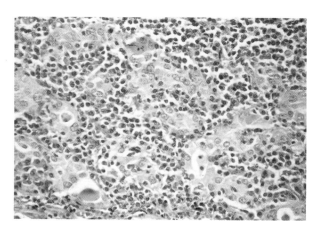

Plate 22 Hashimoto's thyroiditis showing a widespread lymphocytic infiltration in the thyroid and thyroid follicular destruction (original magnification ×400).

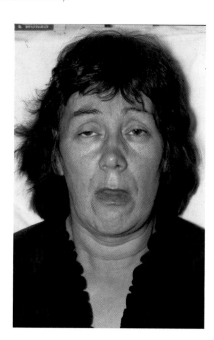

Plate 23 Myasthenia gravis.

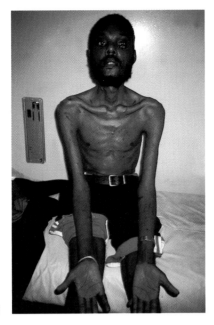

(a)

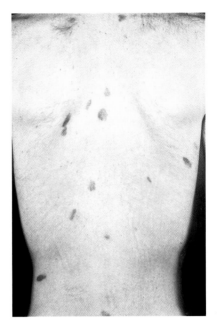

(b)

Plate 24 (a,b) Kaposi's sarcoma (KS) in an East African man with HIV infection (visible as multiple pigmented skin tumours). KS is commonly seen in immunosuppressed subjects and is a tumour derived from cells which normally form blood vessels. Although it has long been suspected to have a viral cause, no virus could be identified in the tumour by conventional techniques. However, using the technique of representational difference analysis (which uses PCR to selectively amplify small amounts of foreign DNA present in diseased, but not in normal, tissue), sequences of a novel human herpesvirus have recently been identified in all cells of KS lesions. It is hypothesized that this new virus may somehow cause KS after it is no longer controlled by the immune response—but the mechanism is as yet unknown.

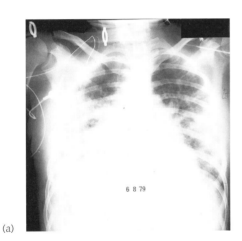

(a)

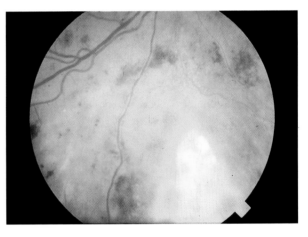

(b)

Plate 25 Cytomegalovirus (CMV) disease and immunosuppression. Cytomegalovirus pneumonitis in a bone marrow transplant recipient (a) and retinitis in a patient with advanced HIV infection (b). Human cytomegalovirus is carried by more than half the adult population, in whom it persists for life without causing disease. However, if subjects have their cellular immune system suppressed (for instance by drugs if they have had an organ transplant, or by HIV infection), primary infection with CMV, or reactivation of CMV they already carry, can produce disease in many organs including the lung and eye as shown. Normal virus carriers have in their blood a high frequency of cytotoxic T lymphocytes capable of killing CMV infected cells: it is believed that it is the loss of this response when immunosuppressed which leads to uncontrolled virus infection and disease.

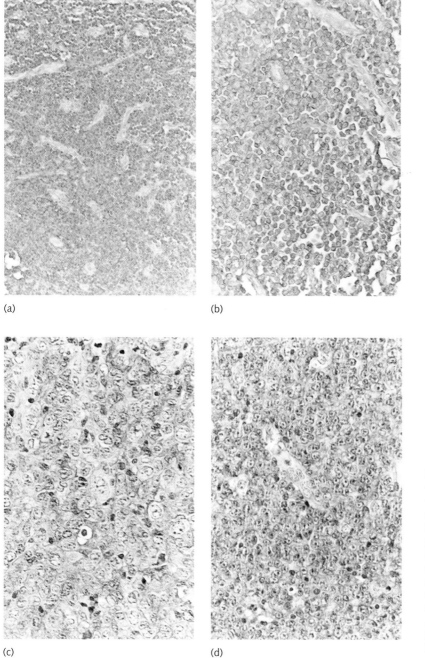

(a)

(b)

(c)

(d)

Plate 26 Paraffin wax sections stained with CAMPATH-1G. (a) Low power view of B lymphocytic lymphoma showing staining of the neoplastic cells. Small vessels are unstained. (b) High power view of B-cell lymphocytic lymphoma. (c) Large cell anaplastic cells showing membrane staining. (d) Adult T-cell leukaemia/lymphoma cells showing staining. The cells of small vessels are unstained. Avidin–biotin complex immunoperoxidase technique with haematoxylin counterstain was used for all sections.

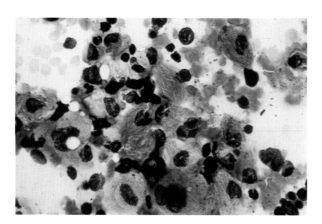

Plate 27 Gaucher's disease. The large cells with blue crinkled cytoplasm are the macrophages characteristic of this lysosomal storage disease, shown here in a stained bone marrow smear.

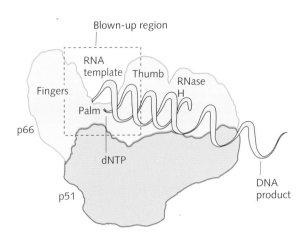

(a)

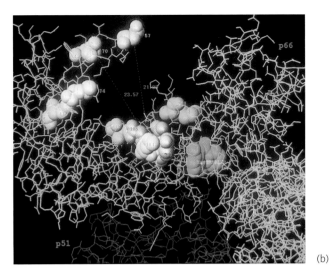

(b)

Plate 28 Crystal structure of HIV reverse transcriptase. (a) This illustrates the general architecture of the molecule which is composed of two subunits p66 and p51 (p51 is an amino-terminal fragment derived from p66). Although p51 contains a subset of the sequence of p66 it adopts a distinct conformation. The active sites are on the p66 subunit which contains two activities: DNA polymerase (which can work off an RNA or DNA template) and RNase H (which destroys an RNA template once it has been used). The template/primer complex lies in a deep cleft enclosed by the 'fingers' and 'thumb', and the active site is in the floor of the cleft: the palm. (Adapted from Kohlstaedt, *Science* 1992.) (b) Detailed picture of the active site of the enzyme determined by X-ray crystallography. A non-nucleoside, green nevirapine, can be seen occupying a hydrophobic pocket under the active site of the enzyme. Also shown are the active site residues 183 and 185 (purple) and a number of residues which have been implicated in resistance to nucleoside analogue inhibitors (residues 41, 67, 70, 215 and 219—resistance to AZT; residue 74—resistance to ddI; residue 184—resistance to 3TC. All shown in yellow). Also indicated is the surprising distance in Ångstroms between residues involved in residance (67 and 70) and the active site. (Courtesy of Dr David Stuart, Oxford University.)

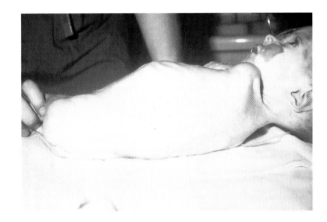

Plate 29 Severe combined immunodeficiency such as occurs in adenosine deaminase deficiency. Children present with recurrent viral, fungal and bacterial infections leading to wasting, diarrhoea and failure to thrive.

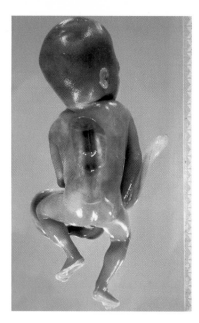

Plate 30 Fetus after termination of pregnancy showing a large thoracolumbar spina bifida (neural tube defect).

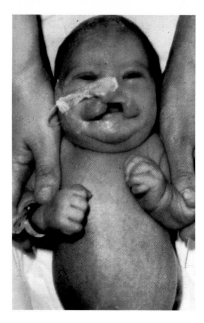

Plate 31 A neonate with Trisomy 13 (Patau's syndrome) showing the typical features of this chromosome disorder, e.g. severe midline facial cleft, microcephaly, polydactyly. (With kind permission from Dr Lynn Chitty.)

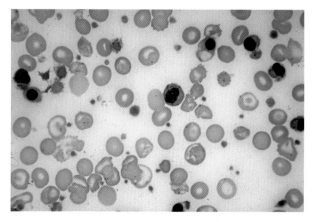

(a)

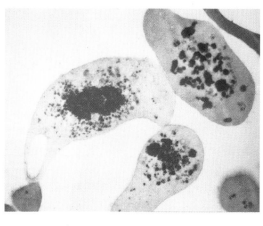

(b)

Plate 32 (a) Blood film from a patient with thalassaemia major showing microcytic, hypochromic red cells and nucleated red cells. (b) Transmission electron micrograph of red cells in thalassaemia major, showing precipitation and unpaired α chains. (With kind permission from Professor Bernadette Modell.)

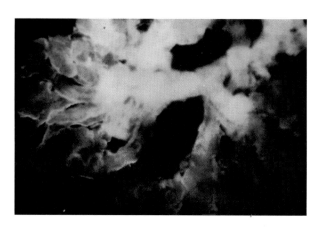

Plate 33 A biopsy of chorionic villi obtained from the placenta by transcervical biopsy forceps. The specimen is clean and shows healthy villi with capillaries and trophoblastic buds.

animals with experimental autoimmune thyroiditis prove that the infiltrate precedes the appearance of class II on thyroid cells.

These facts show that antigen presentation by class II-positive thyroid cells is not an initiating event in autoimmune thyroiditis, although it is possible that, once induced, this aberrant class II expression could amplify and thus perpetuate the response of autoreactive T-cells. However, class II-positive thyroid cells are only weakly able to present antigen to T-cells *in vitro*, and it is difficult to be sure that even these modest responses are not due to contamination by 'professional' antigen-presenting cells, such as macrophages and dendritic cells. At present, there is no firm evidence that thyroid cells can provide a necessary co-stimulatory signal to T-cells (Fig. 11.6). Without this signal, it is possible that aberrant class II expression may in fact result in peripheral tolerization of T-cells which have escaped central (thymic) tolerance in ontogeny.

THE ROLE OF OTHER MOLECULES EXPRESSED BY THYROID CELLS

Thyroid cells in autoimmune glands also express an important mediator of T-cell adhesion, intercellular adhesion molecule-1 (ICAM-1). This is normally confined to cells of the lymphoid system, and binding of lymphocyte function-associated antigen-1 (LFA-1) to ICAM-1 is an important initial step in antigen presentation and in the recognition of target cells by cytotoxic T- and natural killer (NK) cells. A variety of cytokines, including γ-IFN, TNF and IL-1, induce ICAM-1 expression on thyroid cells, which renders them more susceptible to cell-mediated cytotoxicity; blocking ICAM-1 with a monoclonal antibody inhibits thyroid cell killing by T-cells *in vitro*. This inhibition is incomplete, suggesting a role for additional adhesion molecules (such as LFA-3) on the thyroid cell surface. Thyroid cells also secrete IL-6, a pluripotential cytokine that stimulates T- and B-cell proliferation and differentiation. This IL-6 release is stimulated by γ-IFN, TNF and IL-1, which are known to be produced by the lymphocytic infiltrate in thyroiditis, as well as by TSH and TSAb. Therefore the thyroid cells may participate in the autoimmune response by expressing class II molecules and ICAM-1 and by synthesizing IL-6 (Fig. 11.8).

EFFECTOR MECHANISMS

TSAb produce Graves' disease by stimulating the TSH receptor in an unregulated fashion. Transplacental passage of these antibodies results in neonatal thyrotoxicosis, which recovers as maternal antibodies decline in

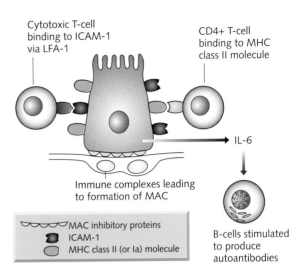

Fig. 11.8 Participation of thyroid cells in the autoimmune response. Cytokines (γ-IFN, TNF) enhance expression of MHC class II, ICAM-1 and MAC-inhibiting proteins by thyroid cells and stimulate release of IL-6. The possible consequences of these phenomena are illustrated.

the baby. Autoimmune hypothyroidism is the result of humoral and cell-mediated injury. Thyroid cells, like many other nucleated cells, are relatively resistant to the lytic effects of homologous complement, in part due to the expression of CD59, a protein which prevents insertion of the membrane attack complex (MAC) into the cell membrane. Thus, complement fixation by TPO antibodies will only result in cell death if the formation of MAC is powerful or sustained. MAC can be demonstrated by immunohistochemistry around the thyroid follicles in Graves' disease and Hashimoto's thyroiditis. Even sublethal amounts of MAC may produce tissue injury; the cAMP response of thyroid cells to TSH is reduced and toxic oxygen radicals, prostaglandins and IL-6 are released under these conditions, which will exacerbate tissue injury.

Multiple sclerosis

This is a demyelinating disease of the central nervous system, characterized by relapses and remissions. It has a lifetime frequency of one in 800 in the UK and is the most common cause of neurological disability in young adults. Epidemiological evidence suggests that an infectious agent acquired at a critical time early in life is aetiologically important. Even so, the production of lesions depends on an autoimmune response. Considerable insight into the pathophysiology of multiple sclerosis has been gained from an animal model, experimental allergic encephalomyelitis (EAE). EAE is induced by immunizing rodents with myelin basic protein (MBP) and adjuvants, and certain forms follow a chronic, relapsing course, with histological features similar to multiple sclerosis. EAE can be transferred to naive animals by CD4+ T-cell clones specific for MBP.

The signs and symptoms of multiple sclerosis are due to focal inflammatory demyelinating lesions within the central nervous system. Initially lymphocytes and monocytes accumulate around venules, leading to oligodendrocyte destruction and loss of myelin sheath. Oligodendrocytes become depleted and finally there is healing with scar formation. Remyelination is unusual and temporary (Fig. 11.9).

Autoantigens in EAE and multiple sclerosis

The predominant protein in central nervous system myelin, MBP, is clearly the initiating antigen in EAE. This antigen is relatively small (about 17 kDa), abundant and easily purified, factors which have inspired extensive studies of its recognition by the immune system in EAE. Initial experiments demonstrated that only the amino-terminal 37 amino acids of rat MBP were required to induce EAE in mouse strains bearing certain MHC haplotypes (H-2u), while the carboxy-terminal 80 amino acids were sufficient in strains of mice with other haplotypes (H-2s). These variations depend on the particular class II genes within the MHC of the mouse, as would be predicted from the MHC restriction of the CD4+ T-cells which mediate this disease.

Not all T-cell clones reactive with rat MBP produce EAE on transfer into mice. Some of these clones do not recognize mouse MBP, which differs from the encephalitogenic amino-terminal fragment of rat MBP by deletion of residues 10 and 11. Other clones do cross-react but appear incapable of inducing disease, possibly through their failure to elaborate appropriate cytokines.

The epitopes on MBP have been further analysed using short, overlapping synthetic peptides. The minimum amino-terminal sequence capable of inducing EAE in PL/J mice (with the MHC H-2u haplotype) consists of amino acids 1–9. The first amino acid, alanine, must be acetylated for maximum potency. A second epitope also exists, from amino acids 9 to 16, spanning the region with deletions in mouse MBP. Non-encephalitogenic murine T-cells can recognize this sequence of rat (but not mouse) MBP. Several T-cell epitopes exist in the carboxy-terminal of MBP; these include overlapping sequences comprising residues

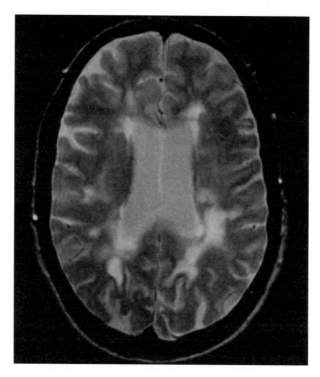

Fig. 11.9 Magnetic resonance imaging (MRI) from a patient with multiple sclerosis. This disease is characterized by inflammation in the central nervous system with episodes disseminated in time and space: there are multiple areas of abnormal signal intensity shown as white within the substance of the brain—especially prominent in the right parieto-occipital region. These represent areas of demyelination of the white matter which normally gives a dark signal in MRI studies.

89–100, 89–101 and 96–109, which are recognized by discrete encephalitogenic T-cell clones from SJL/J (MHC H-2s haplotype) mice.

Is MBP an autoantigen in multiple sclerosis? Peripheral blood and cerebrospinal fluid T-cells from about a quarter of such patients proliferate in response to MBP *in vitro*. Some responses are also obtained in patients with other neurological diseases and even in healthy subjects. It remains possible that a higher proportion of the autoreactive T-cells in the disease plaques may be responding to MBP, or that recognition of particular epitopes on MBP is important in the T-cell response in multiple sclerosis: there is preliminary evidence for two immunodominant regions in human MBP (residues 84–102 and 143–168) recognized primarily by T-cells from multiple sclerosis patients. However, it is also possible that the inconsistent T-cell responses observed are merely secondary to myelin destruction, and that the primary autoantigen remains to be identified. T-cell reactivity has also been demonstrated against two other central nervous system antigens, proteolipid protein and myelin oligodendrocyte glycoprotein, in multiple sclerosis and these are therefore also key candidate autoantigens.

Genetic predisposition

IMMUNOGENETICS OF EAE

The strain specificity of EAE results from T-cell recognition of a particular combination of MBP peptide and class II molecule. Some of these peptides of MBP are presented by I-A molecules (the homologue of HLA-DQ in humans) and some by I-E molecules (the homologue of HLA-DR). Administration of monoclonal antibodies against class II molecules prevents EAE. There is evidence that susceptibility to EAE in certain strains of mice and guinea-pigs is determined by the level of class II expression on antigen-presenting cells: diminished expression is associated with resistance to disease.

IMMUNOGENETICS OF MULTIPLE SCLEROSIS

The concordance for multiple sclerosis in monozygotic twins is around 25%, ten-fold higher than for dizygotic twins, indicating a genetic component to this disorder. As with other autoimmune disorders, however, environmental factors have a major influence, perhaps best shown by epidemiological studies on the non-uniform geographic distribution, the effects of migration and the sporadic epidemics of multiple sclerosis, all of which suggest a role for an unknown infectious agent. This is a polygenic disorder; in keeping with the findings in EAE, the MHC has some role in determining susceptibility, although different alleles appear to predispose to the same disease. In particular, the frequency of HLA-DR2 is increased in northern European patients, DR2 and DR4 are increased in Italian patients, and DR2, DR4 and DRw6 are increased in Japanese patients. DR7 appears to protect against multiple sclerosis. These associations may be explained by particular DQ genes in linkage disequilibrium with the DR alleles; DQw6 (now known as DQB1*0602) confers a particularly high susceptibility in Caucasians. It is possible that certain MHC haplotypes could influence the clinical course of disease, e.g. severity or chronicity.

As in type 1 diabetes and thyroid autoimmunity, the concordance in HLA-identical siblings of multiple sclerosis patients is less than in monozygotic twins, indicating that other genes also determine susceptibility. As discussed below, the receptors used by T-cells to recognize MBP in EAE are remarkably similar. This limited heterogeneity has directed attention to the germ line T-cell receptor genes as possible susceptibility loci in multi-

ple sclerosis. Polymorphisms in the genes encoding the constant and variable regions of both the α and β T-cell receptor chains have been associated with the disease in population and family studies, suggesting that genes in these regions can confer susceptibility. Genetic susceptibility has also been linked to the MBP gene.

Pathogenesis

ANTIGEN PRESENTATION

Brain macrophages (microglia) and endothelial cells can present autoantigens to T-cells; whether other cells have a similar function in multiple sclerosis is unclear. The neurones, oligodendroglia and astrocytes of the central nervous system uniquely do not express either class I or II MHC molecules constitutively. γ-IFN induces MHC class II molecule expression on astrocytes and such cells may then able to present antigens but recent experiments suggest that this does not occur *in vitro*. Rodent oligodendrocytes do not express class II molecules or function as antigen-presenting cells after treatment with cytokines.

RESTRICTED T-CELL RECEPTOR USAGE IN EAE

An outstanding feature of EAE is the limited heterogeneity of T-cell receptors recognizing epitopes of MBP. Thus in PL/J (H-2^u) mice, 80% of encephalitogenic T-cells use a receptor β chain with a variable (V) region encoded by one of a family of genes called Vβ8.2, and 100% of these T-cells use an α chain V region encoded by a member of the Vα4 family. In the B10.PL (H-2^u) strain, 80% of encephalitogenic T-cells utilize Vβ8.2, 60% Vα2.3 and 40% Vα4.2. Surprisingly, in a different species, the Lewis rat, T-cells which recognize a different MBP epitope to these H-2^u strain mice (amino acids 72–86 rather than 1–9) nonetheless use rat homologues of the Vβ8.2 and Vα2 families.

These results are remarkable in showing restriction of the T-cell receptor even though different MBP epitopes are recognized; further work has shown that this extends to MBP peptides presented by either I-A or I-E molecules. The physical nature of this trimolecular interaction, which seems so dependent on particular Vα and Vβ products, is not yet clear. However, such restriction is not a universal feature of EAE. In SJL/J (H-2^s) strain mice, the encephalitogenic T-cells which react with two of the three epitopes in the carboxy-terminal of MBP are polyclonal.

THERAPEUTIC OPPORTUNITIES IN MULTIPLE SCLEROSIS Several novel methods to treat autoimmune disease have resulted from these observations.

Firstly, antibodies which react with the Vβ8 family of T-cell receptors deplete Vβ8+ T-cells when injected into mice and such treatment reverses EAE in H-2ᵘ strain animals. A second approach has been to modify the T-cell epitope such that it blocks T-cell activation. Modified MBP peptides have been constructed which are non-encephalitogenic but nonetheless bind to class II MHC molecules; these prevent presentation of the native peptide. Substitutions in amino acids at position 3 and 4 in the MBP amino-terminal nonapeptide can achieve this, although it is not clear that they prevent EAE by actually blocking the MHC molecule. Instead, such modified peptides could induce suppressor cells. Finally, immunization with synthetic peptides corresponding to unique sequences in the Vβ8 family of T-cell receptors can prevent EAE. The mechanism here seems to be the induction of suppressor cells recognizing encephalitogenic CD4+ cells which are known to be Vβ8+.

These developments are exciting but their application to human disease depends upon the existence of similar restrictions in the receptors used by autoreactive T-cells, but as is apparent from H-2ˢ strain mice, such restriction is incomplete even within the experimental model of EAE. The susceptibility to multiple sclerosis endowed by T-cell receptor genes suggests an important role for T-cells in disease pathogenesis, possibly related to recognition of key myelin antigens by particular T-cell receptor V regions. This is supported by some evidence of (i) limited heterogeneity in rearranged Vα T-cell receptor transcripts in multiple sclerosis plaques and (ii) shared Vβ T-cell receptor usage by lymphocytes responding to immunodominant regions of human MBP. If these T-cells actually are pathogenic, such restriction in T-cell receptors could be utilized to develop relatively specific immunological therapy for multiple sclerosis, along the lines described in EAE.

EFFECTOR MECHANISMS IN MULTIPLE SCLEROSIS
Why demyelination occurs is unknown. A key initial event must be the penetration of the blood–brain barrier by activated inflammatory cells. Once within the central nervous system these can produce cell-mediated cytotoxicity, cytokine secretion, complement activation, prostaglandin release and reactive oxygen metabolite production. There is good evidence that formation of MAC is critical in EAE, as decomplementation ameliorates this disease. MAC have been localized in multiple sclerosis plaques and on oligodendrocyte-derived membrane vesicles in the cerebrospinal fluid. The pathway by which MAC are formed in multiple sclerosis is unknown.

Myasthenia gravis

This is an uncommon disorder caused by autoantibodies against the nicotinic acetylcholine receptor in the neuro-muscular junction. As a result, the striated muscles are weak and readily fatiguable. The patient characteristically has weakness of muscles of facial expression and swallowing; weakness of muscles supplying the eyelids causes them to droop, resulting in ptosis (Plate 23, facing p. 214).

The acetylcholine receptor

The study of myasthenia gravis was greatly accelerated by the discovery of the acetylcholine receptor (AChR) as the key autoantigen. There is an abundant supply of this in the modified muscle tissue which forms the electric organs of certain fish such as *Torpedo* species (the electric rays). By obtaining purified AChR from this source, experimental models of myasthenia gravis could be developed and the structure of the receptor was determined. More recently, it has been possible to determine the amino acid sequence of the homologous receptor subunits in *Torpedo* and in humans. The receptor consists of a transmembrane pentamer comprising two α subunits and single β, γ and δ subunits.

About two-thirds of the AChR antibodies in myasthenia patients are directed against an extracellular region on the α subunit (the main immunogenic region, MIR). Amino acid residues 67–76 are especially important in determining this B-cell epitope. An important feature is the duplication of α subunits in the intact receptor, which will permit cross-linking by autoantibodies binding to the MIR. The T-cell epitopes on AChR reside outside the MIR. Several epitopes have been identified, each recognized by only a limited proportion of patients, and depending on different HLA haplotypes for their presentation.

The Lambert–Eaton myasthenic syndrome

Brief mention should be made of this syndrome which clinically resembles myasthenia gravis but is due to reduction in neurotransmitter release presynaptically. It is often associated with small cell carcinoma of the lung. The syndrome is caused by autoantibodies which down-regulate a subset of voltage-operated calcium channels found on neurones and small cell carcinoma cells.

Immunogenetics

Myasthenia gravis is associated with the HLA-B8, DR3

haplotype in young patients and with HLA-B7, DR2 in those whose disease presents later. Immunoglobulin and T-cell receptor genes may also contribute to susceptibility.

Pathogenesis

AChR antibodies clearly produce this disease, as their transplacental passage results in neonatal myasthenia. AChR antibody binding *in vitro* has a number of effects, including complement activation, accelerated internalization of the receptor and decreased insertion of new AChR into the membrane. Complement attack and formation of MAC may cause loss of receptors by focal lysis of the junctional membrane or as a result of clearance of MAC from the cell surface.

Anti-glomerular basement membrane disease

This rare disease (annual incidence approximately one to two per million) is characterized by the presence of an autoantibody that binds to the glomerular basement membrane (GBM) and certain other basement membranes, notably the alveolar BM of the lungs.

The condition is capable of destroying the kidneys within a few weeks. With modern renal replacement therapy this aspect is rarely fatal; pulmonary haemorrhage, which can be massive, is much more of a problem. This clinical urgency justifies the use of high doses of corticosteroids, which provide rapid anti-inflammatory action. However, corticosteroids have little or no effect on the underlying production of the autoantibody. The alkylating agent cyclophosphamide, which has particular efficacy against B-cells, is therefore given as well. Finally, cyclophosphamide takes at least 1–2 weeks to have a significant effect on autoantibody production. This is clearly too long to wait, particularly when faced with life-threatening pulmonary haemorrhage, and plasma exchange is used to remove autoantibody rapidly.

The Goodpasture antigen

The antigen recognized by anti-GBM autoantibodies is known as the Goodpasture antigen. Anti-GBM antibodies from different individuals appear to recognize the same or a closely related epitope, as the binding of most of them can be inhibited by a single mouse monoclonal antibody. There has been agreement for some time that the epitope resides in the non-collagenous (NC1) domain of type IV collagen. The problem has been that type IV collagen, as defined by its $\alpha 1$ and $\alpha 2$ chains,

is widely distributed amongst basement membranes, whereas anti-GBM antibodies have a much more restricted binding pattern. The solution to this apparent paradox has been provided by recent developments in our understanding of the molecular composition of type IV collagen. It is now clear that there are additional chains which do indeed have the requisite restricted distribution, in particular the $\alpha 3$ and $\alpha 5$ chains. The sequence for the $\alpha 5$ chain is available, and furthermore it has been convincingly demonstrated that a defect in the gene coding for the $\alpha 5$ chain is responsible for Alport's syndrome (X-linked hereditary nephritis and deafness), a condition in which the Goodpasture epitope is apparently absent from the kidney. More recently, the $\alpha 3$ chain has also been characterized, and it now seems clear that it is in fact this chain that bears the Goodpasture epitope. The apparent absence of this epitope in Alport's syndrome is presumably due to a general disorganization of the BM secondary to abnormalities in the $\alpha 5$ chain.

Immunogenetics

Anti-GBM disease is strongly associated with DR2 and to a lesser extent DR4. Sequence analysis has not found a particular disease-associated variant of DR2. Of the class I alleles, B7 is increased in frequency in patients; although this allele is in linkage disequilibrium with DR2, analysis shows that it is an independent risk factor, and in particular that B7 appears to be associated with the more severe cases of anti-GBM disease.

Pathogenesis

In one sense the pathogenesis of this disease is well understood. There is good evidence from analogous animal models, and from direct transfer of human antibodies into animals, that the anti-GBM autoantibody is pathogenic. Such antibodies are almost always of the IgG_1 and IgG_4 subclasses, and IgG_1 antibodies in particular are able to bind to Fc receptors on macrophages and to fix complement. They can thus engage the effector systems previously discussed, and the end result is severe glomerular inflammation. Although the autoantibody is of primary importance, other factors are clearly involved. This is exemplified by pulmonary haemorrhage: the alveolar BM is not as accessible as the GBM, and perhaps as a result significant lung haemorrhage is usually only seen when there are additional pulmonary insults, notably smoking.

The sense in which the pathogenesis is not well understood is our lack of understanding of the factors that trigger production of the autoantibody. The strong MHC associations clearly imply a role for T-cells, as MHC products are involved in their activation and not, in general, in the activation of B-cells (at least directly). Very little is known about T-cells in this disease (cf. sections on myasthenia gravis and multiple sclerosis).

In the future the molecular identification of the Goodpasture antigen, and the fact that most if not all patients' autoantibodies appear to recognize a very similar molecular species, may permit specific immunoadsorption. This would involve coupling of the Goodpasture antigen, perhaps produced by recombinant technology, to a column through which the patient's plasma could be perfused. This should allow specific and rapid removal only of the autoantibody. Clearly a similar strategy can be envisaged for other disease with pathogenic autoantibodies for which the molecular target is known.

Systemic lupus erythematosus and other connective tissue diseases

As well as systemic lupus erythematosus (SLE), diseases considered in this section include mixed connective tissue disease (MCTD), Sjögren's syndrome, dermatomyositis and systemic sclerosis. These conditions are characterized by the production of a wide range of autoantibodies; although some of these are relatively specific for particular disease entities, individual autoantibodies are often found in several of the diseases in this group. Many of the autoantigens recognized by these antibodies are now well characterized at the molecular level, but it is beyond the scope of this chapter to deal with these comprehensively.

The immunogenetic associations are best defined for SLE. As mentioned above, hereditary deficiencies of a variety of complement components are associated with a very high incidence of SLE. This has been extended to more subtle abnormalities of the complement system: at least in certain population groups there is a high incidence of null (non-coding) alleles for complement component C4A. The possible pathogenetic link between these complement deficiencies and the aetiology of SLE has been discussed above. It seems likely that the association between SLE and the class II allele DR3 may be at least partially explained by this, as null alleles for C4A are found on DR3-bearing haplotypes. In some cases, the immunogenetic associations are stronger with a particular autoantibody rather than with a particular disease. Thus patients positive for anti-Ro and anti-La are usually DR3 or DR2 positive, irrespective of whether they are classified as SLE, MCTD or Sjögren's syndrome. Patients with SLE and epidermolysis bullosa acquisita, a bullous skin lesion caused by autoantibodies to type 7 procollagen, are almost all DR2 positive.

As demonstrated by the last example in the preceding paragraph, certain autoantibodies are closely linked with certain clinical manifestations. Other examples include the almost invariable occurrence of inflammatory interstitial lung disease in polymyositis patients with autoantibodies to histidyl tRNA synthetase (anti-Jo-1), and the production of complete heart block in infants by the transplacental passage of anti-Ro. Other antibodies are closely linked with particular diseases. Autoantibodies to topoisomerase I (anti-Scl-70) are specific for progressive systemic sclerosis, and anticentromere antibodies are found almost exclusively in limited systemic sclerosis (CREST syndrome: calcinosis, Raynaud's phenomenon, oesophageal dysmotility, sclerodactyly, telangiectasia).

A further point of molecular interest is the occurrence of certain idiotypes on autoantibodies in SLE. The 16/6 idiotype, which appears to be encoded by germ line sequences unmodified by somatic mutation, is found on certain anti-DNA autoantibodies. The level of 16/6 idiotype in many cases demonstrates a close correlation with disease activity, often better than the correlation with total anti-DNA activity. Remarkably, immunization of healthy (non-lupus-prone) mice with human monoclonal antibodies carrying the 16/6 idiotype appears to induce an SLE-like illness, as does immunization with a murine monoclonal antibody with anti-16/6 specificity. If these observations are confirmed they serve to highlight the potential importance of idiotype–anti-idiotype interactions between antibody molecules in the aetiology and control of SLE.

Rheumatoid arthritis

Rheumatoid arthritis, which affects approximately 1% of the population, is thought to represent an autoimmune attack directed primarily at synovial membranes. The immunogenetics demonstrate an association with the class II alleles DR1 and DR4; this latter is particularly interesting, as there are a number of subtypes of DR4, not all of which are associated with rheumatoid arthritis. Thus the Dw4 and Dw14 subtypes are both independently associated with the disease, whereas the Dw10 subtype is not. Disease-associated DR molecules appear to share an epitope on the β chain of the DR molecule, comprising the sequence glutamine-leucine/arginine-arginine-alanine-alanine from amino acids 70–74. It is possible that this epitope is required for presentation of a critical autoantigen involved in rheumatoid arthritis.

Apart from the immunoglobulin molecule, which serves as the target for rheumatoid factor, little is known about possible autoantigens in rheumatoid arthritis. Synovial T-cells examined early in the course of disease proliferate against mycobacterial heat shock proteins, and reactivity against such antigens may play a role in triggering a cross-reactive autoimmune response. T-cells isolated from synovial fluid, compared with those in the peripheral blood, appear to be enriched for those that use the Vβ14 family of genes in coding for the β chain of their T-cell receptor; indeed, this subset of T-cells appears to be relatively depleted in the periphery, although only a small number of patients have been studied. This has prompted the speculation that exposure to a microbial 'superantigen' (antigens that are capable of activating all the T-cells expressing a particular family of T-cell receptor genes) may be involved in pathogenesis. Experimentally such exposure, after an initial stimulatory phase, does lead to depletion, and it is possible that only those T-cells that happen to cross-react with a synovial antigen will home to the joints and be spared.

Seronegative spondyloarthropathies

This group of conditions is typified by ankylosing spondylitis, but also includes Reiter's disease and the arthropathies associated with psoriasis and inflammatory bowel disease. They have in common a strong association with the class I MHC allele B27, and in fact this was the first MHC-disease association to be described. This situation is relatively unusual as most autoimmune diseases are more strongly associated with MHC class II alleles, with any class I associations probably reflecting **linkage disequilibrium**. One possible explanation follows from an antigenic similarity between certain B27 variants and components of micro-organisms such as *Klebsiella*. There is now direct molecular evidence of this relationship, with a stretch of six amino acids shared between the hypervariable domain of B27 and *Klebsiella pneumoniae* nitrogenase. This may therefore be an example of molecular mimicry. The pathogenic consequences of this mimicry are speculative, but may involve either a reduction in the immune response to the organism, which may then be more pathogenic, or a cross-reactive autoimmune attack on B27-expressing cells.

Further reading

Aitman T.J. and Todd J.A. (1995) Molecular genetics of diabetes mellitus. *Baillière's Clinical Endocrinology and Metabolism*, 9, 631–656.

Bach J.F. (1994) Insulin-dependent diabetes mellitus as an autoimmune disease. *Endocrine Reviews*, 15, 516–542.

Compston D.A.S. (1994) The pathogenesis of demyelinating disease. *Horizons in Medicine 5*, pp. 119–129. Blackwell Science, Oxford.

Coutinho A. and Kazatchkine M.D. (eds) (1994) Autoimmunity. *Physiology and Disease*. Wiley/Liss, New York.

Lachmann P.J., Peters D.K., Rosen F.S. and Walport M.J. (eds) (1992) *Clinical Aspects of Immunology*, 5th edn. Blackwell Scientific Publications, Oxford.

Lechler R. (ed.) (1994) *HLA and Disease*. Academic Press, London.

Oliveira D.B.G. (1992) *Immunological Aspects of Renal Disease*. Cambridge University Press, Cambridge.

Roitt I.M., Brostoff J. and Male D. (eds) (1993) *Immunology*, 3rd edn. Mosby-Year Book, London.

Todd J.A. (1990) Genetic control of autoimmunity in type 1 diabetes. *Immunology Today*, 11, 123–128.

Weetman A.P. (1991) *Autoimmune Endocrine Disease*. Cambridge University Press, Cambridge.

Weetman A.P. and McGregor A.M. (1995) Autoimmune thyroid disease. Further developments in our understanding. *Endocrine Reviews*, 15, 788–830.

Wraith D.C., McDevitt H.O., Stainman L. and Acha-Orbea H. (1989) T cell recognition as the target for immune intervention in autoimmune disease. *Cell*, 57, 709–715.

Chapter 12 Microbial infections

Introduction

Microbial infection, in all its diversity, has been and will remain one of the greatest challenges to human health. The patterns of specific infection vary markedly across different countries, according to their state of 'development' and geographical/biological characteristics; they can evolve rapidly within any community—as the contemporary AIDS epidemic illustrates. Accurate and efficient diagnosis of infection is essential for the deployment of treatment for assessing the value of new treatments and, in epidemiology, for monitoring of infection and assessing the impact of public health programmes. Molecular biology will play an outstanding role in the fight against infection by providing sensitive and specific diagnostic tools as well as information on new targets for prevention and treatment.

Microbes are the principal cause of illness and death in the Third World and provide new challenges in developed countries with nosocomial and opportunistic infections. The range of possible pathogens that may cause respiratory infection in an immunocompromised host presents special diagnostic difficulties. Establishing a microbial diagnosis provides the rational basis for effective treatment and is necessary for assessing the results of chemotherapeutic trials *in vivo* and defining the epidemiology of infections.

For most bacterial pathogens, any advantage in applying molecular biology techniques to obtain a laboratory diagnosis is far outweighed by the ease with which the organism can be cheaply and rapidly cultured, and its identity and antibiotic susceptibility pattern determined. But there are a number of important exceptions for which molecular biology has revolutionized laboratory diagnosis, making it faster, more sensitive or more accurate. For the most part these tests remain the domain of reference and research laboratories but as these techniques become simplified and automated they will increasingly emerge in the routine bacteriology laboratory — provided that key issues such as quality control and cost implications can be resolved.

The greatest impact of molecular biology on clinical bacteriology and mycology has so far been in the development of a vast range of new **DNA-based typing systems**. This rapid evolution in molecular typing systems has significantly advanced our understanding of the **epidemiology** of many infections both in the community and hospitals. The latter has been put to medical use by helping to identify, curtail and prevent hospital outbreaks of both bacterial and fungal pathogens.

Ultimately the greatest contribution of molecular biology to microbiology is likely to be in unravelling the pathogenesis and immunology of these infections. We can now far more easily identify major components of a microbe, elucidate possible functions and so determine whether they may be useful targets for new therapeutics and vaccine design. At the same time we are now in a strong position for developing immunotherapy, in the form of genetically engineered human recombinant antibodies and cytokines, which could usefully supplement antibiotics, particularly for those infections proving resistant to existing chemotherapy.

Each of these areas will be discussed in this chapter with selected examples from bacterial, fungal and parasitic human pathogens.

Diagnosis

Standard microbiological practice identifies microbes in clinical samples either by direct visualization after suitable staining, by isolation after culture or by recognition of a specific host antibody response. Direct microscopy is a useful and simple technique applicable to most bacteria and larger microbes. However some bacteria, such as *Legionella pneumophila*, are demonstrated very poorly by Gram staining, and a range of smaller micro-organisms—including rickettsiae, chlamydiae and mycoplasmas—cannot be readily identified by light microscopy. Some bacteria or larger microbes stain well by Gram, Ziehl–Nielsen or silver stains but are not recognized in available clinical samples such as blood, sputum and cerebrospinal fluid (CSF), because they are present in small numbers. Culture provides a valuable amplification step but is a slow process requiring special media for some organisms. **Routine culture fails as a diagnostic procedure in situations in which the pathogen is difficult or impossible to grow, slow to grow or hazardous.**

Traditionally serology, the measurement of antibody titres or antigen detection, has augmented direct microscopy and culture in the routine bacteriology laboratory. Many such tests are commercially available, subject to quality control, relatively cheap and easy to perform or automatable. However, serology is rarely diagnostic during the acute phase of the disease because of the time taken for the titre of specific antibodies to rise to detectable levels. Consequently, there are many disorders where an infective agent or trigger is strongly suspected but where available microbiological methods hitherto have failed to identify a microbe, e.g. necrotizing vasculitis, sarcoidosis, Crohn's disease and multiple sclerosis. Thus more powerful, but complementary, approaches to microbial identification and characterization would be advantageous. Molecular methods based on DNA/RNA detection now offer great sensitivity and specificity of detection and, with appropriate care, the possibility of wide-ranging and efficient application.

DNA-based pathogen-specific kits, however, are not widely available commercially, have not yet been subjected to rigorous inter-laboratory quality control and standardization, and require relatively expensive reagents, access to suitable equipment and trained staff.

This is not to say that they do not play an invaluable contribution to the diagnosis of certain infections and this is set to expand. But because it is so important that a laboratory diagnosis is accurate and not misleading to the clinician, it is often more appropriate for a specialized, DNA-based test to be performed by a reference or research laboratory with expertise in that area. Such centres may serve on a regional or national basis depending on the demand for the test.

Antibody assays

Antibody assays are commonly used for the serodiagnosis of pathogens which are impossible to grow *in vitro* (such as syphilis), slow to grow and/or identify (e.g. systemic mycoses due to dimorphic fungi) or highly hazardous (e.g. psittacosis) (Table 12.1). Sometimes diagnosis can be made on the basis of a single high positive titre but commonly **paired sera** are required, taken several weeks apart, to look for a four-fold rise in titre which then indicates current or recent active infection. Inevitably this delays diagnosis and for this reason detection of pathogen-specific antigens is generally preferred to antibody assays if culture is problematic. This becomes even more critical if the host is immunocompromised, and therefore unlikely to mount a good antibody response. False positives may arise if the patient has been recently vaccinated or skin tested against the homologous organism or had the same or a cross-reacting infection in the past. Often the titre obtained in these circumstances will not be as high as in acute infection (though this too will give only moderate titres if the peak is missed). Further testing against different antigens or identifying the antibody class (IgM versus IgG) may be helpful. A **good history** from the clinician and informed interpretation of results by the laboratory are both essential.

Table 12.1 Examples of antibody assays available for the serodiagnosis of bacterial and fungal infections.

Antibody assay	Examples of applications
ELISA	Leptospirosis, Lyme disease
Complement fixation test	Mycoplasma, brucellosis, Q fever
Indirect haemagglutination assay	Rickettsia, mycoplasma
Haemagglutination assay	Syphilis
Counterimmunoelectrophoresis	Systemic mycoses
Immunodiffusion (double diffusion)	Systemic mycoses
Immunofluorescence	Syphilis, legionellosis, rickettsia, psittacosis
Bacterial agglutination	Pertussis, brucellosis, rickettsia, leptospirosis
Latex agglutination	Cryptococcosis, streptococcal antibodies
Immunoblotting	Culture-negative endocarditis
Radioimmunoassay	Allergic bronchopulmonary aspergillosis

Despite these limitations, antibody assays have proved particularly useful in collecting **epidemiological data,** such as the prevalence of gastric colonization by *Helicobacter pylori*, the spiral bacterium associated with chronic gastritis and duodenal ulceration. They are also an invaluable guide as to the success of vaccination in inducing a protective antibody response. For example, measurement of pertussis antibodies has been used both on an individual patient basis, to identify seroconversion to acellular vaccine, and in assessing clinical trials.

Immunoblotting has been widely used as a means of analysing the antibody response to multiple components of an organism in a single assay. In cases of culture-negative endocarditis, the pattern of a patient's antibody reactivity against immunoblots of streptococci and enterococci can be used to identify the causative bacterium. A further refinement has been the use of a fusion protein, derived by cloning one of these immunodominant antigens into λgt 11 (a phage expression vector), in an indirect enzyme-linked immunosorbent assay (ELISA) for the serodiagnosis of enterococcal endocarditis.

Antigen detection

Serodiagnosis of systemic fungal infections by the detection of circulating antigens has been the subject of intensive research for over a decade (Table 12.2). This is due to the high mortality of the systemic forms of these increasingly common infections. Earlier initiation of treatment, before cultures become positive, is critical in maximizing chances of survival. Commercially available kits for the detection of *Cryptococcus neoformans* have been successful. These are based on the detection of this yeast's polysaccharide capsule in the patient's serum or CSF by **reverse passive latex agglutination** (RPLA; latex particles coated with specific antibody) or **enzyme-linked immunosorbent assay** (ELISA). These tests are easy to perform and highly sensitive and specific for meningeal and disseminated cryptococcosis. The capsular antigen is stable (facilitating dissociation from bound antibodies), produced in large quantities and has a long serum half-

Table 12.2 Examples of antigen assays used in the diagnosis of fungal infections.

Antigen assay	Examples of applications
ELISA	Cryptococcosis, DC
Reverse passive latex agglutination	Cryptococcosis, DC, invasive aspergillosis
Dot immunobinding	DC
Radioimmunoassay	Histoplasmosis

Table 12.3 Assays which have been used for the serodiagnosis of disseminated candidiasis (DC) by detection of candidal antigens or metabolites.

Antigen or metabolite being detected	Method of detection
Heat-labile cytoplasmic antigen(s)	RPLA (Cand-Tec*)
Mannan	RPLA (LA-Candida*, Pastorex*) EIA (ICON*)
Enolase	EIA (Directigen*)
Hsp90	Dot immunobinding assay
D-Arabinitol	Gas–liquid chromatography Enzymatic fluorometric kit*

* Commercially available (Directigen has now been discontinued).

life. Measurement of antigen titres can help in monitoring response to treatment, and a rise in titre often signals relapse.

For **disseminated candidiasis** (DC) a range of serological tests are now commercially available, but the question of which antigen to target or even the best assay format is unresolved (Table 12.3). There are a number of reasons for the difficulty in establishing a reliable serological test for DC. Firstly, detecting *Candida* in a non-sterile site is not diagnostic since immunocompromised patients who have received broad-spectrum antibiotics often become colonized with *C. albicans* and may develop superficial infections (thrush). Even culturing *Candida* from the blood is not in itself diagnostic of DC since transient candidaemia can occur. Furthermore DC can be acute or chronic (hepatosplenic) and can be due to species other than *C. albicans*, such as *C. krusei* which is resistant to fluconazole, a widely used anti-fungal agent. Therefore ideally a serological test for DC would be more sensitive than blood culture (only about half are blood culture positive), able to distinguish DC from other forms of candidiasis and capable of distinguishing species apart from *C. albicans*. Generally enzyme immunoassays (EIAs) are more sensitive, and less prone to false positives, than RPLA tests directed against the same antigen but the latter are popular because of their speed and simplicity. Mannan-based assays are hampered by an intrinsic lack of sensitivity due to the transient nature of mannan antigenaemia in DC. Variable results obtained with tests directed against the same target probably stem from differences in the quality of the antibody probe, in the patient population (neutropenic versus non-neutropenic), and, most importantly, frequency of serum sampling. Frequent (ideally daily) sampling is critical in maximizing the sensitivity of any of these serological tests.

Detection of the polysaccharide capsule of the pneumococcus has also been used for diagnostic purposes. *Streptococcus pneumoniae* is the most common cause of community-acquired pneumonia in all age groups. Despite the availability of antibiotics to which the organism is exquisitely sensitive *in vitro*, mortality is high, a situation likely to worsen with the emergence of penicillin-resistant strains. Pneumococci produce type-specific polysaccharides and in order to detect the majority of them it is necessary to use a mixture of type-specific antibodies such as that produced by the Staten Serum Institute, Copenhagen, which contains rabbit polyclonal antisera to 83 different serotypes. These antibodies have been used to detect pneumococcal antigen by methods such as counterimmunoelectrophoresis (CIE), latex agglutination and ELISA. These have proved useful in the diagnosis of pneumococcal meningitis when applied to CSF samples, provided positive results are interpreted in the light of other parameters such as cell count and glucose. In the diagnosis of pneumonia, serum has a poor diagnostic yield unless bacteraemia is present. Urine gives higher sensitivity but requires concentration. Quantification of antigen detected in the sputum is desirable to exclude colonization. Such procedures are clinically justifiable in situations in which the patient has received antibiotics, rendering them culture negative, and when life-threatening penicillin-resistant infection is suspected.

Another context in which detection of bacterial antigens is valuable is in the identification of the enterotoxins produced by some strains of *Staphylococcus aureus*. These have long been recognized as responsible for the symptoms of staphylococcal food poisoning, but may also be involved in the pathogenesis of other staphylococcal infections. There are a number of sensitive, commercially available assay systems, of which the double antibody sandwich ELISA (Fig. 12.1) is probably the most popular.

DNA probes

The principle behind the use of DNA probes is that complementary nucleic acid strands bind to form stable double-stranded (hybrid) complexes. For medical purposes DNA probes are most widely used for **confirming the identity** of DNA products amplified by the polymerase chain reaction (PCR), as described in detail below, and typing systems (pp. 230–232), but they are also useful in speciating certain pathogens and identifying virulence factors, such as toxins. This is particularly helpful when identification on the basis of phenotypic charateristics is slow, laborious or unreliable. The first step in developing a DNA-based diagnostic assay is to identify a target sequence which is specific to the genus or species but sufficiently conserved to avoid strains being missed. The sensitivity of the assay is likely to be greater if the sequence is present in multiple copies, such as rRNA genes or repetitive satellite DNA. The format of

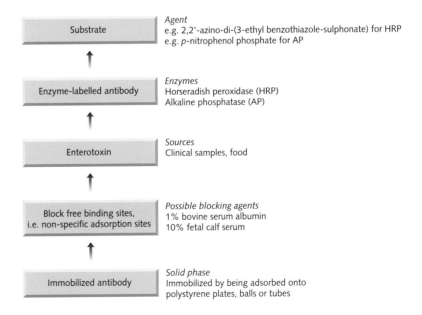

Fig. 12.1 Principles of a double antibody sandwich ELISA.

the assay is also critical. Historically, radiolabelled probes have been used because of their inherent sensitivity, but good non-radioactive labelling systems are now appearing and these are not only less hazardous but also stable, facilitating standardization. Following selection of hybridization conditions, which will determine specificity, definition of the cut-off for positive and negative reactions is required. Finally the assay will need to be assessed on patient specimens in parallel with the current gold standard diagnostic technique.

Commercially available probes are now being used to shorten the time required to diagnose infections due to slow growing organisms. For example the Gene-Probe Corporation (San Diego, California) have probes for the identification of two fungi, *Histoplasma capsulatum* var. *capsulatum* and *Cryptococcus neoformans*. Both fungi are on the increase as causes of serious systemic disease in immunocompromised individuals, including patients with AIDS, and can take several weeks to culture and identify by conventional means. These chemiluminescence-labelled probes are complementary to rRNA sequences. In a recent study both probes demonstrated 100% specificity and sensitivity and significantly reduced the time required for definitive identification.

The recent increase in **tuberculosis** among the homeless, intravenous drug abusers and patients with AIDS, its persistence in the Third World and the emergence of multiply resistant strains has made tuberculosis once again a major health challenge. Not only is culture of *Mycobacterium tuberculosis* slow but speciation by biochemical tests requires a further 2–3 weeks' incubation. Gene-Probe's DNA probe against mycobacterial rRNA is labelled with an acridinium ester. After incubating the probe with the organism, and removing unhybridized probe by chemical degradation, the hybridized, labelled probe is hydrolysed, producing a visible light. Specificity is high but sensitivity is limited by the need to have at least 10^6 organisms/ml. By combining new culture methods with DNA probes organisms can now be both detected and identified within 2 weeks of culture inoculation.

Now that genes are being identified which encode for antibiotic resistance in tuberculosis, probes may soon be used to detect resistant strains. Meanwhile an innovative method of rapid drug testing has been developed. Mycobacteria were infected with phages expressing the firefly luciferase gene. Light production was detectable within minutes of infecting the mycobacterium with phage. When an organism was exposed to a drug to which it was susceptible the light was extinguished, but light continued to be produced from a strain which was resistant.

DNA hybridization remains the gold standard for species identification of members of the genus *Legionella* — *Legionella pneumophila* is the cause of respiratory infections including legionnaires' disease. It is relatively time consuming and technically demanding so alternative approaches are being developed based on DNA fingerprints (p. 230).

In the diagnosis of parasitic infections serology is generally inferior to direct detection of the parasite because often there are cross-reactive antigens, limiting specificity, and discrimination between current and previous or latent infection is poor. Microscopy requires experience, time and a high level of parasites to be sensitive and cannot discriminate between morphologically identical organisms. Therefore DNA-based diagnostics (Table 12.4) have much to offer in this field, though generally amplification of the DNA target by PCR is now preferred because of the increase in sensitivity (Fig. 12.2).

DNA probes have been useful in the identification of

Table 12.4 Examples of DNA probes used in the diagnosis of parasitic infections.

Infection	Species	Target	Comments
Malaria	*Plasmodium falciparum*	21 basepair repeats	Highly species specific but generally less sensitive than microscopy with low levels of parasitaemia
Leishmaniasis	*Leishmania* spp.	kDNA* minicircle	Lack sensitivity and specificity
Chagas' disease	*Trypanosoma cruzi*	kDNA minicircle	Lack sensitivity and specificity
Amoebic dysentery	*Entamoeba histolytica*	Repetitive DNA rRNA genes	Differentiates it from other non-pathogenic amoebae in the gut
Trichomonas	*Trichomonas vaginalis*	2.3 kb fragment	Higher sensitivity than microscopy

* kDNA, kinetoplast DNA (targeted because there are multiple copies per cell).

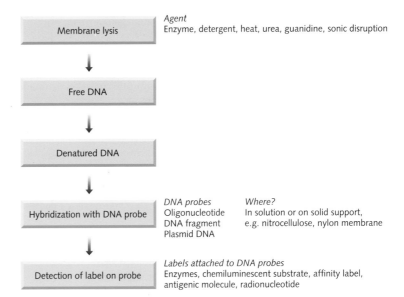

Fig. 12.2 Schematic presentation of the steps involved in the detection of parasites by DNA probes.

Entamoeba histolytica, the cause of **amoebic dysentery** in tropical countries. The intestine can be colonized by several types of amoebae, including several species of *Entamoeba,* of which only *E. histolytica* is pathogenic. Conventional diagnosis, by microscopic examination of faecal material, frequently overestimates the prevalence of pathogenic *E. histolytica* because of the inability to distinguish pathogenic and non-pathogenic strains and the presence of other morphologically similar species. Non-pathogenic *E. histolytica* (which is regarded by some as a distinct species, *E. dispar*) possesses different isoenzyme patterns and contains some distinct DNA sequences which have been used to differentiate between the two (Table 12.4). DNA probes also appear to be superior to microscopy for another protozoan, *Trichomonas vaginalis,* a common cause of vaginal discharge.

Polymerase chain reaction

In certain circumstances PCR has advantages over conventional laboratory diagnosis by culture (Table 12.5). The potential of PCR to detect extremely small amounts of DNA has made it an obvious procedure for attempting diagnoses from tiny samples such as those taken from fine needle biopsies or aspirates. PCR can be performed from less than ten copies of target DNA and can even be applied to archival material such as fixed, paraffin wax-embedded tissue. Its sensitivity is also a major asset when trying to detect a pathogen in a highly diluted environment. For example it detected *Legionella* in

water to a level of 350 CFU/ml—and less than 1 CFU/ml when combined with blot hybridization. But interpretation of a positive PCR can raise its own problems, such as whether or not the organism is viable and what levels are considered significant (Table 12.6).

Pneumocystis carinii is one of the most frequent opportunistic pulmonary pathogens in immunosuppressed subjects such as those receiving cancer chemotherapy and those with AIDS. The confinement of *Pneumocystis* to the pulmonary alveoli and the absence of a culture method for the organism have posed important diagnostic problems and problems relating to targeted therapy. These problems have been addressed by developing a PCR diagnostic that identifies DNA sequences of *P. carinii* obtained from the lungs of experimental animals with immunosuppression. Microbespecific DNA sequences were selected from a genomic library and found by analysis to encode a large subunit

Table 12.5 Situations in which PCR offers considerable benefits over conventional culture.

Problem with culture	Example
Small amount of material	Fine-needle aspirate
High dilution factor	Water testing
Low sensitivity	Invasive aspergillosis, DC
Slow growth or hazardous	Tuberculosis
No growth	Pneumocystis

Problem	Comments
False positives due to contamination	Avoidable through technical improvements
False positives due to the pathogen also being a commensal	May be avoidable by quantification; meanwhile ideally select samples from 'sterile' sites
Cost	Patented PCR technology keeping costs high
Staff time and training	Increasingly easy assay formats available
Clinical interpretation may be difficult, because of e.g. detection of dead bacteria	e.g. Determining whether a *Salmonella* carrier is still a source of infection
Lack of standardization and quality control	Solvable if a sufficient number of labs feel adoption of the test is worthwhile

Table 12.6 Diagnostic difficulties encountered with PCR.

of ribosomal RNA in mitochondria, with sequence homology to mitochondrial ribosomal genes of a red yeast fungus. Ribosomal genes, and particularly those in mitochondria, are likely to be present in many copies thus facilitating their detection by specific diagnostic probes. Based on sequence analysis, priming oligonucleotides for DNA amplification as well as internal oligonucleotide probes to confirm the identity of the amplified products in the PCR were synthesized. Use of these primers in DNA samples extracted from the lungs of infected experimental animals as well as humans allowed specific amplification products from *P. carinii* to be identified — an identity confirmed by hybridization with radioactively labelled oligonucleotides but annealed specifically to the *P. carinii* mitochondrial ribosomal RNA. It was found, using this confirmatory hybridization, that a weak but positive signal could be obtained when the initial sample contained as little as one or two organisms. Potential difficulties arising from contamination of the PCR were overcome by the use of appropriate negative control samples, scrupulous attention to contamination and the use of UV irradiation of all laboratory agents before addition of the sample of template DNA to be tested.

The *P. carinii*-specific method has been tested on different diagnostic samples obtained during multiple episodes of acute respiratory illnesses in subjects known to have AIDS. The results of DNA amplification of bronchoscopic lavage samples were compared with results of conventional silver staining and microscopy for the organism, with diagnosis based on clinical and radiographic features and with now known outcomes to specific treatment. No *P. carinii* DNA was seen in samples from immunocompetent subjects, and weak signals, detectable only by oligonucleotide hybridization of the PCR products, were found in 10 of 46 samples from immunosuppressed individuals not considered on other

grounds to have *Pneumocystis* pneumonia (see Fig. 12.3b).

Thus the PCR test gives strong and specific hybridization signals in bronchoscopic lavage samples and sputum obtained from a majority of individuals who ultimately are shown to suffer from *Pneumocystis* pneumonia. In the occasional individual, strong signals appear to be obtained in the absence of active clinical disease, though in most instances this develops shortly after the *Pneumocystis* organism is detected.

PCR has been successfully applied to the detection of *Aspergillus* species in bronchoalveolar lavage fluids from patients with suspected **invasive aspergillosis**. It can even, in a minority of cases, detect the fungus in urine specimens from infected patients. However further studies have emphasized the problem of false positives due either to cross-contamination or the patient being colonized but not invasively infected. The former has been recognized as an issue with PCR for many years and not only are there well-described technical precautions which should be taken, but also false positives can be detected by judicious use of duplicate samples and negative controls. The latter is a more difficult problem, common with many bacterial and fungal 'opportunistic' pathogens which in immunocompromised patients can cause disease or exist in an asymptomatic commensal state in which they 'colonize' their host. Therefore merely detecting an opportunistic pathogen by PCR does not prove it is the cause of disease (unless it comes from what should be a sterile site, such as CSF) as with detection of a 'primary' pathogen, such as HIV or tubercle, which do not occur as harmless commensals.

Distinction between infection and colonization is conventionally decided on the basis of such factors as whether there is a pure or mixed growth on culture, the latter indicating contamination with resident bacterial flora, and whether the same strain of bacterium is repeat-

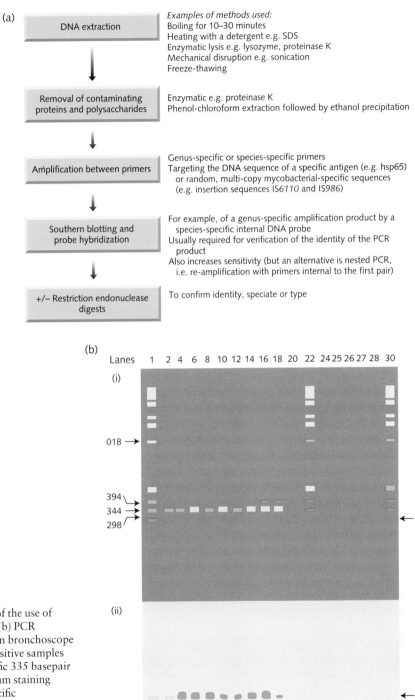

(a)

DNA extraction

Examples of methods used:
Boiling for 10–30 minutes
Heating with a detergent e.g. SDS
Enzymatic lysis e.g. lysozyme, proteinase K
Mechanical disruption e.g. sonication
Freeze-thawing

Removal of contaminating proteins and polysaccharides

Enzymatic e.g. proteinase K
Phenol-chloroform extraction followed by ethanol precipitation

Amplification between primers

Genus-specific or species-specific primers
Targeting the DNA sequence of a specific antigen (e.g. hsp65)
  or random, multi-copy mycobacterial-specific sequences
  (e.g. insertion sequences IS6110 and IS986)

Southern blotting and probe hybridization

For example, of a genus-specific amplification product by a
  species-specific internal DNA probe
Usually required for verification of the identity of the PCR
  product
Also increases sensitivity (but an alternative is nested PCR,
  i.e. re-amplification with primers internal to the first pair)

+/– Restriction endonuclease digests

To confirm identity, speciate or type

(b)

Lanes   1   2 4 6 8 10 12 14 16 18 20   22 24 25 26 27 28 30

(i)

018 →

394 \
344 →
298 /

(ii)

Fig. 12.3 (a) Schematic presentation of the use of PCR in the diagnosis of tuberculosis. (b) PCR diagnosis of *Pneumocystis carinii* from bronchoscope lavage or induced sputum. A set of positive samples (alternate tracks 2–18) with the specific 335 basepair product (arrowed) detected by ethidium staining (upper) and by hybridization to a specific oligonucleotide probe. The tracks with multiple DNA fragments represent markers of defined size, as indicated on the left of the gel.

edly isolated from the same or multiple sites. For antigen-based diagnostics the titre of antigen obtained is often critical in determining its diagnostic significance. Technology for overcoming the problems associated with

quantitative PCR is now being developed (Table 12.7) and it is proving particularly useful in monitoring the disease state of certain viral infections. It has also been applied to the quantification of *Salmonella enteriditis* in

Problem	Some solutions
Variation in the amplification efficiency of different reaction tubes affecting the final concentration of the PCR product	Co-amplification of a predetermined quantity of a competitor template, which must be distinguishable from the target product ('competitive PCR')
The plateau effect which occurs at high cycle numbers	Terminate the number of cycles while still in the exponential phase (but lowers sensitivity)
Loading errors causing inaccuracies in the amount of starting material	Amplification of a second 'housekeeping' reporter gene—then determine target: control products ratio ('differential PCR')

Table 12.7 Technical difficulties peculiar to quantitative PCR.

broth cultures, to distinguish tuberculoid from lepromatous leprosy, and for estimation of the level of parasitaemia in Chagas' disease.

Tuberculosis is an obvious target for diagnosis by PCR. More than 20 different protocols have been successfully applied to the detection of low numbers of the organism in clinical specimens (Fig. 12.3a). In some studies sensitivities have been higher than by culture. While contamination of specimens during amplification, causing false positives, is one possible explanation, culture is well known to be relatively insensitive and therefore PCR may indeed be detecting genuine cases missed by culture. In one carefully conducted study, 80% of clinically diagnosed cases were positive by PCR compared with 67% by culture.

Other species of mycobacteria can also be detected and one group has used PCR to identify all the species and subspecies of mycobacteria encountered in the diagnostic laboratory. There still remains a need to develop robust, simple systems suitable for commercialization. In particular, protocols are required which would more reliably remove inhibitors of PCR (one of the most potent being blood) and avoid false positives due to contamination. Also, since PCR detects both living and dead bacteria, precise clinical interpretation will need to be evaluated.

Preliminary PCR systems have been devloped for the detection of many different parasites but few have been evaluated on large numbers of clinical specimens and/or field conditions. Usually they are more sensitive than DNA probe assays, and can detect the DNA of just one parasite, but to achieve this degree of sensitivity with human specimens will require improvements in methods of extracting DNA while removing PCR inhibitors.

Molecular epidemiology

The development of microbial typing systems is essential to understanding of the epidemiology and spread of infection within the community or hospital environment.

It provides the basis upon which infection can be prevented by instigation of appropriate vaccination programmes or cross-infection control procedures. Traditionally typing systems have relied on the expression of phenotypic characteristics, manifesting as strain-to-strain variation in attributes such as biotype, serotype, phage susceptibility and antibiotic resistance profiles. Increasingly these are being supplemented or replaced by DNA-based 'genotypic' typing systems (Table 12.8).

DNA fingerprinting

Genetic variation between different strains of a microorganism can usually be detected by digesting plasmid or chromosomal DNA with restriction endonucleases. These cut at specific sequences generating DNA fragments the size and number of which vary with the location and frequency with which the restriction site occurs in the DNA. These are then separated by gel electrophoresis and visualized with ethidium bromide, creating a 'DNA fingerprint' of the strain. Intrinsic advantages of most genotypic typing systems are that all isolates can be typed, genetic stability is usually high and the whole genome is in effect screened. The chances of variants being detected is increased if more than one restriction endonuclease is used. An intrinsic disadvantage is that, unless centred around DNA which codes for a critical phenotype such as a virulence plasmid, genotype is unlikely to have any bearing on pathogenicity or spread. In contrast, the serotype of a microbe (e.g. *Salmonella* species, *Haemophilus influenzae*, meningococcus) often gives clinically valuable information as to its virulence or risk of epidemic spread.

Microbial typing systems are classically assessed in terms of their **typability** (the proportion of isolates which yield a type), **reproducibility** (whether the same result is obtained on repeated testing) and **discrimination** (ability to differentiate between strains). DNA fingerprinting systems usually compare favourably with phenotypic typing systems on these criteria (Table 12.9), but the

Table 12.8 DNA-based fingerprinting systems.

Procedure	Comments	Examples of applications
Plasmid fingerprinting	Restriction endonuclease digests of plasmid DNA Robust, rapid, inexpensive technique Plasmid instability a disadvantage	Coagulase-negative staphylococci (CNS), *Yersinia enterocolitica*
Generation of restriction fragment length polymorphisms	Restriction endonuclease digests of chromosomal DNA Stable and often more discriminatory than plasmid fingerprinting Sometimes difficult to analyse because of the number of fragments generated	*Legionella pneumophila, Clostridium difficile, Candida albicans*
Southern blots and ribotyping	Simplifies interpretation—RFLP is transferred (Southern blot) to a membrane and probed with mitochondrial DNA, rDNA (ribotyping), or a randomly cloned DNA fragment. Relatively slow and expensive; may require radioisotopes	*Enterobacter, Acinetobacter, Pseudomonas, Legionella pneumophila,* CNS
Pulsed-field gel electrophoresis	Rare-cutting restriction endonuclease → generation of large DNA fragments → separated by special techniques e.g. PFGE. Slow and expensive	*Bordetella pertussis, Staphylococcus aureus, Candida* (karyotyping)
PCR amplification of a specific variable site	Primers selected so as to amplify a single variable sequence or a consensus sequence with variable distribution; may be followed by restriction endonuclease digests, probe hybridization or DNA sequencing	*Giardia, Naegleria*
Random amplification of polymorphic DNA	PCR performed with a short, arbitrarily selected primer under conditions of low stringency → binding to multiple sites → generation of multiple products of different length. Simple and fast	*Trypanosoma cruzi, Aspergillus fumigatus, Cryptococcus neoformans, Helicobacter pylori, Staphylococcus aureus*

Table 12.9 Comparison of DNA fingerprinting with phenotypic typing systems.

Criteria	DNA fingerprinting	Phenotypic typing
Typability	All isolates typable (with the exception of plasmid fingerprinting)	Variable, e.g. some isolates may be non-typable with phage
Reproducibility	Usually good once technique standardized	Often poor because subject to selection pressures on phenotype
Discrimination	Often good; if not can be improved by using more than one restriction enzyme or combining with Southern blotting	Methods such as serotyping may be highly discriminatory for one species but poor for another
Specialized reagents	Not required	Usually required (e.g. type-specific antisera, phages) and sometimes only available at reference centres
Turn around time	Usually <24 hours but longer if PFGE or Southern blotting required	Very fast (e.g. serotyping) to days or weeks (e.g. biotyping)
Cost	Relatively expensive	Often inexpensive
Staff training	Minimal once familiar with DNA technology; often applicable to other genera or species	Some technically simple and routinely performed; others highly specialized and specific to a particular genus or species

success of a DNA fingerprinting procedure varies widely with the microbe to which it is being applied. Therefore while the techniques themselves are highly versatile, whether or not they will generate a useful typing system for a particular microbe is largely a matter of experimentation. For example the causative agent of whooping cough, *Bordetella pertussis*, when analysed by *Eco*RI-generated restriction fragment length polymorphism

(RFLP), showed a high degree of conservation such that it was impossible to discriminate between strains. In contrast, generation of macrorestriction digests, using a rare-cutting restriction endonuclease, and separation of these much larger DNA fragments by pulsed field gel electrophoresis (PFGE) generated over 22 different DNA types — a far higher level of discrimination than achievable by conventional serotyping.

Macrorestriction digests, which have to be separated by specialized procedures such as PFGE, are often easier to analyse than the RFLPs generated with more frequently cutting restriction endonucleases and separated by conventional agarose gel electrophoresis. But the procedure itself is much more demanding, of time and technical skill, and expensive in terms of the apparatus required. Another means of increasing both the level of discrimination achieved and simpler fingerprints for analysis, is to probe restriction endonuclease-generated digests with one or more DNA probes. This takes considerably more time since the DNA must be transferred onto a membrane (a process called 'Southern blotting') prior to hybridization with the probe. Usually the probes are labelled with radioisotopes which are then visualized through the process of autoradiography, though increasingly these are being replaced with non-radioactive labels which are safer, have a longer shelf-life and are cheaper overall.

PCR has again had a significant impact in this field. In comparison with other DNA fingerprinting systems, PCR-based systems are generally faster, simpler and require less DNA — typically nanogram quantities, a thousand times less than those required for non-PCR techniques. The usual precautions against contamination must be taken. Particularly widely used have been the random amplification of polymorphic DNA (RAPD) or 'arbitrarily primed' PCR (AP-PCR) fingerprinting

systems. These use a single, short, arbitrary primer and conditions of low stringency (low annealing temperature) so that it anneals to multiple sites with varying degrees of mismatch generating polymorphic products. Unlike amplification of a specific variable region this requires no prior knowledge of the DNA sequence being amplified, and scans the whole genome, not one locus. Each primer gives a different PCR profile, so greater discrimination can be increased by using several primers. But while technically simple to perform, several studies have confirmed that the reliability of RAPD is critically dependent on reaction parameters such as reagent concentrations and the model of thermocycler used. The source of *Taq* polymerase can likewise have a significant effect: in one study a 'pseudocluster' of *Aspergillus fumigatus* infections appeared, nine isolates giving similar RAPD fingerprints (Fig. 12.4), but on repeating the analysis with *Taq* polymerase from a different manufacturer there were clearly differences (Fig. 12.5).

This emphasizes the need to rigorously examine new DNA fingerprinting systems on large numbers of isolates, some of which should be indistinguishable from each other (as in an outbreak) and others genetically heterogeneous (unrelated isolates from geographically disparate sources). The new typing scheme should then be assessed by comparison with the established gold standard typing system, in terms of typability, reproducibility and discrimination. Ideally standardization of protocols should lead to multi-centre participation. In practice this is rarely carried through.

Application to a hospital outbreak

DNA fingerprinting of microbes has several clinically useful applications (Table 12.10), of which early identification of hospital outbreaks is one of the most important.

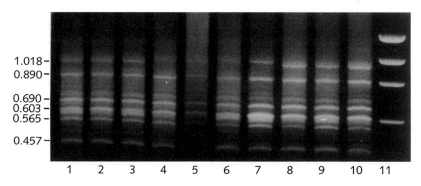

Fig. 12.4 RAPD fingerprints of 10 isolates of *Aspergillus fumigatus*, generated with Bioline *Taq* polymerase—a 'pseudocluster'. Molecular weight marker (*Hae*III-digested ρ x174) in lane 11. Sizes given in kilobases (reprinted with permission from Loudon K.W. *et al.* (1995) 'Pseudoclusters' and typing by random amplification of polymorphic DNA of *Aspergillus fumigatus*. *Journal of Clinical Pathology*, **48**, 183–184).

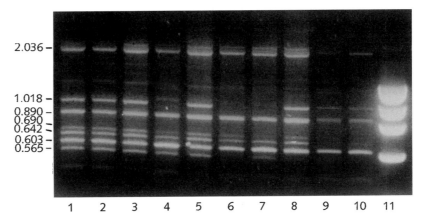

Fig. 12.5 RAPD fingerprints of the same isolates as in Fig. 12.4 generated by Roche AmpliTaq polymerase (reprinted with permission from Loudon K.W. *et al.* (1995) 'Pseudoclusters' and typing by random amplification of polymorphic DNA of *Aspergillus fumigatus. Journal of Clinical Pathology*, **48**, 183–184).

Table 12.10 Clinical applications of DNA fingerprinting.

Clinical application	Examples of where it has been applied
Investigation of outbreaks—early recognition, identifying source, defining size	Hospital outbreaks of methicillin-resistant *Staphylococcus aureus*, *Acinetobacter*, etc.
Elucidating mode of transmission	*Burkholderia* (*Pseudomonas*) *cepacia* in cystic fibrosis patients
Distinguishing relapse from reinfection—the latter is indicated if the strain is a different genotype	*E. coli* K1 meningitis, *Helicobacter pylori*-associated gastritis, *Candida albicans* in AIDS patients
Distinguishing infection from contamination—the latter is indicated by multiple strains	Coagulase-negative staphylococci isolated from blood cultures
Genetic relatedness	Comparison of the mouse-virulent strains of *Bordetella pertussis*, used in vaccine assessment in animals, with clinical isolates

The evolution of DNA fingerprinting systems and their application to nosocomial outbreaks is well illustrated by *Candida albicans*. This yeast is the commonest cause of DC, which has become increasingly frequent in immuno-compromised patients — in hospitals in the US *Candida* species are now the fourth commonest cause of positive blood cultures. DC has a high mortality of 70%, so prevention is particularly desirable. Traditionally DC was attributed to autoinfection by yeasts, colonizing the patient's bowel or intravenous catheters, initiating systemic invasion because of a breakdown in host defence mechanisms. Recognition that DC could also result from the spread of *C. albicans* from one patient to another depended on the development of typing systems. Initially these were based on phenotypic characters (serotyping, biotyping, morphotyping or immunoblot fingerprinting) but these lacked reproducibility or discrimination. The *Eco*RI-generated RFLPs were successfully used to delineate the epidemiology of a series of outbreaks occurring on geographically distinct intensive care units and a peritoneal dialysis unit. The first of these occurred at the Royal London Hospital (Fig. 12.6). An outbreak strain was identified which was far more common in the intensive care unit than in the rest of the hospital. It colonized a proportion of nursing staff, survived better than control strains on nurses' hands, and was more resistant to Hibiscrub, the disinfectant in use at the time. This was changed to povidone–iodine or Hibisol, since the strain proved fully sensitive to these reagents in handwashing studies, and routine prophylaxis with ketoconazole was

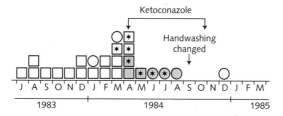

Fig. 12.6 Distribution over time of cases of DC occurring on the intensive care unit at the Royal London Hospital, between July 1983 and March 1984, due to an outbreak strain (□) and a non-outbreak strain (○). Shading indicates patient received prophylactic ketoconazole (given to all patients on the unit from May to October 1984). Existing handwashing reagents were replaced with fungicidal disinfectants in September 1984. *Suspected cases (reprinted with permission from Burnie J.P. et al. (1985) Control of an outbreak of systemic *Candida albicans*. *British Medical Journal*, **291**, 1092–1093).

instigated. Only with the recognition that cross-infection was occurring could such procedures (with their associated cost and risks) be justified.

Now that both PFGE and RAPD have been applied to fingerprinting *C. albicans*, the outbreak has been re-examined by these methods. Phenotypic typing of the outbreak strain had shown it to be serotype A, morphotype A, biotype 0/1,5,5/7 and immunoblot type 1. Using *Eco*RI-generated RFLPs, it was designated type 14, and

18 isolates from 11 patients with DC and two colonized patients had the outbreak strain. But when these isolates were examined by PFGE, five different patterns were revealed, and mixed 'types' frequently occurred among isolates from the same patient (Fig. 12.7). In contrast RAPD fingerprinting (with two primers) correlated well with the results of *Eco*RI-generated RFLPs, correctly identifying the outbreak strain (Fig. 12.8). Southern blotting the PFGE fingerprints and analysis with chromosome-specific probes confirmed that anomalies could result from genetic switching induced by factors such as growth in different media.

This study suggests PFGE is too sensitive as a typing system for delineating *Candida* cross-infections because it picks up unstable variants due to genetic switching. The discovery that a sensitive DNA fingerprinting system reveals differences between two isolates which should be the same strain is not new, and underlines the importance of assessing their clinical value with isolates for which there is a detailed epidemiological history.

New and improved vaccines

Historically a range of highly effective vaccines has been developed using the whole organism (inactivated or alive but attenuated) or some fraction derived from it (subcomponent vaccines). Such vaccines have saved millions of lives, without the need for the identification and devel-

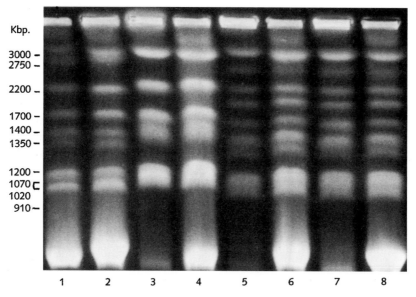

Fig. 12.7 Three isolates (each in duplicate) from a patient with DC from the outbreak at the Royal London Hospital. The PFGE fingerprint of the isolate from the blood (lanes 3 and 4) was different from the PFGE fingerprints of the two isolates cultured from post-mortem material taken at the same time (lanes 5 and 6, and lanes 7 and 8, respectively). Lanes 1 and 2 are duplicates of the PFGE fingerprint of a control strain, *C. albicans* NCTC 3153, showing sizes in kilobases.

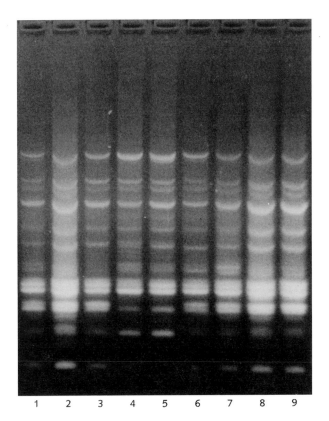

Fig. 12.8 RAPD fingerprints of nine isolates from three patients (lanes 1–3, lanes 4–5 and lanes 6–9, respectively; cultured from various sites) temporally related to the outbreak, showing the same fingerprint occurring from all isolates from two of the patients (lanes 1–3 and 6–9) and a distinct fingerprint for the two isolates from the third patient (lanes 4–5). The three isolates in lanes 1–3 are the same as those shown in Fig. 12.7.

opment of chemically synthesized or recombinant immunogens. But for some pathogens, such as malaria, large-scale production by *in vitro* culture is not feasible and derivation from human blood undesirable because of the risk of contamination by pathogenic human viruses. Alternative strategies based on molecular biology have been crucial to the development of malaria vaccines which are amenable to large-scale, cost-effective production. In other instances, such as the widely used *Haemophilus influenzae* type B (Hib) vaccine, an understanding of molecular immunology has been crucial to the design of immunogenic, protective vaccines. But the fastest growing field in vaccine-related research is now nucleic acid vaccination.

Malaria vaccines

There are over 300 million cases of malaria each year with an estimated 3 million deaths. Naturally acquired immunity is short-lived unless reinforced by frequent reinfection. Therefore to be effective a malaria vaccine must induce more protective, long-lasting immunity than the infection itself. There have been significant advances towards reaching this goal (Table 12.11). Molecular techniques have been the key to the identification and synthesis of specific malarial antigens as recombinant proteins, to mapping the sites to which antibodies bind (epitopes) and in the production of synthetic peptides representing immunodominant epitopes. An important property of the immunogen is that it is antigenically conserved so that all strains are susceptible to the elicited immune response.

Recently, encouraging results have been obtained with the SPf66 vaccine in several clinical trials in South America, including a reported 39% reduction in clinical episodes of malaria in one double-blind, placebo-controlled study. This is a chemically-synthesized 45 amino acid peptide constructed by chemically linked sequences derived from four different proteins of *Plasmodium falciparum* (three merozoite proteins and circumsporozoite protein) that elicit protective immunity to malaria.

Conjugate vaccines

Encapsulated bacteria, such as the pneumococci and *Haemophilus influenzae*, rely on their polysaccharide capsule to evade the host's defensive system. Induction of anti-capsular antibodies by immunization protects against disease by enhancing phagocytosis of the bacteria. The development of a vaccine against pneumococci was complicated by the antigenically distinct capsular serotypes. This was partially resolved by devising a polyvalent vaccine containing purified polysaccharide from the commonest serotypes. However a remaining problem with the current vaccine is that it does not reliably induce protective antibodies in children under 2 years of age—the age group with the highest incidence of invasive pneumococcal infection and meningitis—nor in patients with immunodeficiency disorders or haematological malignancies. This is because polysaccharides are recognized mainly by T-cell-independent mechanisms, which are poor at inducing high-affinity antibodies, particularly in young children. Nor do they induce the T-cell memory required for booster responses. Better responses would probably be induced by covalently linking the polysaccharide to a carrier protein recognized by T-cells, producing a so-called 'conjugated' vaccine.

This was illustrated by the development of conjugate vaccines for **Hib**. The first vaccines against this bacterium, which causes a variety of serious infections in young children including meningitis, consisted of purified

Table 12.11 Landmarks in the development of malaria vaccines.

Landmark	Comments
Vaccinated recipients, exposed to bites from irradiated mosquitoes, became resistant to sporozoite challenge	Proof of concept Method not suitable for mass vaccination
In vitro culture of blood stages of *Plasmodium falciparum*	Allowed characterization of antigens, mode of invasion, erythrocyte receptor. Not a source of parasites for mass vaccination
Simian and rodent malarias	Investigation of immunity in animal models—but sometimes gave misleading results
Key malarial antigens expressed in recombinant bacterial and viral systems	e.g. *Salmonella*, vaccinia
Antigens produced by synthetic peptide chemistry	Definition of T- and B-cell epitopes
CS protein—first synthetic vaccine to undergo clinical trials—an immunodominant B-cell epitope of the CS protein coupled to tetanus toxoid as a carrier	Found on the surface of the invasive sporozoite stage. Only partially effective therefore newer vaccines being developed incorporate multiple T- and B-cell epitopes
SPf66—first blood-stage vaccine to undergo extensive clinical trials	Multicomponent vaccine Early results from several trials encouraging

CS, circumsporozoite.

polyribosylribitol phosphate (PRP), the component of the polysaccharide capsule. However these vaccines were not sufficiently immunogenic in young children — as shown by one study reporting 90% efficacy in children older than 18 months of age, but little protection for younger children. Now several conjugate Hib vaccines are available, linking the polysaccharide hapten to protein carriers such as tetanus toxoid or the outer membrane protein of the meningococcus. These are immunogenic in young children, induce booster responses, and have been shown to be safe and effective in clinical practice. Routine vaccination of all children under 4 years old with conjugated Hib vaccine was launched in the UK in October 1992 and there has been a dramatic decline in the incidence of invasive Hib infections in young children.

Nucleic acid vaccines

Recently, it has become apparent that inoculation of purified genetic material intradermally or intramuscularly can elicit protective immune responses against encoded antigens in mice and other animals. Such nucleic acid vaccines have an intrinsic advantage over synthetic or recombinant proteins for intracellular pathogens, including many viruses and protozoan parasites. They allow presentation of microbial antigens to the immune system in a form, synthesized by the host, similar to that occurring in infection. The antigens syn-

thesized from the injected genetic material within the host cell are directed to the MHC class I and II antigens in the same way as viral antigens during infection (see Chapter 13) and therefore should elicit similar cellular immune responses. Another advantage is that this approach obviates the need for a carrier. Disadvantages include unresolved safety concerns.

An interesting bacterial application has been in the development of potential DNA vaccines against tuberculosis. The current BCG vaccine is far from ideal—efficacy varies from 80% to zero in different parts of the world—therefore better vaccines are highly desirable. A substantial cell-mediated protective response against **tuberculosis** was observed in mice following injection with the gene encoding mycobacterial hsp65.

Drug design and immunotherapy

Up until now, most antimicrobials have been antibiotics empirically obtained by screening soil or microorganisms (often fungi) for substances with antibacterial activity. Molecular techniques are then useful in determining their mechanism of action, the means by which bacteria become resistant, and obtaining derivatives with greater efficacy or safety but that were not used to create the parent antibiotic. Molecular biology has now given us the ability to adopt a very different approach. By using these techniques to better understand the

Table 12.12 Mechanisms of resistance to β-lactam antibiotics.

Mechanism	Example	Comments
Production of β-lactamases	Widespread among bacteria	These enzymes catalyse hydrolysis of the β-lactam ring, inactivating the antibiotic
Alteration in the antibiotic target (ie. penicillin-binding protein, PBP)	Methicillin-resistant staphylococci	Synthesis of an additional PBP, with much lower affinity than normal PBP, so cell wall synthesis continues
Alteration in access to the PBP	Gram-negative bacteria	Mutation in the outer membrane protein channels (porin) decreases permeability to the antibiotic

pathogenesis and immunology of infectious diseases we can rationally design new therapeutics and effective, safe vaccines. Equally important is the ability we now have to develop **genetically-engineered antibodies** and **cytokines** to augment existing antibiotics.

Mechanisms of antibiotic resistance

Probably the best documented example is the genetic and biochemical basis of resistance to the penicillin family (β-lactams). These antibiotics inhibit the sythesis of the bacterial cell wall. Clinical isolates can exhibit any one (or more than one) of three mechanisms of resistance (Table 12.12). The genes encoding β-lactamases are particularly ubiquitous. Of the many different β-lactamases, TEM-1 is the most frequently isolated probably because it is located on transposons, facilitating transmission between bacteria. Recently it has been shown that TEM-1 has a remarkable capacity to cope with the newer, so-called β-lactamase-stable cephalosporins. Bacteria evolved TEM-derived β-lactamases with an extended spectrum of activity which had the ability to hydrolyse these drugs.

This emphasizes the fact that even where the molecular mechanisms underlying antibiotic resistance are well known, bacteria are constantly evolving to meet the challenge of more sophisticated (and more expensive) antibiotics.

Immunotherapy—recombinant antibodies and cytokines

Before the dawn of the antibiotic era in the 1940s, antibodies, in the form of immune sera, were used to treat a variety of life-threatening infections e.g. pneumococcal pneumonia. Such therapy was limited by the risks of serum sickness, viral contamination and cost, but the inexorable rise in antibiotic resistance and advances in

antibody engineering have made use of recombinant antibodies attractive for exploration.

Murine monoclonals induce a damaging human anti-mouse antibody (HAMA) response when given repeatedly to patients. But the modular arrangement of the immunoglobulin molecule into functional domains makes it particularly accessible to protein engineering. The variable domains of the heavy and light chains carry out antigen binding, primarily at the hypervariable complementarity-determining regions (CDR). By combining these domains, or better still just the CDRs, from a protective murine monoclonal antibody with the constant region domains of a human immunoglobulin, the immunogenicity of the rodent monoclonal is reduced (Table 12.13).

More recently it has proved possible to produce short, antigen-binding antibody fragments (single chain Fv or Fab) which are totally human in origin having been derived from the mRNA of antibody-producing human white cells. Using PCR to amplify up variable sequences between relatively conserved primers, heavy and light chain domains are covalently linked together and

Table 12.13 Advances in antibody engineering.

Type of antibody	Construct
Chimeric antibody	Murine heavy and light chain variable domains + human heavy and light chain constant domains
'Reshaped' antibody	Murine hypervariable antigen binding sequences (CDRs) grafted onto human immunoglobulin
Human recombinant antibody fragments	scFv or Fab fragments derived from human lymphocyte mRNA, expressed as fusion proteins on the surface of a filamentous phage

Category	Main sources	Main activities
Interferons, e.g. γ-IFN	Cells which have become virally infected T-cells	Resistance to viral infections
Interleukins (IL-1 to 8)	Most come from T-cells, but some from NK cells, macrophages etc.	Directing specific groups of cells (e.g. T-cells, B-cells, haemopoietic precursors) to divide and differentiate Chemotaxis (IL-8)
Colony-stimulating factors, e.g. M-CSF	T-cells	Directing division and differentiation of bone marrow stem cells and leukocyte precursors
Tumour necrosis factors (TNFα, TNFβ)	Macrophages, lymphocytes	Inflammation, catabolism, fibrosis, etc.

Table 12.14 Main categories of cytokines.

Target	Microbes in which it is associated with protection	Comments
hsp60 (65)	*Mycobacterium tuberculosis*, *Histoplasma capsulatum*	Induces protective cell-mediated immune responses in mice models of these infections
hsp90	*Candida albicans*, *Plasmodium falciparum*	Induces humoral immunity associated with recovery from the infection in animal models; scFv to hsp90 shown to be protective in murine models of DC
PAc	Oral viridans streptococci, e.g. *Streptococcus mutans*	Human studies show antibodies to PAc inhibit development of dental caries (of which *S. mutans* is the main bacterial cause)

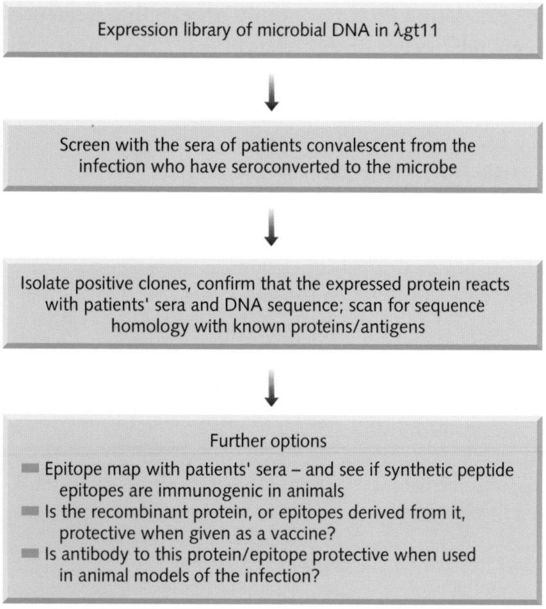

Table 12.15 Some examples of microbial antigens identified through DNA technology which have been associated with the induction of protective immune responses.

Expression library of microbial DNA in λgt11

↓

Screen with the sera of patients convalescent from the infection who have seroconverted to the microbe

↓

Isolate positive clones, confirm that the expressed protein reacts with patients' sera and DNA sequence; scan for sequence homology with known proteins/antigens

↓

Further options

 Epitope map with patients' sera – and see if synthetic peptide epitopes are immunogenic in animals
 Is the recombinant protein, or epitopes derived from it, protective when given as a vaccine?
 Is antibody to this protein/epitope protective when used in animal models of the infection?

Fig. 12.9 Schematic presentation of one approach to the use of DNA technology in identifying immunodominant microbial antigens recognized by infected patients' antisera.

expressed as fusion proteins on the surface of filamentous phage — creating a combinatorial phage display library of antibody fragments. High-affinity human recombinant antibodies can be derived from such libraries. As yet clinical experience with humanized or human recombinant antibodies is sparse. What little data there are have been mainly obtained with humanized antibodies against tumours.

Cytokines are a heterogeneous group of soluble factors involved in signalling between cells during the immune response (Table 12.14). Since they are relatively low molecular weight proteins they are amenable to DNA cloning and expression and a number of recombinant cytokines have been used for tumour therapy, though successes have been few and far between. More recently cytokines seem to have found a clinically useful role in shortening the period of aplasia after bone marrow transplantation or cytotoxic chemotherapy. Clinical trials indicate that macrophage colony-stimulating factor and γ-interferon improve the functional activity of macrophages and leukocytes against invasive fungal infections, augmenting the activity of conventional antifungal agents.

Target identification

Molecular biology has proved particularly fruitful in identifying immunodominant antigens associated with cell-mediated or humoral immunity to bacterial, fungal and parasitic infections (Fig. 12.9; Table 12.15). Often these have proved to be members of the various families of heat shock proteins, such as hsp60 and hsp90, and for some fungal and mycobacterial infections there is now good evidence that this immunity is indeed protective. For example both a murine monoclonal antibody and scFv against the same immunodominant epitope on hsp90 were therapeutic when given to mice with murine candidiasis. The epitope had been identified by epitope mapping C. albicans hsp90 with the sera of patients who had seroconverted during recovery from DC. Extrapolating these observations from animal models to human trials is a major undertaking which itself will depend heavily on the use of DNA recombinant technology.

Challenges for the future

Molecular microbiology has so far had greatest impact

in epidemiological studies and is increasingly important for the rapid diagnosis of infections. In both areas there remain issues of standardization and quality control but these will eventually be resolved. The greatest achievements are likely to be in the prevention and treatment of infections — development of better vaccines and the harnessing of the host's own defence strategies in the form of recombinant antibodies and cytokines. While these aspirations are still some way from being put into clinical practice, the need for a more rational approach to treatment is clear and molecular biology is providing us with the means to achieve this.

Further reading

Hawkey P.M. (1994) The role of the polymerase reaction in the diagnosis of mycobacterial infections. *Reviews in Medical Microbiology*, 5, 21–32.

Howard A.J. (1992) *Haemophilus influenzae* type b vaccines. *British Journal of Hospital Medicine*, 48, 44–46.

Kerr K.G. (1994) The rap on REP—PCR-based typing systems. *Reviews in Medical Microbiology*, 5, 233–244.

Lowrie D.B., Tascon R.E., Colston M.J. and Silva C.L. (1994) Towards a DNA vaccine against tuberculosis. *Vaccine*, 12, 1537–1540.

Malcomson R.D.G., McCullough C.T., Bruce D.J. and Harrison D.J. (1995) The scope of quantitative polymerase chain reaction assays in clinical molecular pathology. *Journal of Clinical Pathology*, 48, M178–M183.

Matthews R.C. and Burnie J.P. (1995) *Heat Shock Proteins in Fungal Infections*. Springer, New York.

Matthews R.C. and Burnie J.P. (1996) Mycoserology. In: *Microbiology and Microbial Infection*, 9th edn (eds L. Ajello and R. Hay), Vol. 4. Edward Arnold, London.

Nussenzweig R.S. and Long C.A. (1994) Malaria vaccines: multiple targets. *Science*, 265, 1381–1383.

Sepkowitz K.A., Raffalli J. *et al.* (1995) Tuberculosis in the AIDS era. *Clinical Microbiology Reviews*, 8, 180–199.

Slack M.P.E. (1995) Invasive *Haemophilus influenzae* disease: the impact of Hib immunisation. *Journal of Medical Microbiology*, 42, 75–77.

van Belkum A. (1994) DNA fingerprinting medically important microorganisms by use of PCR. *Clinical Microbiology Reviews*, 7, 174–184.

Weiss J.B. (1995) DNA probes and PCR for diagnosis of parasitic infections. *Clinical Microbiology Reviews*, 8, 113–130.

Winter G. and Milstein C. (1991) Man-made antibodies. *Nature*, 349, 293–299.

Chapter 13   Viral infections

Introduction

Diseases resulting from virus infections are some of the oldest (e.g. poliomyelitis) and newest (e.g. AIDS) recorded human diseases and include human cancer [associated with e.g. human papillomavirus, Epstein–Barr virus (EBV)]. Knowledge of the molecular biology of viruses and the mechanisms by which they infect cells helps us to understand the way in which they produce disease in the host, how the immune system confers resistance to infection, and how antiviral drugs and vaccines can be designed against viruses.

The study of viruses, the smallest organisms, at the molecular level has often been said to have benefited enormously from the application of molecular biological principles and techniques. However, in fact, there has been a two-way process in which molecular virology has contributed heavily to the whole subject of 'molecular and cellular biology'. A major reason for the contribution of virology to our general understanding of molecular and cellular biology is that viruses have the smallest complete genomes of any class of organisms. Consequently, they were the first genomes to be sequenced at the DNA level and the genome organization of a number of viruses has been extensively studied and manipulated—thus molecular biology is really inherent to the whole of virology. Furthermore, information gained from the study of virus infection, which can be looked on as an intracellular parasitic process and is in the main dependent on host cell machinery, has provided crucial insights into normal cellular physiology.

Viruses are conventionally classified according to: (i) their nucleic acid genome (single- or double-stranded RNA or DNA); (ii) the presence of an envelope; and (iii) morphology of the virus capsid (Table 13.1). In the space available we cannot deal with examples of each of the virus families, details of which are available elsewhere. We will thus focus on one RNA family (picornaviruses)

and an enveloped DNA virus family (herpesviruses), using other examples to illustrate specific points.

Virus structure

Viruses consist of a nucleic acid genome which is surrounded by a virus capsid, itself sometimes encased in an envelope—the **virion** or **virus particle**. Virion structure is classically determined by identification of proteins present in purified free virus preparations, followed by careful electron microscopy to define the nature of their interactions. However, although the resolution of this methodology permits the identification of glycoprotein on the envelope as 'spikes', and with immunoelectron microscopy individual glycoproteins can be identified, details such as the location of receptor and neutralizing antibody binding sites cannot be defined. Additionally, whilst electron microscopy can visualize individual capsomeres in the capsid structure and the symmetry of the capsid, which are important for classification, it has insufficient resolution to determine envelope–capsid–nucleic acid interactions. The more powerful technique of X-ray crystallography has therefore been applied to determine the structure of individual proteins and whole virus particles.

Viral glycoproteins

The first observations using X-ray crystallography were made on influenza haemagglutinin (HA). This molecule is present on the surface of the influenza virus envelope together with another viral glycoprotein neuraminidase (N) (Fig. 13.1). Previous functional studies had indicated that the HA interacted with sialic acid on the surface of the host cell to permit virus entry. The **major neutralizing epitopes**, the region of the protein recognized by antibodies which can prevent virus infection *in vitro*, were present on the HA molecule, whilst N allowed sialic acid

Table 13.1 Classification of human pathogenic viruses.

Virus	Envelope	Example
Single-stranded RNA viruses—positive sense		
Picornaviridae	No	Polioviruses, rhinoviruses, coxsackie, hepatitis A
Caliciviridae	No	Norwalk virus
Coronaviridae	Yes	
Togaviridae	Yes	Rubivirus, rubella, alphavirus, pestivirus
Flaviviridae	Yes	Yellow fever virus, West Nile virus
Retroviridae	Yes	Oncoviruses, HTLV1, spumaviruses, foamy virus, lentiviruses, HIV1 and 2
Single-stranded RNA viruses—negative sense		
Rhabdoviridae	Yes	Rabies
Filoviridae	Yes	Marburg virus, Ebola virus
Paramyxoviridiae	Yes	Mumps, measles, parainfluenza (RSV)
Orthomyxoviridae	Yes	Influenza
Arenaviridae	Yes	Lassa virus
Double-stranded RNA viruses		
Reoviridae	No	Reovirus, rotaviruses
Single-stranded DNA viruses		
Parvoviridae	No	Parvovirus B19, adeno-associated virus
Double-stranded DNA viruses		
Hepadnaviridae	Yes	Hepatitis B
Papovaviridae	No	Papillomaviruses (cutaneous and genital warts), polyomaviruses, BK and JC virus
Adenoviridae	No	Adenovirus serotypes
Herpesviridae	Yes	α herpes (herpes simplex 1 and 2, VZV), β herpes (CMV, herpesvirus 6) γ herpes (Epstein–Barr virus)
Poxviridae	Yes	Smallpox, vaccinia

residues to be more readily exposed on the cell surface. When the crystal structure of HA was described, it was clear that the virus–receptor interaction involved a trimer of the HA molecule. Furthermore the epitopes recognized by neutralizing antibodies were all located some distance from the receptor binding site, and were complex epitopes involving the secondary and tertiary structure of the protein. From a knowledge of this structure two other phenomena were explicable. First, the mechanism of influenza virus entry to the cell cytoplasm: a region within the HA stalk was identified which is strongly hydrophobic and is exposed on acidification by cleavage of the parent molecule to release HA1 and HA2 (Fig. 13.1). After the virus is taken into the endosomal compartment by receptor-mediated endocytosis, acidification in the vacuole exposes this site and allows fusion of the viral and endosomal membranes freeing the capsid to gain entry to the cytosol. Second, the mechanisms underlying viral 'shift' and 'drift' — variations in viral structural antigens, which allow the virus to evade anti-

body immunity and hence persist within the population —became explicable.

Influenza pandemics occurred in 1933, 1957 and 1968, each time caused by strains of influenza virus with major serological differences in the HA molecule and designated the H1, H2 and H3 subtypes, respectively. Although H1 and H3 share significant homology in regions such that the overall structure and binding site of the HA is preserved, considerable numbers of changes are detected in the regions shown in Fig. 13.1. It is probable that this major antigenic change or 'shift' results from influenza acquiring a 'new' HA, possibly from animal orthomyxoviridae by genetic recombination. The result of such a sudden change would be the failure of neutralizing antibodies present in individuals, as a result of natural infection with the previous strain, to inhibit the 'new' virus, resulting in a major pandemic.

However, even between the major pandemics sporadic cases or minor epidemics of influenza A infection occur. These may be accounted for by antigenic 'drift' or the

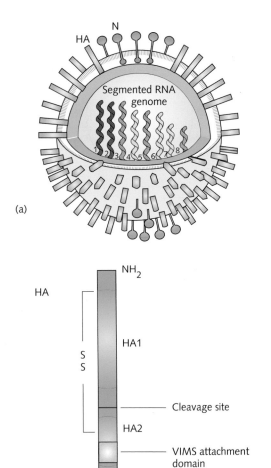

(a)

(b)

Fig. 13.1 (a) The structure of influenza virus is depicted with neuraminidase (N) and haemagglutinin (HA) shown. Each HA spike comprises a trimer of HA molecules. Inside the virus shell is the segmented viral genome comprising eight genomic RNA molecules. (b) The HA molecule is processed after it is expressed in the infected cell by proteolytic cleaveage at the cleavage sight, to generate two polypeptide chains, depicted as HA1 and HA2, which are linked by disulphide bonds. The carboxy-terminus (COOH) of the protein bears the virus attachment protein domain.

accumulation of one or more amino acid substitutions in the HA. Primary DNA and hence protein sequence analysis of a number of viral variants either selected experimentally by monoclonal antibody (escape mutants —viral variants that escape neutralization by antibodies), or from natural outbreaks have been plotted on the HA structure. These substitutions cluster around the major antigenic sites and allow for occasional outbreaks of influenza to occur, although the presence of antibodies

against the other unaffected sites would ensure that in the population most individuals were adequately protected. Monitoring for changes in the structure of HA is of considerable importance in the prevention of future pandemics: the identification of a 'shift' would allow early warning of a major epidemic. In addition, the recognition of where in the HA structure 'drift' has occurred in isolates for the current year, allows the correct mix of HAs from different virus strains to be determined and thus the most effective vaccine for that season to be produced.

X-ray crystallography of virions

Initially electron microscopy can be used to broadly define virus structure which can allow classification, but more detailed analysis requires higher resolution techniques such as X-ray crystallography. This has been applied to picornaviruses in particular (Fig. 13.2), which are especially suitable for such analysis as they form crystalline arrays both *in vitro* and in the infected cell. Previous studies found that the virion is made up of equimolar amounts of four capsid proteins (termed VP1–4). Furthermore, as natural crystals can be formed, the structure of the individual virions must be regular. The four VP proteins form 60 **protomers** that polymerize to make a capsid of icosahedral symmetry. This arrangement was confirmed for each of the picornaviruses studied by crystallography, including, firstly, rhinovirus

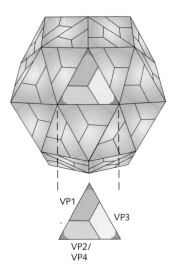

Fig. 13.2 X-ray crystallography has shown that the structure of a typical picornavirus has 60 protomers each made up of four capsid proteins (VP1, VP2, VP3 and VP4) giving a particle with icosahedral symmetry.

14 (a common cold virus), then polioviruses, mengovirus, foot and mouth disease virus, etc. In addition the intermolecular architecture of the capsid proteins forming the protomers was defined.

Although interesting in itself, the structure at this level of resolution has helped understanding of picornavirus infections in a number of other respects. Firstly, as for influenza HA (see above), it was possible to define the position of the major neutralizing antibody binding sites on the capsid of the picornavirus. These sites were found to line the lip of a cleft present in each protomer, termed the 'canyon' (Fig. 13.3), which had a narrow entrance (1.2–3.0 nm), known as the pore, which is too small to permit antibody to enter. By identifying the individual amino acids at the base of the cleft and then making viral mutants by recombinant DNA technology, it was found that the canyon was the receptor binding region on the virion.

These observations, together with the detailed structure of the region, may have practical application in the design of anti-viral agents. Beneath the floor of the 'canyon' is a hydrophobic pocket located in the VP1 protein. A series of arildone-based chemical compounds have been designed to bind to this region. After binding they distort the floor of the canyon such that one-sixth of the depth of the canyon is lost, which blocks attachment of the virus to its receptor or distorts the capsid such that the virus does not uncoat efficiently.

Sequence studies

Viral genomes were the first complete genomes to be

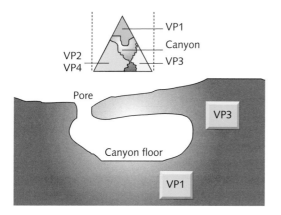

Fig. 13.3 The structure of the protomer generates a prominent cleft or canyon which has a narrow entrance or pore. The canyon floor is known to be necessary for cell attachment during infection.

sequenced, and until very recently the large viral DNA genomes (such as human cytomegalovirus and vaccinia virus) remained the largest contiguous pieces of DNA of any sort to have been sequenced. The techniques used for nucleotide sequencing are described elsewhere, but again it is worth noting that the techniques for rapid DNA sequencing, using random cloning of fragments of the viral genome (so-called shotgun cloning) and computer alignment of the sequenced fragments, were developed on these large DNA viruses and are now being applied to the sequencing of prokaryotic and eukaryotic chromosomes. The principal rationale for chromosomal sequencing is that many genes coding for proteins of as yet unknown function will be identified, and that this is the quickest approach to analysing structure/function relationships. This rationale has already been borne out for viruses: whereas 15 years ago the protein structure of a new virus would be identified by a classical biochemical approach, now a prime goal of research on any new virus is to obtain its genomic sequence. The information which can be derived from a viral genomic sequence is, as with any DNA sequence, manyfold. DNA sequence homology to other viruses can be recognized and may facilitate classification of the virus; identification of homologues of other viral genes and of cellular genes enables function of the products to be predicted; genetic variation or mutation can be identified and related to pathogenesis; and analysis of the genome by deletion and mutation of specific viral genes becomes possible. As noted above, these physical characteristics of the virus are used in the classification of viruses into families, although the widespread use of molecular biology has enabled the additional use of genomic organization, particularly in the classification into subfamilies. This is well exemplified in the case of herpesviruses. These viruses are conventionally divided into three major subfamilies — α, β and γ herpesvirus — based on their tissue tropisms and details of latency/replication, and each subfamily has a characteristic genome structure and orientation of blocks of genes. Two new members of the herpesviruses have recently been identified — human herpesvirus 6 (HHV6) and 7 (HHV7). Before the biology of HHV6 was fully defined it was clear that, by DNA sequence homology and the position and orientation of blocks of viral genes, HHV6 and HHV7 would be members of the β herpesvirus subfamily. Similarly, a recently identified herpesvirus has been found associated with Kaposi's sarcoma, a malignant skin lesion found in older men of Mediterranean origin and also associated with late stages of AIDS. DNA sequencing of this Kaposi's sarcoma-associated herpesvirus (KSHV) has suggested that it is a member of the γ herpesvirus subfamily (Plates 24a and b, facing p. 214).

In the case of small RNA viruses, such as the picornavirus family, 30 or more members, ranging in their tropism from plants, through insects to mammals including humans, have been fully or extensively sequenced (Table 13.1). Overall analysis of the viruses suggests relatedness between virus subfamilies: enteroviruses (including poliovirus) and rhinoviruses (common cold viruses) are closely related but they are closer to encephalomyocarditis viruses of rodents than the apthoviruses of cloven-hoofed animals. Even the individual proteins of picornaviruses have differential conservation and diversity. Non-structural proteins, such as the DNA polymerase, are similar in the plant cow pea mosaic virus and mammalian viruses but there is marked diversity in the structural capsid proteins. This may reflect the immunological selection pressure on the structural as opposed to non-structural proteins.

Virus–cell interactions

The first stage of virus infection is the binding of the virion to a target cell. Viruses can be considered to be obligate intracellular pathogens. Consequently, viral molecular biology is really inseparable from the molecular biology of the cells which they infect. Indeed this close relationship between virus molecular biology and normal cell biology is a principal reason for virology being such a pertinent discipline to the clinical investigator. In the next section we deal with molecular aspects of the interactions between viruses and cells.

Receptor binding and entry

A number of cellular surface structures may act as receptors for viruses. Non-specific structures such as sialic acid, which may be present on a number of different cell surface glycoproteins, bind influenza HA or reovirus-1. Alternatively, viruses may use specific surface molecules as host cell receptors. Consequently, virus entry may be targeted to specific cells (so called **cellular tropism**) in which replication or persistence may be guaranteed. This has a clinical consequence in that the virus tropism may determine the organ-specific clinical disease that is produced. Examples include the use of the cell surface protein, CD4, on T-cells by the envelope glycoprotein of human immunodeficiency virus (HIV), the CR2 complement receptor on B-cells by the EBV glycoprotein gp340, and cell surface intercellular adhesion molecule-1 (ICAM-1) by rhinoviruses. Each of these cell surface proteins is a member of the immunoglobulin gene superfam-

ily and other members of this family are also receptors for poliovirus and echoviruses. The ability to introduce total cellular cDNAs, by DNA transfection, from a cell type susceptible to virus infection into cells not normally susceptible to virus infection has been used to identify the poliovirus receptor. In this situation mouse cells, which are not permissive for poliovirus infection because virus does not enter the cells (that is they lack virus receptors), were transfected with a human cDNA library, and cells which were then recognized by antibodies that specifically protected normally susceptible cells from infection (due to these antibodies recognizing the virus receptor) were analysed for the expression of human cDNAs. From these mouse cells was isolated the human cDNA for the poliovirus receptor (Fig. 13.4). To establish whether the putative receptor was relevant *in vivo*, transgenic mice expressing the receptor in a number of tissues were established. When infected with poliovirus these mice developed paralytic poliomyelitis, implying that the receptor is essential for virus entry *in vivo*, and is itself a major determinant of poliovirus tropism and clinical disease.

Murine cells can permit virus nucleic acid replication even if they lack receptors, as shown by their ability to support replication after introduction of viral nucleic acid into them by transfection. In this case the viral genome, which is RNA, is first converted to a cDNA copy (see Chapter 2) and this cDNA is transfected into cells. However, other cells are not able to support viral replication after their transfection with viral DNA or

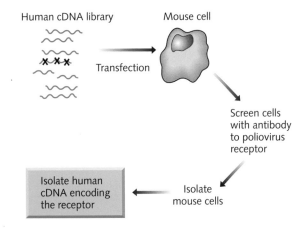

Fig. 13.4 A scheme to clone the poliovirus receptor is shown. A human cDNA library is expressed in mouse cells, which do not express a poliovirus receptor. Transfected cells are screened with specific antibody to the poliovirus receptor and mouse cells expressing the human cDNA encoding the receptor for the virus are isolated. The cDNA is purified from these cells.

cDNA. In the case of poliovirus, viral replication can be supported by cells of mammalian origin or even in mammalian cell extracts (so-called cell-free systems). However, insect cells even if transfected with the virus receptor are unable to support viral replication. Clearly, factors necessary for replication must be absent in these cells. *In vivo* this is mirrored by the differential replication of poliovirus in neurones in humans (where the receptor is constitutively expressed). Viral mutations may alter cellular permissiveness for viral replication. For instance, a number of isolates of poliovirus, isolated from patients developing poliomyelitis after vaccination, were found consistently to have mutations in the 5' untranslated region of the genome compared with the vaccine strain. It was suggested that such a change could alter the secondary structure of the genomic RNA in this region, resulting in the viral genome interacting with specific host cell factors which allowed efficient replication of the virus. Having bound to the cell surface, viruses have to gain entry to the cell cytoplasm to allow uncoating and release of nucleic acid. Enveloped viruses can achieve this by a fusion event after receptor-mediated endocytosis, as has been well characterized in the case of influenza HA (see above). The fusion protein produced often has a hydrophobic region which can insert into the host cell plasma (Sendai virus, measles) or vacuolar membrane (influenza) allowing capsid entry to the cell cytoplasm. In non-enveloped viruses the mechanism of entry is less well established, although adenovirus may have a similar fusogenic region to allow penetration of the vacuolar membrane after endocytosis.

After viral capsid entry, the process of virion uncoating is less well understood and is difficult to study because of the small number of virus particles required to establish productive infection (an infection which replicates and produces more virus), which is probably less than 1% of those which bind to cells. However, in the case of picornaviruses there is some evidence that the disruption of the capsid is not a random but an ordered event — a small capsid protein VP4 is expelled from the capsid first and release of the nucleic acid may be governed in part by an interaction between a viral protein linked to the 5' end of the genome (Vpg) and the capsid.

Transcription

Once a virus has entered a cell and released its genome, it needs to express viral genes and replicate the viral DNA. The strategy for this depends, to a large extent, on the nature of the virus.

DNA viruses

Most DNA viruses transcribe and replicate their genomes in the nucleus. The transcription of viral genes is achieved using the same basal transcription complex as is used for cellular genes, and is dependent on RNA polymerase II (see Chapter 4). However the mechanisms which regulate and control viral gene transcription are critical determinants of the life cycle and pathogenesis of the virus. Many DNA viruses make use of cellular transcription factors to control expression of their genes — the promoter/regulatory regions upstream of those viral genes which are critical for initiating the viral life cycle leading to virus production (the so-called lytic cycle of the virus) contain the appropriate DNA sequences for binding these cellular factors. In many instances expression of viral genes is linked to differentiation of the cells which the virus infects; this differentiation-dependent expression of viruses depends on the presence of cellular transcription factors whose primary function is to induce expression of the cellular genes associated with a specific differentiated phenotype, but which the virus also uses to express its own genes.

In addition to using cellular factors, viruses may also themselves encode genes whose products are transcriptional activators. Examples of this are the E1A gene of adenoviruses, T antigen of SV40, E7 protein of human papillomavirus and some of the so-called immediate early (IE) genes of herpesviruses (expressed immediately the virus infects the cell and before viral DNA replication). Some of these viral proteins (such as adenovirus E1A, SV40 T antigen and HPV E7) are also able to interact physically with cellular proteins which are essential for cell cycle control (such as the retinoblastoma protein), resulting in uncontrolled cell division and neoplastic transformation (see Chapter 8). In the case of the herpes simplex viruses (HSV1 and HSV2, associated with the common cold sore and genital herpes, respectively), a *structural* protein of the virion (VP16) also acts to transactivate expression of the viral *IE* genes: this means the virus itself carries a structural protein which acts as a transcriptional activator protein into the cell, facilitating the rapid expression of viral genes necessary for productive infection. Poxviruses, such as variola which causes smallpox and vaccinia used as the vaccine against smallpox, are DNA viruses which transcribe and replicate their genomes in the cytoplasm, and to do this they carry with them all the necessary enzymes — making them more independent of cellular factors.

We will look in a little more detail at the control of

viral gene expression and the interaction of viral gene products with the host cell using a human herpesvirus, human cytomegalovirus (HCMV), as an example. HCMV is a large (230 kb) double-stranded DNA virus and a ubiquitous pathogen. Although infection *in utero* can result in congenital malformation, the virus rarely causes disease in the immunocompetent. As with all herpesviruses, HCMV is able to establish a life-long latent infection. Reactivation, which is often associated with immunosuppression, can result in severe and often fatal disease, especially in transplant recipients (Plate 25a, facing p. 214) and patients with HIV (Plate 25b, facing p. 214). Like other herpesviruses (see Table 13.1), during lytic infection, HCMV undergoes a regulated cascade of viral gene expression when infecting permissive cells. Three phases of viral gene expression have been defined — so called immediate early, early (E) and late (L) (Fig. 13.5). Immediate early genes of HCMV, like other herpesviruses, are expressed within minutes of infection and do not require any viral gene expression in order for them to be expressed at very high levels in the cell. They are, therefore, dependent on cellular transcription factors and cellular RNA polymerase II for their efficient expression and play a pivotal role in regulating virus infection. Many of the earliest of genes expressed by virtually all DNA viruses on infection have similar characteristics. Not only do they switch on early and late viral genes but they also regulate cellular gene expression in order to optimize the cellular environment for virus production (Fig. 13.5). Two of the most abundantly expressed IE proteins of HCMV are the so-called IE1 and IE2 proteins. Both are expressed from the same region of the viral genome under the control of the same viral promoter/regulatory region—the so-called major IE promoter/enhancer (MIEP). However, these viral proteins have quite specific roles during infection. For instance the IE1 protein positively affects it own expression whereas the IE2 protein negatively autoregulates. Yet both co-operatively activate other later viral genes and other cellular genes associated with DNA replication. Consequently, these IE proteins 'fine tune' viral and cellular gene expression and act as control proteins allowing an ordered progression of viral gene expression at the right time during infection. Similar control proteins are found in the IE proteins of other herpesviruses such as HSV (the ICP0, ICP4 proteins) and EBV (the BZLF1 protein).

Retroviruses

Retroviruses are viruses that have RNA as the viral genome, but upon infection the genome is converted to a DNA copy using a virally encoded reverse transcriptase enzyme. A number of retroviruses are known to cause tumours (see Chapter 8) and are, therefore, sometimes called RNA tumour viruses. A good example of a retrovirus, though not one that results in tumours, which has been extensively studied is HIV. HIV-1 infection results, after a variable asymptomatic period, in a depletion of CD4-bearing T-cells and concomitant immunodeficiency. Upon infection HIV, like all retroviruses, uses virally encoded reverse transcriptase to make a 9.5 kb DNA copy (the so-called **proviral DNA**) of the viral genome (Fig. 13.6). Proviral DNA is integrated into the cell's DNA and is transcribed by cellular RNA polymerase II. Since the HIV genome is an RNA molecule, transcription of full length copies of HIV proviral DNA into mRNA is the actual replication step of the HIV genome. Cellular RNA polymerase II may make millions of RNA copies of the proviral DNA and each full length HIV RNA can eventually be packaged into infectious HIV virions. Cellular RNA polymerase II also transcribes HIV mRNA that can be singly or doubly spliced. Doubly spliced HIV mRNAs encode viral proteins that help regulate the HIV transcription, while unspliced HIV mRNAs encode for retroviral structural proteins and the retroviral reverse transcriptase (Fig. 13.7).

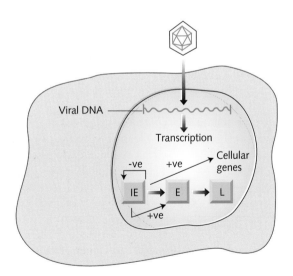

Fig. 13.5 Replication of a typical herpesvirus, such as human cytomegalovirus, is shown. Once in the cell nucleus, the viral genome is transcribed using cellular RNA polymerases in three phases, immediate early (IE), early (E) and late. Viral IE genes, such as *IE1* and *IE2*, are potent transcriptional regulators which affect viral and cellular gene expression both positively and negatively, as depicted by the positive and negative signs.

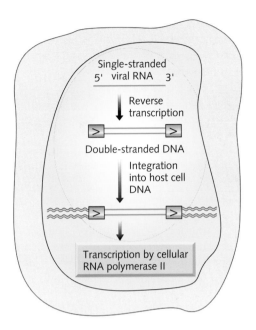

Fig. 13.6 Upon infection with HIV-1, the virus copies its genomic RNA into a double-stranded proviral DNA molecule bounded by long terminal repeats (depicted by arrowed boxes). This integrates into host DNA and is transcribed by cellular RNA polymerases.

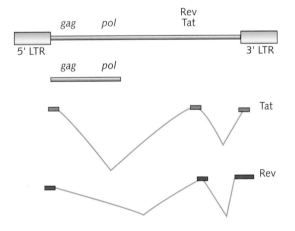

Fig. 13.7 HIV-1 RNA undergoes complex splicing. *gag* and *pol* RNAs are unspliced and encode structural proteins and reverse transcriptase enzyme, respectively. Regulatory proteins such as Tat and Rev are doubly spliced.

After integration of the HIV proviral DNA into the cellular chromosome, the 5′ long terminal repeat (LTR) of the HIV DNA serves as both the promoter and enhancer for transcription of the whole of the HIV genome. This LTR contains a TATA box element, similar to many cellular promoters transcribed by RNA polymerase II, which binds the ubiquitous TATA binding protein (TBP). In addition to a TATA box the HIV promoter contains binding sites for a number of cellular transcription factors including the ubiquitous transcription factor Sp1. Therefore, as with many viruses, the same transcription factors required for transcription of cellular genes are also used by HIV for its own transcription (Fig. 13.8).

The HIV transcriptional enhancer present in the HIV 5′ LTR also contains binding sites for the AP-1 family of transcription factors. Most importantly, the HIV LTR contains binding sites for the transcription factor NFκB. In T-cells, for instance, this transcription factor is localized in the cytoplasm of cells associated with a repressor, IκB. Activation of T-cells by mitogens, antigen recognition, or growth factors results in the dissociation of IκB from NFκB and the translocation of NFκB to the nucleus of the CD4-lymphocyte. Upon translocation into the nucleus, NFκB binds to its recognition sites in the promoter/enhancer of the HIV LTR and activates HIV transcription.

When transcription is initiated from the HIV LTR a number of different mRNAs may be produced. Initially only doubly spliced mRNA is exported from the nucleus into the cytoplasm where it can be translated into proteins. Thus the initial HIV proteins made are Tat and Rev (Fig. 13.9). All HIV mRNAs have a sequence called TAR (transactivation responsive sequence). This RNA sequence, which is located at the 5′ end of every HIV mRNA, can form a double-stranded loop recognized by the Tat protein. When Tat protein binds to the TAR loop transcription of HIV mRNA is increased 1000-fold over the basal levels of HIV mRNA transcription. How the Tat–TAR interaction increases the amount of HIV

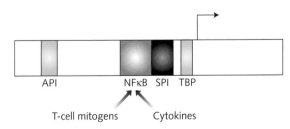

Fig. 13.8 The 5′ LTR of the HIV-1 proviral DNA acts as a strong promoter for viral RNA transcription and is positively regulated by many cellular factors such as NFκB, Sp1 and AP-1. Many of these are increased in the cell by mitogens and cytokines.

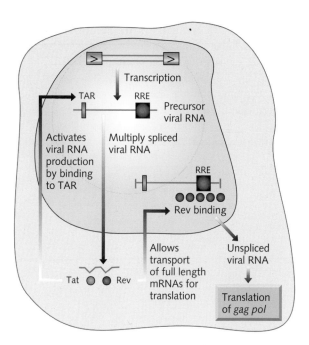

Fig. 13.9 Upon HIV-1 infection, multiply spliced RNAs encoding e.g. Tat and Rev are translated to make Tat and Rev protein. Tat activates viral RNA production by binding to the TAR site on the viral RNA, and Rev binds to the Rev responsive element on the mRNAs and facilitates transport of unspliced mRNAs encoding viral structural proteins and the viral reverse transcriptase.

mRNA is not clear. Perhaps the Tat protein relieves a block to the elongation of HIV mRNA, or after binding of Tat to TAR, the Tat protein attracts more cellular RNA polymerase II to the TATA box of the HIV 5′ LTR.

The Rev protein binds to the so-called Rev responsive element (RRE) on the viral RNA and acts to allow transport of full length unspliced HIV RNAs to the cytoplasm, and so controls the switch from production of mRNAs encoding regulatory proteins such as Tat to genomic RNAs.

RNA viruses

RNA viruses may be divided into two main classes depending on the 'sense' of the RNA genome. RNA viruses whose RNA is able to act directly as mRNA are known as 'positive strand' viruses (see Table 13.1 and Fig. 13.10). Positive strand RNA viruses have a genome that can itself act as the template for replication or as mRNA. In the case of picornaviruses the coding region

of the genome is effectively a single open reading frame which when translated releases a single virus polyprotein. Its subsequent processing to the 11 separate proteins, five structural and six non-structural, that are required for efficient virus replication is governed by specific cleavage sites in the polyprotein and the availability of two virus proteinases which immediately cleave the polyprotein. As these proteinases are specific, that is they cleave at sessile bonds that would not otherwise be susceptible to cleavage by host cell enzymes, they can be targets for specific anti-viral therapy. Several inhibitors of viral proteinases have been described and in the case of HIV, such agents are entering clinical trials.

The 5′ untranslated region of picornaviruses is therefore of critical importance in directing the cell's translation machinery (the ribosome) to preferentially translate viral as opposed to cellular RNA. This region of the virus

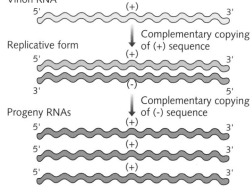

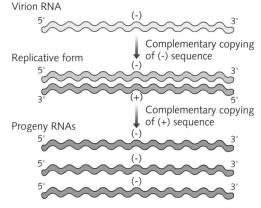

Fig. 13.10 Replication of (a) positive (+) and (b) negative (−) strand viral RNA genomes by RNA-dependent RNA polymerase.

genome lacks a conventional 'cap' structure but has a so-called **internal ribosome entry site** (IRES) which acts to direct initiation of translation by the cell ribosome. This is a complex structure partly dependent on the secondary as well as primary RNA structure in this region. If this IRES is placed upstream of reporter genes, they can then be translated without an RNA cap structure. Mutations in this region may be important in the tropism of picornaviruses, as translation of virus products is also dependent on a number of cellular factors which bind to the IRES and remain to be identified.

The RNA of 'negative strand' viruses (such as influenza and measles) is not able to act as message — these viruses carry an RNA polymerase into the cell with them which enables transcription of a positive RNA strand from the negative strand viral genome from which individual mRNAs can then be transcribed (Fig. 13.10).

Replication

The strategy used by viruses to replicate their genome depends on whether the genome is DNA or RNA and on its complexity. Understanding the mechanism by which viruses replicate is of considerable practical importance —enzymes and other proteins involved in replication are candidate targets for antiviral drugs. In positive strand RNA viruses (such as picornaviruses) the RNA acts as both mRNA and the template from which negative strand RNA is synthesized by a polymerase derived from the viral polyprotein: more positive strand RNA is then made from the minus strand and packaged into the virion. In negative strand RNA viruses the process occurs in mirror image — a positive strand RNA is first synthesized and serves as the template to then synthesize genomic minus strand RNA.

Smaller DNA viruses use the cellular DNA polymerase complex to synthesize new DNA. Larger DNA viruses, such as the herpesviruses, encode more of their own enzymes required for replication, such as the DNA polymerase. Herpesviruses also code for additional proteins involved in DNA synthesis. The ultimate examples of self-sufficiency are the poxviruses which replicate in the cell cytoplasm and encode all the enzymes necessary for their replication.

Retroviruses replicate through a DNA intermediate. Following entry into the cell a reverse transcriptase present in the virion transcribes the viral RNA into DNA which is then integrated into host chromosomal DNA. Transcription of the integrated 'proviral' DNA then gives rise to mRNA for the viral proteins and new viral

genomic RNA. Retroviral reverse transcriptase has become an indispensable tool of molecular biology, used for making complementary DNA copies of RNA, for instance as part of a gene cloning strategy (see Chapter 3).

Hepatitis B virus, which infects hepatocytes and is one cause of viral hepatitis, in contrast, is a DNA virus which replicates through an RNA intermediate: its small, circular DNA genome is first transcribed into full length RNA (as well as mRNA for proteins) from which genomic DNA is synthesized by a virus-encoded reverse transcriptase. This suggests an ancestral relationship between hepatitis B and retroviruses (Fig. 13.11).

Latency and persistence

The term **persistence** is applied to those viruses which are maintained in the host following acute primary infection, usually for its lifetime. For many such viruses, persistence goes hand in hand with their replicative cycle (e.g. the retroviruses and herpesviruses). Some other

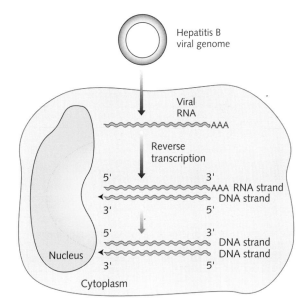

Fig. 13.11 Hepatitis B virus replication. Hepatitis B virus has a small, circular DNA genome which, upon infection, is transcribed into mRNA. The viral mRNA is then reverse transcribed to generate a cDNA copy and the RNA strand of the DNA/RNA intermediate is removed and replaced with a complementary strand of DNA, generating a double-stranded DNA copy of the viral genome. All these replication steps take place in the infected cell cytoplasm.

viruses only infrequently establish persistent infection and it is not an essential feature of their replication (e.g. measles virus, hepatitis B virus). Viruses may replicate continuously during persistence (e.g. HIV) — the term **persistent infection** is sometimes restricted solely to these — whereas others exhibit classical **latency** (e.g. herpes simplex virus) in which no, or very limited, transcription takes place and there is no virus replication. Latent viruses may **reactivate** under the influence of various stimuli. For instance, sunlight is a well-known cause of HSV1 reactivation leading to the ubiquitous cold sore.

The molecular events involved in persistence and latency are complex and not completely elucidated. What is known is that it is likely that latency depends in large part on transcriptional control of the virus exerted by the presence or absence of specific cellular transcription factors. The extent of virus gene expression during persistence is variable: there may be expression of a restricted set of viral genes (so-called latent genes) essential to maintain the viral genome in the infected cell, with a block to transcription of lytic genes which encode viral transcriptional activators, genes coding for structural proteins of the virus and factors needed for replication. This pattern of restricted viral gene expression is seen in EBV, where the so-called Epstein–Barr nuclear antigens (EBNAs) expressed by the virus are true latent gene products required for B-cell immortalization (see Chapter 8) and latent replication of the virus. EBV persists in a small fraction of B-cells. In lymphoblastoid B-cell lines (immortalized B-cell lines) *in vitro*, the EBV DNA exists as non-integrated circles of DNA (episomes) which are maintained at constant copy number as the cells divide, with expression of a limited number of proteins (the EBNAs) necessary for the maintenance of this episomal DNA — there is probably similarly restricted EBV gene expression in the B-cell *in vivo*. EBV also persists in epithelial cells in the oropharynx, but here the later lytic cycle genes are expressed with viral replication and shedding from the oropharyngeal epithelium.

Alternatively, there may be no apparent viral proteins produced at all as seen with herpes simplex virus. The α herpes viruses, such as HSV and varicella zoster virus (VZV), establish latent infection in neuronal cells in sensory ganglia, whence they periodically reactivate and are transported down the axon to infect cells at the nerve ending. There is little or no viral transcription occurring for most of the time. The only viral gene expression detectable during HSV latency in neurones is of the so-called **latency-associated transcripts** (LATs) which are not expressed as protein and whose function is uncertain

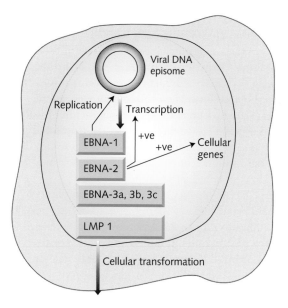

Fig. 13.12 EBV gene expression during latent infection. The viral genome is transcribed to generate the EBNA RNAs encoding EBNA-1, 2, 3a, 3b, 3c and another latent protein, LMP 1. These have various roles during latent infection. EBNA-1 is needed to maintain the viral genome as an autonomously replicating DNA circle, and EBNA-2 regulates viral gene expression and upregulates many cellular genes encoding cell adhesion molecules. Together with LMP 1, EBNA-2 plays a role in cellular transformation.

(Fig. 13.12). The molecular mechanism by which latency is maintained is relatively poorly understood, and is a major area of current study in herpes virology.

Retroviruses integrate their proviral DNA into chromosomal DNA and its transcription and translation then occur in the same general way as for cellular genes, but may depend on the state of activation of the cell. For instance, integrated HIV proviral DNA is transcribed in CD4+ T-cells only when they become activated in response to external signals, such as contact with antigen and interleukin-2.

Most persistent infections are prevented from producing active disease in the normal host in large part by the immune response, and tend to cause disease principally in the clinical setting of immunosuppression. This relationship with the immune response may be complex; it is worth noting that the cellular sites of persistent virus infection frequently include cells which may be less accessible to the immune system, such as epithelial or neuronal cells and the cells of the immune system itself (as in the case of HIV). The 'visibility' of the virus to the immune system in these sites depends on the level of viral gene expression, and hence viral antigen presentation to the B- and T-cells of the immune system. Thus whether neurones carrying latent HSV are susceptible to attack by immunological mechanisms is uncertain but seems unlikely. For EBV the extent to which its two sites of persistence in B-cells and epithelial cells are accessible to the immune response *in vivo* is also uncertain, although it is assumed that the potential of EBV to induce B-cell transformation is somehow restrained *in vivo* by the T-cell response directed against the virus in B-cells.

Assembly and release

Assembly of virion particles varies with different virus families. The formation of the virus capsid has been well studied with a number of plant viruses and picornaviruses. In the latter instance the virion structure has been resolved by X-ray crystallography (see p. 242). Assembly of the virions occurs readily in the infected cell or cytoplasmic extracts of infected cells. This implies that assembly is largely determined by the intrinsic properties of the constituent proteins and that the final capsid structure is the lowest energy state that can be adopted by the subunits, resulting in self-assembly. The first stage of picornavirus assembly is the interaction of three capsid proteins, VP1, VP3 and VP0 (made up of VP4 and VP2), which aggregate into structures, five of which then link to make a pentamer. The pentamers then combine to form an empty capsid, into which viral genomic RNA, coupled to a covalently linked protein (Vpg) at its

amino-terminal end, then enters. It is probable that this is an ordered event but its details are unknown. What is clear is that after genome entry a maturation step is required in order to generate a fully infectious particle: VP0 is cleaved internally to produce VP2 and VP4. Similar maturation cleavages are important in a number of other viruses (e.g. HIV), and inhibition of this event could again be a target for anti-viral therapy.

Virus release is normally effected from the cell by one of two mechanisms: cell lysis or budding. Conventionally it is assumed that release of non-enveloped viruses occurs after cell death and lysis. However, recent studies suggest that this may also occur in an ordered way as some release of SV40 is reported to occur without cell death and can be from only one specific surface of the cell (**polarized**).

In contrast, enveloped viruses are released either by budding from the plasma membrane or into vacuoles that are then transported to the surface. A number of factors may determine the site of budding from the plasma membrane, including regions of the cell where viral glycoproteins localize and exclude host cell glycoproteins. Furthermore, viral glycoproteins also alter the rate of transport of host cell vesicles to the membrane to facilitate virus egress.

Epithelial cells often have differentiated apical and basal surfaces with ordered sorting and transport of cell proteins to one surface or the other (Fig. 13.13). Viruses utilize this polarization; ortho- and para-myxoviruses are budded from the apical whereas VZV and retro-

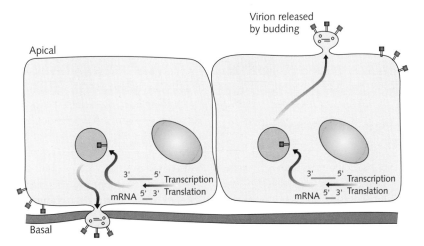

Fig. 13.13 Virus release can be targeted to different parts of the cell. Certain viruses preferentially bud from either the apical or basal surface of polarized epithelial cells. For example, influenza buds from the apical surface and certain retroviruses from the basolateral surface. This preferential budding is determined by initial targeting of the viral envelope glycoproteins to specific regions of the cell membrane. The information for targeting glycoproteins to either surface is contained in the amino acid sequence of the protein.

viruses use the basal surface. This polarity of budding is directly determined by the viral glycoproteins. When the **ectodomains** of individual virus glycoproteins are exchanged, then the expressed polarity of the protein is reversed in some instances. In this context it is worth mentioning that these basic mechanisms of intracellular processing and sorting of glycoproteins in normal cells were first defined by the use of viral glycoproteins (in particular the VZV glycoprotein) as probes.

Use of viruses as vectors

Many viruses have been adapted to serve as plasmid vectors for foreign genes, either for the purpose of achieving high-level expression of the inserted gene in eukaryotic cells to produce protein, or for the purpose of vaccination or gene therapy *in vivo*. The attractions of viral vectors are that genes can be efficiently introduced into cells by the normal infective process and then expressed at high level—something the virus has evolved to do.

The use of viral vectors for gene therapy is covered in Chapter 16, and we do not deal further with this topic here. There are numerous examples of the use of viruses as expression vectors *in vitro*. Baculovirus is an insect virus used as a vector for the expression of genes at very high level in insect cells (up to 70% of all protein synthesis in the infected cell), in order to produce large amounts of recombinant protein *in vitro*. Vaccinia viruses have been widely used as vectors for the expression of foreign genes, particularly with a view to their use as candidate vaccines. So far, recombinant vaccinia virus vectors have been widely used *in vitro* by cellular immunologists as tools to express selected genes in cells that act as targets for the study of cytotoxic T-cell immunity. Although no recombinant vaccinia virus has yet been licensed for use as a vaccine (see p. 257), one expressing HIV gp120 has been used in Phase 1 trials in the USA.

Viral molecular biology—application to infection in the host

An understanding of the molecular biology of virus infection — how the virus targets specific cell types, its entry into the cell and the mechanisms by which the virus controls both viral and cellular gene expression — helps us to understand the disease process and can only help in generating sensible anti-viral strategies.

Immune response

Protection against virus infection in animal hosts depends principally on the production of a specific immune response (although interferon, which can act as a powerful anti-viral by inhibiting viral RNA translation as well as 'natural' non-specific immunity, may also have a role to play). Antibody is required to neutralize virus in the fluid phase, whilst effector T-cell immunity is particularly important for the recognition and elimination of virus-infected cells. In fact the analysis of how T-cells recognize virus-infected cells has been instrumental in revealing the basic mechanism of T-cell recognition.

Antibody

The induction of anti-viral antibody responses, as with other complex antigens, is dependent on the provision of T-cell help to the responding B-cells (see Chapter 10). All classes of immunoglobulin can be produced in response to virus infection — IgG, IgA and IgM. This is partly determined by the site of entry of the virus — whether through a mucosal surface in the gut or respiratory tract or via a parenteral route. The class of the antibody is a major determinant of its biological activity: for example IgG and IgM anti-viral antibodies may bind complement (which enhances neutralization and allows for lysis of virus-infected cells), the Fc portion of IgG may bind to Fc receptors on lymphocytes or macrophages (enabling them to mediate antibody-dependent cell-mediated cytotoxicity), and IgG can transfer protection across the placenta. However, the ability of antibody to neutralize virus particles is probably its main role in the host protective response and the main mechanism of protection induced by anti-viral vaccines.

Viral neutralization requires an interaction of the antibody with the virion particle. Conventionally, neutralization is thought to result from direct inhibition of virus binding to its host cell receptor—thus many epitopes recognized by neutralizing antibodies are closely apposed to, or form part of, receptor binding sites on the virion (Fig. 13.1). The advent of molecular technology has allowed greater understanding of the localization of such epitopes, as well as their variation and escape from antibody responses.

The most frequent approach used in identifying neutralizing epitopes on viral proteins is to develop a series of monoclonal antibodies against a virus, and then to culture the virus in the presence of the antibody. During such culture some viruses will mutate in positions that are a major component of the neutralizing site on the virion, and will grow in the presence of the antibody as 'escape' mutants: the virus genome, or in the case of larger viruses the relevant gene, is then sequenced and mutations identified. Using this approach the major mutations possible in the influenza HA were identified.

This method was also adopted to define the location of neutralizing sites on human rhinovirus 14. Certain mutation positions in the primary structure of this virus, and later poliovirus, were particularly important in that most variation resulting in escape of the virus from antibody neutralization occurred at these sites. The sites were located in two clusters on VP1 and one each on VP2 and VP3. The crystallographic data showed these regions were combined to produce a complex tertiary structure close to the receptor binding 'canyon' on the virion (see p. 243). It is easy to envisage that in such a location the antibody would be able to sterically inhibit receptor binding; however, this explanation is in fact too simple. It has been known for some time that with some neutralizing antibodies virus neutralization is enhanced *in vitro* by the presence of complement. Furthermore, it was found by equilibrium studies, that although human rhinovirus has 60 potential receptor binding sites only four immunoglobulin molecules were needed per virion to inhibit infection; similar observations have been made for other viruses. This indicates that neutralizing antibodies can act by a number of mechanisms in addition to directly blocking receptor binding sites and these include:

1 distorting the whole virion structure such that binding at distant receptor binding sites cannot occur;

2 the virion may bind but the presence of antibody prevents uncoating of the virion;

3 as the number of Fab fragments required for neutralization greatly exceeds the number of whole immunoglobulin molecules, the Fc portion of the immunoglobulin may recruit other effector mechanisms such as complement.

It should be remembered that prevention of binding at the epithelial surface may be of particular importance in virus infection. In this regard the ability to generate an effective, specific IgA response may be of major value. This can often be achieved by using a mucosal vaccine, of which the best example is oral live attenuated poliovirus. Both killed and live polio vaccines are effective in preventing paralytic poliomyelitis, but the live vaccine may block initial entry of the virus to epithelial cells in the gastrointestinal tract, whereas the killed vaccine relies on the induction of neutralizing antibodies to prevent spread of virus after infection of the host. This ability to produce a mucosal immune response may be a particularly important strategy for future vaccine development, especially for viruses which enter the host via the gastrointestinal, genitourinary and respiratory tracts.

Virus-specific T-cells

T-lymphocytes recognize antigen through their T-cell receptor. In its most common form the T-cell receptor consists of γ and β chains, each composed of variable (V) and joining (J) segments [with an additional diversity (D) segment for the β chain]: these segments are encoded by separate genes which undergo DNA rearrangement to give very many different combinations (see Chapter 10). T-cells recognize viral and other conventional antigens not as whole proteins but as short peptide fragments derived from the protein after its processing in the cell (**intracellular processing**). These peptides bind in a groove on the heavy chain of the class I and class II molecules of the major histocompatibility gene complex (MHC). Particular amino acid residues at critical points in the peptide sequence 'anchor' the peptide in the groove, and this interaction is relatively specific for each of the different allelic forms of MHC molecules. Thus it is a complex of peptide and MHC molecule (and the MHC molecule must be the same allelic form as that on the T-cell) which is recognized by the T-cell receptor with consequent activation of the T-cell and expression of its effector functions. The association of peptides with MHC alleles on the one hand, and the diversity of the T-cell receptor on the other, allows T-cells to recognize a huge number of antigens whilst conferring extreme specificity on this recognition — which means that only a small fraction of all T-cells will respond to any given antigen. The molecular details of antigen processing and presentation have been worked out to a large extent using virus systems — which is appropriate given that these mechanisms evolved in large part to combat virus infections. In general, endogenous synthesis of viral proteins within the cell is required for association of their peptides with class I molecules to occur in the endoplasmic reticulum, whereas exogenous viral proteins are processed through the endosomal pathway, and associate with class II MHC molecules (Fig. 13.14).

T-cells are conventionally divided into two broad functional classes, helper and cytotoxic T-cells.

HELPER T (T$_H$) CELLS

T$_H$ cells recognize processed peptides derived from viral proteins and presented to them by antigen-presenting cells — principally dendritic cells, macrophages and B-cells. T$_H$ cells are generally restricted in their recognition of peptides by class II MHC molecules and in humans are CD4+. Virus-specific T$_H$ clones have been studied in some detail *in vitro*, particularly for influenza. It is clear that the peptides predominantly recognized by T$_H$ cells

(a)

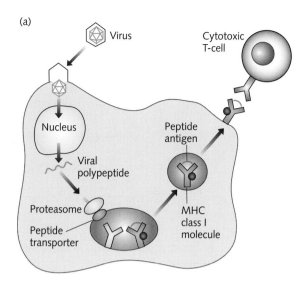

(b)

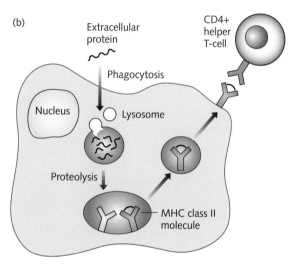

Fig. 13.14 Presentation of peptides by MHC class I or II involves different pathways. MHC molecules act as 'peptide receptors', presenting peptide fragments of proteins to T-cells which recognize peptide + MHC via their T-cell receptor. (a) Proteins which are synthesized in the cell (as in the case of viruses or intracellular bacteria) are processed into peptides by the proteasome, and transported into the endoplasmic reticulum by specific peptide transporters, where the peptides associate with class I MHC molecules and are then exported to the plasma membrane where they are recognized by CD8+ cytotoxic T-cells. (b) Extracellular proteins are digested to peptides in the endosome where they associate with class II MHC molecules and are recognized by CD4+ (mainly helper) T-cells.

ing of peptides on exposed surfaces of the molecule which are recognized by antibody. T_H cells provide help in the form of cytokines/growth factors such as interleukin-2 (IL-2), IL-4, and γ-interferon (γ-IFN) and CD4+ cells may also act as effector cells mediating delayed hypersensitivity (DTH) or cytotoxicity.

CYTOTOXIC T (T_C) CELLS

MHC class I-restricted virus-specific T_C cells have been extensively studied in virus systems, ever since the first description of the MHC restriction of their function in the context of murine lymphocytic choriomeningitis virus infection (Fig. 13.15). Class II-restricted virus-specific CD4+ cells may also be cytotoxic, although the majority (90%) of T_C cells are CD8+. As for other T-cells, virus-specific T_C cells recognize viral proteins as processed peptides bound to MHC molecules. The induction of virus-specific T_C cell memory requires presentation of peptide associated with class I MHC, but the evidence suggests that this presentation can occur on *any* class I MHC-bearing cell, and not just on specialized antigen-presenting cells.

Virus-specific T_C cells are thought to play a major role in the resolution of virus infections and the containment of persistent infections. The evidence for this derives from experimental models where adoptive transfer of T_C cells protects from lethal challenge with viruses in many virus infections (Fig. 13.15). The existence of virus-

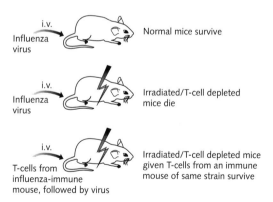

Fig. 13.15 Cytotoxic T-cells can protect against virus infection. Normal mice given a sublethal dose of influenza virus survive. If immunosuppressed by irradiation or other methods of T-cell depletion, the mice die of overwhelming infection. However, if such immunosuppressed mice are given cytotoxic T-cells from an influenza-immune mouse of identical strain (a procedure known as 'adoptive transfer') they survive the virus infection, thus demonstrating the protective effect of cytotoxic T-cells.

are not necessarily the same as those recognized by antibody—thus peptides throughout the influenza virus HA molecule may be recognized by T_H cells, in contrast to the predominantly conformational epitopes, or cluster-specific T_C cells can be shown by *in vitro* techniques in humans but their role is obviously harder to prove.

Virus evasion of the immune response

There is recent evidence from several *in vitro* systems that viruses can modulate the expression of cell surface molecules involved in the induction and effector components of the immune response. This can have clear functional consequences *in vitro*, conferring resistance to the immune response, although it remains to be seen whether the same applies *in vivo*.

For instance, in one of the best known examples adenovirus can downregulate the amount of class I MHC molecules on the infected cell surface, to the point where the cell can no longer be recognized by adenovirus-specific cytotoxic T-cells. Deletion studies have shown that this effect is mediated by a specific adenovirus gene product (encoded in the E3 region), which causes retention of class I MHC molecules in the endoplasmic reticulum on their export pathway to the cell surface.

Similarly, it is now becoming clear that a number of herpesviruses, such as CMV and HSV, also avoid cytotoxic T-cell recognition by encoding genes which downregulate expression of cellular class I MHC molecules, either directly, by altering rates of protein turnover, or indirectly, by preventing their transport through the endoplasmic reticulum (Fig. 13.16).

In addition to the interaction of the T-cell receptor with antigen and MHC molecules, a range of adhesion molecules are also important in antigen presentation and recognition of their targets by effector cells. These include the interactions between ICAM-1 and LFA-1, and between LFA-3 and CD2 (Fig. 13.16). Recent work indicates that expression of these adhesion molecules can be modulated by viruses: for example EBV transformation of B-cells may be associated with reduced expression of LFA-1 — B-cell lines derived from Burkitt's lymphomas show this as resistant to lysis by EBV-specific T_C cells. However, such cell lines only express the EBNA-1 protein and it has also been shown that the EBNA-1 protein of EBV contains amino acid repeats that prevent the protein from being processed and presented in virus-infected cells, by an as yet undefined mechanism.

The ability of viruses to mutate with consequent selection of strains which can escape antibody neutralization has been referred to already. It has been shown that variants of HIV with mutations in a sequence coding for a peptide recognized by T_C cells can emerge *in vivo* in HIV-positive individuals: it is suggested this may represent a corresponding example of a T-cell escape mutant.

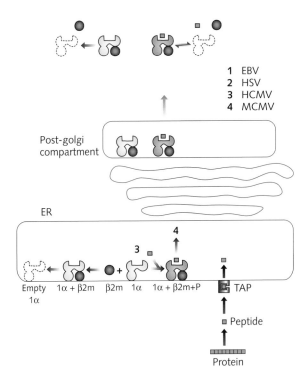

Fig. 13.16 Virus infection can result in changes in cellular gene expression to evade immune surveillance. A number of viruses can reduce the surface expression of MHC molecules which makes it more difficult for T-lymphocytes to recognize the infected cell. The different mechanisms used by herpesviruses to achieve this are shown here. (1) The Epstein–Barr virus nuclear protein EBNA-1 cannot be processed into peptides and transported into the endoplasmic reticulum, making it impossible for its peptides to be presented. (2) The herpes simplex virus protein ICP47 blocks the function of the transporter of antigenic peptides (TAP) which interferes with the assembly of class I MHC molecules. (3) Human cytomegalovirus increases the turnover of class I MHC heavy chain in the endoplasmic reticulum. (4) Murine cytomegalovirus blocks the export of fully assembled MHC molecules from the endoplasmic reticulum.

Pathogenesis

The advances in molecular virology are now also being applied to studies of the mechanisms by which viruses produce disease in the host.

Deletion and mutation analysis in studies of viral pathogenesis

In order to define which virus gene products may be important in the development of viral disease, molecular techniques can be used to generate a series of mutant viruses. Initial studies concentrated on RNA viruses where **genetic reassortants** could be readily produced. In these viruses the viral genome comprises up to 12 individual RNA molecules—a so-called **segmented** genome (Fig. 13.17). Consequently, when virions are produced from cells infected with two different virus strains, individual viruses may contain RNA molecules derived originally from both strains. The best example of this approach is the observations by Fields and colleagues on the role of viral proteins in the pathogenesis of reovirus-1 infection in the mouse. Reovirus-3 produces severe meningoencephalitis on intracerebral inoculation whereas a much milder form of disease occurs in reovirus-1 infection. By taking advantage of the reovirus segmented genome it is possible to 'cross' the two strains of virus to generate chimeric viruses containing combinations of viral RNAs. The pathogenic effect with respect to CNS disease was thus mapped to the σ-1 protein from reovirus-3 which mediates cell attachment. More precise localization to the globular head of the molecule, which interacts with the host cell, was defined by antibody neutralization escape mutants. Further factors contributing to neurovirulence have been identified by reassortants in the outer capsid protein of reovirus-3.

This powerful technique is restricted to those viruses with segmented genomes where such production of reassortants by 'crossing' is possible. In most instances, however, particularly where the viral genome is present as a single DNA or RNA molecule, site-directed mutagenesis (as used for defining poliovirus tropism) or deletion of single virus gene products is required to assess the role of specific genes in pathogenesis. This can be carried out because DNA or, if the virus has an RNA genome, cDNA copies of these viral genomes, can be introduced into cells resulting in their expression and production of infectious virus (so-called **infectious molecular clones**). These infectious molecular clones can be manipulated at the DNA level to alter DNA sequences at specific sites resulting in specific mutants engineered by recombinant DNA technology. However studies of pathogenesis, or the determination of virus attenuation in the development of live virus vaccines, depend on the availability of an animal model of disease. Such models do not exist for all human viral infections and we then have to rely on correlations of sporadic or natural mutations with observed virulence in humans.

Homologous cellular genes

The large-scale DNA sequencing of viral genomes has led to the recognition that some viruses code for proteins with homologies to human proteins, perhaps particularly proteins involved in the immune response. The pathogenetic significance of most of these homologous genes remains to be assessed, but the degree of homology and their retention by the virus suggests they may be 'captured' cellular genes conferring some selective advantage on the virus. Vaccinia virus is particularly striking in this respect, with homologous genes to those for the IL-2 receptor, serine protease inhibitors (serpins) and various complement proteins: the vaccinia protein with homology to the C4 binding protein can inhibit the classical pathway of complement activation. Herpes simplex virus has a glycoprotein (gC) which acts as a C3b receptor. Human CMV has a glycoprotein which is homologous to the class I MHC heavy chain, although whether and how it has any pathogenic function remains to be seen. EBV possesses a gene (*BCRF1*) with homology to a cytokine synthesis inhibitory factor (also known as IL-10) produced by murine T_H2 cells, and which has similar functional activity.

The most direct way experimentally to assess the pathogenetic significance of these homologous genes is to delete them from the genome and assess the phenotype of the deleted virus, as discussed above. However this may be difficult unless there is a good animal model of pathogenesis in which to study the deletion mutant. Using this approach deletion of individual homologous

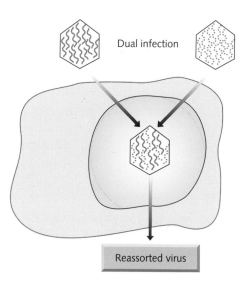

Dual infection

Reassorted virus

Fig. 13.17 Co-infection of cells with two different strains of a virus with a segmented genome, such as influenza or a reovirus, can result in genetic reassortants and can be used to map which of the genomic RNA molecules may encode genes which determine differences in viral pathogenesis.

genes in vaccinia virus has been shown to attenuate virulence in the mouse — although the mouse is not the natural host for his virus. EBV and CMV do not infect experimental animals, so no *in vivo* studies of pathogenesis of deletion mutants are possible.

Impact on therapy

Our slow but steady increase in understanding the molecular mechanisms of virus infections has undoubtedly begun to have an impact on the design of anti-viral strategies.

Anti-viral drugs

This subject is fully covered in Chapter 15. The principal difficulty which for a long time retarded the development of effective anti-viral drugs is the dependence of the viral life cycle on normal cellular functions. This makes it necessary to devise drugs which can in some way discriminate between normal and virus-infected cells, interfering with viral replication or other functions in virus-infected cells without inhibiting the corresponding functions in normal cells. The first really effective anti-viral drug — acyclovir — exemplifies this point: it is preferentially phosphorylated in HSV-infected cells by the virus-specified thymidine kinase, and can only then be incorporated into replicating viral DNA where it then blocks further elongation of the nascent DNA chain. A detailed knowledge of the molecular virology of a given infection is thus an essential prerequisite for designing targeted anti-viral drugs. Thus far all the new anti-viral drugs have been directed to interfering with viral replication, but other classes of anti-virals directed at targets such as the receptor binding proteins, or virus-encoded proteases responsible for processing viral polyproteins (as for HIV), are now being developed. A detailed knowledge of molecular virology and the ability to obtain the genomic sequence of drug-resistant mutants is also crucial for developing anti-viral therapy and to understand and circumvent anti-viral drug resistance.

Soluble receptors

An attractive approach to anti-viral therapy, which is in reality an extension of virus neutralization, is the administration of a soluble form of the natural virus receptor such that it may inhibit binding of virus to the corresponding receptor on the cell membrane. Obviously this approach is only suitable where a relatively specific receptor has been identified. This has been tried in clinical practice with the CD4 receptor for HIV. HIV binds to the outer portion of the CD4 Ig-like structure. A form of the receptor was engineered which did not possess the transmembrane region of the glycoprotein and was modified to allow release from a transfected cell. This material bound to HIV and *in vitro* and *in vivo* had some evidence of efficacy. However, it has so far proved not to be the major advance originally hoped for, because extremely high concentrations of the receptor are required and, as with many viruses, mechanisms of entry may differ with the cell type, e.g. HIV may not use CD4 to enter neurones. It remains possible that this approach may be of value with other infections in the future.

Antibody for therapy and prevention

Antibody has been used for the therapy and prevention of virus infections to a limited extent for some time — examples are the use of immune globulin for the prevention of hepatitis A and B, and of VZV infections. These antibodies are prepared by fractionation of serum from immune donors. However the advent of several new technologies offers the possibility of preparing anti-viral antibodies directed against specific viral epitopes *in vitro*. These include the ability to prepare monoclonal antibodies in large quantities, to genetically engineer the variable regions of rat monoclonal antibodies into a human framework (**humanized monoclonals**), and to select V_H and Fab' immunoglobulin fragments by screening λ expression libraries made from human V_H and V_L sequences. In principle this should enable much higher concentrations of antibody to be used *in vivo* than has hitherto been possible; however the theoretical advantages of antibodies constructed in these ways have yet to be proved in clinical trials.

Impact of molecular approaches on the design of vaccines

The ability to manipulate viral genomes to produce recombinant viruses expressing genes of other viruses, and techniques to enhance production of viral proteins in prokaryotic and eukaryotic expression systems, are leading to new approaches to vaccine design.

Recombinant subunit vaccines

Many of the conventional vaccines are effective in the control of the childhood exanthems, and the widespread and world-wide control of these infections depends as much on adequate production and delivery of existing vaccines as on devising new or improved vaccines.

However, there are still many fundamental problems in developing effective vaccines for persistent virus infections. Often these agents, such as herpesviruses, papillomaviruses and retroviruses, have oncogenic potential and experimental models of infection may not accurately mimic human disease. Furthermore, the generation of a neutralizing antibody response alone may not be sufficient to ensure host protection throughout life, particularly if the virus is capable of being transmitted inside cells where effector T-cell immunity is important in controlling this type of cell-to-cell mediated infection. These problems have resulted in attempts to determine which virus products are the targets for a range of immune responses and then to produce a subunit vaccine which may generate the appropriate response *in vivo*. Production of the relevant viral protein is then achieved by expression of the gene in a system which allows large-scale production *in vitro*. In the case of viral glycoproteins this may mean employing a mammalian cell expression system to permit full glycosylation — as is currently being used for the production of HIV gp120.

In humans, the first vaccine to be produced by recombinant DNA technology, and the most effective and important subunit vaccine presently in regular use, is the hepatitis B surface antigen vaccine. This consists of a short peptide sequence of HBs antigen presented in a circularized form to ensure that neutralizing antibody (the effective response in this instance) is generated.

Engineered live vaccines

Viruses are used as vectors for inserting genes *in vitro* and *in vivo* in experimental studies, and the use of this approach in vaccine delivery and gene therapy is presently under active investigation. Experimentally such recombinant virus vaccines have all the advantages of more traditional live virus vaccination—especially the induction of most types of immune response including effector T-cell responses—but the consequences of using a modified live agent require careful consideration. Their potential effectiveness has been well demonstrated by the use of a recombinant vaccinia virus as a rabies vaccine for animals. This was deliberately released in Belgium, and reduced the frequency of natural rabies infection in the fox population.

Several viruses have the potential for use as live vectors for vaccines. A critical requirement is that the vector itself is non-pathogenic, which means choosing a virus of known low virulence, deleting pathogenic genes, or disabling the virus so it can only undergo limited (or no) replication. In humans, vaccinia is the virus which

has been most studied as a vector, largely because of its successful track record as the vaccine which eliminated smallpox, and its ability to accommodate large DNA inserts. It has the disadvantage of known but rare neurological side effects whilst having the advantages of producing a limited, lytic and localized infection which induces both cell-mediated and antibody responses to inserted sequences — as has been shown in studies of its use in humans for HIV gp120 immunization. Another vector under active study is adenovirus — not least because adenovirus has also previously been used as a live vaccine. In this approach the inserted gene is placed in the E1 region of the virus genome. This region has to be expressed in order to allow virus replication to proceed, and inserting a gene at this site effectively

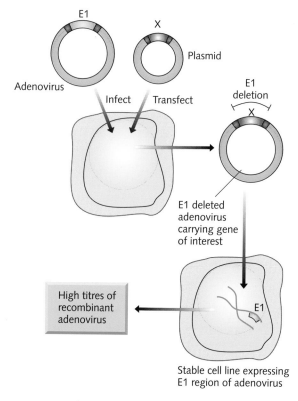

Fig. 13.18 Viral vectors can be used to express recombinant proteins. Adenovirus recombinants, in which the E1 region of the virus has been replaced with a gene encoding an antigenic protein, can be generated by transfecting into cells a plasmid carrying the gene of interest flanked by short homologies to the E1 region of adenovirus. Site-specific recombination occurs generating recombinant virus. Because these virions do not contain the vital E1 region of the adenovirus genome they are defective and do not replicate. Consequently, high titres of the defective virus can only be produced by infecting cells that have been stably transfected with the virus E1 region, allowing good virus production due to complementation of the defective virus with the stably transfected E1 region in the infected cells.

blocks any new lytic virus being produced *in vivo*, whilst the inserted gene is efficiently produced. The vaccine virus itself is grown in complementing cell lines that express the missing E1 protein constitutively: this provision of E1 in *trans* allows full production of the virions which encapsidate the recombinant DNA (Fig. 13.18). In this approach expression is restricted by the viral tropism and it does not allow long-term expression of the inserted sequence — a disadvantage for gene therapy but not for a vaccine. Several other viruses are also being studied as candidate vectors but none is any nearer human trials than the two discussed above.

Peptide vaccines

Hepatitis B vaccine has already been referred to as an example of a polypeptide subunit vaccine. Antigenic epitopes have been identified in other viruses which could potentially be used to generate immune responses. Antibody responses are often less effective if directed against a single epitope and are also susceptible to being evaded by genetic mutation or recombination causing antigenic variation in the pathogen. In theory, T_C peptide epitopes could also be used in immunization to induced protective virus-specific T_C. Unfortunately this approach is limited by the polymorphism of MHC class I and II genes in the population, meaning that no single peptide would be effective for all recipients. Thus at best, even if a multiple peptide vaccine were developed, individuals with unusual MHC haplotypes might be left unprotected. Indeed this problem has already been identified to a limited extent with the hepatitis B vaccine where individuals homozygous for a particular extended MHC haplotype (*B8,SC01,DR3*) are genetic non-responders to the vaccine. A further problem is that peptides may require a 'carrier' protein to induce an effective antibody response. Short peptide sequences may also be expressed in a live virus vector, e.g. poliovirus.

For these reasons it seems unlikely that vaccines based on short peptide epitopes for antibody or T_C will find widespread application.

Other approaches

To date most vaccine strategies require the artificial expression of a particular viral gene product at high levels to achieve immunization. However, other approaches are also possible. In particular, deleting certain genes may make a natural virus less pathogenic — an interesting example of this is the *nef* deletion mutant of simian immunodeficiency virus (SIV) which appears to confer immunity to wild-type SIV without itself producing an AIDS-like illness. This type of targeted molecular virus attenuation based on deleting genes of known pathogenic function is particularly feasible where a good animal model allows attenuation to be proven prior to human use. The construction of viral reassortants or chimeric viruses offers another approach to attenuation. Therapy or inhibition of virus replication by the use of vectors expressing anti-sense RNA (see Chapter 16) may also be possible.

Further reading

Fields B.N., Knipe D.M. and Howley P.M. (eds) (1991) *Virology*. Raven Lippincott, New York.

Chapter 14

Recombinant products for medical use

Introduction

This chapter describes:
• different applications of genetically engineered agents for clinical use, e.g. hormones, growth factors, cytokines, novel antigens for immunization and therapeutic monoclonal antibodies;
• the methods that are used to obtain recombinant gene products and the technology for their expression on an industrial scale;
• examples of use of recombinant products that show advantages of these agents for human therapy.

Developments in molecular genetics and molecular biology have had their most obvious applications in the field of **therapeutic proteins** and **vaccine production**. An astonishing array of products have been approved for clinical use and with an equally broad range of applications. No sooner is a new growth factor or cytokine identified, than it can be explored as a therapeutic agent. Similarly, with the identification of novel epitopes expressed on human lymphocytes, circulating cytokines or other mediators of inflammatory responses, **humanized monoclonal antibodies** can be generated to examine their effects on the course of diseases. Recombinant techniques are also used to synthesize antigens for immunization against microbial diseases. Several of the conspicuous successes of genetically engineered drugs are presented in this chapter.

The benefit of prophylaxis for infectious diseases has been recognized from the time of Jenner with his crude immunization against smallpox by variolation. More sophisticated vaccination against smallpox represents a landmark in public health and has led to global eradication of this disease. Recombinant DNA technology has also made an impact on immunization procedures, elim-inating the need for potentially dangerous live-attenuated vaccines or heat-treated vaccines.

Our understanding of inherited diseases is much more recent. Here, the genetic defect ultimately results in or contributes to the abnormal function of a specific protein. There may, for instance, be a complete lack of an essential protein (e.g. insulin in diabetes mellitus), a mutated protein (e.g. haemoglobin in sickle cell anaemia) or of equal importance, gain of function or loss of regulatory controls of cell proliferation in malignant transformation.

Genetic diseases may be inherited through the germ line or somatically acquired through exposure to a DNA-damaging agent such as tobacco smoke, strong sunlight or dietary factors. Often the changes at the DNA level are comparatively small but the effects are drastic. Table 14.1 lists a few examples of diseases where the genetic disorder has been characterized (these are not necessarily all targets for therapy using recombinant proteins). In a number of these the gene responsible has been cloned and defects within it characterized. In appropriate instances, this allows manipulation of the normal gene using the techniques of **genetic engineering** and production of the protein which it encodes in **recombinant systems**. This has obvious advantages over traditional methods of isolating and purifying biologically active material from large amounts of the appropriate animal tissue. Table 14.2 lists a number of examples of therapeutic proteins now in the clinic which have been produced using recombinant DNA technology.

Recombinant human insulin has replaced that purified from porcine pancreas in the treatment of insulin-dependent diabetes mellitus. Although pig insulin functions well in the treatment of human diabetics there are rare instances of antibody development. A more con-

Table 14.1 Single gene disorders.

Disease	Defective protein	Manifestations
Fabry's	α-Galactosidase A	Accumulation of galactosyl–galactosyl glucosylceramide; renal or cardiac failure, neuralgic limb pain
Niemann–Pick	Sphingomyelinase	Accumulation of sphingomyelin; mental retardation and enlargement of liver and spleen
Gaucher's	Glucocerebrosidase	Accumulation of glucocerebrosides in macrophages; neurological disorders, enlargement of spleen and liver, bone infarction and lysis
Diabetes mellitus	Insulin	Hyperglycaemia, ketosis, vascular disease
Chronic myelogenous leukaemia	Chromosomal translocation 'Philadelphia chromosome'	Proliferation and expansion of myeloid cell series in bone marrow; anaemia, bleeding due to platelet deficiency, infection due to reduced number of neutrophils
Somatotrophic dwarfism	Human growth hormone	Stunted growth and development
Sickle cell anaemia	Single amino acid change in β chain of haemoglobin	Haemolytic anaemia, infarction crises in bones, lungs and brain; predisposition to bacterial infection
Lesch–Nyham syndrome	Guanine phosophoribosyl transferase	Aggressive behaviour, self-mutilation, gout and renal failure due to hyperuricaemia
Phenylketonuria	Phenylalanine-4-monooxygenase	Severe mental retardation
Galactosaemia I	UDP glucose: galactose-1-phosphate uridyl transferase	Liver cirrhosis, mental retardation, growth failure
Galactosaemia II	Galactokinase	Cataracts
Von Gierke's	Glucose-6-phosphatase	Liver enlargement due to excess glycogen, hypoglycaemia, acidosis, enlarged kidneys
Cystic fibrosis	Cystic fibrosis transmembrane receptor	Abnormal mucus secretion causing pancreatic failure, intestinal obstruction in infancy (meconium ileus), bronchopulmonary infection with lung destruction and abscesses

vincing example of the advantages of 'clean' recombinant products compared with material derived from animal or human tissues was well publicized in the media in 1993. Before the use of recombinant human growth hormone (hGH), children with growth defects were treated with hGH derived from the pituitary glands of cadavers. Subsequently, as young adults, about 20 individuals have so far developed Creuzfeldt–Jacob disease, the fatal neurodegenerative disorder, as a consequence of contamination present in the purified hormone. Similarly, the use of unscreened non-recombinant factor VIII from pooled blood led to the infection of thousands of haemophiliacs worldwide with the human immunodeficiency virus (HIV). Even now, despite stringent screening procedures, contaminated non-recombinant blood products are still a potential route of HIV transmission.

The use of recombinant products has major advantages when compared with material purified from tissue sources, particularly in relation to human proteins (e.g. see Box 14.1). Often, large amounts of tissue as a source of the active principle are not available. In addition, the production processes used in making the protein can be more carefully controlled and hence reproducible, ensuring equivalent biological activity in different batches. Finally, once the recombinant system is established as an industrial process, the product will nearly always ultimately be cheaper to manufacture.

A genetic engineering approach to the production of clinically relevant proteins

You will have learnt from Chapter 2 about the basic principles of transcription of DNA to RNA and translation of the RNA to protein. Having an understanding of these mechanisms allows us to design techniques to clone specific genes efficiently in order to direct the **synthesis of recombinant proteins**.

Product	Disease activity*
Human insulin	Diabetes mellitus
Somatotropin	Pituitary dwarfism
Tissue plasminogen activator	Acute myocardial infarction
α-Interferon	Hairy cell leukaemia, chronic myeloid leukaemia, myeloma, hepatitis B, Kaposi's sarcoma in AIDS
β-Interferon	Multiple sclerosis (trials)
γ-Interferon	Anti-tumour agent
Erythropoietin	Anaemia in anephric patients and renal failure
Granulocyte-stimulating factor	Sepsis/neutropenia
Granulocyte–macrophage-stimulating factor	Autologous bone marrow transplant to accelerate regeneration of leukocytes after cytotoxic chemotherapy
Epidermal growth factor	Severe burns
Factor VIIIc } Factor IX }	Haemophilia A and B
Glucocerebrosidase	Gaucher's disease
Interleukin-2	Cancer immunotherapy
Interleukin-3	To improve myelodysplastic cell function and synchronize leukaemic myeloblasts for chemotherapy
Interleukin-4	Immunodeficiency diseases, cancer therapy, vaccine adjuvant
Stem cell factor	To expand haematopoietic stem cells before marrow grafting
Anti-CD3 antibody	Organ transplantation
CAMPATH-1H (anti-lymphocyte antibody)	Rheumatoid arthritis (trial), non-Hodgkin's lymphoma
Anti-endotoxin antibody (monoclonal)	Gram negative bacterial infections
Anti-tumour necrosis factor (monoclonal antibody)	Severe inflammatory states, cerebral malaria, rheumatoid arthritis (trials)

Table 14.2 Therapeutic proteins now used in clinic.

* Includes current and possible trials.

Case study: the use of the CAMPATH-1H humanized monoclonal antibody in the treatment of autoimmune disease and lymphoid malignancies

Introduction

The CAMPATH antigen (now designated CD52) is an abundant molecule distributed on greater than 95% of all human peripheral lymphocytes and monocytes. It is not expressed on granulocytes, platelets, or erythroid and myeloid bone marrow cells. In addition, the antigen is absent from pluripotent and multipotent stem cells. However, CAMPATH antigen is strongly expressed on cells from the majority of B-cell malignancies and at varying levels on T-cell malignancies (see Plate 26a–d, facing p. 214). Because of the specific distribution of the antigen, its presence on B- and T-cell malignancies and its absence on the stem cells required for regeneration of the immune system, the CAMPATH-1H antigen was considered a suitable target for antibody therapy for the treatment of lymphoid malignancies and autoimmune disease. In autoimmune disease, treatment with an anti-lymphocyte antibody would clear self-reactive T- and B-cells from the periphery without destroying the stem cells required for immune regeneration. Treatment of lymphoid malignancies with an anti-CAMPATH-1H antibody would clear disease from the blood, spleen, bone marrow and lymph nodes, again without total immune ablation.

In 1983 spleen cells from a rat immunized with human T-lymphocytes were fused to a myeloma cell line to generate mono-clonal antibody (mAb)-secreting cell lines. Several clones were isolated which produced mAbs that recognized CAMPATH-1 antigen and could lyse T-cells in the presence of human complement. One of these mAbs was designated CAMPATH-1M (a rat IgG1). Subsequently, a class switch variant of an IgG2a mAb to an IgG2b mAb was isolated. This IgG2b mAb, CAMPATH-1G, was the most potent rat subclass for cell depletion *in vivo*, probably because it

Box 14.1

binds to human Fc receptors and can activate the complement system. However, there was considerable evidence that therapeutic treatment with rodent mAbs was likely to be limited by an antiglobulin response, and this problem would be reduced or eliminated by the use of a human antibody. A set of chimeric antibodies was constructed using the rat variable regions of the CAMPATH-1G antibody and different human constant regions. Human IgG1 subclass antibodies were shown to be superior for both lytic ability with complement and with human effector cells. A reshaped 'humanized' version of the rat antibody was subsequently constructed using the hypervariable regions of the rat antibody and human framework regions based on known antibody structures. The first of the reshaped antibodies had significantly lower binding affinity compared with the parental antibody but this was fully restored by a small modification to one of the human framework regions. Finally the reshaped heavy chain variable region was joined to a human IgG1 constant region to gener-

ate CAMPATH-1H. The genes encoding the heavy and light chains of the humanized antibodies were cloned into expression vectors of the type described later in this chapter and large amounts of protein were synthesized and purified from recombinant Chinese hamster ovary cells. This antibody was subsequently used in a number of small-scale clinical trials.

CAMPATH-1H in autoimmune disease—rheumatoid arthritis

Rheumatoid arthritis is a common progressive crippling disease: because of its association with HLA and its response to a number of therapies such as lymphoid irradiation and cyclosporin, there is good evidence that T-cells have a crucial role in its pathogenesis.

Previous studies with rodent mAbs had shown limited success due to variable affinity for antigen and, importantly, an antiglobulin response. The 'humanized' CAMPATH-1H minimized this

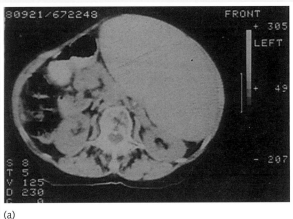

(a)

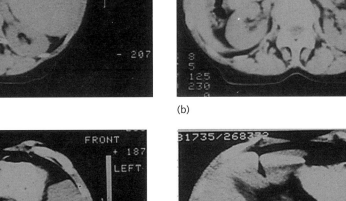

(b)

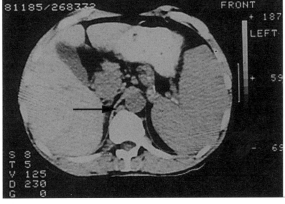

(c)

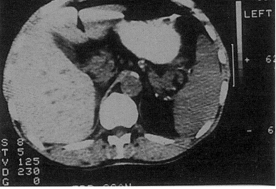

(d)

Fig. A Computed tomography scans showing affected spleens and lymph nodes of two patients with non-Hodgkin's lymphoma, (a) and (c) before treatment; (b) and (d), 7 weeks after treatment with CAMPATH-1H. Note the decrease in spleen size (large organ on right of figure representing left side of abdomen) and para-aortic and other lymph nodes (arrow shows a retrocrural node) (from Hale *et al.* (1988) with permission).

Continued on p. 264

Box 14.1 *Continued.*

response although anti-idiotype and anti-allotype responses could still occur. A number of patients at different centres were recruited and varying dosing regimens were administered. In one study by Isaacs, Waldmann and co-workers at Cambridge, most patients showed impressive, sustained responses by a number of therapeutic measures including reduction in joint swelling and improvement in joint thermography. Duration of remission varied from 12 weeks to 8 months. Selected patients were given second doses and over 70% continued to show therapeutic benefit up to 200 days after retreatment. No significant anti-globulin response was detected. The side effects observed in these studies were transient and were described as acceptable bearing in mind the improvement in the quality of life produced by therapy. Adverse effects were short lived following the first dose and were of the type associated with cytokine release (nausea, fever, etc.). Apart from occasional oral ulceration, infective complications were rare, despite aggressive anti-T-cell therapy, perhaps because the antibody does not bind to and clear neutrophils and monocytes.

Clinical investigations using CAMPATH-1H are currently in progress in a number of other indications with autoimmune involvement, such as systemic vasculitis, psoriasis and multiple sclerosis.

CAMPATH-1H in lymphoid malignancies—non-Hodgkin's lymphoma

Non-Hodgkin's lymphoma (NHL) refers to a family of T- and B-cell malignancies which are characterized by the early stage of lymphocyte development at which neoplasia occurs. NHL includes lymphoblastic lymphoma, lymphocytic lymphoma, lymphoplasmacytoid, T-zone lymphoma and follicular centre tumours such as Burkitt's lymphoma. Patients usually succumb to bone marrow failure and massive infection due to the flooding of the lymph nodes with clonal, non-activating lymphocytes. This makes it an ideal candidate for treatment with an anti-lymphocyte antibody. Malignant cells are cleared from the blood and other sites but progenitor cells that do not express CD52 remain to re-establish the immune system.

In similar small-scale clinical trials to test the efficacy of CAMPATH-1H in this indication, the response in advanced disease was site specific. Clearance or partial clearance of disease was observed in blood, bone marrow and spleen but generally not in the lymph nodes, which may indicate different accessibility of the antibody or associated effector cells to tumour cells in the different compartments of the body. Overall response rates were disappointing, particularly in patients with bulky nodal disease. However, in patients with the T-cell form of prolymphocytic leukaemia, which primarily involves the blood and bone marrow, responses were good with several complete remissions. Adverse effects associated with cytokine release, particularly following the first dose, were common. Anti-idiotype responses were very rare, possibly because of the greater degree of pre-existing immune suppression in these patients.

Recombinant humanized antibodies offer significant clinical potential over other therapies. The cloning and production methods allow large quantities of pure protein to be produced. The reagents may be potent immunomodulators or highly effective in lysing target lymphocytes, and perhaps most importantly their specificity means that they can be targeted to diseased cells or subsets of cells (Fig. A). This has clear advantages over traditional cytotoxic drugs or radiotherapy. Although problems such as anti-idiotype and anti-allotype antibodies and side effects observed on first dose remain to be addressed, and the reagents need to be tested in patients at earlier stages in their disease progression, humanized monoclonal antibodies represent an example of a genetically engineered recombinant protein that will have a major impact on medicine over the next decade.

Box 14.1 *Continued.*

Cloning of the gene of interest

Typically a mammalian cell contains in the region of 10 000 different mRNA species. Some of these are highly expressed (i.e. abundant), others are scarce with perhaps only a few copies per cell. Ultimately the proteins which these mRNA molecules encode determine the differentiated state and properties of the individual cell.

Because most eukaryotic genes contain regions termed introns between the coding sequences, the size of the gene impedes the isolation and retrieval of functional information from the cloned sequence. Fortunately, this problem can be readily circumvented by manipulating the transcribed copy of the gene or mRNA because all the introns are spliced out and the sequence represents only the coding information of the gene. However, because mRNA is difficult to manipulate, in order to isolate or clone the gene of interest, complementary DNA (cDNA) copies of each mRNA species from the appropriate cell or tissue are generated. This process is referred to as making a cDNA library. The steps involved in making a cDNA library are summarized in Fig. 14.1. First, the total cellular mRNA is isolated and copied into cDNA sequence using the reverse transcriptase enzyme that can be primed using short oligonucleotides that bind either randomly or specifically to the poly(A) tail at the 3' end of mRNA molecules. This mRNA/cDNA hybrid is converted into double-stranded DNA by incubation with the enzyme DNA polymerase I which synthesizes the complement to the first strand cDNA molecule. In this form, the DNA can be ligated into replicating cloning vehicles such as plasmids or bacteriophage to generate the final cDNA library that is propagated in a bacterial host.

Remember that a cDNA library should represent the entire spectrum of RNA molecules being transcribed within the cell at the time of isolation. Thus, to identify a specific cDNA clone, the library has to be screened using

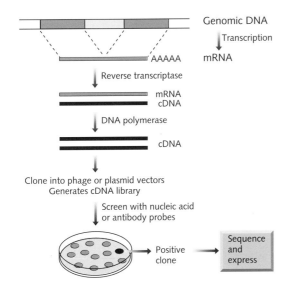

Fig. 14.1 Steps involved in making a DNA library.

a specific nucleic acid or antibody probe. If a partial amino acid sequence is available for the protein, it is possible to convert this information to a consensus nucleic acid sequence and prepare corresponding short DNA probes (oligonucleotides) which can be radioactively labelled and used to screen the library by selective hybridization. Alternatively, antibodies can be raised to the required protein and used to screen a phage **expression library**. Expression libraries are based on the ability of the cloned cDNA to direct the synthesis of protein in the host bacterium so that the cDNA is transcribed under the control of a suitable bacterial promoter present in the phage vector (see below). These are the usual ways to identify a cDNA clone, but with the breadth of molecular techniques now available, there are alternatives. Whichever protocol is used, once the required cDNA is isolated it can be sequenced, thus allowing the protein sequence to be deduced and confirmation of the identity of the cloned gene.

Expression systems for recombinant proteins

Many expression systems are available and much effort has gone into optimizing them to achieve high yields of protein. Generally, the choice of expression system is determined by the particular properties of the protein to be expressed and the purpose for which it is intended. If the protein is a complex multimeric molecule which is extensively post-translationally modified (e.g. a monoclonal antibody), a mammalian expression capable of carrying out the processes will be preferred. Conversely, if a prokaryotic protein is to be produced (e.g. tetanus toxin proteins for a vaccine) then expression in a bacterial expression system would be preferred.

Expression vectors

Whether a eukaryotic or prokaryotic expression system is chosen, the vectors for each all have a number of features in common. These are summarized in Fig. 14.2 and described as follows.

Origin of replication

Virtually all cloning vectors are based upon modified bacterial plasmids which contain a bacterial *ori* (origin of replication). This sequence allows the plasmid to replicate to high copy number without integration into the host bacterial chromosome — a feature that allows production of large amounts of pure DNA for further manipulation. If expression is to be carried out in a mammalian cell, the vector may also contain a viral-based *ori* sequence such as that derived from the simian virus 40 (SV40). If the mammalian host cell (e.g. COS cells, derived from monkey kidney cells) or vector also directs the expression of the appropriate replication-specific protein for this *ori*, in this case the SV40 large T-antigen, then high-copy episomal replication can occur in these cells for several days. This is referred to as a transient mammalian expression system and is useful for the production of small quantities of the recombinant protein for initial studies.

Promoter

This element is positioned immediately upstream of the gene to be expressed and it is responsible for the specificity and efficiency of transcription. The promoter acts as an entry site for RNA polymerase which forms part of the multimeric transcription complex and begins transcribing the cDNA insert into mRNA. The promoter often constitutes the major determinant for the degree of expression levels obtained and, by the correct choice, it is possible to express genes either constitutively or inducibly at low or high level. An additional key feature of the promoter region is a series of unique restriction enzyme-cloning sites placed at its 3′ end. This bank of sites, or polylinker as it is known, enables the cDNA to be inserted into the correct position and orientation for transcription.

General structure

(a)

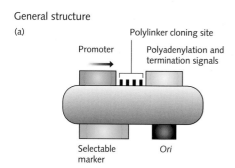

(b)

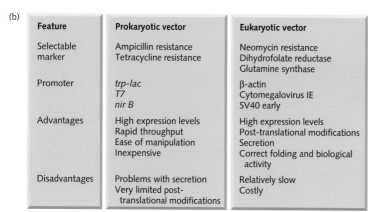

Feature	Prokaryotic vector	Eukaryotic vector
Selectable marker	Ampicillin resistance Tetracycline resistance	Neomycin resistance Dihydrofolate reductase Glutamine synthase
Promoter	*trp-lac* T7 *nir B*	β-actin Cytomegalovirus IE SV40 early
Advantages	High expression levels Rapid throughput Ease of manipulation Inexpensive	High expression levels Post-translational modifications Secretion Correct folding and biological activity
Disadvantages	Problems with secretion Very limited post-translational modifications	Relatively slow Costly

Fig. 14.2 (a) General structure of expression vectors; (b) features of expression vectors.

Termination signals

The termination of transcription, processing and stability of mRNA is dependent upon the addition of specific sequences at its 3′ terminus. These are provided from termination blocks, and in the case of mammalian expression systems, are responsible for tailing the mRNA with the characteristic poly(A) 3′ sequences. The combination of the promoter, cloned gene and termination signals is often referred to as an 'expression cassette'.

Selectable marker

In either prokaryotic or eukaryotic systems, the process of introduction of DNA is known as transfection and is a relatively inefficient one. The identification of those cells which have successfully taken up the foreign DNA can be enhanced considerably by incorporating a selectable marker (constituting a separate expression cassette), either directly into the expression vector or by co-transfecting with another plasmid containing the marker. The selectable marker cassette usually codes for a protein which confers drug resistance, or corrects a mutation in a metabolic pathway of the host or allows the host to metabolize a toxic agent. In a number of

instances, it also allows the copy number of the gene of interest to be increased in response to the selective agent. This process is known as amplification and is fundamental to most mammalian expression systems. Whichever marker is chosen, the end result is selective death of the non-transfected host cells and the enrichment and propagation of the host cells which express the transfected DNA as stable integrants.

Other considerations

Despite much knowledge about the behaviour of expression systems, it is often found that two different genes in the same cell line in the same vectors are expressed at greatly different levels. This is accounted for by several factors, some of which can be predicted and standardized.

Before cloning the gene into expression vectors, it is practice to remove as much 5′ and 3′ untranslated region (UTR) from the cDNA as possible. The 3′ regions may contain signals for RNA degradation. Clearly, if the RNA is rapidly degraded, expression is likely to be low. The 3′ regions also contain large poly(A) tracts. Because expression vectors already contain poly(A) signals, the resulting transcripts will have tandemly repeated poly(A) regions which may cause instability. The stability of the protein is determined by its primary amino acid sequence, and as such, is difficult to manipulate without altering characteristics of the product. If the protein is to be secreted, the secretion signal can be optimized using genetic engineering techniques and site-specific mutagenesis. The expression of some proteins to high levels can be toxic to the cell and this will cause problems in maintaining viability over the many cell divisions required in the manufacturing scale-up procedure. There are reports of single amino acid changes to a protein which completely remove this toxicity, although it may be necessary to use a different approach to expression if this problem is encountered. It is clear that a detailed understanding of the process of gene expression allows us to develop systems which usually produce cell lines expressing high levels of heterologous proteins. Occasionally though, despite all of the optimization procedures described, some genes have inherent properties that lead to low-level expression in heterologous systems. In these instances, manufacturing process and scale have to be adjusted accordingly.

Expression of recombinant proteins in transfected mammalian cells

Selection of a transfected cell line

Although there are a variety of expression systems available, many of the therapeutic proteins in clinical use are expressed in stable, amplified mammalian systems and it is these that are discussed here.

Once a plasmid, containing expression cassettes with the gene of interest and the selectable marker, has been transfected into the eukaryotic cell, the growth conditions are changed in order to select specifically for cells stably expressing the genes encoded by the plasmid DNA. Often, the cells harbour a mutation in a vital metabolic pathway and selection for cells expressing plasmids can be effected by growing the cells in conditions under which the defect is not complemented so that the cell does not survive. The gene required to metabolize appropriate precursors and complement the cellular defect is provided in the vector as the selectable marker so that only transfected cells are able to propagate. (Those cells that are not stably expressing the plasmid-encoded marker gene are unable to grow in the selective medium and die.) This initial selection can generate clones expressing quite high levels of protein (up to 15 μg recombinant protein/million cells/24 h).

The actual level of expression from an individual transfected clone of cells will depend upon the efficiency of transcription of the expression cassette. This, in turn, will depend upon the promoter used but also the position of plasmid DNA integration into the host cell chromosome. Because DNA integration is an entirely random process, the DNA may integrate at a region of the chromosome that is normally highly transcribed or may contain active enhancer elements. Clones of this sort are likely to express recombinant proteins at higher levels than those where the DNA has integrated at a transcriptionally silent region.

Alternatively, expression vectors containing a selectable marker and gene of interest may be based upon viral origins of replication. These can be introduced into cells together with genes encoding viral gene products which maintain the episomal maintenance of the plasmid, such as is seen for Epstein–Barr virus (EBV)-based vectors (Fig. 14.2a). This results in high numbers of replicating plasmids with correspondingly high levels of expression of any genes on the plasmid vector.

Amplification of expression levels

Protein expression can be increased further by increasing the number of copies of the expression cassette within the cell—amplification. In amplification, the cells from the selection process are grown in the presence of a toxic agent which interacts with, and effectively titrates out, the protein produced by the selectable marker. An example of this would be the toxic drug methotrexate and the selectable marker dihydrofolate reductase (DHFR), an essential enzyme in the pathway of folate biosynthesis. Folate is required for pyrimidine biosynthesis and thus DNA replication by dividing cells. Thus, if the transfected cells are to survive this additional selection, they must synthesize more of the DHFR protein. To do this, they expand many-fold the region of the chromosome containing the selectable marker gene. Because the gene encoding the protein to be expressed is adjacent to the selectable marker by virtue of being linked in the transfected expression vector, it is also amplified. By using appropriate levels of selective drug, the number of copies of the integrated DNA can be increased by up to 100-fold. This process of amplification will generate clones expressing up to 50 μg recombinant protein/million cells/24 h, which remain stable in culture for many generations.

Industrial-scale production

Once a stable cell line has been established, it can be scaled up for bulk production of the protein. This involves the generation of a master cell bank: a store containing hundreds of frozen samples of an individual clone for use in industrial-scale production fermentation. An individual sample will contain about 1 million cells in 1 ml of culture medium. This has to be scaled up through increasingly large volumes to perhaps an 8000 litre 'fermenter' containing between 1 and 2 million cells/ml, and hence the requirement for stability becomes obvious. Clearly the choice of cell type influences the production process. Ideally the transfected cell will grow rapidly in the serum-free suspension conditions of the fermenter. The integrated DNA should be stable in these conditions and expression should be maintained at a high level throughout the production process. This may require progressive adaptation of the clones from the conditions used for the initial production to those used in the production process, with careful monitoring of expression levels at each stage.

Choice of expression system

As stated, each expression system has certain advantages and disadvantages (Fig. 14.2). Prokaryotic (i.e. bacterial) systems are generally quick, cheap, easy to manipulate and are somewhat simpler to use. The expression cassette can be maintained in the cell episomally by growing in the presence of a selective agent such as an antibiotic. Bacteria grow readily to very high cell densities in suspension in comparatively simple media. However, they are not suitable for proteins that require secretion and modifications such as glycosylation or lipidation because they lack the necessary post-translational machinery. Conversely, eukaryotic (principally mammalian) systems can post-translationally modify and secrete proteins. In some instances this is required for activity and clearly, secretion of a protein significantly simplifies purification procedures. In contrast to prokaryotic systems, it takes much longer to generate clonal lines of eukaryotic cells capable of expressing high levels of recombinant protein. Eukaryotic expression systems are generally more costly because of the complex conditions they require for optimal growth.

Generally, production of therapeutic proteins is carried out either in stable, amplifiable mammalian systems or bacteria, depending on the protein expressed. However, other systems are sometimes used. Yeast expression systems can be used and have some of the advantageous properties of mammalian and prokaryotic systems. They are able to carry out some limited post-translational modifications found in mammalian cells and in some instances can secrete very large amounts of protein. In addition, they grow readily in suspension to high cell density in simple medium and can be transfected with episomal expression vectors.

Another class of expression vectors are the viral systems, the most common being baculovirus-infected insect cells. In this system, the gene of interest replaces a viral gene polyhedrin, that is not essential to the lytic life cycle of the virus. The recombinant virus can now be used to infect host insect cells that can produce very high levels of recombinant protein. The infected cells modify the protein post-translationally but secretion is limited. The system is rapidly established, relatively easily manipulated and insect host cells adapt well to growth as a suspension in serum-free medium. The disadvantage of both of these systems is that although they are able to carry out most post-translational modifications, they may not be identical to the original protein. This is particularly true of the last modifying steps of glycosylation, which may induce unexpected difficulties related to antigenicity as well as survival in the bloodstream, when administered to the patient.

Characterization and quality control of the recombinant protein for clinical use

Once an appropriate expression system has been established, much work will be needed before the protein produced is suitable for clinical use. The protein must be pure before being used in human therapy. All contaminating proteins must be removed to prevent unwanted immune reactions to proteins from the host cell or from the culture medium. This often requires complex and costly purification procedures. The non-specific toxicity of the protein must be assessed in a variety of laboratory animals and ultimately in human volunteers (e.g. see Box 14.2). The protein must also be thoroughly characterized and its biochemical activity compared with the native protein. The stability, pharmacology, tissue distribution, excretion and bioavailability of the recombinant product are determined and each batch of material is subjected to a rigorous quality assurance to ensure that the specific activity of each batch is reproducible. This is obviously important when designing dosing regimens. Once all these preliminary data have been gathered, the protein is ready to be used in clinical trials. This requires approval from regulatory licensing authorities and ethical committees. Following this, the protein is ready for the lengthy clinical trial process (Fig. 14.3). In 1988, it was estimated that the overall cost incurred in the development of each successful product, including the failures, was of the order of £100–200 million.

Case history: the use of recombinant-derived human erythropoietin to treat the anaemia of chronic renal failure

One of the first patients in the world to be treated with recombinant human erythropoietin (r-HuEPO) was a 26-year-old printer with Alport's syndrome, in 1986. In 1982 he had developed chronic renal failure and had started regular haemodialysis. A renal transplant in that year had failed, leaving him highly sensitized and difficult to retransplant. He was dependent on regular blood transfusions and by the time r-HuEPO treatment became available, had had 64 units in 4 years. His ferritin was 3400 µg/l. He was breathless and without energy in the 10 days before his transfusions when his haemoglobin reached 5 g/dl. He was treated with escalating doses of r-HuEPO and his haemoglobin rose to 15 g/dl. He no longer required transfusions, no longer felt the cold and regained his energy. The only complication was clotting of his arteriovenous fistula which was surgically restored. In the summer of 1988 he and another home haemodialysis patient treated with r-HuEPO cycled from Land's End to John O'Groats to raise money for research.

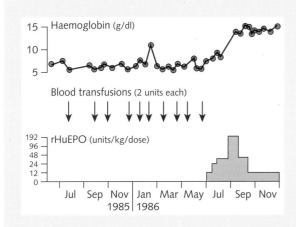

Fig. A See box text for explanation. (Figure supplied courtesy of Dr C. J. Winnearls.)

Box 14.2

Summary

Clearly the use of recombinant proteins will have an increasingly important role to play in the treatment of human disease. More products, some with novel activities which have been approved for use in the clinic, are coming into the pharmaceutical market place and a number of examples are given in Table 14.2. Whilst the potential for the production of proteins by recombinant technology is obvious, the clinical value of such products is under rigorous scrutiny, especially in relation to mammalian proteins that are post-translationally modified by the addition of sugar residues. This glycosylation plays an important role in the structure and hence presentation to the immune system. Since glycosylation is cell type, tissue type and species specific, proteins expressed in heterologous systems may differ in their glycosylation profile from the native human protein. Where multiple doses of the protein are required, adverse reactions may be expected and represent an important challenge for the future exploitation of this technology.

As the genetic basis for disease becomes increasingly understood, the number of instances whereby a recombinant protein can be used to effect a useful clinical response looks set to increase dramatically. A notable recent advance has been the use of modified human glucocerebrosidase for the treatment of the lysosomal storage disorder, Gaucher's disease (Plate 27, facing p. 214). Administration of tissue-derived human glucocerebrosidase, modified to reveal terminal mannose residues (alglucerase, 'Ceredase') alleviates the manifestations of this disorder — which is due to the deficiency of the enzyme primarily in cells of the mononuclear phagocyte system. It appears that modification of the native enzyme enhances its uptake by macrophages and targets the product for lysosomal complementation. Latterly the supply of human placentas has limited production of

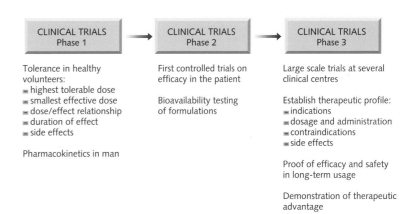

Fig. 14.3 The clinical trials process.

the drug and a suitably modified recombinant product, with comparable efficacy, Cerezyme, has been manufactured from Chinese hamster ovary cells.

In the future, the impact of gene therapy (Chapter 16) coupled with data from the human genome sequencing project will greatly increase both our understanding of disease processes and our opportunity for clinical intervention at the molecular level and allow us to tackle the major medical challenges of diseases such as cancer and AIDS.

Further reading

Bebbington C.R. and Hentschel C.C.G. (1987) *DNA Cloning,* *Vol. 3, A Practical Approach*, Ch. 8, pp. 163–188. IRL Press, Oxford.

Cooper D.N. and Krawczak M. (1993) *Human Gene Mutation*, Appendix 1. BIOS, Oxford.

Hale G., Dyer M.J.S., Clark M.R., Phillips J.M., Marcus R., Reichmann L., Winter G. and Waldmann H. (1988) Remission induction in non-Hodgkin lymphoma with reshaped human monoclonal antibody. CAMPATH-IH. Lancet, **ii**(Dec), 1394–1399.

Old R.W. and Primrose S.B. (1994) *Principles of Gene Manipulation*, 5th edn. Blackwell Scientific Publications, Oxford.

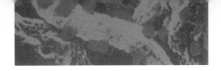

Chapter 15 Drug discovery

Introduction

In the past, the search for new drugs relied heavily on chance, using molecules randomly tested with little hope or expectation that they would have any useful biological activities. The advent of molecular biology has added a new dimension to the drug discovery process and has made possible a far more rational approach to the problem. Nowhere has this impact been greater than in the area of infectious diseases and in virology in particular. In this chapter we will look at the many contributions molecular biology is making, both to our understanding of current drugs and to the discovery of new ones. Many of the examples used will be from the area of AIDS research, since the serious medical problems posed by this disease and the willingness of governments, private institutions and the pharmaceutical industry to invest heavily in the search for a cure has led to an unprecedented level of research activity. However, it should be remembered that many of the principles described here can be applied in any other disease area. There are still many unsolved diseases where drugs could have a significant impact, and the approaches now being developed provide real hopes that the future may not be left totally to chance.

Identification of drug targets

Drugs act by interfering in the pathways which lead to disease, inhibiting an enzyme, preventing the interaction of a molecule with its cellular receptor, and by other potential mechanisms. If we wish to adopt a rational approach to the drug discovery process our first task is to identify the precise point in the pathway at which we would like to intervene. This involves first having a clear understanding of pathogenesis, the processes which lead to the development of the disease. Fortunately for the virologist who is interested in those diseases caused by

viruses, it is reasonable to work on the assumption that if we block multiplication of the virus in the tissues of the infected host (the patient) we are likely to arrest disease progression and thus improve the outcome. We can therefore narrow down our target to a protein whose function is essential for virus replication. However, the biggest difficulty faced is that viruses multiply inside the cells of the host organism, and the ideal drug is therefore one which can penetrate the cell, interfere in the virus multiplication process but have absolutely no effect on the delicate and complex machinery of the cell.

Although viruses are **intracellular parasites** and use the machinery of the host cell in their replication, a virus also encodes its own complement of genes, many of which are absolutely required for multiplication. Some will encode **structural proteins**, the building blocks required to construct new virus particles; others, more importantly from the perspective of potential anti-viral drugs, will encode proteins essential for replication of the virus's own genetic material (**the genome**); and yet others may encode proteins involved in the regulation of the cellular machinery, allowing the virus to use that machinery efficiently to serve its own needs. Amongst these virus-specific protein products we can find appropriate targets for our drugs.

Some virus-coded proteins may be similar in function to cellular proteins. For example, a virus whose genome has its genetic information encoded in a DNA molecule will have to produce replicas of that DNA molecule in the infected cell in order to build new virus particles. This requires the activity of an enzyme which can catalyse the synthesis of DNA, a **DNA polymerase**. Normal cells possess several **DNA polymerases** involved in various aspects of **DNA synthesis** and the virus could, in theory, use one of these enzymes for its own replication, as indeed happens with some viruses. However, most DNA viruses encode their own **DNA polymerases** and these are all suitable anti-viral targets. The problem, of course, is that any inhibitor of this virus enzyme must be able to distinguish between the virus enzyme and that of the host.

By far the most attractive targets are those functions that are unique to the virus-infected cell, since it is those which offer the greatest chance of selectivity. Viruses often use somewhat bizarre mechanisms during replication, and these can provide the 'Achilles heel' the drug hunter is looking for. A simple example can be seen in the influenza viruses.

The genome of **influenza** is composed of eight fragments of RNA. However, these RNA molecules cannot themselves be translated by the machinery of the host cell to make virus proteins, they must first of all be copied into **complementary strands** which then act as mRNAs. Normal mRNA has a complex 'cap' structure on its 5′ end comprising methylated nucleosides, and this is generated by a group of specialized host cell enzymes. However, instead of using host cell enzymes to generate the **cap structure**, influenza employs the rather underhand technique of stealing the caps from newly made cellular mRNAs (Fig. 15.1). This achieves the primary function of capping the influenza mRNA, but also has the secondary effect of inactivating host cell transcripts, thus freeing up the translation machinery to make only virus proteins. Clearly such an unusual process would make an excellent drug target. The question is, are similar unusual functions encoded by other viruses?

Fortunately most viruses have a relatively restricted complement of genes (in the range 10–100) and with most pathogenic human viruses we have a good idea of the functions of many of them. One starting point in the search for unusual functions will be the sequence of the virus genome itself.

Since viruses encode only a handful of genes, they were the first organisms to have their genetic information completely defined. The first virus genome, that of the bacterial virus ϕx174, was sequenced in 1976, and since then we have seen the determination of the genomic sequences of most pathogenic human viruses. The most dramatic example is that of the **human immunodeficiency** virus (HIV), the causative agent of AIDS, where there was a gap of only 2 years between the first description of the virus in 1983, and the publication in 1985 of the complete nucleotide sequence of the 9000 bases in its RNA genome, although even this achievement pales somewhat when compared to the mammoth task of sequencing the genomes of the **human herpesviruses**, each of which contains between 100 000 and 200 000 basepairs.

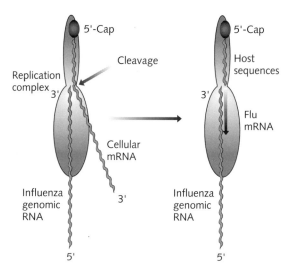

Fig. 15.1 Cap-stealing in influenza transcription. The negative sense genomic RNA segments of influenza virus are transcribed by a complex of three virus encoded proteins. Rather than generate its own 5′-cap structures, a feature of most cellular mRNA species, influenza virus steals ready-made caps from nascent host cell mRNA molecules. Host mRNA is bound to the replication complex and a 5′ fragment including the cap and the first dozen or so nucleotides is clipped off. The 3′-end of this fragment is then used to prime influenza mRNA synthesis. Influenza mRNA species therefore have a short non-translated segment composed of host sequence at their 5′ end. This novel, virus-specific process should obviously provide a highly specific anti-viral target.

Nevertheless we do have the complete sequences of three of the human herpesviruses, **varicella-zoster**, **herpes simplex** and **human cytomegalovirus**. Analysis of the sequence data allows the identification of the possible **open reading frames** (uninterrupted strings of codons encoding amino acids) which define for us the polypeptides encoded by the virus.

The next task is to assign function to the protein products, and here again molecular biology has made a valuable contribution. Knowledge of the **replication strategies of viruses** built up over the years, often using laborious genetic and biochemical techniques, has provided many clues to the functions required by viruses for replication. For example, all must inevitably encode a number of structural proteins. These are often the easiest to identify and the best characterized proteins, but unfortunately they are probably the least useful as drug targets. There are two other categories of protein which provide better targets, the enzymes involved in genome replication and **regulatory proteins**. However, these non-structural proteins are often more elusive and difficult to tie down.

In the absence of existing knowledge, one approach which may sometimes give a quick idea of function is to compare the amino acid sequence of the putative virus protein with the sequences of other proteins of known function, a process which is made possible by the existence of accessible comprehensive databases and powerful computer programs designed to do the job. If we are lucky this approach will pick up small **motifs** (runs of a few amino acids) represented in both the viral and a nonviral protein. If the function of the motif in the non-viral protein is known, this may provide clues to the functional role of the virus protein.

This kind of approach was used, for example, to identify two putative **protein kinases** encoded by herpes simplex virus, enzymes capable of phosphorylating other proteins of either the virus or the infected cell. Since the cellular counterparts of these **protein kinases** have been replaced in many important **regulatory processes**, these are obvious candidate virus **regulatory proteins**. It has also been used to identify **proteases** encoded by a number of different viruses, including herpes viruses, HIV, hepatitis C and many others. These are enzymes which cleave other protein molecules and which are again involved in regulating protein function or, in the virus field, allowing **particle maturation**.

The characterization process is of course simplified if we know what we are looking for. For example, as we have seen already, the **replication strategies** of some viruses involve biochemical processes rarely if ever seen in the uninfected cell. All viruses which have RNA genomes, such as influenza, polio or HIV, fall into this category since they must either encode enzymes which can replicate RNA or, in the case of **retroviruses** such as HIV, they must encode **reverse transcriptase**, an enzyme which is able to copy the RNA genome into DNA form. Often these nucleic acid polymerases can be recognized by telltale motifs. However, the final proof of function is often obtained only when the suspect gene is hooked to an appropriate promoter, expressed in a heterologous system, purified and shown by biochemical techniques to possess the expected activity.

The final important question is whether the gene product is essential for virus multiplication, since this is another key characteristic required of a target protein. Genetic approaches can help to answer this question.

There are a large number of virus mutants which have been isolated either spontaneously or following **mutagenesis** of the virus, which have been called **conditional lethal mutants**. The feature of these variants is that they will grow under normal conditions but if exposed to selective pressure — this could be for example a higher than normal temperature — they fail to replicate. The breakdown in the replication process is due to a failure of the mutant protein to function under the selective or **'non-permissive'** conditions. A more recent approach is to delete the gene of interest from the virus. If this results in the failure of the virus to grow in normal cells then this is clear evidence that the gene product is essential (Fig. 15.2). Therefore, if a lesion in a particular gene is known to result in a **conditional lethal variant**, then the gene product is required for replication and is thus a potential target.

If the virus has a DNA genome, molecular approaches may be useful for telling us which proteins we should avoid as drug targets, proteins whose functions are not absolutely necessary for multiplication. If the protein product is not required for replication, its gene can generally be deleted from the virus genome without compro-

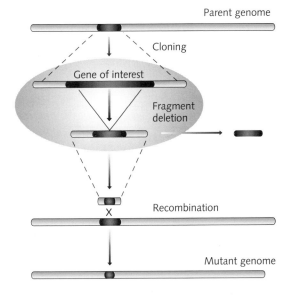

Fig. 15.2 Deletion of a virus gene. A good way of demonstrating that a virus gene is essential, and therefore an appropriate anti-viral target, is to show that deletion of the gene renders the virus non-viable. The gene of interest along with flanking sequences is cloned into a suitable vector system and a fragment of the gene is then deleted. The gene carrying the deletion is introduced back into virus by recombination with the parent. This recombination is carried out in a cell line engineered to express the gene of interest so that the recombinant carrying the deletion is able to grow, and the recombinant is isolated in the same complementing cell line. Finally the viability of the recombinant is tested in normal cells. If the recombinant grows in complementing cells but not normal cells, this shows that the deleted gene is essential.

mising the replication process. This approach can be illustrated using the **thymidine kinase** gene of **herpes simplex virus** as an example. **Thymidine kinase** is an enzyme which phosphorylates thymidine to thymidine monophosphate. This is the first stage in the conversion of the nucleoside to its triphosphate which is the building block used for DNA synthesis. To attempt to construct a virus lacking this function, a fragment of the genome containing the kinase gene is first of all isolated as a plasmid clone. Next a portion of the gene is deleted from the clone using a pair of appropriate **restriction enzyme sites**. The resulting fragment is introduced into a cell along with intact DNA derived from the parent virus using any one of a number of transfection techniques. DNA from the wild-type virus is infectious but during replication it will **recombine** with the deleted fragment. The result of such a **recombination** event is the appearance of a new genome with an internal deletion in the gene of interest, thus precluding expression of the active product from the mutant genome. If such a variant is viable it will grow and can be isolated as a pure clone from the virus population. The isolation of such a recombinant tells us that the thymidine kinase encoded by the virus is not required for replication and is thus unlikely to be a satisfactory drug target. Using this kind of approach it has been possible to show that many viruses encode a significant number of non-essential gene products not required for multiplication. It should be pointed out that these products are not without value but their effects are often seen only in animal models of the disease process.

Using a combination of the techniques outlined above, a picture of the genetic composition of a virus can be built up. Its genes can be identified, in many cases the functions of the products can be assigned, and those which are absolutely required for virus replication can be distinguished from the 'luxury' functions. This can readily be illustrated for HIV, where in the past few years it has been possible to assign function to all of the 15 open reading frames identified in the sequence (Fig. 15.3).

Having identified the genes and their functions, we can consider how we might select appropriate anti-viral targets. Again we can take HIV as the example.

Molecular targets in HIV

If we look at the proteins expressed by HIV, they fall very clearly into the three classes that we have discussed already: **structural proteins**, **regulatory proteins** and **enzymes**. What are their relative merits as potential targets?

Structural proteins

The structural proteins are of two types, the so-called **gag proteins** which form the core of the virus and which are capable of aggregating in a regular array to form a protective shell around the virus nucleic acid, and the **env proteins**, **glycoproteins** which are associated with the lipid membrane which surrounds the core (Fig. 15.4). The glycoproteins are responsible for attaching the virus

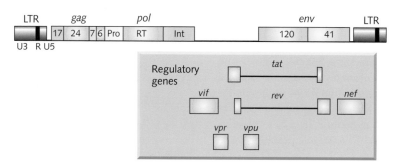

Fig. 15.3 Genome organization of HIV. In common with all retroviruses, HIV has three major groups of genes. The *gag* region encodes the structural proteins of the virus core, p24 being the major structural protein. The *pol* region encodes the enzymes activities required for virus replication; Pro is an aspartyl protease involved in processing the gag-pol precursor polypeptide by proteolytic cleavage, reverse transcriptase encodes a bifunctional enzyme having both reverse transcriptase and ribonuclease H activities, and Int is a protein involved in the integration of the HIV provirus into the host

cell chromosome. The *env* region encodes the surface glycoproteins, gp120 which binds to the CD4 receptor on the cell surface, and gp41 which is involved in membrane fusion. Finally, there is a series of genes unique to the lentiviruses (of which HIV is a member) which have been termed the 'regulatory genes'. These are involved in controlling a number of virus–host interactions. Each end of the HIV genome (in its DNA form) is composed of the LTR (long terminal repeat) sequence which is manufactured during reverse transcription of the RNA genome.

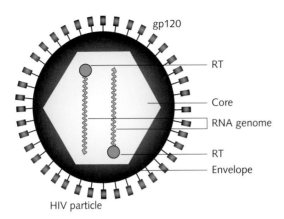

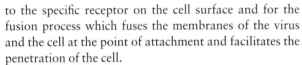

Fig. 15.4 The HIV particle. The main features of the HIV particle are an outer envelope into which the glycoprotein, gp41, is embedded (the second glycoprotein, gp120, is complexed with gp41 but there are no strong covalent bonds and so it is only loosely attached to the particle), and an inner core which contains two copies of the RNA genome along with the reverse transcriptase.

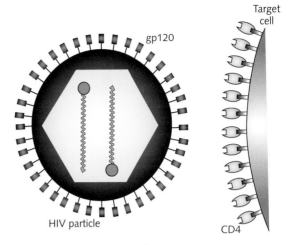

Fig. 15.5 Attachment of HIV to a cellular receptor. The initial recognition of a susceptible host cell by HIV is mediated through an interaction between the surface glycoprotein, gp120, and the cell surface receptor CD4. Multiple interactions are required to bind the virus to the cell surface. Subsequently the virus and cell membranes fuse and the virus core penetrates the cell.

to the specific receptor on the cell surface and for the fusion process which fuses the membranes of the virus and the cell at the point of attachment and facilitates the penetration of the cell.

The only process mediated through the structural proteins which has been attacked with any success has been the interaction between the **glycoprotein gp120** and the **cellular receptor**, the **CD4 molecule** (Fig. 15.5). It was reasoned that since gp120 must bind to the extracellular portion of CD4, if the CD4 receptor itself could be obtained in a soluble form, this material could be used as a decoy to saturate the gp120 protein and thus prevent the attachment of the virus to the target cell. This was achieved by taking a clone of the whole CD4 molecule, removing its carboxy-terminal **membrane anchor domain** and expressing the remaining fragment in *Escherichia coli*. The soluble product could indeed be shown to block virus attachment in tissue culture systems (Fig. 15.6), but results with this product in the clinic have been disappointing.

There appear to be several reasons for the failure of this approach. Firstly, although laboratory-adapted virus strains were exceptionally sensitive to inhibition by this protein fragment, when isolates from patients were looked at they appeared far less sensitive. Secondly, there is the simple logistical problem that there are a large number of gp120 molecules on the virus surface and it is necessary to smother the particle with CD4 to prevent attachment, a process requiring a very high concentra-

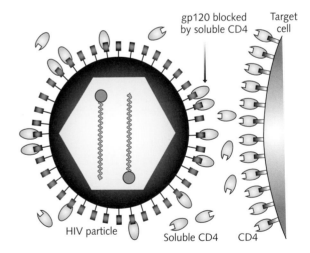

Fig. 15.6 Soluble CD4 blocks attachment of HIV to the cell. One approach to blocking the interaction between the HIV glycoprotein, gp120, and its receptor on the cell, CD4, is to introduce large quantities of soluble CD4 (soluble CD4 is produced by expressing a fragment of CD4 with the transmembrane anchor removed). The soluble protein binds to the virus surface and prevents interaction with the cell-surface CD4 molecules. Although this approach was shown to work in principle in the laboratory it has not so far proven useful in the clinic.

tion of the product. Finally, it transpired that **soluble CD4** was fairly rapidly degraded in the relatively hostile environment of the human body.

An interesting development was to try to use the CD4 molecule to target not the virus itself, but the infected cell. One of the consequences of virus multiplication in the infected cell is that the virus glycoproteins appear on the surface of the cell. If the CD4 molecule is linked to a powerful **toxin** such as **ricin** or the *Pseudomonas* toxin, the toxic species can be targeted specifically to the virus-infected cell which will be killed. This 'magic bullet' approach is one which certainly works *in vitro* but there are still many problems in translating it to use in patients.

Regulatory proteins

HIV, in common with many other viruses, encodes proteins involved in the regulation of events in the infected cell. Of these, two have attracted particular attention as potential drug targets. The product of the *tat* gene (**transactivator of transcription**) is a small protein which cranks up the level of virus transcription in the infected cell. Unlike many host cell transcription factors which bind to specific sequences in DNA, *tat* is unusual in that it binds to a sequence in messenger RNA precursors, the so-called **TAR sequence**. The second regulatory protein is the product of the *rev* gene. This product also binds to RNA, at the **RRE element**. Its function seems to be to block the splicing of the mRNA of the virus, which is required for the expression of the structural proteins of the virus.

In both cases the important interactions of these proteins are with short RNA sequences and also with other transcription and translation factors. There is some doubt about the absolute requirement for *tat* expression in the infected cell, which may make *rev* the better target, but in any case although there has been considerable progress in understanding the functions of these proteins we are still a long way from designing effective inhibitors.

Enzymes

The only other proteins encoded by HIV are a group of enzymes, the products of the *pol* gene. There are three proteins encoded by this region, **reverse transcriptase**, **protease** and **integrase**. The least well characterized of the three is the integrase, which is involved as its name suggests in the integration of the **proviral DNA** into the **chromosome** of the cell (see Chapter 13). The other enzymes have both been the focus of intense activity

which has led to the discovery of a number of potent inhibitors of the virus and which will be discussed in more detail later.

Once the molecular targets have been identified, we then have the immense problem of discovering effective and selective inhibitors, but before this can be tackled we need to generate supplies of the proteins and we need to establish simple assay systems in which we can look at their functions.

Heterologous expression

One of the severe limitations to the study of virus proteins has been that many of them, especially the enzymes and regulatory proteins, are made in the infected cell in extremely small quantities. However, with the advent of techniques for the expression of gene products in **heterologous systems** under the control of powerful **promoters** (see Chapter 4) this has ceased to be a major problem with most virus proteins. There is a bewildering array of possible cell systems that can be used, bacterial, yeast or eukaryotic, with a variety of methods of introducing foreign genes into the cell. The approach which is normally adopted is to use the simplest system which will provide an adequate supply of the active protein.

The first system to be tried is usually **transformation** of a bacterial cell with a **plasmid** carrying the required gene. The outcome cannot be predicted, as can be easily illustrated using HIV **reverse transcriptase** and HIV **protease** as examples. **Reverse transcriptase** is a large complex protein and problems with expression would not be surprising. However, this protein can be made in large quantities in *E. coli*. It is produced as a native, soluble product which can be readily purified. In contrast, **protease** is a small simple protein which might be expected to be an ideal candidate for bacterial expression. The opposite is the case. The first problem is that HIV protease is extremely toxic to the cells and so in order to grow cells carrying this gene the gene must be turned off. A **promoter** which requires induction must be used and when not induced there must be no leakiness. When cells have reached an appropriate density the promoter can be turned on, the protein expressed — and the cells die.

Our problems are not over when the protein has been expressed to high levels in the bacterial cell since the product is nearly all contained in **inclusion bodies** in an insoluble form. This problem can be solved either by growing very large quantities of cells and purifying the very small quantity of soluble protein, or with this protein it is possible to recover the denatured product from the inclusion bodies and to refold the protein into its native, active form.

Each protein to be expressed will have its own unique problems, but it is fair to say that if there is sufficient incentive to obtain the product these problems will normally be soluble.

Once the gene and its product are isolated, if we are to seek inhibitors we must establish assay procedures which allow us to look at the activity of the protein. In fact, once such assays are in place they can themselves be used to search for inhibitors among existing chemical compounds. This can be done in the traditional random fashion, looking at all compounds available, but it is more likely to be successful if it is done more rationally. Since we know the function of the target protein, and specifically the types of molecules with which it normally interacts, we can restrict our searching to those molecules in our libraries which bear a structural resemblance to the natural **ligands**. The hope is that such molecules might bind to the protein but in some way interfere with function.

Normally with an enzyme it will be possible to establish a simple assay in the test tube. The ideal assay is generally one which generates a coloured product from colourless precursors, or a readily measured radioactive product. If the assay is to be used for screening compounds it will need to be automated and with high throughput, preferably in a 96-well format. Increasingly, robotics are being introduced to carry out the many repetitive and, for the human operator, boring tasks involved in this type of operation.

A high throughput assay is less important if it is used primarily to assess compounds which have been made as a result of drug design efforts, since in this case it will be the time taken by the chemist to generate the compounds which will be rate determining.

A biochemical assay is a 'must' if the objective is to design drugs, but if we simply require an assay which measures gene function this can sometimes be developed in virus-free cellular systems. This is a considerable advantage if you do not want to work with a dangerous pathogen or if the virus of interest is unable to grow in conventional tissue culture systems (such as **papillomavirus** or **hepatitis C**).

The basic idea behind all the cell-based assays is essentially the same. The gene of interest is introduced, usually by **transfection**, into an appropriate cell. Also in the cell there is a 'reporter' gene, a gene whose product is easily measured, and the system is arranged so that expression of the **reporter gene** requires the function of the virus gene product. A simple example would be systems which have been developed to look at the HIV

regulatory gene *tat* (Fig. 15.7). The normal function of *tat* is to turn on expression of HIV genes through an interaction with the TAR sequence. If the TAR sequence is hooked up to the reporter gene its expression becomes dependent upon *tat* function. So, if *tat* is expressed in the same cell the **reporter gene** will also be expressed. However, if an inhibitor of *tat* is introduced into the system the **reporter gene** is turned off. The **reporter gene** would normally encode an enzyme not found in the eukaryotic cell such as **LacZ** or **secreted alkaline phosphatase**.

There are a number of potential pitfalls with assays of this type. In the example of the *tat* assay discussed above, it would not only be *tat* inhibitors which would turn off synthesis of the reporter gene product, but also any compounds which are general inhibitors of transcription or translation, and so very careful controls have to be

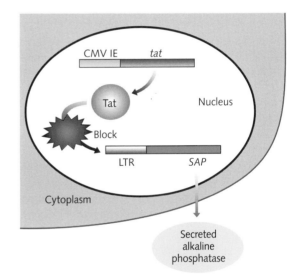

Fig. 15.7 Cell-based assay of *tat* function—*SAP* reporter gene. A cell-based assay is illustrated which allows the testing of potential inhibitors of the HIV transcription activator, Tat. A reporter gene, in this case secreted alkaline phosphatase, is linked to the HIV LTR. Expression of the reporter gene requires transcriptional activation of the LTR, and this is achieved by the parallel expession of the *tat* gene under the control of the strong 'immediate early' promoter of human cytomegalovirus. Expression of SAP can be readily monitored by a colorimetric reaction using extracellular fluids. Inhibitors of *tat* function which are able to penetrate the cell block activation of the LTR and thus excretion of *SAP*. The difficulty with this type of assay is that it generates 'false positives', since inhibitors of other stages in the transcription and translation pathways also block *SAP* expression. These alternative mechanisms need to be tested through appropriate controls.

designed to take this into account. Nevertheless, these assays do provide powerful tools for identifying inhibitors and they have the advantage over strictly biochemical assays in that they will only detect those compounds which are able to penetrate the cell.

With a supply of the protein, appropriate assays in place and an understanding of the mode of action we are in a position to take a more rational approach to drug discovery. However, there is one other area which needs to be investigated in some detail to provide the final piece in the jigsaw, and that is the three-dimensional structure of the protein.

Virus protein structure

If we are able to see the surface architecture of the protein and, in particular, how the various substrates bind to that surface and the molecular interactions involved, we will have valuable additional information to feed into the design process. We can, for example, attempt to design inhibitors which fit comfortably into a site normally occupied by a substrate, or take advantage of nooks and crannies in the surface to achieve even tighter binding. While this type of information can be used to attempt to design inhibitors from scratch, its real power lies in the ability to see how weak binding inhibitors latch on to the target protein. This information can then be used to drive new chemical synthesis to enhance the binding.

The technology used to determine the structure of large macromolecules such as proteins or nucleic acids is **X-ray crystallography**. Ironically, the virus proteins which until recently were best characterized were structural. This was simply because large quantities of material are required for crystallographic studies and virus particles could often be prepared in sufficient quantities and could also form the regular crystalline arrays required for crystallography. In fact, one of the earliest applications of crystallography in this area was to work out the mode of action of a number of related inhibitors of **polio and rhinoviruses**.

There is a 'family' of inhibitors of these viruses that are classified as 'capsid binders' which bind to the particle itself. It had long been known that, following **attachment** of the virus particle to the cell, a second event involving a change in the **conformation** of the particle was required for **penetration**, and capsid binders appeared to block this process. Once the structure of the virus particle with the inhibitor attached had been solved, it was clear that the inhibitor was in fact occupying a large hydrophobic pore or pocket just beneath the surface of the particle. It is believed that the ability to block penetration is due to the prevention of the **conformational change** required during penetration, simply by preventing the 'breathing' of the molecule. In other words, they behave rather like a small piece of grit in a well-oiled and complex machine.

As well as the structures of complete virus particles, the two envelope proteins of **influenza virus** have also been structured, but by rather different techniques. Influenza has two glycoproteins on its surface. One of these, haemagglutinin, facilitates the binding of the virus to its cellular receptor, sialic acid. The second is an enzyme, neuraminidase, which is able to remove sialic acid from the cell surface and is probably involved in the escape of new virus particles from the infected cell. Although the haemagglutinin structure has been known for some time, there has been little progress in designing inhibitors of its function. In contrast, the structure of **neuraminidase** has been used to design analogues of the **sialic acid** substrate, which are extremely potent and selective inhibitors of both the enzyme and the virus itself, and these compounds are undergoing clinical evaluation.

An important contribution of molecular biology has been to make **non-structural** virus proteins, usually made in minute quantities in the infected cell, available in large quantities for structural studies. We will use HIV **protease** as an example to show how biochemical and structural data can be used in the drug design process.

De novo drug design—HIV protease

Initially it was knowledge of the biochemical activities of **HIV protease** which provided the lead into drug design. **HIV protease** plays a key role in the **assembly** and **maturation** of the virus particle. Both the **core (gag)** proteins and the enzymes in the *pol* region are synthesized not as individual proteins but as components within a large **polyprotein**. This polyprotein has to be broken down by a series of specific **proteolytic cleavages** during the maturation of the virus to generate the individual functional proteins. It is **HIV protease**, which is itself a component of the large polyprotein, which is responsible for these cleavages. The enzyme could be recognized from **sequence motifs** at its active site to be a member of a large family of proteases known as the **aspartyl proteases**, so-called because of the two catalytic aspartic acid residues in the active site. This immediately raised the issue of **selectivity**, since any inhibitor would be required to distinguish between the virus enzyme and its cellular counterparts which included such important enzymes as renin and cathepsin.

Biochemical approaches

The first information that was required if a biochemical approach was to be used was the nature of the cleavage site recognized by the **protease**. As it turned out, there was not a single cleavage site but rather the enzyme recognized a number of different sites. From these it was possible to build a picture of the residues most commonly represented in the cleavage region, the so-called **consensus site** (Fig. 15.8). However, it was not so much the nature of the **consensus sequence** itself which attracted the attention of the drug designers, but rather the fact that the enzyme was able to cleave at a site flanked on one side by an aromatic amino acid and on the other by a proline residue. The proline residue was particularly important because no other aspartyl protease was able to tolerate a proline residue in this position.

Further biochemical studies showed that the enzyme handled very effectively **peptide substrates** containing as few as six amino acid residues. This then was the starting point for the drug design exercise. Initially, hexapeptide substrates were made which contained a central Phe-Pro dipeptide which was cleaved by the enzyme. This showed that the peptide fits snugly into the active site with the Phe-Pro dipeptide properly positioned relative to the catalytic aspartyl residues. There was a considerable background expertise in building inhibitors of the cellular proteases by replacing the cleaved peptide bond with any one of a number of non-cleavable linkages, some of which mimicked very closely the tetrahedral reaction intermediate.

By this approach it proved relatively straightforward to design potent and selective inhibitors of the enzyme. However, these inhibitors illustrate one of the common problems in drug design or discovery: inhibitors of a target protein do not necessarily make good drugs. A good drug must have many additional properties if it is to work in humans in the disease situation. The basic flaw in **peptide mimetics** is that it is very difficult to deliver them in sufficiently high concentrations and they lack biological stability. The human body is amply endowed with enzymes capable of digesting peptides since they form part of our staple diet.

It was obvious that some further development of these molecules was required. In several groups a similar strategy was adopted, and that was to attempt to modify the peptide arms on either side of the cleavage site mimic, both reducing their bulk and attempting to eliminate their peptide bonds. This met with some success and several extremely potent and selective inhibitors were designed, although all suffered to a degree from a lack of **bioavailability**. In the main, the modifications made were guided by the intuition of the medicinal chemist who attempted to produce mimics of the natural peptides. However, as this work progressed another power-

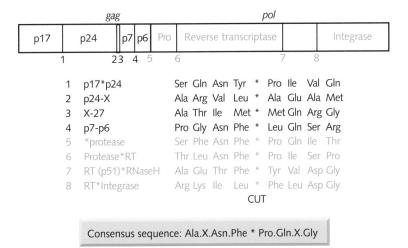

Consensus sequence: Ala.X.Asn.Phe * Pro.Gln.X.Gly

Fig. 15.8 Cleavage sites in the p160 gag/pol precursor. The gag/pol region of HIV is expressed initially as a polyprotein which is subsequently cleaved by the aspartyl protease encoded in the *pol* gene. There are eight cleavage sites and these are illustrated. Comparison of the sites reveals a number of similarities and these can be used to construct a consensus cleavage site. In the example shown, the amino acid chosen for each position in the consensus site appears in at least three of the eight sites examined.

ful tool was introduced into the drug designers' arsenal, as the **three-dimensional structure** of the enzyme was solved by X-ray crystallographers (Fig. 15.9).

Structural approach

The structure of the enzyme itself was extremely informative, but real insight came when the structure was analysed with many different **peptide mimics** bound into the active site (Fig. 15.10). It was then possible to see the deep groove in the surface into which the substrate bound and distinct pockets into which each of the amino acid side chains bound. This information then helped the design of more effective side arms on the inhibitors. Furthermore, it also became clear that the groove into which the peptide bound was essentially symmetrical around the active site. This observation led to the design of a series of novel inhibitor types with a two-fold axis of symmetry around the cleavage site.

Although several of these inhibitors have been tested in the clinic, none so far appears to possess all the characteristics required in a successful drug so this inevitably poses the question, 'where next?' The answer may be in totally novel molecules designed using knowledge of both biochemical properties of the enzyme as well as highly refined information on its structure. Already we are seeing reports of non-peptide inhibitors designed in this way which appear to resemble more closely more

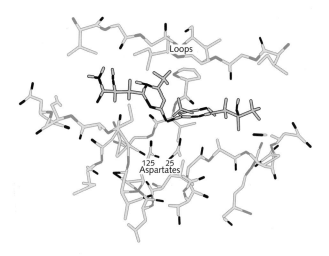

Fig. 15.10 High-resolution structure of the active site of HIV protease with an inhibitor bound into the active site. In this representation, atomic detail can be seen with the positions of all atoms (except hydrogen) defined. Both the peptide backbone and the positions of the amino acid side chains can be clearly seen. Carbon atoms are pale blue in protein and grey in the inhibitor. Nitrogen atoms are dark blue; oxygen is black.

traditional pharmaceutical products. **HIV protease** is leading the way towards truly **rational inhibitor design**, and although there are still many sceptics both within and outside the pharmaceutical industry who believe the only way to discover good drugs is by accident, it may be that the intense efforts on this enzyme will finally lay this dogma to rest. This can only be for the good, as it will clear the way for similar approaches with many other targets of therapeutic importance.

Anti-viral drug resistance

The major focus of this chapter has been the search for new anti-viral drugs. Little has been said about existing drugs and what we can learn from them about the needs of the future. In fact, anti-viral agents have been around for the past 30 years or so, although it was only with the discovery of the anti-herpes nucleoside analogue, acyclovir, in 1974 and its clinical investigation throughout the 1980s that it became clear for the first time that anti-viral drugs can be truly selective. Until that time it had been thought that the intracellular site of replication and the dependence of viruses on host functions would inevitably mean that all anti-virals would be toxic.

With the advent of AIDS there was an explosion of interest in anti-virals, and although I have used the HIV

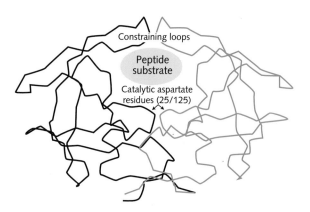

Fig. 15.9 The structure of HIV protease revealed by X-ray crystallography. The figure shows the positions of the α-carbon atoms in the peptide backbone of the molecule. The molecule is composed of two identical polypeptide chains of 99 amino acids. The catalytic region, where cleavage of polypeptides occurs, encompasses amino acid residues 25 and 125 (equivalent aspartic acid residues on each polypeptide chain). The target polypeptide lies in the deep cleft formed by the main body of the protein and is held in position by the loops which fold over above the substrate.

protease as an example to illustrate the processes of rational drug discovery, it was in the area of **nucleoside analogues** targeted at the **reverse transcriptase** that the first real successes were gained with the discovery of the anti-HIV activity of **AZT** (2′,3′-dideoxy-3′-azidothymidine), and the subsequent description of the **dideoxynucleosides** such as **ddI** (2′,3′-dideoxyinosine) and **ddC** (2′,3′-dideoxycytidine). This was soon followed by the discovery of a whole family of **non-nucleoside inhibitors** of reverse transcriptase, found by screening compounds against the recombinant enzyme. Experience with these drugs is pointing the way to the future, particularly knowledge gained in the field of **drug resistance**.

As experience was gained with the anti-herpes drug acyclovir, one of the questions at the back of many minds was whether we might see the emergence of drug resistance similar to that seen with antibiotics. In fact, this fear was largely unfounded. Resistant variants have emerged in treated patients, but only in the severely immunocompromised such as transplant recipients or AIDS patients. Although many millions of **immunocompetent** patients have been treated for conditions such as **cold sores**, **genital herpes**, **shingles** and other related conditions, resistant strains have rarely been observed. The situation changed dramatically when the treatment of HIV infection began in the mid 1980s.

Nucleoside inhibitors of HIV

The first licensed drug for the treatment of AIDS was the **nucleoside analogue AZT**. It soon became apparent with this drug that although treated patients derived benefit from treatment with the drug, that benefit, in patients with advanced disease, was relatively short-lived. Shortly afterwards it was shown that drug-resistant variants were emerging in treated patients. With the application of molecular technology the events leading to resistance have gradually been unravelled.

Since the target of this drug is reverse transcriptase the first question was to ask that was going on at the level of the reverse transcriptase gene itself. Through a careful comparison of the nucleotide sequences of reverse transcriptase genes derived from resistant viruses compared with their parent strains, a number of mutations were identified which it was felt might play a role in **resistance**. The work was complicated by the inherent **genetic variability** of HIV which results in significant sequence differences even in multiple isolates taken from the same patient at the same time. However there were a group of **mutations** which were frequently seen, but only in the **reverse transcriptase** genes derived from **resistant variants**. These appeared likely candidates to have been selected by the drug. The proof that these **mutations** were implicated in resistance was derived using molecular manipulation techniques in a series of elegant experiments performed by Larder and colleagues at the Wellcome Research Laboratories.

If a DNA copy of the HIV RNA genome is introduced into a suitable cell by transfection, expression of the genome results in the production of infectious virus. If mutations are introduced into the DNA by **site-directed mutagenesis** prior to **transfection**, mutant virus will emerge from the cell and its properties can be investigated (Fig. 15.11). Using these techniques it was confirmed that there are five specific mutations in the **reverse transcriptase** gene which are involved in **resistance**, and that as they accumulate in the gene the virus becomes gradually more resistant to the drug. From these studies and also careful monitoring of clinical isolates, it also

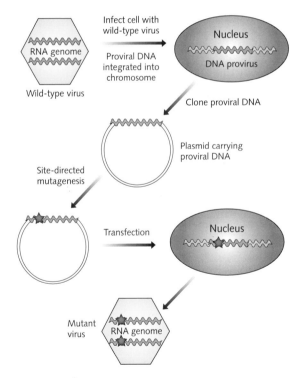

Fig. 15.11 Introduction of specific mutations into HIV. Following infection of a cell with HIV, the virus RNA genome is converted to a proviral DNA copy which is integrated into the chromosome. This genomic copy can be cloned into an appropriate vector and the plasmid then manipulated by site-specific mutagenesis to introduce specific mutations. The DNA can then be introduced into a susceptible cell such as a T-lymphocyte and the cell will then produce infectious virus carrying the required mutation. The phenotypic effects of the mutation can be investigated by comparing the properties of the mutant virus with those of its parent.

appears that there is an ordered acquisition of these mutations.

Subsequently, experience has been gained with other nucleoside analogues, particularly the dideoxynucleosides, and all appear capable of selecting resistant variants.

Non-nucleoside HIV reverse transcriptase inhibitors

Great excitement was generated when several laboratories described the discovery of a series of unrelated compounds which were potent inhibitors of the reverse transcriptase and of HIV-1 itself. These are known generically as the 'non-nucleoside reverse transcriptase inhibitors'. Initial high hopes for these compounds soon diminished when it was shown that growth of the virus in the presence of these drugs resulted in the rapid emergence of resistant variants. They were further diminished when it was shown that in the clinic in treated patients the same phenomenon was seen.

By techniques similar to those described for AZT it was soon shown, both in the case of the dideoxynucleosides and the non-nucleoside reverse transcriptase inhibitors, that single mutations in reverse transcriptase were sufficient to cause the emergence of resistant virus.

So where does this leave us in relation to treatment of this immensely threatening disease? It seems clear that if single agents are used against this virus we must expect to see the emergence of resistance. Historically, drug combinations have been used in both cancer and infectious diseases to tackle the drug resistance problem, and traditionally the approach has been to use agents directed at different targets. This is certainly an approach which should and is being investigated in HIV disease, but consideration is also being given to the merits of using combinations of drugs targeted to the same enzyme.

Combination therapy

The usual reasons for discounting the use of drugs in combination directed to the same target are the possibilities of cross-resistance, of similar side effects resulting in unacceptable toxicity, and of interference at the target site. The first two considerations can be discounted by careful selection of the combinations, for example, we see little evidence of cross-resistance between AZT and the other dideoxynucleosides or with the non-nucleoside reverse transcriptase inhibitors (although cross-resistance is seen to varying degrees in pairs of non-nucleoside inhibitors), and quite distinct side effect pro-

files are seen with these drugs. The third possibility, interference at the active site, could under certain conditions be viewed as a positive benefit.

The first indication of this possibility came when it was shown that, if patients who had been on AZT for some time and who had acquired AZT-resistant virus were switched to ddI treatment, this could result in the emergence of ddI-resistant virus but the loss of resistance to AZT. Subsequent molecular studies showed that these variants retained the mutations which in the normal situation conferred AZT resistance, but that their effect was suppressed by an additional mutation which conferred ddI resistance. This phenomenon is not restricted to the combination of AZT and ddI but is seen with others too, including combinations with non-nucleoside inhibitors. These observations should not be over-interpreted, but they do suggest that it may become increasingly difficult for mutations in reverse transcriptase to allow the enzyme to escape the inhibitory attentions of multiple drugs targeted to it.

The holy grail of drug design would be to design drugs which in combination eliminate the possibility of drug resistance. This ideal may be as unattainable as the holy grail itself, but recent work on the structure of the enzyme and its drug interactions is providing some insight.

Structure of reverse transcriptase

Although reverse transcriptase was readily produced in bulk in heterologous systems and was relatively easy to crystallize, the determination of its structure has been very slow. However, from the work of Steitz at Yale and Arnold at Rutgers University a picture of the structure of the enzyme is at last emerging (see Plates 28a and b, facing p. 214). From more recent studies it is clear that the non-nucleoside inhibitors all bind in a common hydrophobic pocket close to the active site but in a location distinct from that occupied by the non-nucleosides, presumably a location involved in nucleotide binding.

Although we are still a long way from understanding the mechanisms by which this complex enzyme operates, it is hoped that the structural studies will shed some light on the mechanisms of drug resistance and point the way forward to new and more effective drugs.

Inhibition of virus gene expression by antisense and ribozymes

A number of other strategies for anti-viral therapy also exist. These include:

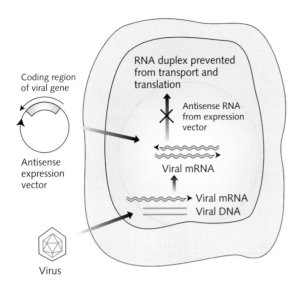

Fig. 15.12 Antisense inhibition can be used to prevent expression from specific viral genes. If a viral gene is cloned into an expression vector in the 'incorrect' orientation with respect to its coding sequences, an mRNA complementary to the viral mRNA of that gene is expressed when introduced into cells by transfection. This antisense RNA will anneal to the viral mRNA expressed on virus infection due to complementarity, and the RNA/RNA duplex is not correctly transported out of the nucleus for translation. This results in an inhibition of expression of this specific virus RNA at the protein level.

1 antisense inhibition;
2 RNA with enzymatic activities.
The annealing of DNA and RNA by complementary basepairing can be experimentally manipulated to inhibit specific gene expression, resulting in so-called **antisense inhibition**. Addition of a synthetic single-stranded DNA, which contains DNA sequences complementary to specific HIV genes — so called **antisense oligonucleotides** — to cells in culture is able to inhibit virus replication. This occurs because the synthetic oligonucleotides anneal to the HIV mRNA preventing its transport from the nucleus and/or its translation on the ribosome. Similar procedures have been used to prevent infection and viral gene expression with a number of viruses.

Obviously, the successful use of such novel therapies will depend heavily on the development of technology to target high levels of the antisense oligonucleotides specifically and stably to sites of virus infection. Stability of the antisense DNA can be ensured by the use of DNA derivatives such as phosphothiorate DNA derivatives, but targeting the antisense molecules is more difficult. To these ends, techniques to deliver plasmid vectors expressing high levels of RNA complementary to a target gene have been developed. These so-called **antisense vectors** (Fig. 15.12), often based on viruses (see Chapter 16), have been shown experimentally to inhibit the expression of a number of viral and cellular genes. However, the clinical use of such technology is still some way off.

Alternatively, expression vectors (again more often than not based on virus vectors) have been used to express RNA molecules which are able to catalyse the cleavage of other specific RNA molecules. Such **ribozymes** have been used successfully to prevent HIV infection of cells in culture by targeted cleavage of a number of HIV mRNAs. However, as with antisense expression vectors, the use of such novel therapies still requires extensive evaluation for efficacy and safety (see Chapter 18).

Summary and future prospects

The aim of this chapter has not been to provide a comprehensive review of the field of drug discovery, but rather to use examples derived from the anti-viral area to illustrate how molecular biology is contributing to drug discovery and design. The leaning has been towards the more rational approaches but I had no intention of discounting the traditional tried and tested methods. Rather, the newer technology should be used in addition to and side by side with the older methods.

We are not in a position where, having identified a potential drug target, we can sit down and design the perfect drug — in fact we may never be in that position. However, molecular techniques can provide insights into disease processes, pinpoint potential target proteins, assist in the study of these targets and guide our thinking about potential inhibitors. It would be extremely short-sighted to ignore their potential. Many of the approaches described are equally applicable to other infectious diseases, to cancer or to pharmacological targets, and we will certainly see their increasing application in the future.

Chapter 16 Gene therapy

Introduction

Tomorrow's physicians will be molecular surgeons. In the same way that today's high-tech aseptic surgical techniques evolved from battlefield amputations with no anaesthesia or antibiotics, the hitherto crude manipulation of genetic material currently pursued in scientific laboratories is slowly giving birth to a sophisticated new medical technology. There is no doubt that despite the formidable problems still to be overcome, selective manipulation of malfunctioning genes, replacement of defective genes and inhibition of unwanted genes (in malignant tissue or invading organisms) will become the common practice of the next century. That this will proceed smoothly is highly unlikely: there have been and will be false starts, inflated claims, occasional (hopefully) medical disasters and gratifying triumphs. There will be widespread debate among scientists, physicians, moralists and the general public about the ethics of tampering with the genetic material of an individual and possibly his or her descendants. Whether or not as a qualified doctor one is directly involved in the practical administration of gene therapy, it is going to be critical to its wise implementation that doctors in all disciplines, and scientists alike, are fully informed of the consequences and limitations of gene therapy.

Is gene therapy new?

If one defines gene therapy as treatment of a disease by genetic manipulation, then doctors have been performing this for many years. Treatment of an individual with thyroid hormones for hypothyroidism, or with steroids to damp down inflammation in asthma or colitis, all result in different genes in different tissues of the body being turned up or down or switched on or off. A number of gene therapy protocols under consideration involve no more radical a change in the body's functioning than this. The essential difference is the introduction into the individual of new genetic material.

Whilst common perceptions of gene therapy may be that it is limited to treating rare inherited disorders, those in the field already see genetic manipulation of the human genome and of pathogenic organisms as being a discipline which will leave untouched very few fields of medicine.

Somatic cell and germ line gene therapy

Gene therapy falls neatly into two categories, so-called somatic cell gene therapy and germ line gene therapy. In the latter, all cells in the body have their genetic make-up altered because the germ line cells, the sperm and ova, have been genetically altered. Thus, any change introduced will be passed on to one's descendants. Somatic cell gene therapy aims to treat an individual and perhaps a single organ or tissue in that person, without affecting their germ cells. Lack of intent does not always coincide with lack of effect, and therapies aimed to be 'somatic' should ideally be positively engineered such that they *cannot* enter the germ line. This point is often missed by groups claiming to be developing only somatic cell gene therapy. For the moment, however, let us assume that when the term somatic cell gene therapy is described, it only involves treatment of the individual.

With any new therapy several questions need to be asked.
1 Is it necessary?
2 Is it effective?
3 Is it practical?

4 How much does it cost?

Gene therapy scores well in some of these; in others it is too early to tell.

Necessity

For the individual born with a single gene defect the prospects are not encouraging. Unless one is fortunate enough to have inherited a disease like phenylketonuria (Box 16.1), in which scrupulous avoidance of phenylalanine-containing substances is compatible with normal growth and development, one's quality of life is likely to be severely impaired. Even haemophiliacs, where replacement therapy with purified clotting factor proteins is now routine, can hardly be described as living a normal existence. Surveys on single gene disorders have estimated that current treatments, at their best, lead to a normal life span in only about 15% of cases. In only 11% of conditions does the individual have a normal reproductive capacity, and in only 6% are patients judged as living a normal, fully socially adapted life.

For single gene disorders there is a strong argument for a better treatment aimed at correcting the defect. For diseases other than this, is the case compelling? Certainly if gene therapy was useful in cancer treatment, few would doubt its value. While patients with early stage Hodgkin's or testicular teratomas now have a favourable outlook, the same cannot be said for patients presenting with small cell carcinoma of the lung or virtually all patients with metastatic disease.

Infections may not appear the most obvious target for a genetic approach to treatment. For many infections this is true, and the impressive armamentarium of powerful anti-bacterial and anti-fungal drugs will continue

---

Adenosine deaminase deficiency

This is an autosomal recessive defect, resulting in absence of adenosine deaminase. This causes accumulation of deoxy-ATP, specifically in T-lymphocytes. The severe form causes severe combined immunodeficiency characterized by recurrent viral fungal and bacterial diseases with wasting, diarrhoea and, if untreated, early death (see Plate 29, facing p. 214).

Box 16.2

to be pivotal in treatment. For viral diseases, and particularly persistent viral infections, the results to date are less promising. AIDS may be taken as an example. Drug treatment of HIV infection can best be described as disappointing. However, a virus which can remain latent, is passed on vertically from cell to daughter cell, and which has an enormous capacity to mutate is a desperately difficult target to hit using pharmacological agents and, if latent, the virus is 'invisible' to the immune system. Drugs targeted against the viral enzyme, reverse transcriptase, are met by the virus with mutation to produce resistance and a vaccine approach has been similarly hampered by the mutability of the viral envelope. HIV, HTLV-1 (the virus causing adult T-cell leukaemia and a demyelinating spinal disease) and, possibly, hepatitis B, all of which integrate into the host genome, are diseases which, in the long term, will be most effectively treated genetically.

Effectiveness

The simple answer to the question of effectiveness is that it is too early to judge. In those cases where gene therapy has been carried out, such as adenosine deaminase (ADA) deficiency (Box 16.2), the results are very impressive and superior to anything previously tried. The real test will come when gene therapy is used in conditions where there are other treatments having a moderate success rate where direct comparison can be made.

Practicality

Despite intensive research and the mass of knowledge accumulating daily on the molecular biology of the cell and gene transfer, the two problems which confront gene therapy are the delivery of DNA to the cell and control of expression of that DNA once in the cell. Since several million years of evolution have been at work to try and ensure that the only genetic material surviving within a cell is that of the host, it is not a trivial problem to fool

---

Phenylketonuria

Incidence

One in 14 000 (USA).

Characteristics

Autosomal recessive disorder characterized by failure of conversion of phenylalanine to tyrosine, due to a defect in the enzyme phenylalanine hydroxylase. Causes mental retardation and hypopigmentation.

Treatment

Low phenylalanine diet.

Box 16.1

the cell into accepting extraneous DNA and maintaining it intact. However, as discussed later (p. 289), considerable success has been achieved and at its most basic, as in direct injection of DNA, gene therapy is comparable in simplicity to other parenterally delivered treatments.

Cost-effectiveness

In a medical paradise this would not be a concern. Any effective treatment would be delivered no matter what the cost. Health resources, unfortunately, are not a bottomless pit, as politicians insist on reminding us. In gene therapy we have, as yet, few examples by which to judge. Heroic efforts to correct genetic defects in the liver have entailed enormous expense, whereas treatment of ADA deficiency which is performed on an out-patient basis is undoubtedly cheaper than prolonged in-patient stays caused by the patient's immunodeficiency leading them to contract multiple infections. It seems unlikely that gene therapy will be any more expensive than treatment for haemophilia or for Gaucher's disease, as currently practised. For many diseases it is likely to be cheaper. Those considered as candidates for gene therapy are listed in Table 16.1.

What do we mean by gene therapy?

In the world of science fiction, the patient with the genetic defect caused by a single base mutation would have that single base corrected. Alternatively, a gene defect such as a large deletion in the gene structure would be cured by having the offending part removed by molecular excision and replaced with a perfect new copy. Sadly we are far from this. The types of gene therapy practically envisaged at present fall into several groups.

Gene supplementation

In the case of a disease caused by lack of a gene product (haemophilia, muscular dystrophy), where the cause is not an absence of the genetic material but a mistake within the native gene, the aim is to introduce an extra new functioning copy into the cell.

Gene suppression

Overexpression of some genes is clearly deleterious. Uncontrolled expression of oncogenes leading to cancer might best be stopped either by introducing a physiological tumour suppressor gene such as the retinoblastoma gene product, or by interfering with the expression of the gene which is out of control by antisense or ribozyme technology.

Dominant negative approaches

In some diseases a mutant protein interferes with the functioning of its normal counterpart. This can be turned to our advantage in diseases such as infections where it would be beneficial to interfere with the assembly of an infectious organism. Introduction of a mutant viral protein into a cell might disrupt the function, assembly or polymerization of the normal counterpart. Because a small number of mutants is able to disrupt a large number of normal proteins, this is called a dominant negative effect.

Autolytic destruction

Much conventional therapy, particularly in the cancer field, is aimed at destroying cells. Chemotherapy and

Table 16.1 Gene therapy candidates.

Disorder	Frequency	Regulation
Haemoglobinopathy	Up to one in 600	Required
Lesch–Nyhan, ADA, NPD deficiency	< One in 10^6	No
Phenylketonuria	One in 12 000	?
Urea cycle disorders	One in 30 000	?
Glycogen storage I^A	One in 100 000	?
α_1-Antitrypsin deficiency	One in 3500	?
Haemophilia A + B	One in 10 000 males	?
Lysosomal diseases	One in 1500	Required
Familial hypercholesterolaemia	One in 500	Required
Cystic fibrosis	One in 2500	?
Duchenne	One in 3000 males	?
Huntington's disease	One in 20 000	Required

radiotherapy aim to kill off cancerous cells and, with varying degrees of success, do so whilst sparing normal tissue. Together with specific monoclonal antibodies, targeting suicide genes to tumour cells or cells infected with a dangerous pathogen, like HIV, is probably as close as we will get to the fabled 'magic bullet'. It is certainly relatively easy to kill cells, once again the problem is targeting the destructive moiety and controlling its expression.

In the future we may look forward to genuine gene replacement. Genetic repair processes within the cell are capable of restoring discontinuity in genes by taking a copy from the other one of the chromosomal pair, and exchanges between sister chromatids occur during cell division. This gene reassortment contributes to the diversity of the species. Site-specific 'cutting and pasting' of genes is the aim for the future by manipulating some of the known repair processes in the cell. The specificity of some restriction enzymes and site-specific recombinases means this is not a completely fictional proposition.

Gene transfer—the problems

The problems of gene transfer may be broken down into four areas: (i) purifying (cloning) the DNA you want; (ii) understanding the control sequences; (iii) obtaining enough target cells to put it in; (iv) getting it in. The first two of these are described elsewhere. Obtaining enough target cells may mean extracting bone marrow from an individual and separating off haematopoietic stem cells or removing hepatocytes and transducing those, or, ideally, targeting gene therapy specifically to a certain cell type such that on a simple injection sufficient of the material ends up in the appropriate cells.

Finally, getting the DNA in. Introducing DNA into cells is a routine procedure in the laboratory, where there is a diversity of physical methods of varying efficacy and toxicity. As a general rule, the more efficient the technique for getting DNA into the cells, the more cells it kills in the process. DNA can be precipitated with calcium phosphate or dextran so that it sticks to the surface of cells and is taken up. Electric currents can be fired through cells, such that the negatively charged DNA on its way to the anode perforates the cell and gets caught up inside. For experimental purposes single cells can be micro-injected with DNA directly into their nucleus, undoubtedly the most certain and by a long way the least practicable of techniques for somatic cell human gene therapy. DNA can also be coated on colloidal particles and fired, shotgun-like, at the cell, hoping that those cells receiving sublethal wounds will submissively take up the foreign DNA. It is fair to say that there is little scope for any of these methods in human gene therapy, although they are of immense value in laboratory studies on transformed cell lines. More sophisticated delivery methods are required for getting DNA into primary human cells. These involve a variety of targetable or non-targetable viral or non-viral vectors.

Whilst laboratory scientists struggled with the concept of forcing foreign genes into cells, it became clear that viruses were already doing this extremely efficiently and had been doing so for millions of years. Thus, the strategies to hijack viral particles as genetic delivery systems began. Several viruses have proved themselves amenable to having their own genetic material substituted by foreign genes. Those of particular value have been vaccinia, adenovirus, adeno-associated viruses, herpesviruses and retroviruses. A brief summary of these viruses follows and appears in Table 16.2.

Viral vectors

Retroviruses

Retroviruses have been an obvious choice for gene delivery. Despite carrying an RNA genome in the virus, they convert this to a DNA copy when in the cell and integrate this into the chromosomes of the host cell. Here it is processed in the same way as the other host cell DNA, and it is essentially undetectable by the cell. Retroviruses package their own RNA because they recognize special

Table 16.2 Candidate viruses for gene delivery.

	Nucleic acid	Integration into chromosomes	Gene-carrying capacity (kb)	Cytopathicity of vectors
Adenovirus	DNA	No	4–8	Low
Herpesvirus	DNA	No	20	High
Adeno-associated virus	DNA	Yes	<4	Low
Retrovirus	RNA	Yes	Up to 4–8	Low
Vaccinia	DNA	No	25–75	High

folded segments of the RNA, so-called packaging signals. This probably occurs by basepairing between different bases in the single RNA genome strand, forming a double-stranded and then a folded structure. Removing the packaging signal from the RNA does not affect its ability to act as a normal messenger RNA and to code for the proteins of the virus, as these signals usually occur in non-coding regions of the genome. Thus, by skilful and specific deletion of small parts of the virus genome, one can engineer a virus which is capable of producing all the viral proteins and assembling viral particles, but whose RNA is incapable of entering the

assembled structure. Rather obviously one then must engineer the appropriate packaging signal into the RNA that one wishes to get into the virus particle and express this in the same cell. Thus, a cell line producing empty virus particles will be turned into a vector-producing cell line where the virus particles have become Trojan horses (Fig. 16.1). The main advantages of retroviruses are, first, the ability to produce high-titre virus, so that many cells can be transduced with the appropriate gene; second, in general, they are not dangerous and they can be engineered to be minimally or non-pathogenic; third, they will integrate into the target cell. There are theoreti-

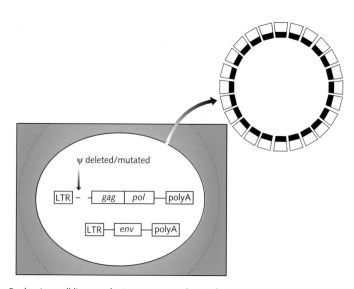

Packaging cell line producing empty viral particles

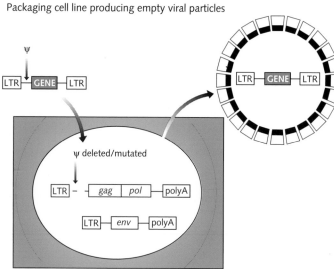

Vector with packaging signal encapsulated

Fig. 16.1 Using retroviruses to transfer genes. The retroviral genes encoding the structural proteins of the virus are stably expressed in the cell (*gag*, *pol* and *env*). With deletions in encapsidation signals these will produce viral particles which contain no viral RNA. Introduction into the cell of a vector containing a packaging signal (ψ) will allow encapsidation of the vector RNA into the virus particles and delivery to the cell for which the virus normally infects.

cal disadvantages, of course, to integrating into the chromosome and it is conceivable that one could disrupt a normal cellular gene and cause cell damage. Although integration of retroviruses is said to be random, in practical terms insertional mutagenesis is an extremely rare event in the retroviruses which have been used for gene transfer. In some experimental models in animals up to 10^8 cells are transduced by a retroviral vector. If integration were random, this would equate to approximately one integration every hundred bases in the genome. Despite this no insertional mutagenesis has been seen in these models. Another good thing about retroviruses is that they are a complete, self-contained integration units. The virus carries with it all the enzymes required to turn the RNA within it to DNA and then to integrate it into the chromosome. All that needs to be provided is an appropriate nucleotide sequence with the correct ends and a signal sequence which allows the start of the RNA to DNA conversion. Although retroviruses are one of the smaller viral vectors, the potential carrying capacity of between 4 and 8 kb of nucleotide sequence (depending on the virus) is enough in the majority of cases to carry a DNA copy of a messenger RNA (a cDNA). Most cDNAs will fit into a retrovirus vector. Most retroviruses currently in use have the limitation that they can only integrate their genome into cells which are dividing. This appears to be due to an inability to penetrate the nuclear membrane. Lentiviruses (a subgroup of retroviruses, including HIV) *can* integrate into non-dividing cells and identification of the gene products responsible for this capability means that chimeras can be constructed between different viruses containing the best qualities of both.

Adenoviruses

Adenoviruses have larger genomes, and deletions can be made to render them replication defective and to make room for heterologous genes. They are very infectious, have a high titre, and they can infect non-replicating cells. Despite this, they have disadvantages in that they will not integrate their DNA into the host cell and the vectors still contain a number of adenovirus proteins and genes whose products might trigger an immune response, or even possibly transform the target cell. They may have specific applications for gene delivery to epithelial cells, particularly the respiratory and gastrointestinal epithelium. This takes advantage of their normal airborne or oral route of infection. For gene therapy approaches in which a single burst of high level gene expression is required for a limited period of time, such

as in a gene therapy vaccine, adenoviruses may be the ideal delivery system. Recent evidence also suggests that, despite failing to integrate, long-term (months) expression of genes in brain tissue may be achievable using adenovirus vectors.

Adeno-associated viruses (AAV)

AAV is another front runner in the gene therapy field. Its limitation is its very small genome and thus its restricted gene-carrying capacity (less than 4 kb). The big advantage it has is the ability to integrate its genome into non-dividing cells. At first this appeared to be perfect, because there is a specific site in chromosome 19 into which AAV always integrates, without affecting cell function. This however appears to be the case only when all the AAV genes are present. When the genetic material has been substituted by heterologous genes, integration still occurs but no longer into a single specific site. Integration into a resting cell is clearly an advantage when one is targeting tissues which are not actively mitotic, such as hepatocytes or neuronal cells.

Herpesviruses

As with many gene vectors, it was the scientists working on the virus who were quick to identify potential advantages of their own vector. Herpesviruses, such as herpes simplex and varicella-zoster, are neurotropic and thus gene delivery to the nervous system is a real possibility. Herpesviruses also can establish a latent state and persist indefinitely in neurological tissue. Many disease targets, particularly single gene defects and some infections, are ones in which nerve tissue is affected, and these combined properties of penetration into the CNS and persistence have given herpesviruses a potentially unique niche in the gene therapy repertoire. They have a large genome and much can be deleted to accommodate large DNA segments. To date the only major disadvantage has been that attempts to attenuate the virus have met with limited success. Although low pathogenicity herpesvirus vectors have been made which are replication defective, they are still often lytic to the cells to which the gene is delivered.

Vaccinia viruses

For short-term high-level expression of genetic material, vaccinia has proved to be a valuable resource, particularly in immunological studies where recombinant vaccinia viruses containing heterologous genes can make large numbers of cells express these genes at high level for a short period of time. The size of the genome unfortunately means, as with herpes, that a cumbersome procedure of recombination is required to insert the gene of choice into the vaccinia genome. Vaccinia is also highly cytopathic. Very major modifications will have to be made to vaccinia before it is likely to be a gene vector with significant advantages over its competitors for gene supplementation. As a tool for delivery of genes to elicit an immune response, the virus which gave its name to vaccination may turn out again to be a valuable tool to protect against other infections.

Non-viral delivery of genetic material

Apart from the physicochemical and electrical methods outlined above, a number of molecules and structures have been used to deliver DNA to cells. The senior citizen in this field is probably the liposome. Liposomes are small, spherical 'bubbles' with a wall made of lipid micelles. These micelles fuse readily with the cell membrane and discharge the contents of the liposome into the cell. Liposomes can be targeted to some extent by size and by altering the lipids in the wall such that the charge on the surface favours cell fusion. Liposomes are already in use as a delivery modality for certain drugs like amphotericin, as this can avoid targeting the drug to undesirable sites such as the kidney where the major toxic side effect occurs. Liposomes are somewhat difficult to handle and really have not made the impact in gene therapy which one might have predicted.

Some clever complexing of molecules has been performed in an attempt to create a hybrid 'gene vector' molecule which both binds DNA and can deliver it specifically to a cell. One of the best studied of these is the asialoglycoprotein–polylysine molecule. Polylysine is positively charged and acts as a binding region for plasmid DNA, and the asialoglycoprotein (ASGP) takes advantage of the fact that liver cells have a receptor for proteins which have lost their sialic acid (and which are probably senescent) and can take these up specifically. ASGP–polylysine DNA conjugates can be shown in experimental animals to target DNA to the liver (Fig. 16.2). What happens subsequently to the DNA is more of a problem, as ideally one would like to integrate it or keep it in a stable episomal form. Perhaps the most surprisingly obvious methodology is direct DNA transfer. Naked DNA which is injected into muscle can enter the cell and the genes encoded may be expressed for a year or more. This is unlikely to be a method of correcting genetic muscle defects, but the muscle can act as a source

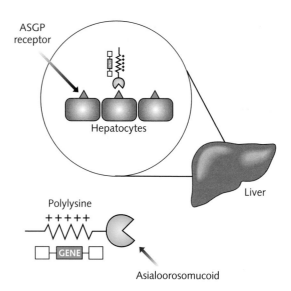

Fig. 16.2 Targeting DNA using complex macromolecules such as the asialoglycoprotein (ASGP) asialoorosomucroid conjugated to polylysine. The complex will bind DNA and deliver it to hepatocytes which carry an ASGP receptor.

of secreted protein required elsewhere. Thus defects such as haemophilia might be appropriately treated this way. Mixing and matching useful components with non-viral vectors is being exploited as well. Thus, the ability of adenovirus capsids to disrupt lysosomes and protect against lysosomal degradation is being used to protect a DNA/DNA binding complex, bound to irradiated adenovirus capsids. Viral 'spare part surgery' may be critical in developing efficient vectors in the future.

Artificial chromosomes

Much work has concentrated on transferring small genetic units such as cDNAs. The capacity of the vectors has placed limitations on the level of control sequences upstream and downstream of the gene which can be included. For some genes the control elements are situated at a considerable distance, and for the genetic unit to function completely physiologically, it would be preferable to transfer the complete chromosome fragment into a cell. Some progress towards this has been made using artificial chromosomes. These are currently based on the yeast artificial chromosome into which can be engineered human genes. More recently mammalian artificial chromosomes have been developed, and progress in understanding the different structural features of the chromosome, such as the centromere and telomere, mean it is likely that in the near future large

DNA segments, 'human artificial chromosomes', will be available for gene transfer. Delivery of such large segments of DNA is likely to require the use of non-viral vectors.

Controlling expression of the genes

With transfer of large DNA fragments on artificial chromosomes, it is likely that sufficient of the control elements are there, such that they will simply slot into the ongoing cellular processes and be controlled like the original physiological gene. Cells are quite efficient at switching off genes, and a common stumbling block in gene therapy experiments is that having finally achieved the goal of delivering DNA into a cell and integrating it into a safe portion of the chromosome, it promptly becomes transcriptionally inactive and useless. One can consider genes in cells as falling into two categories: those which are expressed in all cells, sometimes termed housekeeping genes, and those which are expressed in one or a restricted range of tissues, such as haemoglobin, keratin, etc. — tissue-specific genes. There are a number of ways in which one could keep a gene active. Firstly, one could deliver it to a tissue under the control of the tissue-specific promoter. The α-fetoprotein promoter is one such example which will keep a gene transcriptionally active inside hepatocytes (Fig. 16.3). Alternatively, one can put a gene under the control of a housekeeping promoter. The expectation then is that whichever cell the gene is delivered to it will be transcriptionally active. If tissue-specific expression is required, cell targeting of the vector will be essential. Thirdly, one can use a completely non-mammalian promoter such as a virus promoter. These can be inducible or constitutive: the immediate

early region promoter from cytomegalovirus is a powerful constitutive promoter, and the HIV long terminal repeat is a promoter inducible by the HIV *tat* protein, and a variety of other viral and cellular stimulants.

The extra level of sophistication provided by inducible promoters is appropriate if controlled switch-on and switch-off of the gene is required, or if there are concerns about the level of expression of the gene. One model is for a gene to be inserted into a cell under the control of a drug-sensitive promoter such as the corticosteroid response element, and then to be able to give the patient a dose of corticosteroids by mouth or injection which will switch on the gene when it is required. Conversely, one can use such systems to eliminate unwanted cells or organisms. Marking a toxic gene inducible by a specific viral protein will mean that the gene will only be expressed in the cells which are infected with that virus. Infected cells will theoretically be eliminated with greater than surgical precision leaving uninfected cells unharmed. However, most inducible promoters are unfortunately idiosyncratic in their handling and may be induced by a number of different inducers. Inappropriate activation of the suicide gene may then occur.

Targeting one gene to a region of the chromosome which is transcriptionally active is a double-edged sword, in that it is more likely to do damage if it inserts into an important functional site, however it is less likely to be switched off inadvertently. Some viruses appear to favour integration in transcriptionally active chromatin, although the mechanism is unclear.

Non-integrated DNA

Cells in general do not tolerate DNA which is not part of their chromosomes. It is degraded, eliminated or lost during cell division. Once again viruses have provided an answer to this through necessity of survival and some, such as Epstein–Barr virus (EBV), manage to maintain their own DNA outside of the chromosomes (episomally) where it can apparently persist and divide at cell division, being transmitted to daughter cells. In EBV a small segment of the viral DNA has been identified as being responsible, and this 'origin of replication' can be incorporated into a gene therapy construct to maintain the DNA in a stable episomal form.

Not all cells are as inhospitable to foreign DNA. Muscle cells, for example, appear to have a reduced ability to rid themselves of injected DNA. They may continue to harbour episomal DNA for many months and allow it to be transcriptionally active.

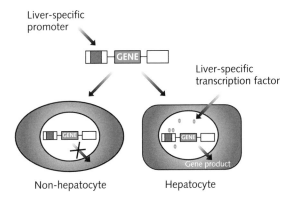

Fig. 16.3 Using tissue-specific promoters to allow expression of a gene in the target tissue and prevent expression in other cells.

Endogenous substitute genes

Until now we have concentrated on introducing new copies of a gene into a cell to substitute for one that is missing or damaged. In some cases, however, there are acceptable substitutes which are transcriptionally silent within the cell. One good example is the fetal γ-globin gene. This is transcriptionally silent in adults, but attempts are being made to reactivate it to substitute for the defective globin gene in sickle cell disease (Box 16.3), thalassaemia (Box 16.4) etc. Where a gene responsible for elimination of a toxic substance is defective, it may be possible to enhance alternative salvage pathways. This has been as yet relatively unexplored.

Site-specific gene insertion

The human cell has a number of methods of self-repair of defective genetic segments. Recombination between different chromosomes can lead to swapping of a genetic segment or repair of a defective segment using the correct homologue as a template. The process of homologous recombination can be turned to our advantage by introducing into a cell a DNA with a corrected region. In some cases the cell will identify the sequence and do a neat repair job, inserting the correct gene into the defective locus. The sickle haemoglobin gene has been corrected *in vitro* by such a method of gene targeting. As yet the efficiency with which this process occurs is extremely low, and experiments involving homologous recombination usually involve the addition of a special selectable marker to the DNA, inserted to either positively select the corrected genes or negatively select the uncorrected genes or both.

Target cells for gene therapy

The major considerations in deciding on target cells for gene insertion are whether one is trying to correct a defect within that target cell population, or use those cells as a source of secreted protein for correction of a

---

Thalassaemia

Thalassaemia is due to reduction or absence of a globin chain species, e.g. β-thalassaemia is due to absence of β-globin. Inheritance is autosomal recessive. Disease depends on the individual lesion and individual chain affected. It may cause intense chronic haemolytic anaemia, growth deformities, etc. Much of the pathology is caused by an excess of the normal retained complementary globin chain precipitating in cells.

Box 16.4

---

systemic defect. An obvious example of the former would be thalassaemia, where one wishes to produce erythrocytes containing the correct haemoglobin and so gene therapy should be aimed either only to transduce erythrocyte precursors or only to be activated within cells of the erythrocyte lineage. Haemophilia is a disease falling into the latter category in which, although restoring the synthetic capacity of hepatocytes to produce normal factor VIII would be ideal, some benefit would undoubtedly be gained by providing factor VIII from any cell, providing it was then accessible to the circulation. A variation on this is where one is using gene therapy to try and provoke an immune response. This might be against an infectious organism or against a tumour antigen. Once again, it would not matter greatly which cell was targeted to present the antigen, providing an efficient immunogenic stimulus was given, although the cell expressing the gene is likely to be eliminated as well.

Gene therapists are, on the whole, pragmatic individuals and much work has focused on that most easily accessible target cell, the lymphocyte, which can be easily harvested from the peripheral blood and then reinjected. Lymphocytes have been taken from patients with ADA deficiency, which causes a severe combined immunodeficiency picture with an absence of cell-mediated and humoral immunity. The ADA gene has been inserted into lymphocytes using a retroviral vector and the cells then reinjected. Apart from diseases directly affecting lymphocytes, these cells are also involved in the control and elimination of tumours and infectious organisms. It would be useful to make these lymphocytes more 'aggressive' against their appropriate targets. One attempt at this has been to clone and expand lymphocytes which are found invading malignant tumours, 'tumour-infiltrating lymphocytes' (TIL).

As yet, no one has used gene therapy to alter the antigenic specificity of the T-cell to try and direct its activity against a specific pathogen or tumour. In the long term, however, tumour and infection-specific T-cells are likely

---

Sickle cell disease

Sickle haemoglobin (HbS) results from a point mutation in β-globin. Heterozygotes display reduced susceptibility to malaria. Homozygotes have abnormal HbS which polymerizes on deoxygenation, producing distorted 'sickled' erythrocytes. This causes haemolytic illnesses and vaso-occlusive disease.

Box 16.3

to be produced in the same manner as monoclonal antibodies.

Many single gene defects affect the haemopoietic system. The search has been on to find the ultimate precursor totipotent haemopoietic stem cell from which all other cell lineages derive. Much progress has been made in this area, both in experimental models and in humans. In mice, for example, one can narrow down a specific subpopulation of circulating cells which express the CD34 antigen, such that single figure quantities of these are able to completely reconstitute a syngeneic mouse whose marrow has been completely ablated by irradiation. With a tiny target cell number such as this, it becomes more practicable to insert genes which are required to be expressed in some of the downstream lineage. The control of these genes in the correct cell population is, however, still a thorny issue.

The massive and diverse synthetic capacity of the liver means that it is inevitably the focus of a number of genetic defects. Introducing genes into hepatocytes is an attractive option. Evolution, however, has designed the liver to be a particularly awkward tissue in which to make genetic alterations. First, it is physically difficult to access. Second, the average human hepatocyte only divides once or twice during the complete life span and, hence, vectors which rely on cell division to integrate have a rather small susceptible target cell population. Third, there is an impressive network of cells of the reticulo-endothelial system in and around the liver sinusoids capable of taking up and degrading particles targeted at hepatocytes. In experimental animals these problems have been overcome by performing a partial hepatectomy, culturing the excised hepatocytes, transducing them in their mitotically active state and then reinfusing them into the regenerating liver, whereupon they become incorporated into the newly reconstituted organ (Fig. 16.4). Rather more remarkably, this has also been achieved in humans and is described later (p. 294).

The skin is an attractive target for gene transfer. Apart from its obvious accessibility, it is the largest organ in the body. Outward shedding of the skin means that genes expressed in superficial layers will soon be lost, however, transduction of basal mitotic layers of the skin has been achieved and there is some evidence of secretion of gene products in an inward direction into the bloodstream. Keratinocytes can also be grown in rafts in cell culture and applied to a suitably prepared area of the body in the form of a skin graft.

In animals, it has been possible to transduce cells such as those lining the vascular endothelium by inserting complex catheters which can isolate a section of blood vessel using inflatable balloons at either end, then intro-

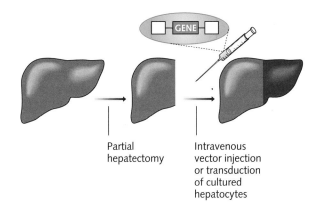

Partial hepatectomy

Intravenous vector injection or transduction of cultured hepatocytes

Fig. 16.4 Vectors which require cell division can be introduced into non-dividing cells such as the liver by removal of a liver segment and incorporation of vector into the regenerating hepatocytes.

ducing viral vectors into the lumen between them. Expression of marker genes, such as β-galactosidase (which gives easily detectable blue staining of cells), has raised hopes that this may be a useful target cell population, either to transduce directly for treatment of vascular disease or as a source of gene products for secretion into the circulation. Epithelial cells of the pancreas and the airway would be the preferred target for correction of diseases such as cystic fibrosis.

Tumour cells have been an early target for gene transfer. On the one hand it has been the aim to try and render a tumour cell more immunogenic and break the apparent immunological tolerance which a malignancy induces in its host. To this end, tumour cells have been transduced with immunostimulatory molecules such as the B7 protein complex, which is involved in antigen presentation and may make a tumour cell a more tasty target for the immune system. The second purpose of tumour cell transduction has been to put toxic genes within them to try and eliminate them, and this is discussed later (p. 296). Labelling of tumour cells to indicate the origin of tumour relapse has also been used.

Diseases for treatment

As will be obvious by now, there are a number of different categories of disease target for gene therapy, including single gene defects, malignancy and infection.

Single gene defects

With at least 4000 single gene defects described, the field for therapy seems wide. The ideal condition to treat is one in which the gene is cloned, sequenced and the control of its expression is understood. It should ideally fit into a convenient vector. Control of expression of the gene should not be critical, in other words, low level expression should be beneficial and overexpression should not be harmful. Lastly, the gene-transduced cells should have some selective advantage over their non-transduced counterparts. There are possibly three conditions which would fulfil these criteria: ADA deficiency, purine nucleoside phosphorylase (PNP) deficiency and (hypoxanthine-guanine-phosphoribosyl-transferase HXGPRT) deficiency (Lesch–Nyhan syndrome).

ADA deficiency is an extremely rare condition in which the enzyme adenosine deaminase is poorly or non-functional. The defect leads to a toxic accumulation of deoxy-ATP (dATP), which because of salvage pathway constraints affects particularly the T-lymphocyte series. Severely affected patients thus suffer a selective destruction of their T-lymphocytes leading to an immunodeficiency against all forms of invading pathogen, so-called severe combined immunodeficiency (SCID). Despite the rarity of this condition, it is somewhat celebrated, having been the key condition which was first treated by a number of therapeutic strategies, e.g. bone marrow transplant. The critical features are that expression of only a small proportion of the normal level of ADA is sufficient to protect T-cells, whereas overexpression to the level of 50 times normal can be found in some individuals who are apparently completely normal, apart from a slight tendency to haemolysis. Thus, the level of expression of the gene is not critical. With the corrected gene in place the cells should be able to detoxify dATP and should thus have a growth advantage over uncorrected cells.

Moderate forms of the defect can be treated with a precipitated form of the ADA enzyme by intravenous infusion. More severe cases do not respond well to this, and in the handful of cases which have been treated by gene therapy there was evidence of decline in physical state despite this enzyme replacement. In the two cases treated first in the USA, both individuals had leukopheresis performed on a regular basis and a retroviral vector containing the ADA gene was used to transduce peripheral blood T-cells. Up to 10^{11} cells were treated each time, and the results have been impressive. The patients showed evidence of immune reconstitution with return of immune responses against skin test antigens and a decline in the number of infections. The gene-corrected cells increased in the peripheral circulation until they numbered 25–30% of the total T-cell population, and they were shown to have a longer half-life than the non-gene-corrected counterparts. The treatment was conducted on an out-patient basis, and despite the complexity of the manoeuvres involved in transducing such a large number of cells, this can be judged a therapeutic success.

PNP deficiency in theory holds the same attractions, yet it is as rare as ADA deficiency and as yet there has been no attempt at genetic correction. Similarly Lesch–Nyhan syndrome will undoubtedly be one of the early targets for single gene defect correction.

Familial hypercholesterolaemia due to defects in the low density lipoprotein (LDL) receptor (see Chapter 7) has also been treated in a small number of individuals. The animal model of this, the Watanabe rabbit, was extremely useful in demonstrating improvement in serum cholesterol after gene transduction of the human LDL receptor into the rabbit hepatocytes. Sustained lowering of the blood cholesterol was noted. In recently published work patients with LDL receptor deficiency were treated. Because it was necessary to introduce the gene into hepatocytes and because hepatocytes are non-dividing cells, the patients underwent a partial hepatectomy and the hepatocytes from the receptive specimens were plated out into tissue culture plates. Gene transduction with a retroviral vector containing the LDL gene was performed and the gene-transduced hepatocytes were then reinfused into a catheter which had been left in the portal vein. Thus the regenerating liver incorporated into itself gene-transduced hepatocytes which, because they were dividing, had stably acquired the retroviral vector. A measure of the Herculean nature of this treatment was that for each patient 800 Petri dishes were required to plate out the liver cells. Gene transduction of the LDL receptor was demonstrated, however the fall in blood cholesterol was slightly disappointing and did not reduce to a level near the normal range.

Because of its prevalence and ultimately poor prognosis, cystic fibrosis has been a major target for gene therapy. Another factor has been that much of the pathology relates to the lung and there are a number of efficient methods of delivering gene constructs to epithelial surfaces. With the cloning of the *CFTR* gene there have already been attempts using adenovirus vectors and cationic liposomes to deliver the *CFTR* gene to cells of the respiratory epithelium. The early results are moderately encouraging with gene expression detectable for up to 6 weeks.

α_1-Antitrypsin deficiency will be another early target and haemophilia will follow soon afterwards. Gene defects in the haematopoietic system are candidates and this has been encouraged by the success of treatment with bone marrow transplantation in which over 30 genetic diseases have been corrected. It is now proving practicable to isolate stem cells from peripheral blood in experimental animals and this is soon likely to become practicable in humans. Gene correction can then be done into a self-replicating progenitor population which will affect all the cell lineages from the bone marrow. There are a number of enzymatic defects which fall under the heading lysosomal storage diseases, in which there is a toxic accumulation of products which are normally broken down by the body, but in the absence of a critical enzyme this cannot occur. In a number of these, bone marrow transplantation has been shown to be effective in correcting the storage defect in the peripheral blood and in the somatic organs, but there has been no correction of the storage disorder within the central nervous system and, tragically, the brain disease has progressed. It is in defects such as this that targeting the correct gene to both brain cells and cells outside the central nervous system will prove to be a dramatic advance. The first therapeutic trial for treatment of Gaucher's disease has been approved in the USA, and a number of others will no doubt soon follow, including both glycogen and lipid storage disease.

It will have become apparent that all the defects so far mentioned are caused by a recessive mutation. Diseases caused by autosomal dominant mutations will require a more sophisticated approach aimed at either switching off the damaging dominant mutant protein or sequestering it away from the site at which it causes damage. There are a number of single gene defects in which gene therapy is still a long way from providing an answer. The haemoglobinopathies provide one such example. Although major advances have been made recently in identifying the control regions for globin genes, it remains difficult to restrict expression of such gene constructs exclusively to the erythroid lineage. In a protein such as haemoglobin where co-ordinated expression of two subunits, α- and β-globin for example, is required, damage may be caused not by the lack of expression of one but by the overaccumulation of the normal gene product. Gene therapy is a long way from being able to accurately introduce a gene and co-ordinate its expression with one which is already present.

Muscle diseases will be similarly difficult to treat. Here the problem will be the practicability of getting gene correction into every muscle cell. Despite the useful characteristic of muscle cells in allowing persistence of episomal DNA for a considerable length of time, the current approaches to treat inherited muscle diseases by transduced myoblasts or direct injection are as yet little more than demonstrations of micro-injection techniques on a slightly larger scale.

Treatment of cancers

Cancer presents two enigmas. First, what series of events has transformed the cell into one which is free of the normal regulatory constraints on cell division? Second, how does it escape immunological surveillance and clearance by the highly efficient cytotoxic T-cell system and other specific and non-specific immunological mechanisms? Gene therapy has looked at these questions and tried to devise methods to counteract the two aberrations. Delivering genes to cancer cells specifically will remain problematic until specific tumour cell markers, to which vectors can be targeted, are available. Thus elimination from without is an unlikely goal. Elimination from within by making the tumour more immunogenic is more hopeful. Tumour cells can be transduced with genes expressing immunostimulatory molecules, such as the B7 protein which mediates interactions between antigen-presenting cells and T-cells. In animal models removal of tumour cells, followed by transduction of B7 and reimplantation, has been shown to break tumour abnormal tolerance and, in developing immunity to the B7-transduced cells, the animal also can develop immunity against the parental tumour cells and clear them.

There are a number of variations on this theme, all of which are designed to make the tumour more 'visible' to the immune system. The efficiency of immunological clearance will always be greater than that of chemotherapeutic methods and this is likely to be a major form of cancer chemotherapy in the future. Stimulating the immune system itself by removing tumour-infiltrating lymphocytes (TILs) and expanding these in culture for reinjection approaches the same problem from a different stand point. Early experiments showed that, by gene marking these cells using a retroviral vector, they could be shown to retarget to the tumour when reinjected. This has led to some early studies using TIL cells which have been transduced with various genes to enhance their immune capacity, such as the interleukin-2 gene. There have undoubtedly been a number of dramatic clinical regressions using these, however, the treatment is currently under intense scrutiny and re-evaluation.

In one specific scenario tumour cells can be targeted in preference to normal tissue. This occurs with malignancies of the central nervous system. Here the tumour presents a dividing cell population in the midst of essentially mitotically inactive cells. Advantage has been taken of this by introducing directly into the tumour cell mass a cell line producing retroviral vectors (Fig. 16.5). These retroviral particles contain a construct which codes for a conditional lethal gene. The best example is the thymidine kinase (TK) gene, which is harmless inside a cell

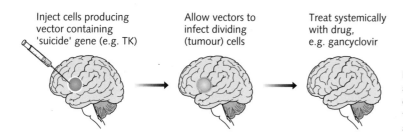

Fig. 16.5 Treatment of brain tumours, taking advantage of the fact that normal brain tissue does not divide and will, therefore, not take up vectors carrying a conditional lethal gene such as thymidine kinase (TK).

unless the cell is exposed to the kinase substrate acyclovir or gancyclovir. The kinase phosphorylates these drugs and this leads to cell death. Injection of the vector-producing cell line into the tumour leads to release of vector particles into the vicinity of the tumour which will be taken up and incorporated into tumour cells as these are dividing. Treatment of the patients with the appropriate drug then leads to toxic elimination of all the vector producer cells and any cells which have taken up the vector. This work is in early-stage clinical trials at present and there are some promising results. Some of the tumour cell clearance seen is in excess of the number of cells which might have been expected to take up the vector, and it is likely that death of vector-transduced cells also leads to some bystander cell death by mechanisms such as interruption of blood supply. In another context the TK gene can be used to provide an added degree of autodestruct control on cells transduced with other genes after they have been reintroduced into the patient.

Gene marking in cancer therapy

Treatment of some cancers involves removal of bone marrow, treatment of the patient with highly toxic doses of chemo- and radiotherapy, then haematological rescue by infusion of the previously stored marrow. In patients with some leukaemias relapse may occur, and it is then difficult to know whether the recrudescent cancer cells have arisen because the therapy was not adequate or because there were residual tumour cells in the reinfused marrow. Gene marking has been helpful here. The bone marrow cells are transduced with a harmless marker gene and then if the tumour relapse contains this gene it must have arisen from the reinfused marrow. Elegant studies have shown that this indeed may occur and have strengthened the case for stringent 'purging' of the marrow prior to reinfusion.

Infections

Analogous to malignancy, one can approach infection

with genetic strategies designed either to immunize an individual against a pathogen or to directly interfere with the pathogen's replication. Genetic vaccines may have a wide application, however, in the near future at least, gene therapy will be restricted to diseases with a poor prognosis and for which current conventional treatment is unsuccessful.

Direct introduction of genetic sequences coding for an immunogenic part of a pathogen has been established in the animal model of influenza. Injection of DNA coding for the nucleocapsid gene triggered a T-lymphocyte response which was then able to protect the animal from lethal challenge with the virus.

Actively interfering with the replication of a pathogen can be approached in a number of ways. The advantage of gene therapy is that there are more targets in the pathogen's life cycle which are amenable to gene therapy than are accessible to conventional chemotherapeutic agents. Infection with HIV is a good example of an infectious condition for which gene therapy will soon be in use, and it serves to illustrate the principles (Fig. 16.6). Interfering with virus entry can be attempted by expressing a soluble form of the virus receptor in the circulation (soluble CD4), such that this receptor protein will bind to the surface of the virus and prevent it from infection cells. The enzymatic processes involved in converting viral nucleic acid through RNA to DNA (in the case of retroviruses) and then in transcribing the DNA to produce messenger RNAs for viral protein production are all amenable to intervention. Antisense RNAs and ribozymal sequences which will cleave target RNAs can be designed to interfere with a number of these steps. Similarly, dominant negative modalities can be used to introduce mutant regulatory or structural proteins into a cell which can be expressed when the pathogen itself is present (Fig. 16.7). These will interfere either with the functioning of the regulatory protein or with the assembly of the structural parts of the pathogen. Another alternative is to introduce anti-viral genes such as interferon into cells which are infected by viruses such as HIV and put them under the control of an HIV-inducible promoter. Thus the cell will function normally until the

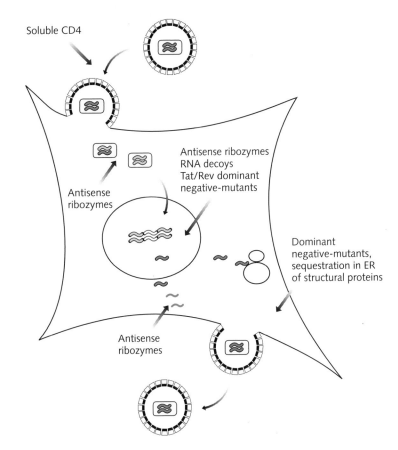

Soluble CD4

Antisense ribozymes
RNA decoys
Tat/Rev dominant
negative-mutants

Antisense
ribozymes

Dominant
negative-mutants,
sequestration in ER
of structural proteins

Antisense
ribozymes

Fig. 16.6 The life cycle of a retrovirus such as HIV, indicating the large number of steps at which gene therapy can be used to interfere with virus replication.

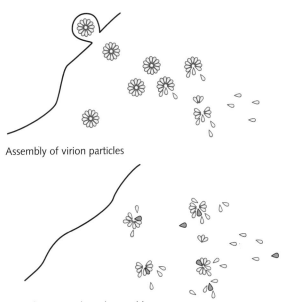

Assembly of virion particles

Intereference with viral assembly
by dominant negative-mutant

Fig. 16.7 How a dominant negative mutant protein can be used therapeutically to interfere with replication of a pathogenic micro-organism.

pathogen enters, at which point it will switch on the anti-viral gene which will either cause inhibition of viral replication or perhaps autolytic destruction of the cell, preventing it becoming a focus for spread of the pathogen to other cells.

Summary

This chapter has attempted to give a flavour of how medical practice may be altered by gene therapy in the next century. Gene therapy protocols have already begun and the number of approved studies is increasing by the month. As yet, somatic cell therapy is the only acceptable form of treatment and germ line gene therapy is considered unsafe. This relates both to our level of ignorance of the molecular biology of the cell and also the paucity of conditions for which germ line gene therapy really is an arguable therapeutic modality. As with every other branch of medicine, there are areas where gene therapy is appropriate and will be effective and others where it is not. As techniques improve, gene therapy may come to be applied to conditions which are currently treated by other methods, and judgements will have to be made as to the risks and benefits of this approach for each disease.

Chapter 17 Prenatal diagnosis

Introduction

Hereditary diseases and fetal malformations account for approximately 20% of perinatal deaths. Prenatal diagnosis is now part of antenatal care and it has four main aims.

1 To relieve the genetic 'roulette' which some families who are carriers of an abnormality face when embarking on a pregnancy.

2 To provide reassurance (in most cases) that the fetus is not affected.

3 To plan treatment when there is an abnormality which may be treated antenatally (rhesus disease and some renal tract abnormalities).

4 To detect abnormalities in what would otherwise be considered a low risk pregnancy.

Clearly prenatal diagnosis cannot guarantee a normal child; common handicaps causing spasticity such as cerebral palsy may result from antenatal events and genetic defects that escape antenatal screening. **Fetal karyotyping** was first carried out in 1964, 8 years after the normal human karyotype had been determined. Rapid progress has been made and new methods of diagnosis continually enter the list of disorders that are amenable to prenatal diagnosis. In particular, the ability to investigate parts of the fetal genome directly by analysis of DNA has influenced the practice of prenatal diagnosis.

Non-invasive methods such as **ultrasound** and biochemical testing of maternal blood can be considered as 'screening tests' in that they can be offered to all pregnant women without risk to the pregnancy. Invasive methods are used to obtain a sample for diagnostic analysis and cause some interference within the fetoplacental unit and to that pregnancy. They are usually only offered in cases where there is a known risk of a significant abnormality, possibly as a result of a positive screening test, and are performed only after further consideration and counselling. The criteria for invasive testing are shown in Table 17.1.

Some pregnancies are considered 'low risk', i.e. where there is no history of an abnormality and the mother is young; others are 'high risk', e.g. where there has been a previous congenital abnormality, or the mother is older (>35 years) when **Down's syndrome** is more likely, or when there is history of genetic disease. At the outset, accurate dating of a pregnancy is important. Certain structural abnormalities may not be identified in early gestation and biochemical screening tests rely on accurate assessment of gestational age: each invasive test has its gestation limits. An ultrasound scan performed between 8 and 11 weeks, measuring the **fetal crown–rump** length (Fig. 17.1), can date a pregnancy to within a few days. This, therefore, is an important component of any 'screening programme'.

Antenatal care is based on identifying early abnormalities, including alterations in fetal growth and amniotic fluid volume. In cases of reduced amniotic fluid (oligohydramnios), placental insufficiency or a fetal renal tract abnormality may be present, among other causes, and where there is increased amniotic fluid (polyhydramnios) other structural abnormalities such as fetal gut atresias may be present. Underlying karyotypic abnormalities such as Down's syndrome may also be associated with oligo- or polyhydramnios.

Screening programmes

Maternal serum α-fetoprotein screening for neural tube defects

α-Fetoprotein (AFP) is a glycoprotein synthesized in the fetal liver, yolk sac and gastrointestinal tract. It is not usually present in the adult circulation except in cases of rare tumours. Its concentration rises in the maternal

Table 17.1 Criteria for invasive testing.

- The disorder suspected is sufficiently severe to warrant investigation
- No treatment is available (except in some circumstances—see text)
- Termination of an affected pregnancy is acceptable to the couple, although this certainly is not a prerequisite for testing
- An accurate test for the condition is available
- The risk of an abnormality being present is sufficiently high to warrant the risks associated with testing

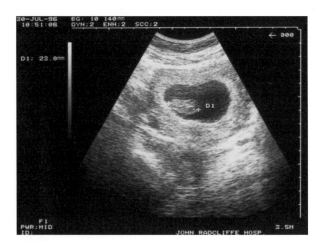

Fig. 17.1 Ultrasound picture showing fetal crown–rump length, at 8 weeks' gestational age.

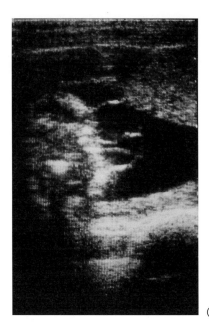

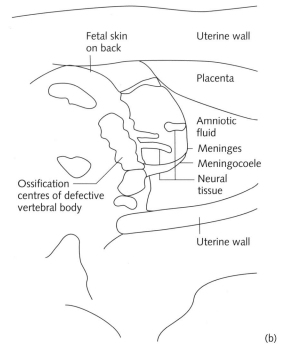

Fig. 17.2 Spina bifida. (a) Ultrasound picture of cross-section of fetal trunk at level of the fifth lumbar vertebra, showing myelomeningocoele. (b) Diagram of ultrasound picture.

blood from the end of the first trimester (12 weeks' post-menstrual age) until 34 weeks' gestation. It is raised still further in association with structural abnormalities, e.g. **neural tube defects** and anterior abdominal wall defects including exomphalos and ectopia vesicae. The mechanism for this rise is not understood.

An abnormally elevated concentration of maternal serum α-fetoprotein (MSAFP), taken in the 16th week of pregnancy, has been used since the mid-1970s as a screening test for neural tube defects. The introduction of high-resolution ultrasound scanning in obstetric units as a routine has however reduced the need for this test, as 98–99% of spina bifida cases can be detected by ultrasound (Fig. 17.2; Plate 30, facing p. 214). A cut-off for normal MSAFP has been taken as 2.5 MoM (multiples of the median), which in a unit not providing routine anomaly scanning but only an MSAFP programme, would mean that approximately 10% of the obstetric population would be recalled for further tests to identify the one to two per 1000 pregnancies complicated by a neural tube defect.

Before the advent of high-resolution ultrasound,

examination of the amniotic fluid for AFP and acetyl-cholinesterase (AChE) was carried out. There are, however, many causes of a raised amniotic fluid AFP ranging from major neural tube defects to minor skin blemishes. In current practice, amniotic fluid would only be sampled for AFP analysis if ultrasound examination was equivocal.

Maternal serum screening for Down's syndrome

More recently a 'triple screen' using AFP, human chorionic gonadotrophin (hCG) and unconjugated oestriol concentrations in the maternal blood, in combination with maternal age, weight and gestational age, has been used to estimate the risk of Down's syndrome (trisomy 21) in the fetus.

The incidence of Down's syndrome increases with maternal age. Hitherto amniocentesis for definitive diagnosis has been offered to older women (>35 or 38 years of age) or those who have had a previous Down's syndrome child, where the risk of the test roughly equals the risk of the abnormality being present. This approach at best would only lead to the detection of 30% of all Down's syndrome fetuses, since most are born to the much larger proportion of younger mothers. Using the triple test in all women over 30 years, it is estimated that 60% of cases of Down's syndrome would be identified, with amniocentesis only being required in 5% of women including those who are younger.

At present screening can only be performed in the second trimester (16–18 weeks), but attempts are being made to identify markers which would allow screening to be carried out in the first trimester. Pregnancy-associated placental protein A (PAPP A) may prove to be just such a marker. It is produced by the placenta, but its function is unknown.

Screening for fetal anomalies using ultrasound

Ultrasound scanning was introduced into obstetric practice in the 1950s. Originally the equipment gave static images of limited information. Although images now obtained are still two-dimensional, the ability to observe movement and to have high-resolution images continually updated in 'real time' enables us to make a comprehensive survey of the fetus for structural abnormalities and for tone and breathing movements. Technology to provide three-dimensional images is currently under development.

The use of ultrasound routinely allows accurate dating and assessment of fetal growth and gives reassurance to most pregnant women with a normal fetus. The fetal organs and structures that are routinely examined are shown in Fig. 17.3. Where an abnormality is suspected, ultrasound assists in invasive sampling techniques which may be required to clarify the diagnosis. Currently many life-threatening anatomical defects can be diagnosed before birth. Similarly, structural abnormalities may indicate an underlying chromosomal abnormality, in particular trisomy 21 (Down's syndrome), trisomy 18 (Edwards' syndrome) or trisomy 13 (Patau's syndrome) (Plate 31, facing p. 214). Frequently further investigation by fetal sampling and karyotyping is required, especially in hydrocephaly, omphalocoele, duodenal atresia, urinary tract abnormalities and cardiac defects. The aetiology of most malformations is still entirely obscure, but developments in the molecular analysis of morphogenesis are likely to lead to increased understanding of developmental processes and how they may be deranged.

Other screening programmes

Within any obstetric population there are ethnic groups who may carry specific genetic diseases associated with their country of origin. The ethnic population amounts to 6.5% of the general population in the UK. Screening programmes aimed at reducing the incidence of a disease must be able to detect the carrier state in order to identify 'at risk' couples. Ideally carrier screening would be carried out before conception (prospective carrier screening) but antenatal clinic screening, or screening after the birth of an affected infant are, at present, the more common approaches. There has been resistance to the introduction of selective carrier screening for some diseases (e.g. sickle cell disease) since targeting of ethnic minorities brings with it the natural fear of racial stigmatization. However, failure to provide such programmes might be considered as an abdication of responsibility.

Screening for carriers of the haemoglobinopathies

The haemoglobinopathies are the commonest genetic diseases worldwide and have autosomal recessive inheritance. The thalassaemias are characterized by ineffective erythropoiesis (Plate 32a and b, facing p. 214), whereas in sickle cell disease there is abnormal haemoglobin. People from the Mediterranean countries and of Asian descent are at particular risk for the thalassaemias. Similarly those of African or Afro-Caribbean origin are at risk of sickle cell disease. Screening is technically easy and inexpensive with the Sickledex test for sickle cell carriers and examination of the mean cell volume for thalassaemia, or haemoglobin electrophoresis for both.

DATE OF SCAN:		LMP:	GA by LMP:	GA by U/S:

BPD:	WKS	DAYS	MSAFP:
OFD:			DATE OBTAINED:
HC:			VALUE:
AC:			DOES SCAN GA = GA BY LMP? yes/no
FL:			IF NO, IS REVISED MOM NORMAL? yes/no

	NORM	ABN		NORM	ABN	
CRANIAL VAULT			KIDNEYS + BLADDER			
CEREBRAL VENTRICLES			LIMBS			
CEREBELLUM			FACE			
NECK AND SPINE			FETAL TONE			
4 CHAMBER VIEW OF HEART			A.F. POCKET DEPTH			
STOMACH + ANT. ABDOM. WALL			FETAL MOVEMENTS			

PLACENTAL SITE:

COMMENTS:

Signature ---

Fig. 17.3 Checklist for fetal anomaly scanning.

Prenatal diagnosis is readily available but the acceptability of this procedure varies within the different ethnic groups.

Many carriers of haemoglobinopathies are identified by incidental screening at routine blood tests for other procedures, e.g. surgery, although in obstetric practice **antenatal testing** is still the most common method of identification. **Community screening** and counselling followed by prenatal diagnosis if both parents are carriers is the ideal and has achieved a dramatic reduction in the incidence of β-thalassaemia in Cyprus, Sardinia and other areas of Greece and Italy.

Screening for carriers of Tay–Sachs disease

A total of 3–5% of Ashkenazi Jews are carriers of **Tay–Sachs disease**, together with 0.5% of the non-Jewish population. Carrier screening, by hexosaminidase-A estimation, is available and prenatal diagnosis is accurate. Uptake of screening is, however, low. The birth rate of affected individuals has not so far been altered significantly by the introduction of selective population screening, and although testing is still available on request, routine screening has been abandoned.

Screening for carriers of cystic fibrosis

Cystic fibrosis is the most common recessively inherited disease of children in most Western countries including the UK. It is estimated that as many as one in 20 of the population are carriers. Although prenatal diagnosis has been available for some time it is only recently that identification of the gene has allowed detection of carriers. Most affected individuals have a trinucleotide deletion at the F508 codon in the CFTR protein, but the remainder (>30%) may have many other mutations. The selection of appropriate probes enables the identification of most, but not all carriers. Risk assessment and counselling therefore raise complex issues. There is still debate over how and when screening should be performed, whether people want it and whether it should be provided by the State.

Potential difficulties of carrier screening

Some of the pitfalls encountered with screening programmes are shown in Table 17.2.

Screening programmes for recessive disorders have distinct advantages for couples who are known to transmit the disease, since early identification of affected children is possible and termination of pregnancy after prenatal diagnosis is an option. Many antenatal screening procedures are, however, carried out without adequate explanation, consent or information regarding the implications of a positive screen test result. It is important to involve primary health care workers in screening programmes so that further verbal explanation can be added to written information given at the time of testing. Movement towards community screening is an ideal, as this would enable considered decisions to be made before pregnancy occurs rather than during the anxious first few weeks of pregnancy.

Screening for carriers of dominant disorders presents a special difficulty, since the identification of a carrier amounts to a preclinical diagnosis. In disorders such as **Huntington's disease** where there is no effective treatment there are profound implications of making such a diagnosis, because the carrier herself or himself is informed that they will have a distressing illness with death at 40 or 50 years of age. Counselling before testing is critically important and counselling and support after the test result becomes available are also needed. Although there is a place for such screening programmes, they not widely available at present and the advantages they offer to affected families await clarification.

At present, unless there are population-based screening programmes, such as those introduced into areas with a high carrier rate (Cyprus for β-thalassaemia), antenatal clinic screening remains the usual approach. This has the disadvantage that the pregnancy may already be well advanced before it is discovered to be at

risk, and then hurried decisions have to be made if further investigation is to be instituted.

Isolation of fetal cells from the maternal circulation

It has long been known that although the fetal and maternal circulations are separate, small 'leaks' occur between the two even in normal pregnancy thus allowing alloimmunization to occur in rhesus-negative mothers. New work in this field has enabled fetal cells to be isolated for analysis directly from the maternal circulation.

Small numbers of fetal nucleated erythrocytes, lymphocytes and syncytiotrophoblast cells have been identified in the maternal circulation. It is possible to use techniques based on the **polymerase chain reaction (PCR)** to amplify sequences of fetal DNA specifically from these cells, and also to obtain signals by **hybridization** *in situ* with chromosome-specific probes. This raises the possibility of prenatal diagnosis without any interference to the fetus. Currently little is known of the extent and time at which transfer of fetal cells occurs. Usually the cells are destroyed when they express incompatible ABO blood group or HLA antigens, but in the future methods for optimizing their recovery and purification from maternal blood may enable non-invasive diagnostic analysis to be carried out for many inherited disorders during pregnancy.

Diagnostic fetal interventions

Obtaining fetal cells

Leonardo Da Vinci, among many of his far-sighted ideas, imagined ways in which we might gain access to the growing fetus. It was many years before this dream could be achieved with the techniques now used. The techniques and samples obtained are summarized in Table 17.3.

Amniocentesis

Amniocentesis involves removal of 10–20 ml of fluid from the amniotic cavity. It is employed between 16 and 20 weeks' gestation for investigation of genetic diseases, but can also be used in the second and third trimesters for the investigation of rhesus albimmunization. The culture of cells from amniotic fluid and therefore the result takes between 2 and 3 weeks.

Before the advent of ultrasound, amniocentesis was performed 'blind'. The clinician relied on his or her clini-

---

- To whom should screening be offered, when and by what means?
- What is the sensitivity, specificity or predictive value of the test that is offered?
- How might false positive and negative results be communicated?
- Is screening desirable and who requests or requires it?
- Is screening 'cost-effective'?
- Is effective treatment available?
- How can the public and health professions be educated about the condition and the screening programme?

Table 17.2 Potential pitfalls in the screening of carriers.

Table 17.3 Techniques and fetal samples obtained for prenatal diagnosis.

Technique	Gestational age (weeks)	Sample	Possible analysis	Estimated additonal risk of fetal loss (%)
Amniocentesis	15+	Amniotic fluid	Cytogenetics Biochemistry Enzyme activity DNA	0.5–1.0
Chorion villus sampling	10+	Placenta	Cytogenetics Biochemistry Enzyme activity DNA	2–4
Fetal blood sampling	18+	Blood	Cytogenetics Biochemistry Enzyme activity DNA	1–2
Liver biopsy	18+	Liver	Enzyme activity	1–2
Skin biopsy	15+	Skin	Histology Electron microscopy Immunofluorescence	1–2
Muscle biopsy	20+	Muscle	Immunofluorescence	1–2
Tumour biopsy	20+	Tumour	Histology	1–2
Fluid collections (cysts or urine)	?16+	Fluid	Histology Cytogenetics Biochemistry	1–2

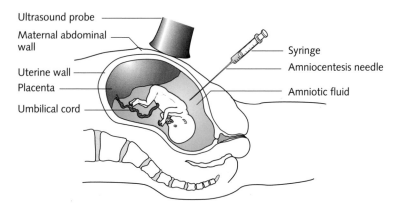

Fig. 17.4 Diagrammatic representation of technique of amniocentesis.

cal skills to identify the lie of the fetus and probed with a large needle into the area around the fetal limbs. In terms of fetal loss, injury and the incidence of failure or haemorrhagic aspirations the risks associated with this procedure were high. Ultrasound has rendered amniocentesis a relatively safe procedure since it allows the needle to be guided accurately into the amniotic cavity (Fig. 17.4). Experienced practitioners lose less than one in 200 fetuses; the main complications of the procedure are spontaneous abortion, persistent leakage of amniotic fluid, sepsis and interference with fetal lung development.

Chorion villus sampling

Termination of pregnancy for abnormality in the second trimester by induction of labour is particularly distressing and the aim of prenatal diagnosticians has been to develop rapid methods which may be used in the first trimester. **Chorion villus sampling** (CVS) is such a test but it is not without hazard. The first attempts at CVS were made in 1968, in women who had decided to terminate pregnancy, using an endoscope which was passed through the cervix to biopsy the chorion frondosum. Diagnostic procedures were not performed, as the complication rates were unacceptably high and samples were obtained in only 50% of cases.

In 1975 a Chinese group reported the recovery of

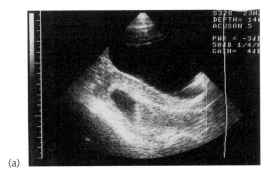

(a)

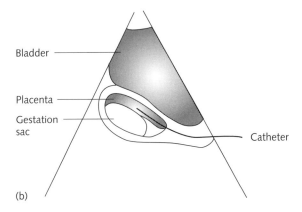

(b)

Fig. 17.5 (a) Ultrasound picture and (b) diagrammatic representation of technique of transcervical chorion villus sampling.

chorionic villi by transcervical aspiration in continuing pregnancies using a metal cannula inserted 'blindly' through the endocervical canal. The success rate (for fetal sexing) was high with only a 4% fetal loss rate but later the procedure was banned. In the West, advances in the molecular diagnosis of the haemoglobinopathies stimulated obstetricians to develop techniques for sampling fetal tissue during early pregnancy. A flexible polyethylene catheter was passed through the cervix and into the placenta under ultrasound guidance, allowing villi to be aspirated. This method, introduced in 1982, has been widely used. Since then various other aspiration systems and biopsy forceps for both transcervical and transabdominal CVS have been developed (Figs 17.5 and 17.6). Fetal loss rates vary and depend on the degree of operator experience, but in general they are 2–4% greater than the spontaneous rate of loss. More recently doubts have been cast upon the safety of CVS because of a suggested link between very early sampling (before 9 weeks' gestation) and limb reduction abnormalities. Difficulties also occasionally arise in the culture and analysis of the samples, as discussed later (p. 307).

Fetal blood sampling

Fetal erythrocytes for prenatal diagnosis of the haemoglobinopathies were first obtained in 1974 by blind needling of the placenta. The chorionic plate was punctured repeatedly allowing blood-stained amniotic fluid to be aspirated. In about 15% of cases only maternal and no fetal cells were obtained and the risks to the pregnancy were high. This early procedure was rapidly superceded by puncture of the vessels under direct vision using **fetoscopy**, and the success rates and fetal loss rates improved. Later developments in ultrasound technology led to the replacement of this technique by fine-needle puncture of various sites to obtain fetal blood under

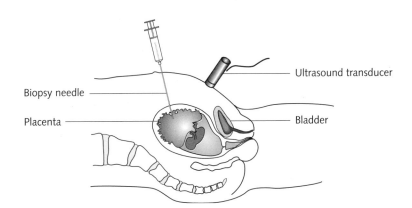

Fig. 17.6 Diagrammatic representation of technique of transabdominal chorion villus sampling.

ultrasonic guidance. The **umbilical cord vein** (Fig. 17.7) at either the placental or fetal insertion, the intrahepatic portion of the umbilical vein, and even the heart may be punctured, according to their accessibility.

There has been a shift in the indications for fetal blood sampling (FBS). It was used mainly for prenatal diagnosis of the haemoglobinopathies and haemophilia but these conditions are now diagnosed in the first trimester by CVS and DNA analysis. FBS is now mainly used in the further investigation of fetal malformation where there is an increased risk of chromosome abnormality.

The indication for sampling also affects the risk related to the procedure. For example, if the fetus already has growth retardation or is being investigated for an abnormality which makes it likely that it will die before birth, such as hydrops fetalis, the losses will appear to be high. In general there is a 1–2% increased risk of pregnancy loss as a result of FBS in the second trimester, where there is an otherwise uncompromised fetus.

Fetal liver biopsy

Until recently, prenatal diagnosis of enzyme deficiencies of the urea cycle (e.g. ornithine carbamyl transferase (OCT) and carbamyl phosphatase synthetase (CPS) defi-

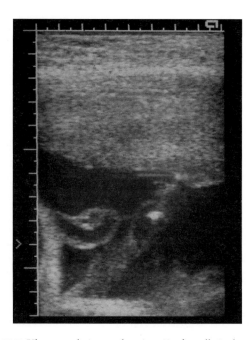

Fig. 17.7 Ultrasound picture showing tip of needle in the umbilical vein for fetal blood sampling. The needle has been guided under ultrasound control through the anterior placenta into the base of the cord at its attachment to the placenta.

ciency) required biopsies of fetal liver to be taken. Now that the underlying molecular pathology of these enzymatic defects is known, because linked markers have been identified, diagnostic procedures based on DNA analysis of chorionic tissue have emerged. **Fetal liver biopsy** is practised in very few specialized centres and as the need for it diminishes, fewer centres will maintain their level of expertise. Like FBS, liver biopsy was originally performed under direct vision using fetoscopy, but now sampling by aspiration through a double needle under ultrasound guidance is preferred. The needle is inserted into the parenchyma and a small core of tissue aspirated for enzymatic or histological study.

Fetal skin biopsy

Fetal skin sampling is used to diagnose inherited skin diseases in affected families. Although from 15 weeks' gestation there is cornification, the normal keratinization of skin does not usually occur until the 24th week of gestation and therefore disorders of keratinization come to light later. Some require specific or multiple sampling sites, such as Hallopeau–Siemens dystrophic epidermolysis bullosa which requires a sample from the sacral area. Junctional epidermolysis bullosa is the most common indication for skin biopsy and this can be diagnosed as early as 15 weeks, using fluorescence-labelled monoclonal antibodies to the basement antigens. Fine ultrasound-guided forceps are used to obtain biopsies leaving few marks or blemishes. Fetal skin biopsy has been welcomed by pregnant women in families at risk from life-threatening disorders such as harlequin ichthyosis or junctional epidermolysis bullosa.

Fetal muscle biopsy

Although rarely employed, fetal muscle biopsy has been used in a few cases to make the diagnosis of **Duchenne muscular dystrophy** by immunofluorescence of **dystrophin**. This has been necessary when DNA studies have not been informative and CVS was, therefore, not appropriate.

Fetal tumour biopsy

Abnormal solid masses detected within the fetus by ultrasound can be sampled as for liver biopsy for diagnostic analysis. This technique has been successfully employed for **congenital adenomatoid malformation** of the lung and fetal teratomas.

Sampling of abnormal fluid collections

Many abnormal fetal fluid collections have been sampled in an attempt to improve diagnosis, for karyotyping and also for treatment. Unfortunately, although they are easily accessible, few are of diagnostic or therapeutic use. Fluid obtained from the distended renal tract, i.e. urine, is, however, important if invasive therapy is contemplated. Biochemical analysis provides information about kidney function. Fluid from cystic hygromas is the only fluid collection which has yielded cells for chromosome studies.

Embryo biopsy and pre-implantation diagnosis

With the development of techniques for *in vitro* fertilization and embryo transfer has come the possibility of **pre-implantation diagnosis**. To date, in a handful of human pregnancies, **sexing of embryos** to allow transfer of only female embryos in X-linked disorders has been achieved. It is now possible to study **chromosomes, enzyme activity, metabolites** and **DNA** from pre-implantation embryos. Techniques are also being developed to analyse the **polar body** in unfertilized eggs so that embryo manipulation may be unnecessary. This would avoid the ethical difficulties that arise from biopsy procedures in human embryos. Using a micromanipulator, embryos can be biopsied in two ways:

1 at the blastocyst stage by splitting the zona pellucida opposite the inner cell mass and removing a few trophoectoderm cells;

2 at the 4–8 cell cleavage stage by aspirating a blastomere with a micropipette.

Attempts to obtain blastocysts by uterine lavage are usually unsuccessful and blastomere biopsy is a more promising procedure, although more experience is needed before the safety and success of this procedure can be properly judged.

Fluorescence *in situ* hybridization (FISH) employing chromosome-specific probes can detect numerical chromosome aberrations and can be used to sex embryos by using a Y-chromosome-specific probe. The PCR can be used to amplify specific DNA sequences from a **single cell** and is a generally applicable method for pre-implantation diagnosis. Allele-specific PCR procedures are readily used to detect mutations responsible for genetic disorders. Biochemical assays of embryonic cells are dependent on the level of expression of a given gene under investigation in the pre-implantation stages, and on the availability of assays with sufficient sensitivity for the analysis of minute quantities of active material.

Studies performed on fetal cells

Cytogenetics

AMNIOTIC FLUID

Amniocytes survive in refrigerated amniotic fluid for up to 2 days, but ideally they are sedimented for culture immediately after sampling. The supernatant fluid can be analysed for AFP, bilirubin or other substances. The pellet is resuspended in culture medium and left undisturbed for 7 days, after which the cells settle and form colonies. The colonies can be subcultured to extend the cell line and maintain colony growth. However, subculturing of amniocytes, unlike fibroblasts, is limited to a few passages so that cultures cannot be maintained indefinitely. Cells are harvested after 8–14 days of seeding and arrested in metaphase by the addition of colchicine. They are examined by light microscopy after staining to show specific banding of the chromosomes. The morphology of the cells found in amniotic fluid is varied. Cells from the amnion, skin, urogenital tract, respiratory tract and alimentary systems may be present, but in the absence of mosaicism or a culture artefact all will exhibit the same karyotype. Maternal cells rarely contaminate amniotic fluid culture as they have limited survival and are sensitive to trypsin treatment which is routinely used for cytogenetic examination.

CHORIONIC VILLI

The aim is to obtain vascularized and budding villi (Plate 33, facing p. 214) from the chorion frondosum (placenta). This sample requires immediate attention, unlike amniotic fluid, to ensure that it is free from decidual (maternal) contamination. If a sufficiently large sample has been obtained, it is divided to provide **'direct' preparations** and **long-term cultures**.

'Direct' preparations (48-h culture) are performed in conjunction with long-term culture (approximately 7 days) because the information obtained from the former is less reliable than the latter. If only a small sample is obtained a long-term culture is preferable. Colchicine may be added to the washed villi so that cells in metaphase in the cytotrophoblast at the time of sampling can be fixed for examination. Cytogenetic information may be available within a few hours but if the mitotic index is low many cells will be disrupted and chromosome material is lost.

Long-term cultures of chorionic villi, as with amniotic fluid, contain many cell types but undifferentiated fibroblasts derived from the mesenchymal core of the villi often predominate: these grow rapidly in culture. If the villi are inadequately cleaned maternal cells may overgrow and lead to a mixed culture. Chorionic villus cells may be harvested for analysis after 8–14 days, depending on the rapidity of growth.

Unfortunately **mosaicism** is more common in villi obtained from normal pregnancies than in amniotic fluid and this may lead to difficulties in diagnosis in about 2% of cases. Mosaicism is found more often in 'direct' preparations in cells derived from the cytotrophoblast. **Tetraploidy** and **trisomies** 2, 3 and 20 occur in culture and since these abnormalities are incompatible with intra-uterine life, they probably represent artefacts. The occurrence of **other trisomies** (8, 9 and 15) creates diagnostic difficulties and fetal blood sampling or amniocentesis is required to resolve the matter decisively unless early abortion is requested.

FETAL BLOOD

Lymphocytes obtained from fetal blood can be readily induced to undergo mitosis in culture and provide an excellent source of cells for accurate karyotyping. There are several ways in which fetal blood can be processed: microculture, 24-h culture of whole blood, and culture of separated blood. Lymphocytes divide rapidly, and because these degenerate within 48 h, fresh samples are usually required for examination. There is a lag phase before mitotic activity starts in lymphocytes. The cells are best harvested on the third day, but in cases of urgency they may be examined earlier.

Most cytogenetic procedures for prenatal diagnosis are carried out to exclude trisomy and this can be achieved with conventional staining followed by light microscopy. Other staining techniques are required for the examination of individual chromosomes and for detection of inversions, deletions and insertions. **G-banding**, the most commonly used procedure for prenatal diagnosis, is carried out after treating slides with a protease and exposure with Giemsa stain. Each chromosome can then be examined for symmetry and compared with the normal karyotype. In **Q-banding** quinacrine, which binds to DNA, is added: this is useful for studying specific regions of chromosomes (e.g. centromeric regions of chromosomes 1, 9 and 16) and may assist in the detailed analysis of the Y-chromosomes. Other techniques are available for the investigation of specific abnormalities, for example the 'fragile sites' in the fragile X syndrome. The indication for testing will determine the particular staining technique that is employed.

Biochemical tests

About 80 genetic metabolic disorders are caused by enzyme deficiencies that can be detected directly in cell cultures from amniotic fluid or villi, or indirectly by the analysis of accumulated metabolites. **Direct enzyme assay** is possible for many metabolic disorders using homogenates of chorionic villus cells. As a consequence, a result may be available the same day. In some inborn errors of amino acid, organic acid and purine metabolism, incorporation of a radioactive precursor into cultured cells is investigated. Quantitative studies are then possible, for example measuring $[^{14}C]CO_2$ production after $[^{14}C]$leucine incorporation as a test for maple syrup urine disease.

Table 17.4 indicates the many disorders that are amenable to prenatal diagnosis by direct biochemical assay.

Molecular analysis of human genes

Methods for the molecular analysis of DNA enable the genotype rather than the phenotype to be determined. DNA obtained from any somatic tissue is representative of that individual; this has the advantage that prenatal diagnosis does not depend on the phenotypic expression. The methods used are critically dependent on the state of knowledge of the molecular pathology of the disease that is under investigation. **Fetal DNA** can be extracted from either chorionic villi or amniotic fluid fibroblasts. The

Table 17.4 Genetic diseases amenable to prenatal diagnosis by biochemical analysis.*

Carbohydrate disorders	Sphingolipidoses
Galactosaemia	Tay–Sachs disease
Pompe's disease	Sandhoff disease
Leigh's disease	Gaucher's disease
	Niemann–Pick disease
Mucopolysaccharidoses	Krabbe's disease
Hurler's disease	Anderson Fabry disease
Hunter's disease	Farber's disease
Sanfilippo's disease A and B	
Morquio A disease	Other lipidoses
	Wolman's disease
Aminoacidopathies	Mucolipidoses Type I and II
Homocystinuria	Fucosidosis
Cystinosis	
Phenylketonuria	Purine disorders
OCT deficiency	Lesch–Nyhan disease
Citrullinaemia	
Maple syrup disease	
Organic acidaemias	
Propionic acidaemia	
Glutamic acidaemia Type I and II	

* This list is not exhaustive.

former source, being more cellular, is preferred since it yields more DNA. A diagnosis can be made directly if the mutation causing the disease affects a known restriction site, as in sickle cell disease. Alternatively, the use of mutation-specific oligonucleotide probes either by filter hybridization or amplification refractory mutation system (ARMS) enables a direct diagnosis to be made where there is a defined range of genetic lesions responsible for the disorder. In most cases linked markers shown by **restriction fragment length polymorphisms** (RFLPs) or **short repeat sequences** may be used. Increasingly PCR is being used to amplify cDNA or subgenomic fragments of DNA that encompass the genetic lesion; this greatly enhances the sensitivity of detection of lesions in minute quantities of input DNA.

The first group of disorders to be diagnosed antenatally by these techniques were the **haemoglobinopathies**. This group represents the most common inherited single gene defect world-wide. There remain families in whom molecular diagnosis is not possible and who require FBS combined with globin chain synthesis studies, as in the past, but in most cases early diagnosis by chorion villus sampling and DNA analysis is possible. DNA is usually obtained from family members so that the appropriate means for analysis can be decided upon before the diagnostic sample of chorionic villi is obtained.

The **α-thalassaemias** are often related to deletions on chromosome 16. There are two α genes on each chromosome so that large deletions may be found in severely affected pedigrees. α_+-Thalassaemia results from the loss of only one active gene, whereas in α_0 both functional genes are lost on each chromosome so that no α chain synthesis can occur. This is not compatible with life and the fetuses develop **hydrops** and die *in utero*.

β-Thalassaemia differs in that there are many diverse molecular defects, ranging from point mutations or small deletions in the β-globin gene cluster on chromosome 11. Although β-thalassaemia major is now compatible with life, affected children require regular monthly blood transfusions combined with chelation therapy to remove excess iron and their quality and expectancy of life is markedly reduced. When the mutation causing loss of gene function is unknown, alterations in contiguous DNA sequences that are linked to that mutation may be found: these give rise to characteristic RFLP markers. When these markers are close to the gene, the likelihood of crossover at meiosis is remote, so that RFLP analysis can be used for prenatal diagnosis. Sickle cell disease results from a point mutation leading to an A → T transversion and leads to substitution of a valine for a glutamate at codon 6 of β-globin. This modifies a recognition site for the restriction enzyme for

*Mst*II. The mutation is thus readily amenable to restriction mapping and Southern blotting or analysis of amplified β-globin gene fragments using PCR combined with endonuclease digestion and agarose gel electrophoresis of the cleavage products.

Many other genetic diseases can be diagnosed prenatally using DNA techniques. Some of the more common ones are Duchenne muscular dystrophy, myotonic dystrophy, Huntington's disease, cystic fibrosis, haemophilia A and B, congenital adrenal hyperplasia, α_1-antitrypsin deficiency, phenylketonuria and fragile X syndrome.

Consequences of prenatal diagnosis

There are three possible outcomes of prenatal diagnosis, continuation of the pregnancy, **termination of pregnancy** or spontaneous abortion, the latter either caused by the procedure or resulting directly from the condition of the fetus. The pregnancy may continue because prenatal diagnosis has not identified an abnormality or because in the end, the couple do not wish to terminate the pregnancy despite the presence of a confirmed abnormality, or because treatment can be offered for the affected infant. Not all couples wish to terminate when a significant abnormality has been identified and they need or request support for the consequences of this decision. Arrangements for immediate postnatal care may need to be put in place, particularly if the infant is likely to die shortly after birth, or require ventilatory support or surgery.

At present few abnormalities are amenable to treatment *in utero*, but as knowledge increases and as new techniques are developed this may change. Evaluation of techniques such as 'shunting' of abnormal collections of fluids is under way. Shunting of **hydrocephalus** was one of the first applications of the procedure but this has now been abandoned because the eventual outcome did not improve. Perhaps the most successful intervention *in utero* has been in the treatment of **rhesus disease** and other blood disorders, such as **alloimmune thrombocytopenia**, by means of **intravascular transfusion**. Decompression of obstructive abnormalities of the urinary tract by shunting and the drug treatment of **fetal tachyarrhythmias** are also instances where intra-uterine therapy of the unborn infant has been successful in selected cases. In the future, different approaches to fetal therapy may be adopted. These may include **stem cell transplantation** and gene manipulation. However there is, and doubtless will continue to be, ethical controversy surrounding such innovations. Few would argue that stem cell transfusion or manipulation of somatic cells might not be beneficial to the individual infant, but the resources that are needed and concerns about artificial genetic selection by effects on the germ line raises sensitive issues that are akin to those that surrounded the quest for the 'Ubermensch' or 'super race' amongst Nazi geneticists.

Termination of pregnancy

For many couples, the decision to terminate a pregnancy is an extremely painful one. For some parents, to have a child born alive that will die soon after birth is preferable to termination. The child has been given the chance of a life and the parents would not themselves be responsible for its death. For some, those few hours of life are precious and memories of a live child are more tangible than those of a terminated fetus with whom no physical contact has been made beyond the experience of fetal movements in the uterus. Other parents do not wish to prolong the life and possible suffering of the fetus unnecessarily, and to bring into the world a child that is destined to die or be handicapped. For them, this course of action would cause more guilt than termination. This is especially true of parents who have had first-hand experience of a child affected by a serious defect that has been inherited. Their desire for a normal pregnancy outcome can be readily understood and the anxieties surrounding prenatal diagnostic testing are often very great.

As our abilities to detect minor abnormalities improve and some defects are detected later in gestation, we are left with difficult decisions as to what period of gestation constitutes viability, and what defects can be classified as life-threatening. Because of improvements in neonatal care, infants born at 23 and 24 weeks' gestation may now survive. In the UK at present termination of pregnancy is legal even after 24 weeks' gestation provided the condition of the mother or the abnormality in the fetus are serious and life-threatening. What benefit do we achieve by making the diagnosis of an abnormality such as cleft lip and/or palate which, although disfiguring, is treatable and does not jeopardize life? It can be argued that forewarned is forearmed and that parents may be helped to face the birth and the later complexities of treatment and educational difficulties that may arise when they know what to expect beforehand. For some, however, the knowledge of an abnormality alienates them from the pregnancy and interferes with the emotional bonding that would develop with the infant after delivery.

If we detect an abnormality are we morally obliged to

inform the parents or should we withhold some information, and face possible legal recrimination later? There can be no simple guidelines for dealing with any particular abnormality. Each predicament has to be judged individually, allowing parents and clinicians to act as they feel appropriate—albeit within the law. A woman's right to choose and be informed has to be uppermost in our minds, although this may leave doctors and parents with almost unresolvable dilemmas. Care must be taken that the fundamental principles of the patient's rights to autonomy and confidentiality are observed. The fetus, a third party, has also to be considered, even though the fetus is not autonomous and cannot be consulted. Moreover, the **legal status of the unborn fetus** has yet to be defined; however, in the future legal dictates as to the rights of the fetus may yet emerge.

Conclusions

Some issues in prenatal diagnosis are straightforward. There is a burgeoning list of inherited conditions that are amenable to antenatal detection. The risks of inheriting a particular disorder have to be balanced against the risks to the pregnancy from invasive procedures that are required for its diagnosis.

With continuing innovation in the technology of ultrasonic investigation of the gravid uterus, we are able to identify minor structural abnormalities that are not life-threatening and which may be amenable to curative treatment *in utero*.

Difficult questions may arise as to who is in ultimate control, parents, the doctor or, through the law, society as a whole. No completely satisfying policy has been drawn up to establish how much we should interfere with natural outcomes of 'imperfect' pregnancies. At present, the issues are usually settled pragmatically in relation to specific cases, each of which is the focus for individual debate and discussion between at least one parent and, one hopes, a doctor and other counsellor who are trusted and experienced in this field.

Further reading

Brock D.J.H., Rodeck C.H. and Ferguson-Smith M.A. (eds) (1992) *Prenatal Diagnosis and Screening*. Churchill Livingstone, Edinburgh.

Modell B. and Modell M. (1992) *Towards a Healthy Baby*. Oxford University Press, Oxford.

Weatherall D.J. (1991) *The New Genetics and Clinical Practice*. 3rd edn. Oxford University Press, Oxford.

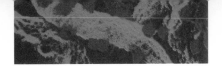

Chapter 18 Molecular biology and the future of medicine

Molecular medicine in a changing world

As in the past, the care of the sick will forever challenge our best minds and the charity of our most civilized societies. Because the burden of sickness is placed on the whole of society, the solutions to moral and economic questions posed by illness in the modern world will need, in part, to be political but ideally will be arrived at by debate within an informed, realistic — and compassionate—public.

Despite our new scientific understandings, therapeutic revelations have been disappointingly few in the history of medicine: without the public health measures and anti-microbial drugs that have been introduced into medical practice this century, we would continue to face infectious plagues and the low expectation of life that characterized the lot of the common person from medieval to Victorian times. The era of molecular biology has created an **atmosphere of expectation** in contemporary medicine, but the early application of its discoveries is occurring at a time of radical political change. In developed countries, governments perceive an unending appetite for health care and research spending: as a result, goal-orientated research, with a marketable product, is encouraged at the expense of secure funding for 'blue skies' science in the disinterested pursuit of knowledge.

In medical practice, ever more expensive and technology-based palliative treatments are being developed for the repair of pathology. Hospitals appear to have assumed the role of technocratic palaces and those who work in them seem to some as devoid of human feelings. Dissatisfaction and the **unrealistic expectations of medical care** has led to calls for better education of medical students and doctors in the arts of medicine. In response to this, governments are intervening in the allocation of resources and the introduction of health plan-

ning independently of the profession to gain better **value for money**. Consumer pressure is being exerted and a marketplace ideology is being introduced. There have been calls to provide medical students with an education containing a basic 'core curriculum' in science with greater emphasis on ethical problems, on communication skills and on palliative care. Without wishing to enter further into this educational debate, one might just point out that there will be always disputes about what really does constitute the essential core of a medical curriculum (one lecturer's 'essential' will be another's 'optional module'). Molecular biology is seen as the apotheosis of the **reductionist approach** to medical science which has spawned an inadequate high-tech medicine that is bringing the economies of rich countries to near bankruptcy and, at the same time, ignoring our humanitarian needs. Rationalist views have led to loss of interest in religion or a rise in an anti-intellectual evangelistic reaction to the evolution of ever more secular societies.

It is salutary to examine modern medicine with a global perspective. Whilst in developed countries life expectancy is rising (Fig. 18.1), in fact only a minority of the world's population can expect to live more than three score years and ten. Ageing and its associated medical disorders such as Alzheimer's disease can be regarded as an artefact of civilization. Bacterial, viral and protozoal infections combined with malnutrition cause premature death in at least a third of the population. Public health measures have failed: the global population expansion and the rise in cigarette smoking that accounts for escalating deaths from cancer, heart and respiratory disease; infantile diarrhoea, malaria and tuberculosis remain, as always, major killers (Table 18.1).

The world population is rising (Table 18.2) and several governments have attempted to limit this expansion by the introduction of measures to control the birth

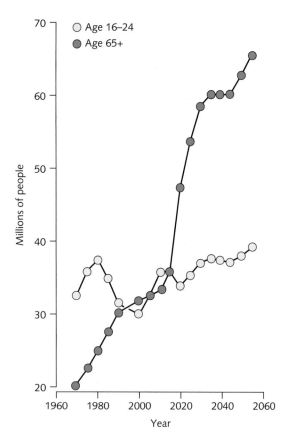

Fig. 18.1 The changing age structure of the US, more or less characteristic of all industrialized nations. For the foreseeable future, the age group 16–24 will remain rather constant in numbers, whereas the number of senior citizens (greater than age 64) will increase dramatically (from Neel (1994)).

rate. In the absence of improvements in infant mortality, voluntary measures, despite various incentive policies, have been disappointing. The fiscal policies of birth control introduced in China have, despite much criticism in the West of their interference with personal choice and freedom, been effective in regulating **population growth**. It seems likely that many countries will be obliged to introduce effective policies to limit their population growth in the near future. Should this occur, the natural wish of parents to have healthy offspring will be in conflict with the natural occurrence of disease and especially unexpected genetic disease in their children. Here genetic counselling linked to prenatal diagnosis and abortion where necessary may in part meet the need for reassurance that, say, the two offspring allowed can be reasonably be expected to survive to healthy adulthood. The introduction of these measures would raise ethical questions that involve whole populations and an agreed (or

perhaps enforced) contract with government. They are measures that may be relatively easy to prescribe, but difficult to accept. Nonetheless, it is likely that stringent mass birth control will be introduced by legislation in several countries within the next decade, and the role of predictive DNA testing and prenatal diagnosis will be greatly expanded.

We have seen that scientific revelations in medicine are all too few, but they have been sufficient in 300 years to provide some understanding of disease. It has been pointed out recently that Robert Boyle, discoverer of the gas laws and bioluminescence and a major figure of the scientific revolution of the seventeenth century, would treat his fevers by placing toads, arsenic, virgins' menstrual blood and emeralds in containers around his neck. These measures sought to address the inbalance of humours that were thought to account for illnesses since the time of Galen. The Public Health Act of 1875, and 70 years later the award of the Nobel Prize for Medicine for the discovery of penicillin, gives some indication of the pace of improvement in our therapeutic approach. Hitherto, the era of molecular biology in medicine has been accompanied by some disillusionment with a lack of progress; but it is premature to expect the diseases that puzzle us so much already to have been eradicated. Ultimately, we will understand the **interplay between genes and environment** in many degenerative disorders, in cancer and perhaps in disordered immunity. In global terms, there has been insufficient time to mount successful attacks on the common infectious causes of death and disease; but the development of recombinant vaccine for hepatitis B—a major cause of liver disease and cancer in Africa and China—is one landmark achievment. There are reasonable expectations that within the next decade, chemotherapeutic agents for vaccines for mass immunization of populations stricken by malaria, HIV and other infectious agents will become available through the study of microbial genetics and the molecular basis of immunity in their host.

Historical examination indicates that our high expectations of medicine are recent; indeed they were probably raised by the emergence of **chemotherapeutic agents** such as Salvarsan, Prontosil and **penicillin**. A thousand years before that, our ancestors were surrounded by the threat of death, usually from infection. Until recently, infant mortality of 25% had been endured for centuries, reflecting old medical practices, poor understanding of microbiology and the absence of any experimentally tested understanding of disease processes.

When we consider these concepts in relation to the industrialized world, where moral principles and human dignity are particularly threatened by the technology-

Table 18.1 Death rates and percentage of total deaths for the leading causes of death, 1900 and 1988 (from *Monthly Vital Statistics Report*, National Center for Health Statistics, **39** (7), supplement, 28 Nov. 1990).

1900		1988	
Cause of death	Deaths per 100 000	Cause of death	Deaths per 100 000
Cardiovascular–renal disease	345.2	Diseases of heart	311.3
Influenza and pneumonia	202.2	Malignant neoplasms, including neoplasms of lymphatic and haematopoietic tissues	197.3
Tuberculosis	194.4	Cerebrovascular diseases	61.2
Gastrointestinal disease	142.7	Accidents and adverse effects	39.5
'Senility'	117.5	Chronic obstructive pulmonary disease and allied conditions	33.7
Accidents	72.3	Pneumonia and influenza	31.6
Malignant neoplasms	64.0	Diabetes mellitus	16.4
Diphtheria	40.3	Suicide	12.4
Typhoid fever	31.3	Chronic liver disease and cirrhosis	10.7
Complications of pregnancy	13.4	Nephritis, nephrotic syndrome and nephrosis	9.1
All causes	1719.1	All causes	882.0

based approach to body repair, we can again identify the potential for molecular biology in medicine. How else are we going to understand autoimmunity, hypertension, psychiatric disease, vascular and neurological degeneration? We need to understand the interactions between our constitution and environmental factors now that these are changing — the relationship between our immune constitution and our new microbial environment may well be altering as the selective pressures of nutritional and the old infectious diseases recede. The identification of somatic mutations in cancerous cells may allow specific targets unique to the cancerous cell to be identified for the treatment of particular malignant diseases. At present, chemotherapeutic regimens seem appallingly crude and expensive: for a slight improvement in outcome figures compared with the natural course of malignant disease, patients are brought practically to the brink of death and require intensive medical support while their tissues recover from the mutagenic insult, hopefully uncontaminated by surviving neoplasm. Cytotoxic chemotherapy delivered by today's oncologists strikes many as unspecific, empirical and showing few signs of innovation.

Impact of the Human Genome Project

Although the official inauguration of human genome projects in the United States and other participating countries was in 1990, the scientific planning of this initiative long preceded this. The project has widespread support from diverse funding agencies in the United States such as the Department of Energy and the National Institutes of Health. Collaborative agencies in the UK, France, Italy, Canada and Japan provide input so that the effort into high-resolution genome mapping and sequencing projects has become a highly coordinated international venture.

Application of information provided by the Human Genome Project combined with the ever-burgeoning bank of known expressed sequences in the nucleotide and protein databases is improving the overall efficiency of cloning strategies for the identification of human disease loci (see Chapter 6). At the time of writing, it seems likely that those regions of the genome that have been physically mapped to the highest density will be subject to direct DNA sequencing using large-scale automated nucleotide sequence analysis. Greater emphasis on sequence analysis will act catalytically to refine the development of physical gene maps for chromosomal regions. Thus future progress in the characterization of disease genes will rely increasingly on their identification by the dual 'positional–candidate gene' approach.

Recognition of the remarkable evolutionary conservation of eukaryotic genes, especially those that are found in vertebrate genomes, has enabled human molecular genetics to develop into a discipline that will provide unparalleled insights into molecular physiology. This development stems partly from the expansion of computer-based **genetic informatics** and partly from the emergence of new biological techniques in the experimental science of **transgenesis**.

When an investigator isolates a given candidate gene sequence from human DNA, it can now be scrutinized for likely open reading frames (i.e. coding sequences that are transcribed *in vivo* into mRNA) in all six possible phases and compared with DNA or protein sequences from all the known genes and their products from all the micro-organisms, plants and other animals that hitherto have been 'logged-in' to the vast computerized bioinformatic repositories to which all universities, biotechnology and pharmaceutical companies and research institutes have access. Homology searches, regions of sequence identity, functional protein domains and other detailed comparisons within molecular biology databases can be accomplished within minutes. Every day, investigators are able to recognize structural relationships between their putative gene or protein of interest and thereby establish functional relationships. It is clear

Table 18.2 Estimates of world population by regions, 1650–1950 (United Nations, 1953).

Series of estimates and date	Estimated populations in millions							
	World total	Africa	North America§	Latin America¶	Europe and Asia (exc. USSR)**	Asiatic USSR**	Oceania	Area of European settlement††
Willcox's estimates*								
1650	470	100	1	7	257	103	2	113
1750	694	100	1	10	437	144	2	157
1800	919	100	6	23	595	193	2	224
1850	1091	100	26	33	656	274	2	335
1900	1571	141	81	63	857	423	6	573
Carr–Saunders' estimates†								
1650	545	100	1	12	327	103	2	118
1750	728	95	1	11	475	144	2	158
1800	906	90	6	19	597	192	2	219
1850	1171	95	26	33	741	274		335
1900	1608	120	81	63	915	423	6	573
United Nations estimates‡								
1920	1834	136	115	92	997	485	9	701
1930	2008	155	134	110	1069	530	10	784
1940	2216	177	144	132	1173	579	11	866
1950	2406	199	166	162	1242	594	13	935

* Willcox, *Studies in American Demography* (1940), p. 45. Estimates for America have been divided between northern America and Latin America by means of detailed figures presented on pp. 37–44.
† Carr–Saunders, *World Population* (1936), p. 42.
‡ United Nations, *Demographic Yearbook 1949–50* (1950), p. 10; and United Nations, 'The past and future growth of world populations . . .' (1951), Table II; the 1940 figures are unpublished estimates of the United Nations.
§ United States, Canada, Alaska, St Pierre and Miquelon.
¶ Central and South America and Caribbean Islands.
** Estimates for Asia and Europe in Willcox's and Carr–Saunders' series have been adjusted so as to include the population of the Asiatic USSR with that of Europe, rather than Asia. For this purpose, the following approximate estimates of the population of the Asiatic USSR were used: 1650, 3 million; 1750, 4 million; 1800, 5 million; 1850, 8 million; 1900, 22 million.
†† Includes North America, Latin America, Europe, the Asiatic USSR and Oceania.

that most genes present in yeast, the fruit fly *Drosophila*, the nematode worm *Caenorhabditis* and the tetraodontoid fish *Fugu* are represented in the human genome. These relationships are useful for defining evolutionary significance and for recognizing the core properties of homologous gene products. Such an approach for example was essential to the identification of the cystic fibrosis transmembrane regulation protein and the Wilson's disease gene product: these are members of a family of distinct membrane transporters with ATPase activity that had previously only been recognized in microbes and was unknown in mammals.

In the UK, the human genome mapping project research centre was set up by the Medical Research Council and is now based in the Hinxton Genome Campus near Cambridge, together with the Sanger Centre and the European Bioinformatics Institute. As with other major national resources, the UK centre makes available genomic yeast artificial chromosome (YAC) libraries and hybridization series, panels of monochromosomal somatic cell hybrids, cDNA libraries and comparative mapping resources using the interspecific back-cross service for fine mapping human DNA markers onto the mouse genome. A further important aspect of comparative mapping will be access to genomic resources from the genome of the puffer fish, *Fugu*. This vertebrate genome whose structure has been investigated in pioneering studies by Sydney Brenner and colleagues in Cambridge, possesses essentially the same complement of expressed genes as the human genome, but with a genome one-eighth of the size, largely due to the reduction in repetitive DNA. Not only do studies of this compact genome allow the identification of human homologues, but the overall presence of intra-exon boundaries will greatly facilitate full characterization of the overall human gene structure. Finally the centre provides computing services through the networks, allowing access to the full range of biological information systems. All these resources are available to registered human genome mapping project users. Registration is granted to anybody working within human genetics and the services are provided free to all academic users in the UK and the European Union.

Molecular medicine cannot be a panacea either, but the information explosion that will come from the Human Genome Project will certainly have an impact on society through future applications in medicine. Given the conceptual and economic bankruptcy associated with much contemporary 'high-tech' medicine, we would be better to place our confidence in a long-term view of the rewards that should ensue from understanding disease in terms of cell and molecular biology. Such

confidence would not absolve us from a rational examination of expenditure and of ethical issues in the allocation of resources. We need also a collective appraisal of the means for research support by governments that represent society. Ethical issues will emerge in relation to genetic research — but this is not a time to have misgivings about scientific applications. The human immunodeficiency virus has for one been no respecter of national, economic or cultural boundaries.

To avoid disillusionment we need an element of realism about our expectations of molecular medicine and the Human Genome Project in particular. Even with the monogenic disorders, where one can demonstrate high penetrance and a cause and effect relationship between mutations at a given genetic locus and the development of a clear human phenotype, time is needed to reap the benefits of this information. In some cases, identification of the genetic locus improves the possibilities for diagnosis by direct analysis of genomic DNA, and this can be applied to unborn children where there may be the offer of abortion or early introduction of therapy as a result of prenatal diagnosis. The polymerase chain reaction has greatly aided these approaches. Samples of hair, dried blood spots obtained by population screening at birth, and circulating fetal cells in blood obtained from a pregnant woman can be used as the template for analysis and thus avoid invasive biopsy procedures. However, therapeutic advances may take many years to follow on from the identification of the molecular pathology at a disease locus. For example, the full characterization of sickle cell anaemia as a molecular disease caused by a single amino acid substitution in the β-globin polypeptide by Ingram in 1956 led to few changes in the management of the affected patient for nearly 40 years. Novel therapies using hydroxyurea or butyrate to stimulate compensatory synthesis of γ-globin chains have emerged recently through the bold application of unrelated studies on haemoglobin regulation in murine erythroleukaemia and on methylation in the control of gene expression.

As already shown in previous chapters, defining the genetic basis for a disorder may ultimately lead to the development of somatic cell gene therapy or, occasionally, to the development of a therapeutic drug (e.g. recombinant human factor VIII$_c$ for haemophilia; see Chapter 1); more often than not it leads to a whole chain of experiments to investigate and assess the role of the locus in the development of the disease itself. Thus we must suppress our intellectual greed: identification of the *BRCA1* locus that is responsible for 5% or so of breast cancers in women will not immediately yield a novel treatment for cancer.

Transgenics and the solution of biological problems in medicine

The comparative study of molecular physiology has entered a new phase of experimental revelation with the advent of **transgenesis**. Hitherto, genetics had been based on the characterization of rare mutants. Muller's experiments with X-rays and later work using chemical mutagens, as well as with the transposable elements of maize and *Drosophila*, increased the frequency of experimental mutation, but it remains a largely random process. To investigate the underpinning function of defined loci in the physiology and development of whole organisms is a goal of human molecular genetics, but one that has largely depended upon the study of rare diseases and has followed the Harveian tradition of 'experiments of nature'.

It is possible to use the techniques of homologous recombination or transgenic overexpression to manipulate the genome of the embryonic stem cell for later injection into the developing embryo (see Chapter 3). Thus either a wild-type or mutant human gene can be transferred to the mouse genome or a murine locus can be disrupted selectively to generate animals that have been rendered deficient in the gene product by breeding—the so-called 'knockout' mouse. The ability to generate animal models of disease for experimental purposes represents a new departure in genetics and will provide an invaluable resource for testing the effects of treatments, including gene therapy protocols, on the natural course of human disorders. The cystic fibrosis CFTR knockout mouse is a notable example of this application.

Transgenics depends upon the insertion or deletion of specific DNA sequences into the germ line of experimental organisms so that interspecies comparisons of the function of selected genes can be made. Special insight into human molecular pathology depends upon the transfer of the altered genome into developing mice but there is no theoretical limit to the ultimate host species. The presence of the altered locus from an early embryonic stage permits the effects of the genetic manipulation to be assessed during development and in the whole living animal. Germ line transmission in mice is predicted on the demonstration by Martin Evans that certain undifferentiated cells derived from murine embryos, 'embryonic stem cells' or primitive chorioncarcinomas, can, when injected by microscopic procedures into the inner cell mass of early blastocysts (that are later reimplanted in the uteri of pseudopregnant virgin host animals), repopulate all the tissues, including gonads, of the developing animals.

In some instances there has been disappointment with transgenic knockout mice: selective disruption of a locus of interest has sometimes led to the development of animals that are indistinguishable from wild-type mice despite clear evidence of a complete deficiency of the gene product. The inference here has been that there is considerable redundancy built into the system for many genes, and that enhanced expression of other proteins can often compensate for the absence of one partner, especially when this has been absent from the tissues of early embryos. Although this has, on occasion, been a perplexing outcome to one or two years of hard experimental work, it might be argued that many critical systems would have an inbuilt fail-safe mechanism to compensate for failure of a single component. The unnerving possibility that organisms may have more genes than they might require has provoked much thought, since the observation raises questions about evolutionary 'commitment'.

From the expanding collection of knockout mice it is clear that high organisms do possess some degree of genetic redundancy or in other ways have multiple means to attain their developmental and functional endpoints. Experimental manipulation of the genome of yeast has also shown that several genes can be deleted without any discernible phenotypic effect. Sydney Brenner has urged caution about the way we view redundancy in complex organisms; their very complexity brings with it the risk of a 'signal failure' and it may be that alternative pathways have evolved to compensate. However, as Brenner points out, this is a teleological argument and while natural selection may exert its effects to improve reliability in a system, it could not do this to protect against genetic errors. The evolution of the diploid genome, which provides two copies of every gene in complex animals and plants, provides protection against inactivating mutations.

Quite often environmental challenge, such as the experimental exposure of apparently normal mice lacking an essential component of the NADPH oxidase of phagocytes to pathogenic organisms that cause the equivalent human disease, chronic granulomatous disease, is required to 'bring out' the predicted phenotype. Alternatively, it might be necessary to out-cross the mutant animals with mice of other laboratory strains to examine the effects of gene disruptions in other backgrounds. It is often possible to reveal the effects of epistatic factors present in different strains that influence the phenotype.

The systematic analysis of different heritable contributions to phenotypic expression is the stuff of classical genetics, but it promises much in the investigation of human disease susceptibility when it can be used to study controllable models that can be bred in the laboratory. The future of transgenic experimentation lies in the more refined use of genetically manipulated organisms, and in relation to human disease, the temporal control of the disruption event. Methods are emerging to introduce specific disease-associated mutations into the mouse germ line to investigate genotype–phenotype correlations. It is also possible to disrupt a locus by homologous recombination in selected tissues after embryonic development. These techniques will also allow the function of a given locus implicated in disease to be defined at critical stages of maturation and growth in the whole organism.

The biological pathways that relate pathological phenotype to gene and then back to biological function will present the main intellectual challenge for molecular biology in the future — at least as far as medicine is concerned.

New and old ethical issues

We are familiar with ethical issues in medicine. They permeate all aspects of medical treatment, from decisions about resuscitation; about acceptance of patients on **transplantation** or **haemodialysis programmes**; about **mass immunization** and **genetic screening**. However, with increasing knowledge about genes, there can be no denying that there have been justified calls for increased monitoring. This applies as much to human molecular genetics in clinical practice as it does to the use of live vaccines and the release of genetically-modified organisms into the environment. The popular concept of the genetic blueprint implied by genetic information has focused on the role of statutory bodies to regulate genetic research and especially gene therapy. An uninformed public is probably almost as frightened of a public network of genetic fingerprinting as it is of the Frankensteinian nightmare of germ line manipulation and embryo research.

Ethics establishes principles that allow actions to be judged as good or bad and, by inference, morally right or wrong. These principles impinge on the practice of medicine, such that good clinical practice adheres to stringent ethical precepts. It is a principle that medicine should always seek to provide benefit in psychological or physical terms and, at the same time, avoid harm. International guidelines set out in the Declaration of Helsinki in 1964 provide guidance for medical personnel in the conduct of research; this guidance has been subsequently extended and reviewed periodically by the world medical assemblies. To some extent these initiatives reflect responses to political interference in medical

activities and, regrettably, participation by doctors in the violent activities of repressive governments. Nonetheless, the guidelines establish a general set of accepted moral values for the modern practice of medicine that have an international currency.

Developments in human molecular genetics have been monitored by statutory bodies and ethics committees with the belief that there should be increasing input from members of the public without special qualifications in the medical profession. It is felt that this will provide a more sound assessment of the rights and wrongs of medical research and exploration in the area of human genetics. Apart from one or two conspicuous examples of unethical behaviour by medical scientists, the level of monitoring and sensitivity of institutions to public opinion is such that transgressions have so far been minimized. As we now approach the field of gene therapy, public input into ethics committees and other regulatory bodies may expand so that a collective responsibility is taken for policies that involve ethically complex areas. The importance of balanced *and* informed public representation cannot be exaggerated if societal issues are to remain properly within the ambit of democratic decision-making processes.

Scientists themselves have a key role in being able to assess the relative merits and disadvantages of a particular protocol for an individual who is being offered a novel therapy. Here the assessment of known risks has to be balanced against possible advantages: professional input will always be critical to ensure that a predictable risk does not exceed a possible gain. Given the potential dangers of genetic manipulation of organisms and the pace of cognate medical research, there is a clear need to evolve a corporate policy in society as a whole and to ensure that a scientifically literate public can act independently of sensational journalism and contribute to informed judgement.

Predictive genetics and medical ethics

The issues of genetic screening for pre- and postnatal diagnosis for inherited conditions are particularly relevant. Diagnostic and screening procedures are set up to answer questions raised by parents and families who have experienced or are threatened by the risks of either developing a genetic disorder themselves or bearing affected children. Clinical genetic services help to define the risks in terms of the probability that a given disorder will occur and to assess the potential burden to which the disorder can give rise. As described in detail in Chapter 17, prenatal diagnosis has been possible through improving methods of enzymatic, cytogenetic, haematological and imaging services for many years. Advances in molecular genetics (especially the polymerase chain reaction) and their application to carrier detection as well as prenatal diagnosis, have given greater precision and a wider range of testing. It is possible to test not only for serious single gene defects such as cystic fibrosis, Duchenne muscular dystrophy and the haemoglobinopathies, but also genetic disorders that come to light later in life such as haemochromatosis, hereditary cancers and Huntington's disease.

Prenatal diagnosis

The implications of prenatal diagnosis are far-reaching and bear upon religious and social attitudes. They impinge also on women's issues, especially in relation to pregnancy termination. The generality of opinion is not known but it is clear that a significant minority of mothers would not consider having amniocentesis for severe defects even if they were at risk, for religious or moral reasons. It is also the case that the perspective of individuals who are themselves affected by serious genetic disorders such as cystic fibrosis or thalassaemia is very variable: certainly not all would wish that their parents had undergone prenatal diagnosis and pregnancy termination. A practical point remains that is often ignored: namely the confidence with which a particular outcome or disease severity can be predicted. There is enormous variation in the clinical expression and penetrance of mutant genes and simple genotype–phenotype correlations simply may not hold for most hereditary diseases. The frequent lack of certainty has crucial significance for predictive testing, counselling and standards of good medical practice. It would be wrong to offer prenatal diagnosis where no certain clinical outcome can be guaranteed. Were it possible to identify the pregnancy at risk where there had been no previous experience of the genetic disorder on the part of the parents, then the issues are far more complex and place particular demands on the ability of the clinical genetic services to provide appropriate counselling.

It is widely believed that counselling should be as objective and as non-directive as possible to give a view that is entirely unprejudiced about a genetic disorder. This is particularly true where advances may change the quality of life for a disorder, or where there is marked variability in clinical behaviour, e.g. in the thalassaemias which can range from mild anaemia to the severe manifestations of transfusion-dependent disease with gross iron storage. The practical complexities of biochemical analysis and testing DNA, of course, require the interac-

tions of many individuals in the laboratory and in the clinic; but it is essential that counselling is provided by informed professionals with sufficient experience and depth of knowledge to present the issues. This level of expertise is most unlikely to be held by a single person and the value of information dissemination through professional networking in this field cannot be overemphasized.

In some countries there has been an astonishing growth of laboratories that offer commercial diagnostic kits for DNA analysis for use by private obstetric clinics. As a result of the availability of testing in this way, it is possible that an increasing number of parents will be faced with a prenatal diagnosis and then a consideration of pregnancy termination. Ultimately pressure may be placed on individuals to know more about their genetic status and use this to inform their choice of mate. The social and ethical implications of these developments are very real and it is clear that governments will need, sooner or later, to make recommendations that would prevent indiscriminate prenatal diagnostic testing especially where the predictive power of DNA-based tests cannot possibly be sustained in practice. A good example is that of intelligence. Certain inherited and acquired conditions cause a level of mental disability. It will be difficult for society, or for individuals, to decide at what level of IQ a gene therapy approach is appropriate to improve the person's mental functioning. Leading on from this grey area will be the equivalent of plastic surgery using genetic means. Much plastic surgery at present is involved with important functional improvements, but some is purely cosmetic. Gene therapy, likewise, will ultimately be able to enhance certain genes. Altering those which affect intelligence or musculature or skin coloration would all be in the bounds of possibility. At present this is not an issue; however, it is important to keep in mind that medical advances often move faster than do moral debates and questions such as these will need addressing sooner rather than later.

Religious attitudes vary between countries as well as within and between ethnic groups in a single country. There is likely to be a huge variation in the degree to which genetic testing, and prenatal diagnosis in particular, is accepted by groups influenced by Papal or Islamic authorities, for example. Samuel Johnson believed that the civility and sophistication of a country may be judged by the way care is provided for the sick and the infirm, as well as the needy. Although the availability of abortion on demand would save on health care provision, surely it is not acceptable to provide it until assessments of quality of enjoyable life can be properly judged for those individuals with inherited disorders? These are going to be issues for societal debate and will reflect, to a large extent, the character of the societies in which they are considered: the extent to which a handicapped person is supported by their community already varies greatly between countries and global regions. The extent of this support will continue to be influenced by traditional and religious beliefs as well as economic factors.

Genetic screening

Genetic screening requires that those who are to be screened for genetic disorders understand the basis and reasoning behind the process. It is clearly incumbent upon legislating authorities to ensure that no mandatory programmes are established without a full debate about their worth. It will be necessary to ensure that screening programmes are conducted in an atmosphere of confidentiality and consent and that due weight is given to the implications of genetic information that relates to the whole family. **Confidentiality issues** are, of course, paramount in the conduct of medicine and although the duty of confidentiality must be strongly guarded there are occasions when disclosure is either required or justified in the light of what may be found in relation to genetic analysis. For example, the finding of an important genetic defect in one individual might be important for relatives and their life plans, known health risks and their own decisions about parenthood, of the issues of data protection and what it is reasonable to disclose in the light of current knowledge. There are forthcoming technical developments to facilitate screening for genetic disorders. Many are currently under study and may or may not be introduced as part of genetic services. These include antenatal and preconception screening for haemoglobinopathies such as sickle cell disease, neonatal screening for cystic fibrosis, and carrier screening for Tay–Sachs disease. There are moves, for example, to introduce screening programmes for the detection of cystic fibrosis carriers prenatally in the population, but there are important questions to be raised about the desirability of this before it is introduced generally.

The following are key points about the introduction of screening.

1 The severity of the disorder, its mortality, prognosis and burden should be fully understood as well as its mode of inheritance. Its frequency should be estimated.
2 The availability of interventional treatment should be understood; should the condition affect different ethnic groups the possibility of stigmatization is raised.

3 The acceptability of screening for a particular disorder in communities, taking into consideration stigmatization and the acceptability to particular individuals, should be considered.
4 The means of screening must be acceptable, reliable and sensitive and ideally should be inexpensive in relation to the benefits which will accrue.

In a recent national enquiry it was proposed that screening should be regulated according to the following ethical principles:
1 to conserve the concept of freedom of choice as to whether screening is undertaken;
2 this choice should be informed by knowledge of the significance of screening for health benefit, including reproductive outcome, and for possible disadvantages;
3 confidentiality should be preserved.

For many years mass screening programmes for the newborn population have been established to detect **phenylketonuria** and **congenital hypothyroidism**. These disorders, which occur with a frequency of approximately one in 15 000 and one in 4500 live births, respectively, ably fulfil the criteria laid down to justify screening, since intervention at the presymptomatic stage avoids their development. It is notable, however, that **screening is mandatory** and no freedom of choice is offered to the parents of newborn children; blood for sampling on Guthrie cards that are used for detection is obtained routinely by pricking the heel shortly after delivery.

Genetic screening for presymptomatic disease

Presymptomatic screening offers the clear benefit of excluding risk of disease and may offer (especially in the inherited cancer syndromes) the advantage of early diagnosis which should lead to prolonged survival and improved quality of life. The removal of uncertainty to improve insurance profile and future plans is clearly important but needs to be balanced against the possibility of increased long-term anxiety. Presymptomatic diagnosis may also lead to difficulties with employment and health insurance premiums for what might be an incurable disorder. Presymptomatic screening that results in a bar to health insurance or employment clearly might outweigh all possibile benefits from the screening procedure, and it also demands a high degree of reliability and predictive power.

Conditions where presentation of disease in adult life can be predicted by diagnosis at birth or in the unborn child pose particular ethical issues. In a condition, such as haemochromatosis, where the disorder is usually not manifest until middle age and may be prevented by simple intervention, better methods for population diagnosis would be welcomed. Clearly, where (as in haemochromatosis) it is known that early treatment can restore life expectancy to normal, the benefits exceed the costs. On the other hand, in a condition such as Huntington's disease, stark ethical issues are raised. As described in Chapter 6, Huntington's disease is a severe neurodegenerative disorder inherited as an autosomal dominant trait. Beyond the age of 40 years the penetrance of the condition approaches 100% but is low during the reproductive period. Psychiatric disorders, combined with dementia, as well as restlessness and involuntary movements characterize the condition. Psychiatric abnormalities and behavioural disturbances with social degradation are frequent, and the condition progresses until generalized motor impairment causes death after an interval of up to 20 years from the onset. The detection of expanded trinucleotide repeats (CAG) in the *huntingtin* gene now allow confident prediction of disease in presymptomatic individuals at risk either of developing the disease or of passing the gene on to children.

To individuals at a low risk for Huntington's disease presymptomatic testing has a good chance of relieving anxiety, but the serious implications for those found to carry the condition would have to be endured for many years before even the first symptoms become apparent. There are then the difficulties of investigating a family where the index case is already suffering the effects of dementia. This individual would not be able to give informed consent for any study. Difficulties thus arise in approaching other members of the family for confirmatory molecular analysis, which would require the intervention of an appointed legal guardian with the consent and knowledge of spouse or other relatives. It is also important to consider what the direct benefits to the index patient would be from pursuing such a course of action. Other issues which arise quite frequently in Huntington's disease stem from disclosure of non-paternity in relation to potential risk. This is because the early psychiatric manifestations may involve temperamental and personality changes that alter sexual behaviour and are associated with promiscuity in the patient and sometimes infidelities by their partner. Under these circmstances, the need to allow freedom of testing and bring about practical benefit must be balanced against the need for confidentiality. An important advantage but potential danger of DNA testing in general is that it can be conducted at any age: again, the responsibilities must be extended to potentially affected offspring who might be tested and their ability to give consent before the age of 18 years of age.

Huntington's disease provides a vivid example of the difficulties in offering presymptomatic testing to individuals at risk for genetic disorders. The International Huntington Association, a disease association formed by relatives and patients affected by the condition, together with the World Federation of Neurology, have set out a policy statement identifying the ethical issues which arise in this condition and which provides very useful guidelines for similar DNA diagnosis of related disorders.

When DNA testing is used astonishing benefits can occur from the analysis of archival material either in the form of stored biopsy or *post-mortem* samples (see Chapter 6), blood samples or even dried blood spots collected on Guthrie cards as part of the population-based mass neonatal screening programmes. A conspicuous example of this came to light when it was proposed to obtain samples of DNA from dried blood on a garment worn by President Lincoln at the time of his assassination. The analysis of this DNA for the presence of mutations in the fibrillin gene that might be responsible for the suspected Marfan's disease in the deceased President did pose questions that were subject to legal debate. One group, curious to establish whether or not the President suffered from Marfan's syndrome, felt there were no legal or ethical issues involved; others questioned this invasion into the privacy of an individual, albeit long after his death and with no surviving descendants. The outcome of this study is, at the time of writing, not known.

Forensic applications of DNA analysis: the population archive—a state-run data bank?

In many countries the banking of blood taken at birth on the Guthrie card is mandatory and is used for neonatal screening for certain defined conditions. The question arises as to whether such blood can be used to test for other disorders and, indeed, whether access can be given to Guthrie card DNA in any subsequent legal questions of identification. Clearly it is an ethical question as to whether this information should be provided to determine the frequency of genetic disorders in the population at large that are not currently tested for. This relates to privacy, anonymity and confidentiality and it would be important to have policy statements about the use of such material for genetic profiling and other potential activities of interest to the state.

The applications of DNA testing for forensic diagnosis, using determination of the size of alleles of variable number tandem repeat (VNTR) markers that show independent segregation, have received much attention.

These involve the use of minisatellite DNA patterns, where variants are detected at one locus by the presence of repeats that either create recognition sites for a restriction endonuclease or do not. The repeats can be amplified in the polymerase chain reaction and the units occurring within the locus can then be classified into one or other group by the digestion patterns with the specific enzyme. This enables the minisatellite repeat variants to be digitalized giving a individual locus identification or 'DNA fingerprint'. Whereas this method has clear forensic applications, the ethics of digital DNA typing as applied to population archives will relate very much more to legislative pressures from the state than to the restricted area of medical genetics.

General issues

As explained elsewhere in this book, it is now clear that the rapid pace of development in molecular genetics is having an impact at many levels of contemporary life: in agriculture, forensic investigation, in the biological sciences generally — and especially in relation to medicine. Its incorporation into some aspects of medical practice will be far-reaching and will include recombinant products, anti-viral agents and the development of gene therapy. Molecular genetics is beginning to enhance diagnostics, the prediction of genetic disease, our understanding of development, and promises to identify important alleles at loci that predispose towards the development of common conditions such as coronary heart disease, stroke and cancer. These changes have occurred on a background where radical implementation of different funding methods for health care provision and changes in professional training are occurring in medicine. Medical practice itself is increasingly perceived as going too far in the 'high-tech' repair of degenerative diseases rather than in public health measures for prophylaxis; the explicit development of what is known as a holistic approach for the whole patient and their human and emotional needs, rather than the tacit acceptance of this axiom, is a sign of this disenchantment.

Some are disappointed in the apparent failure of molecular biology to generate novel therapeutic goods. However an epoch has been reached where the science has the capacity to change our understanding of disease processes completely and point our endeavours towards more rational development. It would be desirable if public interest were diffused from the particular and its confidence placed in more genuine scientific tenets than sporadic news reports. Clearly there must be a realistic perspective of what can be achieved; this can so easily be bedevilled by media emphasis on the few striking successes so far achieved. Of course, society needs more than medicine and molecular medicine to keep it healthy and we must be cognisant of pervasive social and ethical questions still to be faced. Nonetheless, 'real diseases', for example the infectious ones caused by **hepatitis** and **herpes viruses** as well as **lentiviruses**, are widespread; there is an epidemic of **cervical cancer** and other cancers related to **papillomaviruses**; **toxigenic** *Escherichia coli*, **rotaviruses** and **respiratory syncytial viruses are the main causes of infant mortality** — there are scientific limits to medicine and even with the best possible molecular understanding of pathological processes, the clinical battlefields in which medical research wages its war against human disease will be constantly changing.

Without new knowledge that lies ahead we cannot hope to improve our lot. A distinguished paediatrician has vividly illustrated this point by drawing an analogy with the poliomyelitis epidemic of the 1950s when children's wards in hospitals contained many patients receiving mechanized support for respiratory failure — the 'iron lung': if it were not for the introduction of poliomyelitis vaccines, we might still be trying to improve the performance of these cumbersome old machines without changing the profile of this epidemic and all its attendant suffering. Francis Bacon, the English philosopher and advocate of utility and progress, can perhaps best goad us for lack of confidence: '**they are ill discoverers that think there is no land when they can see nothing but sea**'.

Further reading

Brenner S., Elgar R., Sandford A., Macrae B., Venkatesh S. and Aparicio S. (1993) Characterisation of the pufferfish (*Fugu*) genome as a compact model vertebrate genome. *Nature*, 366, 265–268.

Harper P.S. (1993) *Practical Genetic Counselling*, 4th edn. Butterworth-Heinemann, Stoneham, MA.

McKusick V.A. (1992) Human genetics: the last 35 years, the present and the future. *American Journal of Human Genetics*, 50, 663–670.

Murray T.H. (1991) Ethical issues in genome research. *FASEB Journal*, 5, 55–62.

Neel, J.V. (1994) *Physician to the Gene Pool: Genetic Lessions and Other Stories*. John Wiley and Sons, New York.

Weatherall D.J. (1995) *Science and the Quiet Art. Medical Research and Patient Care*. Oxford University Press, Oxford. (This book articulates fully and elegantly many of the views about contemporary medical practice, education and professional ethos that have been summarized in this chapter.)

Glossary

Adenine a purine base of DNA and RNA.

Adaptors short double-stranded synthetic oligonucleotides that can be ligated on to the ends of double-stranded DNA fragments to generate known restriction enzyme sites at each end.

Allele alternative forms of a gene occupying the same locus on homologous chromosomes.

Amber mutation a mutant nucleotide sequence of AUG that causes premature termination of protein synthesis.

Aminoacyl-tRNA a tRNA molecule carrying an amino acid which is to be used to extend a growing polypeptide chain during protein synthesis.

Amphipathic containing both hydrophobic and hydrophilic properties.

Anaphase a stage of mitosis during which sister chromatids separate to the spindle poles.

Anti-codon a sequence of three nucleotides in transfer RNA that is complementary to a codon on mRNA.

Apoptosis programmed cell death involving nuclear DNA fragmentation.

Amplification refractory mutation system (ARMS) a PCR system which, due to the primer used, will allow amplification of a single specific allele.

Auto-antibodies antibodies produced by an individual against antigens present in that individual.

Auto-antigen antigens that elicit auto-antibodies.

Auto-immune disease disease resulting from the generation of auto-antibodies.

Autonomously replicating sequence (ARS) a DNA sequence that allows a plasmid DNA molecule to replicate in yeast.

Autoradiography detection of radioactively labelled molecules on X-ray film.

Autosome any chromosome that is not a sex chromosome.

Bacteriophage (phage) a virus that infects bacteria.

Basepair (bp) a pair of complementary nucleotide bases in a duplex DNA or RNA molecule.

Blunt ends ends of a duplex DNA molecule that have no overhangs due to restriction with an enzyme that generates blunt ends or due to removal of the overhangs by single-strand specific nucleases.

Cap structure at the 5′ end of mRNAs containing a methylated guanine residue.

Capsid the outer protein coat of a virus.

Chromosome walking sequencing cloned DNA fragments directionally along a chromosome.

Chromatid one-half of a replicated chromosome.

Chromatin protein–DNA complexes that make up chromosomes.

Clone a population of cells or DNA molecules which came from a single progenitor.

Codon the DNA or corresponding RNA sequence of three basepairs that codes for a particular amino acid or termination signal.

Concatemer multiple copies of a DNA sequence covalently joined together in tandem arrays.

Concordance members of a twin pair exhibiting the same trait.

Consensus sequence a DNA or amino acid sequence that specifies the most commonly found DNA base or amino acid at each position in a sequence of similar DNA or amino acid sequences.

Complementary DNA (cDNA) a DNA copy of a messenger RNA generated by reverse transcriptase.

Cos site cohesive ends of a phage genome.

Cosmid a plasmid DNA containing Cos sites to enable it to be packaged into phage particles.

Cytoplasm contents of a cell outside the nucleus.

Cytosine a pyrimidine base of RNA and DNA.

Cytoskeleton network of microtubules that support the cellular structure and are used for directed transport of many cell constituents.

Degenerate when referring to the genetic code it refers to the fact that more than one codon can specify a particular amino acid.

Diploid refers to a cell or organism containing two complete sets of homologous chromosomes.

Discontinuous replication refers to synthesis of DNA in short fragments (Okazaki fragments) which are eventually joined together to form a complete DNA strand.

DNA polymerase an enzyme that adds nucleotides to a growing chain of DNA in a 5′ to 3′ direction during DNA replication using a DNA strand as a template to copy from.

DNase footprinting a technique which allows the detection of a region of DNA that is complexed with proteins because the proteins protect that region of DNA from DNase digestion.

Domain in a protein this refers to a discrete region of the protein which has a specific function associated with it.

Dominant allele the allele which is observed in the phenotype of a heterozygote.

Dominant negative mutation a mutation generating a mutant gene product whose characteristics are dominant over the wild-type product.

Duplex a complex of two complementary strands of nucleic acids.

Endoplasmic reticulum continuous membrane network within the cytoplasm of cells.

Enhancer DNA domain in the regulatory region of a gene which acts to increase transcription independently of its orientation or site in the promoter.

Epitope the part of an antigen that binds to the antigen binding region of an antibody.

Euchromatin chromatin that is poorly condensed so allowing transcriptional activity.

Eukaryote an organism comprising cells that have a true nucleus.

Exon the segment of a gene which is present in the fully mature RNA after transcription.

Excision repair a system that allows the removal of a damaged piece of single-stranded DNA from a DNA duplex and replacement with a repaired DNA sequence copied from the undamaged DNA strand.

Fluorescence-activated cell sorting (FACS) technique to separate cells from a population on the basis of their expression of specific antigens.

Farwestern blot a technique which transfers protein molecules, after size fractionation on gels, to filter papers to analyse their interaction with other protein probes that are not antibodies.

Fluorescence *in situ* hybridization (FISH) technique to visualize locations on chromosomes which hybridize to specific nucleotide probes.

Frame shift refers to a mutation that shifts the reading frame of triplet codons in a gene during translation of mRNA.

G-banding technique to visualize the band patterns of chromosome on staining with Giemsa.

Gene a unit of heredity that specifies an RNA or mRNA. A gene will also contain intronic regions and regions that control transcription.

Gene mapping the construction of a map of different genetic loci based on their physical position with respect to each other.

General transcription factors (GTFs) proteins that are required to allow RNA polymerase to transcribe a gene at the basal level of transcription. This level of gene expression is then further activated by tissue-specific transcription factors.

Genotype the actual genetic make up of a cell or organism.

Guanine a purine base of RNA or DNA.

Haploid refers to a cell or organism containing only one copy member of a homologous chromosome pair.

Heterochromatin chromatin regions that are condensed and so generally transcriptionally active.

Heterogenous nuclear RNA (hnRNA) the primary transcript generated from transcription of a gene prior to splicing etc. associated with maturation.

Heterozygote refers to a diploid cell or organism that contains different alleles of a gene at one locus on homologous chromosomes.

Hemizygote refers to a diploid cell or organism that contains only one allele of a gene due to loss of one chromosome of a homologous chromosome pair.

Heterodimer a complex of two non-identical moieties, e.g. proteins.

Histones a group of conserved basic proteins that structure DNA in the eukaryotic cell into basic chromatin structure.

Homodimer a complex of two identical moieties, e.g. proteins.

Homologous recombination genetic recombination between nucleic acid sequences that have extensive regions of identical sequence.

Hydrophilic effectively interacts with water.

Hydrophobic ineffectively interacts with water.

Hybridization refers to the ability of complementary single-stranded DNA or RNA molecules to form a duplex.

Immunogen a compound able to elicit an antibody response.

Immunoglobulin a family of proteins that function as antibodies.

Imprinting a change in gene function which occurs early on in development in the egg or sperm such that maternal and paternal copies may differ.

Interphase period of the mitotic cell cycle between one mitosis and the next.

Introns the segments within the coding region of a gene which are not present in the fully mature RNA after transcription due to removal by splicing.

Karyotype the number and characteristics of the full chromosome set of an organism.

Kinase an enzyme that phosphorylates a substrate.

Klenow the largest fragment of the *Escherichia coli* DNA polymerase complex which only has polymerase activity.

Knockout the ability to remove a specific gene in a cell or organism by molecular techniques.

Lagging strand refers to the strand of newly synthesized DNA that is made up from joining of Okazaki fragments.

Leading strand refers to the strand of newly synthesized DNA that is continuously synthesized during DNA replication.

Leucine zipper a leucine-rich domain of a protein that allows protein–protein interaction.

Ligase an enzyme that joins the ends of two duplexes of DNA.

Linkage the tendency for two genes in close proximity on a chromosome to be inherited together.

Liposome small vesicle made up of a lipid bilayer.

Locus the position of a gene on a chromosome.

Logarithm of the odds score (lod) a value for the likelihood of two loci being within a measurable distance from each other.

Long terminal repeat (LTR) the direct repeats at the ends of the proviral DNA.

Lytic cycle the events associated with virus infection during a productive infection.

Major histocompatibility complex (MHC) a family of genes that are involved in mediating T-cell immune responses.

Maternal inheritance preferential carriage of a gene by the maternal parent.

Meiosis eukaryotic cell division during which two sequential divisions generate cells containing a haploid complement of chromosomes.

Messenger RNA (mRNA) the mature transcript from a gene transcribed by RNA polymerase which specifies the order of amino acids during mRNA translation to protein.

Metaphase a stage in mitosis when the parental and newly synthesized chromosomes are maximally condensed but prior to their segregation to opposite spindle poles.

Microtubules filamentous protein structures that make up the cytoskeleton of the cell.

Mitosis the mechanism by which a cell undergoes nuclear division to generate two identical daughter cells with equal complements of chromosomes.

Mobility shift assay technique to analyse the interaction between known DNA sequences and protein.

Monosomy a condition in which one member of a chromosome pair is missing.

Monozygotic genetically identical due to originating from the same fertilized cell.

Mutation a transmissible change in nucleotide sequence which leads to a change or loss of normal function encoded by that nucleotide sequence.

Non-disjunction the process by which duplicate chromosomes fail to separate during cell division resulting in one daughter cell containing both duplicate chromosomes.

Nonsense mutation a mutation resulting in the premature termination during protein synthesis.

Northern blot a technique which transfers RNA molecules after size fractionation on gels to filter papers for hybridization to specific probes.

Northwestern blot a technique which transfers RNA molecules after size fractionation on gels to filter papers for hybridization to specific protein probes.

Nucleosome a subunit of chromatin comprising a core of histone proteins with approximately 146 basepairs of DNA wrapped around.

Okazaki fragment short segments of DNA synthesized during lagging strand DNA synthesis.

Oncogene a mutated gene which is normally involved in the correct control of cell division such that disruption of the normal gene function leads to cell immortalization and transformation.

Open reading frame a series of triplet codons in the coding region of a gene that lie between the signals to start and stop translation.

Organelle a membrane-bound compartment of a eukaryotic cell.

Origin of replication a specific site on DNA at which DNA replication starts.

Pulsed field gel electrophoresis (PFGE) electrophoretic technique to separate very large molecules of DNA by periodically altering the direction of the electric field through which the samples are migrating.

Phenotype the observable characteristics of a cell or organism resulting from the expression of the cell's genotype.

Plasmid a circular DNA molecule capable of self-replication in a cell.

Plaque the clear area on a lawn of bacteria or cells due to virus infection.

Polyadenylation addition of tracts of polyadenylic acid to the ends of transcribed RNA molecules.

Position effect refers to the differences in levels of expression of a gene due to its position in chromatin.

Primer a short nucleotide sequence that provides the starting point for polymerases to copy a nucleotide sequence and make a double strand.

Prokaryotes cells that lack nuclei and membrane-limited organelles.

Promoter a DNA sequence that targets RNA polymerase to a gene for transcription.

Proto-oncogene a normal gene involved in controlling cell division which, when mutated, becomes an oncogene.

Pseudogene a duplicated gene that has become non-functional.

Polymerase chain reaction (PCR) a technique to amplify a target DNA sequence by multiple rounds of DNA synthesis.

Provirus the double-stranded DNA copy of a retrovirus.

Purine an organic base containing two heterocyclic rings that occurs in nucleic acids.

Pyrimidine an organic base containing one heterocyclic ring that occurs in nucleic acids.

Q-banding technique to visualize the band patterns of chromosome on staining with quinacrine.

Quiescent refers to a cell that has exited the cell cycle and is resting.

Reading frame any one of three ways that a specific nucleotide sequence can be read in triplets.

Recessive allele the allele which is masked by the dominant allele in a heterozygote due to the absence or comparative inactivity of the product of the recessive allele.

Replication forks region of DNA resulting from DNA replication in which the parental DNA strands are displaced and DNA polymerase copies the parental template.

Reporter gene a gene which encodes a product which can be easily measured when introduced into cell by transfection.

Restriction enzyme enzymes that cleave DNA at specific sites.

Restriction fragment length polymorphism (RFLP) refers to heritable differences in the length of DNA fragments from a specific region of DNA generated by restriction enzymes due to DNA sequence differences.

Retrovirus an RNA virus that replicates by first converting its RNA genome to a double-stranded DNA copy using reverse transcriptase.

Reverse transcriptase enzyme used to make a DNA copy of RNA.

Reverse transcription–polymerase chain reaction (RT-PCR) amplification of RNA by PCR after copying of the RNA to cDNA by reverse transcription.

Ribosome organelle used for translation of mRNA to protein.

Ribosomal RNA (rRNA) an RNA component of the ribosome.

RNA polymerase an enzyme that makes an RNA copy of a DNA template.

RNA splicing removal of introns from transcribed RNA to generate a mature mRNA.

S phase stage of the eukaryotic cell cycle at which DNA synthesis occurs.

S1 nuclease an enzyme that specifically degrades single-stranded DNA molecules.

Semi-conservative replication the generation of daughter duplexes of DNA which contain one parental and one newly synthesized strand of DNA.

Signal sequence a short amino acid sequence that targets a protein to a specific cellular localization.

Silencer element DNA domain in the regulatory region of a gene which acts to decrease transcription independently of its orientation or site in the promoter.

Somatic cell a cell other than a haploid sex cell.

Somatic cell hybrid a fusion between two different cell types.

Southern blot a technique which transfers DNA molecules after size fractionation on gels to filter papers for hybridization to specific probes.

Southwestern blot a technique which transfers protein molecules after size fractionation on gels to filter papers to analyse their interaction with DNA probes.

Spindle a microtubule structure of the nucleus that is involved in organizing replicated chromosomes during cell division.

Stop codons DNA triplet codons that terminate translation of an mRNA into protein.

TATA box DNA sequence found in many eukaryotic promoters that binds the TATA binding protein in order to recruit RNA polymerase for transcription.

T-cell receptor membrane protein complexes that are expressed on T-lymphocytes and recognize specific antigens when associated with MHC molecules.

Telophase final stage of cell division when the nuclear membrane re-forms around replicated chromosomes.

Tolerance reduced ability to mount an immune response to specific antigens.

Transcription process by which a DNA template is copied to RNA by RNA polymerase enzyme.

Transcription factor proteins, other than RNA polymerase, that are required for transcription of all genes.

Transfection the introduction of DNA into cells in culture.

Transfer RNA (tRNA) small RNAs that function to transport specific amino acids to a growing polypeptide chain on the ribosome during translation.

Translation the mechanism by which mRNA is used as a template to synthesize protein on the ribosome.

Tumour suppressor gene a gene that negatively regulates cell division such that mutation in these genes results in uncontrolled cell division and tumour progression.

Uracil a pyrimidine base that replaces the DNA base thymine in RNA molecules.

Vector a DNA molecule in which DNA sequences can be cloned.

Variable number tandem repeats (VNTR) variations in numbers of tandem repeat DNA sequences found at specific loci in different populations.

Western blot a technique which transfers protein molecules after size fractionation on gels to filter papers for analysis with antibodies.

Wobble hypothesis refers to the ability of a tRNA molecule to recognize more than one codon by relatively free pairing between the third base of the codon and first base of the anti-codon.

X-inactivation refers to the inactivation of one of the X-chromosomes in female somatic cells.

Yeast artificial chromosomes (YACs) plasmid DNA which contains DNA sequences that allow plasmid maintenance in yeast cells and allow cloning of very large regions of DNA.

Index

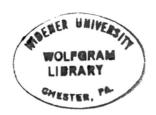

WIDENER UNIVERSITY
WOLFGRAM
LIBRARY
CHESTER, PA.